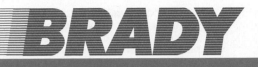

Essentials of Emergency Care

A Refresher for the Practicing EMT-B

Daniel Limmer
Bob Elling
Michael F. O'Keefe

Contributors
Chip Boehm
Rick Buell
Edward T. Dickinson, M.D.

Medical Editor
Edward T. Dickinson, M.D.

BRADY
Prentice-Hall
Upper Saddle River, New Jersey 07458

Library of Congress Cataloging-in-Publication Data

    Essentials of emergency care: a refresher for the practicing EMT-B /Daniel Limmer, Robert Elling, Michael O'Keefe; medical editor, Edward T. Dickinson.

       p. cm.

    Includes index.

    ISBN 0-8359-4963-X

      1. Medical emergencies. 2. Emergency medical technicians. I. Elling, Robert. II. O'Keefe, Michael. III. Title.

    [DNLM: 1. Emergency Medical Services—United States. 2. Emergencies.   WX 215 041e 1995]

RC86.7.038 1995

616.02'5—dc20

DNLM/DLC

for Library of Congress   95-19433

                                          CIP

Publisher: *Susan Katz*

Managing Development Editor: *Lois Berlowitz*

Development Editor: *Terse Stamos*

Editorial Assistant: *Carol Sobel*

Marketing Manager: *Judy Streger*

Director of Manufacturing & Production: *Bruce Johnson*

Manufacturing Buyer: *Ilene Sanford*

Managing Production Editor: *Patrick Walsh*

Production Editor: *Cathy O'Connell*

Editorial/Production Supervision: *Elm Street Publishing Services, Inc.*

Cover Designer: *Laura Ierardi*

Cover Photograph: *© Mitch Kezar/Phototake NYC*

Interior Design: *Lorraine Mullaney*

Managing Photography Editor: *Michal Heron*

Assistant Photography Editor: *Maura McGloin*

Photographers: *Steve Agricola, George Dodson, Michael Galitelli, Michal Heron*

Composition: *Elm Street Publishing Services, Inc.*

Color Separator: *The Clarinda Company*

Printer/Binder: *Metropole*

© 1996 by Prentice-Hall, Inc.
A Simon & Schuster Company
Upper Saddle River, New Jersey 07458

10 9 8 7 6 5 4 3 2 1

ISBN 0-8359-4963-X

PRENTICE-HALL INTERNATIONAL (UK) LIMITED, *London*
PRENTICE-HALL OF AUSTRALIA PTY. LIMITED, *Sydney*
PRENTICE-HALL CANADA INC., *Toronto*
PRENTICE-HALL HISPANOAMERICANA, S.A., *Mexico*
PRENTICE-HALL OF INDIA PRIVATE LIMITED, *New Delhi*
PRENTICE-HALL OF JAPAN, INC., *Tokyo*
SIMON & SCHUSTER ASIA PTE. LTD., *Singapore*
PRENTICE-HALL DO BRASIL, LTDA., *Rio de Janeiro*

NOTICE ON CARE PROCEDURES

It is the intent of the authors and publishers that this textbook be used as part of a normal EMT-Basic refresher program taught by qualified instructors and supervised by a licensed physician. The procedures described in this textbook are based upon consultation with EMT and medical authorities. The authors and publisher have taken care to make certain that these procedures reflect currently accepted clinical practice; however, they cannot be considered absolute recommendations.

The material in this textbook contains the most current information available at the time of publication. However, federal, state, and local guidelines concerning clinical practices, including without limitation, those governing infection control and universal precautions, change rapidly. The reader should note, therefore, that the new regulations may require changes in some procedures.

It is the responsibility of the reader to familiarize himself or herself with the policies and procedures set by federal, state, and local agencies as well as the institution or agency where the reader is employed. The authors and the publisher of this textbook and the supplements written to accompany it disclaim any liability, loss or risk resulting directly or indirectly from the suggested procedures and theory, from any undetected errors, or from the reader's misunderstanding of the text. It is the reader's responsibility to stay informed of any new changes or recommendations made by any federal, state, and local agency as well as by his or her employing institution or agency.

NOTICE ON GENDER USAGE

The English language has historically given preference to the male gender. Among many words, the pronouns "he" and "his" are commonly used to describe both genders. Society evolves faster than language, and the male pronouns still predominate in our speech. The authors have made great effort to treat the two genders equally, recognizing that a significant percentage of EMTs are female. However, in some instances, male pronouns may be used to describe both males and females solely for the purpose of brevity. This is not intended to offend any readers of the female gender.

NOTICE RE "ON THE SCENE"

The names used and situations depicted in "On the Scene" scenarios throughout this text are fictitious.

Brief Contents

Detailed Contents

Chapter 17

Operations *333*

Chapter 18

Hazmat Awareness *373*

Chapter 19

Advanced Airway Management *387*

Appendix A

National Registry Skill Sheets *417*

Appendix B

Appendix C
Answer Key

Patient Assessment Highlights

Photo Skill Summaries

Preface

Essentials of Emergency Care is a new concept in an EMT textbook. This book is designed for experienced EMTs who are beginning, or about to begin, an EMT (now called EMT-B) refresher program. Traditionally, to complete a refresher program, EMTs used their original EMT text, or a subsequent edition. Such texts are designed to present information to a person without experience or training in EMS. However, the authors of this text recognize that the refresher student is different.

The authors acknowledge and respect that you, as an experienced EMT-B, have regularly applied the skills and knowledge learned in your original coursework to your work in the field. Such skills and knowledge are easily remembered, and expansive coverage of this material is not needed in a refresher text. For example, since you have probably had much field experience in bleeding control, this text does not cover it in as much detail as your original text. However, skills and knowledge used less frequently require some "brushing up" before you take a recertification exam. Therefore, such topics are covered in concise, to-the-point presentations.

Not only has material been condensed in this text, but chapters have been combined to correspond to the formats of refresher or recertification programs. For example, the chapters on bleeding and shock have been combined with soft-tissue injuries, much as in your recertification training. If you do not take recertification classes, the book will still be helpful for exam preparation or simply to learn the new curriculum for transitional programs.

The 1994 EMT-B Curriculum

This text also serves as a transitional manual for the U.S. DOT 1994 Revised EMT-Basic National Standard Curriculum, meeting all objectives of this revised curriculum.

While there are new parts of the curriculum, much is simply an adaptation of what you are currently practicing. For example, the patient assessment process, formerly the traditional primary and secondary surveys, is now a series of assessments called scene size-up, initial assessment, focused histories, detailed assessments, and ongoing assessment. Intuitively, you probably recognize that the steps outlined in the 1994 curriculum are not dramatically different from the skills in your primary and secondary surveys. Instead of presenting this as a "whole new" patient assessment process, we help you integrate the sequence into your current practice.

The curriculum does include some newer elements, such as pharmacology and medical direction. These will be new to many currently certified EMTs, and for that reason are covered in greater depth.

When writing this text, we kept several objectives in mind:

- To help you pass the test! Obviously, any textbook must present the information you will need to pass your recertification exams.

- To respect your experience. You may be tackling your first recertification or your tenth. As experienced EMS providers, we have gone through this process ourselves. We recognize the need for a textbook that presents the entire EMT-B curriculum in a clear and concise manner.

- To present the 1994 U.S. DOT Revised EMT-Basic National Standard Curriculum as well as the 1994 EMT-Basic Transitional Program in a manner that will help you easily integrate skills and knowledge into your current practice.

Features of the Book

- **Making the Transition** Each chapter opener has a section called "Making the Transition," a brief listing that reviews how the material in each chapter is presented in the 1994 curriculum. A complete chapter-by-chapter listing is given on pages xv–xvii.

- **DOT and Transitional Curriculum Objectives** Each chapter begins with a listing of all DOT EMT-B and Transitional Curriculum objectives that apply to its content. Each objective is referenced to the page(s) in the chapter where the topic is covered.

- **On the Scene Scenarios** A real-life scenario serves as an introduction to each chapter and integrates elements of the 1994 curriculum, such as the patient assessment steps.

- **Topic Coverage** Although condensed, topics are presented in an easy-to-read format and are often accompanied by illustrations that enhance understanding and maximize coverage.

- **Pediatric Highlights** This feature calls out topics important to pediatric emergency care. It reflects the importance of pediatric patient care and emphasizes the increased attention given to this topic throughout EMS and in the 1994 curriculum.

- **Preceptor Pearls** The experience of the recertification student is mentioned frequently throughout this text. Therefore this feature acknowledges the experienced EMT-B's role as a preceptor, mentor, or trainer. Throughout the text, Preceptor Pearls point out important topics to share with new EMT-Bs, emphasize ways to get your point across, and highlight when and how to mentor the new EMT-B.

- **Skill Summaries** To assist in review of important skills, many chapters contain visual Skill Summaries of important skills.

- **Review Questions** Each chapter ends with Review Questions to test your knowledge on the material you have just completed. An answer key at the back of this book indicates text pages where answers can be found or supported.

- **National Registry Skills Sheets** Each of the skills tested by the Registry in its performance-based skills exam is included.

- **Practice Exams** The text contains two 100-question practice exams. Designed as pre- and posttests, these exams allow you to judge your preparedness for your certification exams. Answer keys are provided for each exam at the back of this book.

A note to instructors: We are offering an Instructor's Resource Manual to accompany the *Essentials* text. The manual presents specific strategies that will help you teach with this textbook. The manual also provides slide references to your existing *Emergency Care* 7th Edition Slide Set. Since most refresher students are tested based on all the DOT EMT-B objectives, the Workbook that accompanies *Emergency Care* 7th Edition is designed to prepare students for test-taking as well.

Comments and Suggestions

We encourage you to comment on the text. Comments and suggestions will help us improve future editions of the text. Please send comments to:

> Judy Streger
> Marketing Manager, Brady
> Prentice Hall
> One Lake Street
> Upper Saddle River, NJ 07458

Additionally, the authors may be reached via E-mail:

> Daniel Limmer: danlimmer@aol.com
> Bob Elling: ellinrob@hvcc.edu
> Mike O'Keefe: mikeokvt@aol.com

We wish you the best of luck in your continued endeavors in EMS!

Daniel Limmer
Bob Elling
Michael O'Keefe

Transition Highlights

Below is a summary of emphases and approaches presented in the 1994 U.S. DOT Revised EMT-B National Standard Curriculum. The summary below briefly outlines how this knowledge is integrated into the text.

Chapter 1 Introduction

- EMTs are now called EMT-Basics, or EMT-Bs.
- Medical direction has an increased role for the EMT-B.
- Quality improvement is included in the curriculum.

Chapter 2 The Well-Being of the EMT-Basic—Emotions and Stress, Scene Safety

- Scene size-up is a formal part of the patient assessment process.
- Size-up is performed before the initial assessment and includes determining BSI needed, scene safety, mechanism of injury/nature of illness, and the number of patients.

Chapter 3 Infection Control

- EMT-B's requirements under OSHA 1910.1030 and the Ryan White CARE Act are explained.
- Proper BSI and PPE required during all phases of an ambulance call are considered.
- Changes in EMT-Bs' attitudes regarding blood and other potentially infectious materials are emphasized.

Chapter 4 Airway

- Importance of BSI is emphasized.
- Use of the two-person bag-valve-mask technique is encouraged.
- Use of a flow-restricted, oxygen-powered ventilation device (FROPVD) is explained.
- Assisting with endotracheal tube placement is recommended.
- Simplified approach to oxygen therapy is included.

Chapter 5 Patient Assessment—Medical Patient

- The initial step in detecting and treating immediate threats to life is now called the initial assessment instead of the primary survey.
- The next steps in the assessment depend on the category into which a patient falls: medical or trauma; responsive or unresponsive; significant mechanism of injury or no significant mechanism of injury; adult, child, or infant.
- Re-evaluate stable patients every 15 minutes, unstable patients every 5 minutes.

Chapter 6 Patient Assessment—Trauma Patient

- The trauma patient with a significant mechanism of injury should receive a limited physical exam (the rapid trauma assessment) at the scene and prompt transport.
- During the physical exam, you should search for DCAP-BTLS (deformities, contusions, abrasions, punctures/penetrations, burns, tenderness, lacerations, and swelling).
- If a trauma patient is complaining of pain in the pelvis, do not compress it. You will cause the patient a great deal of pain without gathering any additional useful information.

Chapter 7 Communication and Documentation

- The 1994 curriculum describes the information you should transmit in a radio report and the order in which you should transmit it.
- A minimum data set describes the minimum information each EMS system should collect.
- Special situations require alterations in the usual manner of documenting incidents.

Chapter 8 General Pharmacology

- Medications carried on the ambulance are explained.

- Medications the EMT-B may assist the patient in taking with medical direction's approval are discussed.

Chapter 9 Medical Emergencies—Cardiac

- The emphasis in EMT-B courses has changed from distinguishing among the different causes of cardiac problems to management based on the patient's signs and symptoms.
- When your patient has chest pain, an adequate blood pressure, and his own nitroglycerin, you can now assist him in taking it.
- As an EMT-B, you are expected to be able to operate an automated external defibrillator.

Chapter 10 Medical Emergencies—Respiratory, Allergic Reactions, Environmental

- The term "breathing difficulty" is used to describe a group of previously diagnosed respiratory conditions.
- How to assist patients with the use of prescribed inhalers and epinephrine auto-injectors is explained.
- Instead of trying to decide whether a patient has heat stroke or heat cramps, the EMT-B should use skin temperature to determine the proper treatment.

Chapter 11 Medical Emergencies—Diabetes, Poisoning and Overdose, Behavioral

- Treatment of the medical emergencies involving diabetics, poisoning/overdose, and behavioral problems is driven by assessment findings.
- EMT-Bs are now able to administer oral glucose and activated charcoal.
- Dilution of some ingested poisons is recommended.
- Scene-safety is stressed before an EMT-B treats a behavioral emergency.

Chapter 12 Trauma—Bleeding, Shock, Soft Tissue

- Shock is defined as hypoperfusion.
- Pneumatic anti-shock garment (PASG) is recommended for use in the presence of pelvic instability, for controlling bleeding and shock (hypoperfusion), and for stabilizing pelvic, hip, femoral, and multiple-leg fractures.

- Early recognition and transport of patients with life-threatening conditions are emphasized.

Chapter 13 Trauma—Musculoskeletal, Head and Spine

- The assessment and emergency care of a painful, swollen, or deformed extremity are explained.
- The use of the PASG as a splint is described.
- The procedure of rapid extrication and when it is used is described.

Chapter 14 Pediatric Patients

- Developmental differences between the five pediatric age groups are described.
- Differences between pediatric anatomy and physiology and that of an adult are explained.
- Recognizing and managing pediatric respiratory emergencies are emphasized.
- Treatment of special needs of pediatric patients at home is explained.

Chapter 15 Obstetrics and Gynecology

- There are no significant changes in the procedures involving childbirth.
- The EMT-B may call on medical direction for assistance in normal and abnormal delivery situations.
- The curriculum includes identification of and treatment for meconium (fecal matter) in amniotic fluid.

Chapter 16 Lifting and Moving Patients

- Use of proper body mechanics during lifting and moving is explained.
- Safe lifting, reaching, pushing, and pulling are emphasized.
- Emergency, urgent, and non-urgent moves are classified.

Chapter 17 Operations

- Carrying the right equipment to the patient's side to ensure proper initial assessment is emphasized.

- Ambulance collision risk factors are explained.
- Medical incident command is explained in detail.

Chapter 18 Hazmat Awareness

- Ongoing education of EMT-Bs should include hazmat first responder awareness level of training in compliance with OSHA regulations.

Chapter 19 Advanced Airway Management

- How to prepare for an intubation is explained.
- How to insert and assure the proper placement of an endotracheal tube are described.
- How to perform orotracheal suctioning is explained.
- How to use an indirect advanced airway such as an EOA or EGTA is described.

Acknowledgments

The authors wish to thank many people and organizations for their effort in writing and producing this textbook. First, to our families for their support to us all through yet another textbook project, we thank you.

The team at Brady has worked diligently on this text as well. We would like to thank our Publisher, Susan Katz for her support of this project. As usual, Lois Berlowitz was instrumental in the details of making this book a success and we thank her. We would also like to thank Patrick Walsh and the production team, as well as Judy Streger, Judy Stamm, and Carol Sobel for their input and work throughout the process.

Terse Stamos was the editor for the textbook. Editing takes a tremendous amount of work and organization for which Terse performed admirably. Thank you!

The photography work for this text was coordinated by Michal Heron. Michal did for this text what she has done for our others—a wonderful job and we thank her. Steve Agricola, George Dodson, and Michael Galitelli shot some photographs with Richard Beebe, BSN, REMT-P, as a technical advisor.

Reviewers

A textbook relies on reviewers for shaping the content as well as checking its accuracy. When writing a textbook that is a relatively new concept, this input is even more essential. We thank our reviewers for their hard work and detailed comments.

Beth Lothrop Adams, M.A., R.N., NREMT-P
ALS Coordinator, EMS Degree Program
Adjunct Assistant Professor of
Emergency Medicine
The George Washington University
Washington, DC

Ralph Backenstoes
Emergency Health Services Federation
New Cumberland, PA

Marianne J. Barry, M.A., EMT-P
Allied Health/EMMT
Lee College
Baytown, TX

John L. Beckman FF/PM Instructor
Lincolnwood Fire Department
Lincolnwood, IL

Kerry Campbell, NREMT-P
Lakeshore Technical College
Cleveland, WI

Robert Glover
Virginia Beach Fire Department
Virginia Beach, VA

Sgt. John Hannon
EMS Coordinator
Foxborough Police Department
Foxborough, MA

Debby Hassel, NREMT-P, B.S.
Denver Fire EMS Division
EMS Educator
Denver, CO

J. Kevin Henson
State EMS Training Coordinator
New Mexico EMS Bureau
Santa Fe, NM

Sgt. David M. Johnson, MICP
Emergency Services Unit
Montville Township Police
Montville, NJ

Jackie McNally, MICP
MICU Clinical Coordinator
Chilton Memorial Hospital
Pompton Plains, NJ

Greg Mullen
Director of EMS Education
HealthONE EMS
Littleton, CO

Ed Scheidel
Davenport College
Center for the Study of EMS
Grand Rapids, MI

Douglas Stevenson
EMS Department Head/Northwest College
Houston Community College System
Houston, TX

Brian J. Wilson, NREMT-P
Education Coordinator
Dept. of Emergency Medicine
El Paso, TX

Rhoda R. Woodard, R.N., NREMT
Chairperson EMT 1+1 Paramedic
Nursing Allied Health Center
Hinds Community College
Jackson, MS

Photo Acknowledgments

Photo Sources Photos are credited as follows: Figure 15–5, Custom Medical Stock Photo/SIU; Figure 17–5, Charly Miller; Figures 2–1A, 17–9 and 18 On the Scene, Robert J. Bennett; Chapter 18 Opener, RMC Medical, Philadelphia, PA; Figure 19–13, Edward T. Dickinson, M.D.

Companies We wish to thank the following companies for their cooperation in providing us with photos: Ferno, Inc., Wilmington, OH; Laerdal Medical Corporation, Armonk, NY; Marquette Electronics, Inc., Milwaukee, WI; Nonin Medical, Inc., Plymouth, MN; PhysioControl Corporation, Redmond, WA; RMC Medical, Philadelphia, PA; Road Rescue, Inc., St. Paul, MN; SpaceLabs Medical, Inc., Redmond, WA; Wehr Engineering, Fairland, IN; and Westech Information Systems, Inc., Vancouver, BC.

Organizations We also wish to thank the following organizations for their assistance in creating the photo program for *Essentials:*

Colonie Department of EMS, Colonie, NY; Hudson Valley Community College, Troy, NY; Montgomery County Public Service Training Academy, Rockville, MD; North Bethlehem Fire Department, North Bethlehem, NY; Riverdale Fire Department, Riverdale, MD; Rockville Fire Station #3, Rockville, MD; Sandy Spring Volunteer Fire Department, Sandy Spring, MD; Suburban Hospital, Bethesda, MD; Shady Grove Adventist Hospital, Shady Grove, MD; Town of Colonie Police Department, Colonie, NY; Town of Guilderland EMS, Guilderland, NY; Western Turnpike Rescue Squad, Albany, NY; and Wheaton Volunteer Rescue Squad, Wheaton, MD.

Technical Advisors Thanks to the following people for providing technical support during the photo shoots:

Mark T. Beall, EMT-P Instructor, Career Firefighter, Paramedic
Maryland State EMS Instructor

Richard W.O. Beebe, B.S., R.N., EMT-Paramedic Instructor, EMS Program
Hudson Valley Community College

Gloria Bizjak, EMT-A, Curriculum Specialist
Maryland Fire and Rescue Institute

Steve Carter, Manager, Special Programs
Maryland Fire and Rescue Institute

Gail Collins, NR-EMT, EMT Instructor

Michael Collins, EMT-P

Ann Marie Davies, EMT-P

Bob Elling, MPA, REMT-P

Lt. Willa K. Little, EMS Training Officer
Montgomery County Public Service Training Academy

George Morgan, Industrial Training Specialist
Maryland Fire and Rescue Institute

Bruce Olsen, B.S., RRT, EMT-P
Paramedic Program Coordinator
Hudson Valley Community College

Jonathan Politis, B.A., EMT-P
Director, Emergency Medical Services
Town of Colonie

Jay Smith, EMT Class Coordinator
Montgomery County Public Service Training Academy

Christine Uhlhorn, EMT-A, EMT Instructor
Maryland Fire and Rescue Institute

Linda Zimmerman, EMT-A, EMT Instructor
Maryland Fire and Rescue Institute

About the Authors

Daniel Limmer, EMT-P,
is a paramedic and police officer in the Town of Colonie, New York. He has been involved in EMS for over 15 years. He is an instructor for the Hudson Valley Community College Institute for Prehospital Emergency Medicine in Troy, New York, and is a co-author of *Emergency Care,* 7th Edition and *First Responder: A Skills Approach,* 4th Edition.

Bob Elling, MPA, REMT-P,
is the Program Coordinator for the Hudson Valley Community College Institute for Prehospital Emergency Medicine in Troy, New York. He is also a senior flight medic with the Town of Colonie, EMS Department, and a consultant with Synergism Associates, Ltd. Bob has served as a paramedic for NYC*EMS, Associate Director of the NY State EMS Program, Coordinator for Emergency Medical Update, and is the author of the Workbook that accompanies *Emergency Care,* 7th Edition.

Michael F. O'Keefe, REMT-P,
is the Training Coordinator for the Vermont Department of Health's EMS division. He has been active as chairperson of the National Council of State EMS Training Coordinators and with the development of various national EMS curricula. He was a member of the curriculum development group for the national standard first responder curriculum. He co-authored *Emergency Care,* 7th Edition.

About the Contributors

Chip Boehm, R.N., EMT-P, is Education and Quality Improvement Officer for the Portland, Maine Fire Department. He is a voting member for the National Council of State EMS Training Coordinators, served as an outside reviewer for the revised 1994 EMT-Basic National Standard Curriculum, and has worked on several projects for its implementation. Chip is both a volunteer and per diem paramedic with two EMS services.

Rick Buell, EMT-P, is Washington State EMS Education and Training Coordinator, Department of Health, Office of Emergency Medical Services and Trauma Prevention. He has been active as a paramedic, EMT, and fire captain.

Edward T. Dickinson, M.D., NREMT-P, is an assistant professor and Director of EMS for the Albany Medical Center's Department of Emergency Medicine and Medical Director for the Town of Colonie Department of Emergency Medical Services. He began his career in EMS in 1979 as an EMT-firefighter and remains active in hands-on prehospital patient care. An emergency medicine physician, paramedic, researcher, and instructor, he has been involved in EMS for the past 16 years. As our medical editor, Dr. Dickinson brings broad experience and perspective to his work on this text.

CHAPTER 1

Introduction

The U.S. Department of Transportation 1994 EMT-Basic National Standard Curriculum brings some changes to the way you will practice as an EMT. There are also many parts that remain unchanged or are changed only minimally. This chapter combines some new topics with many important old topics. It discusses the Emergency Medical Services (EMS) system, the role of the experienced EMT-B as a preceptor, quality improvement (QI), and a topic that will be used

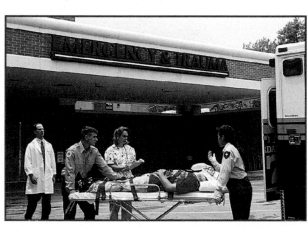

frequently in the new curriculum: medical direction.

The various medical/legal aspects of providing care are also worthy of review and are included in this chapter. Concepts such as scope of practice, consent, negligence, confidentiality, and other legal principles are covered to assist you in your daily activities as an EMT-B, as well as to prepare you for your recertification exam. In addition, the EMT-B's responsibilities at a crime scene are reviewed.

MAKING THE TRANSITION

- EMTs are now called EMT-Basics, or EMT-Bs.
- Medical direction has an increased role for the EMT-B.
- Quality improvement is included in the curriculum.

OBJECTIVES

The numbered objectives below are from the United States Department of Transportation 1994 EMT-Basic National Standard Curriculum. Objectives with colored bullets that follow in italics are from the EMT-Basic Transitional Program.

■ KNOWLEDGE AND ATTITUDE

At the completion of this lesson, you should be able to:

Introduction to Emergency Medical Care

1. Define Emergency Medical Services (EMS) Systems. (pp. 5–6)
2. Differentiate the roles and responsibilities of the EMT-B from other prehospital care providers. (pp. 6–9)
3. Describe the roles and responsibilities related to personal safety. (pp. 6–7)
4. Discuss the roles and responsibilities of the EMT-B towards the safety of the crew, the patient, and bystanders. (p. 7)
5. Define quality improvement and discuss the EMT-B's role in the process. (pp. 9–10)
6. Define medical direction and discuss the EMT-B's role in the process. (pp. 10–11)
7. State the specific statutes and regulations in your state regarding the EMS system. (p. 12)
8. Assess areas of personal attitude and conduct of the EMT-B. (pp. 8–9)
9. Characterize the various methods used to access the EMS system in your community. (p. 6)

Medical/Legal and Ethical Issues

1. Define the EMT-B scope of practice. (p. 12)
2. Discuss the importance of Do Not Resuscitate [DNR] (advanced directives) and local or state provisions regarding EMS application. (pp. 12–13)
3. Define consent and discuss the methods of obtaining consent. (pp. 12, 14)
4. Differentiate between expressed and implied consent. (pp. 12, 14)
5. Explain the role of consent of minors in providing care. (p. 14)
6. Discuss the implications for the EMT-B in patient refusal of transport. (pp. 14–15)
7. Discuss the issues of abandonment, negligence, and battery and their implications to the EMT-B. (pp. 14, 16)
8. State the conditions necessary for the EMT-B to have a duty to act. (p. 16)
9. Explain the importance, necessity, and legality of patient confidentiality. (p. 16)
10. Discuss the considerations of the EMT-B in issues of organ retrieval. (p. 16)
11. Differentiate the actions that an EMT-B should take to assist in the preservation of a crime scene. (pp. 16–18)
12. State the conditions that require an EMT-B to notify local law enforcement officials. (p. 17)
13. Explain the role of EMS and the EMT-B regarding patients with DNR orders. (pp. 12–13)
14. Explain the rationale for the needs, benefits, and usage of advance directives. (pp. 12–13)
15. Explain the rationale for the concept of varying degrees of DNR. (pp. 12–13)

- *Compare and contrast the revised 1994 EMT-Basic curriculum with the old curriculum. (pp. 3–5)*
- *Define the purpose of the transitional program (if you are taking a transitional refresher course). (pp. 3–5)*
- *Explain the rationale for a relationship between the EMT-B and medical direction. (pp. 4, 10, 11)*
- *State the components of the minimum data set. (p. 12)*
- *Support the rationale for medical direction. (pp. 9, 10–11)*
- *Serve as a model for other EMTs and prehospital care providers. (pp. 4, 8–9)*
- *Explain the rationale for serving as an advocate of the revised assessment-based curriculum. (pp. 3–5, 8–9)*

You receive a call from your Emergency Medical Dispatcher (EMD) about a 69-year-old male patient with chest pain. The EMD reports that the patient is conscious and breathing and has a medical history of cardiac problems. The patient's wife will make him comfortable and meet you at the door.

You arrive at the scene and perform a **scene size-up.** You do not observe any hazards before you exit the ambulance or as you approach the house. The patient's wife meets you at the door and escorts you in. You have considered body substance isolation. There appears to be only one patient but you keep in mind that you may need to request ALS backup.

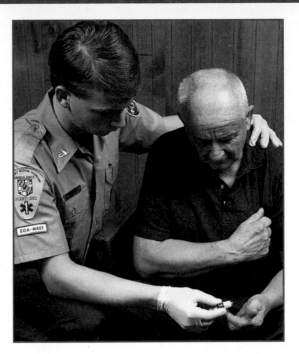

As you approach the patient, you introduce yourself. Mr. Seaver asks that you call him "Mike." You perform an **initial assessment,** which reveals the patient can speak in full sentences and appears oriented. You find that the rate and depth of Mike's breathing are adequate and his pulse is strong, regular, and within a normal range. You observe that he is sweaty and pale. He holds his hand firmly at his chest to describe his chief complaint: severe chest pain. Your general impression is an unstable patient who has severe chest pain, necessitating a high-priority transport and ALS backup.

You carefully screen for clues that may indicate trauma, such as loss of consciousness or a fall. The patient has a medical complaint so you move into the **focused history and physical exam** for a medical patient, which relies heavily on the patient's history. You partner has already placed the patient on oxygen and begins to take a baseline set of vitals while you perform a history using the SAMPLE mnemonic. The patient tells you that the pain came on while he was raking leaves and that it has lessened since he came in and sat down, although it is still a "5" on a 1 to 10 scale. The patient has nitroglycerin tablets that were prescribed when he had his last episode of chest pain, but he has never had to use them and therefore forgot to take one of the tablets.

You obtain Mike's vital signs from your partner: BP 136/88, P 88 strong and regular, R 20 and adequate. Mrs. Seaver hands you the nitroglycerin. You observe that it is Mr. Seaver's prescription, dated about four months ago. Your local protocols allow you to assist patients in taking their prescribed nitroglycerin once you obtain permission from the medical control physician at the hospital's emergency department. While your partner prepares the patient for transport, you speak to the on-line physician on the Seaver's telephone. After your brief report, she approves the use of two nitro administrations while en route, spaced 5 minutes apart, as long as the chest pain continues and the patient's systolic blood pressure remains above 110 mmHg.

En route to the hospital, Mike is reassessed after each administration of nitroglycerin. An **ongoing assessment** that includes a repeat of the initial assessment, vital signs, chief complaint, and your patient's reaction to intervention is performed at least every five minutes on an unstable patient.

You radio and advise the hospital of the patient's status and response to the nitroglycerin. Your ETA is now 8 minutes. After completing a final ongoing assessment, you arrive at the emergency department and turn over your patient after giving the nurse a verbal report of your findings and out-of-hospital management. ∎

∎ AN ASSESSMENT-BASED CURRICULUM

You have, undoubtedly, treated patients such as Mr. Seaver. As you read the scenario, you probably noticed a difference in the approach to assessment and care. This new approach was designed to help you better assess and treat the patient. While assessment and care will be discussed in depth throughout this text, breaking down the On the Scene scenario will help explain some of the philosophies behind the new curriculum.

Note that the information relayed by the dispatcher was more in depth than it probably was in the past. This is because more and more dispatchers are being trained as Emergency Medical Dispatchers (EMDs). This training usually qualifies the dispatcher to obtain more information from the patient as well as provide pre-arrival instructions to the patient and family members. This information includes telephone instruction in CPR. Depending on how long you have been certified and the dispatch system in use in your area, you may or may not be familiar with EMDs.

Upon arriving at the scene, the EMTs (EMT-Bs in the new curriculum) were concerned with several things: safety, infection control, the type of emergency, and number of patients. The new curriculum takes what we have already been practicing and formalizes it into the **scene size-up.**

What was formerly called the "primary survey" is now the **initial assessment.** This step is still a treat-as-you-go process for life-threatening problems found when checking the ABCs and when checking for spinal injuries. A step called **forming a general impression** is added to help you set priorities and gain direction early in patient care.

The next step in the old curriculum normally would be obtaining a history and vital signs. There were always some differences between the assessment of a trauma patient, in which the care is largely hands-on, and the medical patient, in which the history plays a large part in assessment. The new curriculum follows this trend as well with the **focused history and physical exam** and **baseline vitals and SAMPLE history.** There are now two different focused history and physical exams: one for the medical patient and one for the trauma patient.

Many of us were originally trained in the AMPLE method of history determination. SAMPLE retains the AMPLE information and adds "Signs and Symptoms" to the mnemonic.

Perhaps the largest change in the new curriculum, and one that may take experienced EMT-Bs a bit of getting used to, is the switch from diagnosis to assessment-based thinking. In the past, the EMT would have looked at the patient's signs and symptoms and, based on the onset and relief, would have determined that the patient was suffering from angina pectoris. True, the patient had an onset during exertion which subsided during rest, but the old curriculum asked us to diagnose conditions that even emergency depart-

ment physicians may not have been able to diagnose without specific tests. Furthermore, would our care change if the patient had angina pectoris, myocardial infarction, or heartburn? No.

This new approach to the assessment and care of patients has left some EMT-Bs feeling shortchanged, feeling as if something valuable has been taken away. Another example is the term "fracture." The curriculum has limited the use of the term fracture and replaced it with "painful, swollen, deformed extremity." The principle behind this move was that EMT-Bs should treat every injury that may be a fracture as a fracture. Attempting to distinguish between a sprain and a fracture could be counterproductive to care. Again, sophisticated diagnostic equipment is being used in the hospital to make a determination which EMTs had been taught to differentiate with only their senses.

Another dramatic change in the new curriculum is that it allows the EMT-B to give additional treatments. **Interventions,** such as assisting the patient with his nitroglycerin, are new and potentially beneficial. Interventions include assisting patients with medications such as nitroglycerin, Epi-pens®, and inhalers. While oxygen has always been carried on the ambulance, now other medications, such as activated charcoal, can also be carried.

Previously, the main radio communications carried out by an EMT would be the call to the emergency department advising about the patient's condition and the ETA. Medical advice was traditionally given only to advanced-level EMTs such as Intermediates and Paramedics. Now the same medical direction will be made available to the EMT-B in many systems. The exchange of information and advice about patient care has the potential to benefit the EMT-B, the patient, and the hospital personnel.

A **detailed exam** is performed next, if necessary and if time permits. This exam would usually be performed en route to the hospital for a trauma patient with a significant mechanism of injury. The detailed exam is an expanded version of the focused history and physical exam and is performed only when time permits, so that transport to the emergency department is not delayed. Medical patients will usually not receive a detailed exam. As previously stated, **ongoing assessment** is also performed en route to the hospital. It repeats the initial assessment and vital signs at least every 5 minutes for unstable patients and at least every 15 minutes for stable ones.

The assessment process will be discussed in detail later in the text. This chapter introduces the general concepts behind the new curriculum's philosophy of emergency care.

■ THE EMERGENCY MEDICAL SERVICES SYSTEM

As an Emergency Medical Technician going through an update or refresher, you have undoubtedly experienced most if not all the components of the Emergency Medical Services (EMS) system (Figure 1–1). The EMS system includes the following components:

Bystanders

Bystanders or other persons on the scene are responsible for activation of the EMS system. Bystanders may also initiate CPR or other emergency care measures prior to the arrival of EMS units.

Emergency Medical Dispatchers

Dispatchers take incoming emergency calls, obtain important information from callers, assign response priorities, and provide pre-arrival instructions to lay people at the scene.

First Responders

These people may include fire, police, or EMS units that respond from a location close to the scene and arrive first, providing emergency care until arrival of the ambulance. First Responders may be public, private, industrial, or otherwise.

Emergency Medical Technician-Basic (EMT-B)

The EMT-B may function in many areas, the most common of which is on an ambulance. EMT-Bs continue care started by First Responders and provide transportation of the patient. Additional training is available above the EMT-B level. EMT-Intermediates and EMT-Paramedics are considered advanced EMT-Bs (AEMTs).

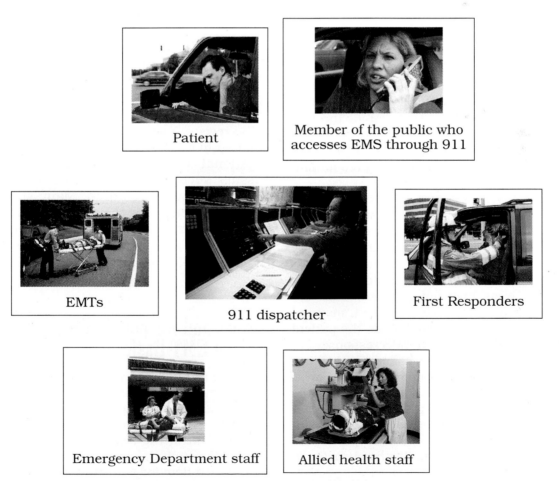

Patient

Member of the public who accesses EMS through 911

EMTs

911 dispatcher

First Responders

Emergency Department staff

Allied health staff

FIGURE 1–1 The Emergency Medical Services system.

Emergency Department Staff

The emergency department staff receives the patient and continues care using hospital resources. Serious trauma cases may pass quickly through the emergency department to the operating room where surgical correction of life-threatening injuries may be performed.

Specialty Centers

Many hospitals are also designated as specialty centers who care for all patients but have special resources and training for patients such as trauma centers, burn centers, pediatric centers, and poison centers.

Allied Health Personnel

During the course of treatment, a patient may be seen by allied health personnel such as therapists, technicians, and other specialists.

System Access

When many EMTs began their initial training, 911 communications was simply a vision. Now, many communities have **911 access** to a centralized communication center for emergency police, fire, or EMS calls. This number, made public through advertising campaigns and television shows, is important because it is easily remembered. In the future, it will be the only number required nationwide to obtain help in an emergency.

Studies have shown that the earlier CPR is started, the greater the chance of survival. The 911 number, by allowing easy and quick access to the EMS system, decreases the time it takes to get to the patient. However, not all areas have 911. These areas are called **non-911 systems.** Dialing 911 in these areas may not be ideal. Calls are routed to operators who, while trained, may not even be in the same city or region as the patient and thus may cause delays in EMS response.

Enhanced 911 (sometimes called "E-911") is a system set up so that the number and location of the person who dialed 911 is displayed on the screen for the emergency dispatcher. This is beneficial in cases in which the patient loses consciousness or is unable to speak or perhaps a small child is making the call. This has benefits in police emergencies as well.

Levels of Training

In 1992, a group of EMS professionals representing many national organizations convened to discuss the direction of EMS levels of training. Currently, different states have different definitions for a First Responder, EMT-B, or Advanced EMT (AEMT). In some states and regions, some levels of training are advanced, while other states allow minimal use of skills for their providers.

The **National Emergency Medical Services Education and Practice Blueprint** was developed to outline what skills should be performed by each level and is an attempt to standardize levels of training. While there will always be some differences in training among states and regions, the following are levels of training according to the blueprint:

- First Responder
- Emergency Medical Technician-Basic
- Emergency Medical Technician-Intermediate
- Emergency Medical Technician-Paramedic

The **National Registry of Emergency Medical Technicians** is an organization which provides a means of nationally registering First Responders and all levels of Emergency Medical Technicians. The registry uses a written and practical examination to qualify candidates for registration. The National Registry is also active in many EMS issues such as curriculum development, standardization, and research. Many states use the national registry for their final examinations and for license reciprocity. Having National Registry certification may make it easier to relocate to other states or regions.

Roles and Responsibilities of the EMT-Basic

After performing the job of an EMT for a period of time, one might think that the roles and responsibilities you are bound by would be relatively obvious. Since the roles and responsibilities are spelled out in the DOT 1994 EMT-B curriculum and differ from the previous curriculum, they are presented here for your information.

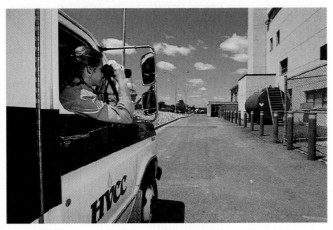

Personal Safety

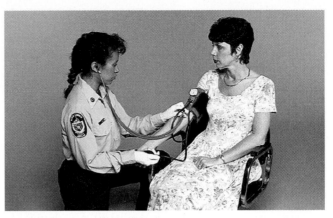

Patient Assessment

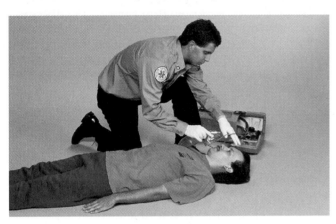

Patient Care

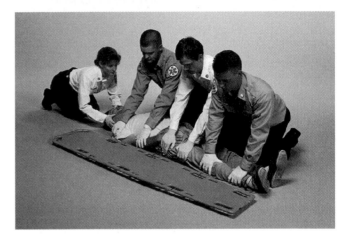

Lifting and Moving

FIGURE 1–2 Some roles and responsibilities of an EMT-B.

- *Personal Safety.* The new document stresses safety in several areas, most notably in the scene size-up portion of the assessment. Safety issues include hazards from chemicals, violence, traffic, natural forces, and others. (Figure 1–2)

- *Safety of the Crew, Patient, and Bystanders.* Continuing the emphasis on safety, the EMT-B must also look out for the safety of others. Emergency scenes are dynamic events. Untrained personnel may act in unusual ways when in emergency situations.

- *Patient Assessment.* In the new assessment-based curriculum, you will perform a patient assessment on every patient you encounter. This will enable you to make appropriate treatment and transport decisions. Assessment procedures continue throughout the call.

- *Patient Care.* Based on your assessment, you provide patient care.

- *Lifting and Moving Patients.* Since EMS treatment almost always results in transportation to

a hospital, lifting and moving the patient safely and effectively becomes very important. Improper lifting and moving not only can injure the patient, but can worsen the patient's condition and injure the EMT-B.

- *Transport/Transfer of Care.* Once moved to the ambulance, the patient must be safely delivered to the hospital. Once at the hospital, the patient and the patient information you have gathered must be turned over to hospital personnel.

- *Record Keeping/Data Collection.* While some may not consider completion of a run report as record keeping, this report *is* a legal document and must be completed neatly and accurately. As EMS grows, research will be needed to determine trends and information that will help improve EMS care. Thus accurate and thorough record keeping and data collection can contribute to improving patient care.

- *Patient Advocacy.* This responsibility is a relatively new listing. In the time you spend with your patient you learn a great deal about his or her condition and needs. An advocate does more for the patient than textbook emergency care. Looking after the patient's needs you may find that he or she has a special concern that you can bring to the attention of hospital personnel that will comfort the patient. Performing this significant task can make a tremendous difference to a patient.

Professional Attributes of an EMT-B

Several professional attributes that are desirable for an EMT-B include a neat, clean appearance, positive image, maintaining up-to-date knowledge, and *safely* placing the patient's needs above your own. For example, a patient who is experiencing chills on a hot day would not want the ambulance's air conditioner running full force. You should turn the air conditioner off because it is in the best interest of the patient.

The EMT-B as a Preceptor

Since you (or your instructor) chose this book, you most likely have some experience as an EMT. This book takes a slightly different look at the EMT-B curriculum in several ways. Most notably, it presents the material that covers the objectives in an abbreviated form since you have been taught much of the material earlier in a full course.

The second way this text differs is that it realizes that you will be an example for new EMT-Bs as they finish their training. In the past, being a trainer has not been considered a major part of the roles and responsibilities of an EMT.

Try to recall your first few months or years as an EMT. You most likely had some good and bad experiences as you learned the trade. Some experienced EMTs were extremely helpful and supportive; others may have actually helped you learn *the wrong information.*

The receipt of an EMT-B card is not the end of EMS learning—it is the beginning. As an experienced EMT, you will be called upon to teach new EMT-Bs, both formally when giving orientation sessions, and informally by example. This section discusses ways you can help teach the new EMT-B through your everyday role as a preceptor, or mentor.

Webster's Dictionary defines "mentor" as "a wise and trusted counselor and teacher" and "preceptor" as "tutor." These definitions capture the essence of what you are called to do when working with new EMT-Bs. Remember that the EMT-B course is primarily classroom and lab work with minimal field experience. Students emerge from the course with a considerable amount of new knowledge but with little experience applying that knowledge in the field. The transition from classroom to field application is neither smooth nor easy. The first calls of a new EMT-B are critical for developing confidence that will form the basis of a successful EMS career.

Even before you begin to teach skills such as assessment or splinting, you can provide some important, practical insight to EMS:

- Let new EMT-Bs know that their EMS education is a life-long commitment. It does not stop with their EMT-B training. Show the new EMT-B you mean it by participating in continuing medical education (CME) and other available training. Stimulate the newcomer by quizzing or offering challenging situations for him or her to solve.
- Since EMS is not all excitement, help the new EMT-B understand this. People who are led to believe that EMS is all emergencies are disillusioned when they learn the truth. Cultivate a life-long provider rather than a flash-in-the pan!
- Encourage the qualities of loyalty, reliability, and good judgment in a new EMT-B.

While it's important to recognize that not all people are cut out for EMS, it is equally important to recognize that we lose talented people because they are never "broken in" properly. They never see good examples or work with those who can act as mentors.

Preceptor Pearl

A disservice is done to new EMT-Bs when they are told "forget what you learned in the classroom ... you're on the street now." This is damaging and confusing. Help integrate classroom knowledge into the field. Even shortcuts in assessment and care can confuse new EMT-Bs. Allow the newcomer to cement a foundation of knowledge and skills before providing new "tricks." ❖

This "Preceptor Pearl" feature is used throughout the remainder of this text. The feature is designed to remind you of your role as a preceptor and to provide pearls that are important to pass along to students.

It is very difficult to determine just how much freedom to give a new EMT-B. While many agree that it is improper to allow the newly trained

Support	Coach
Delegate	Direct

CHART 1–1 Situational Leadership Model II

person to be crew chief, there are more subtle issues that are extremely important. Some experienced people never allow the newcomer to participate, while others allow the new EMT-B to perform tasks that are above his or her current capabilities. The resultant failure erodes the confidence of the student.

The Situational Leadership II Model[1] provides some insight into mentoring new EMT-Bs (Chart 1–1). How you choose to lead an EMT-B will depend on his or her capabilities. An EMT-B may have excellent assessment skills, but may never have applied a traction splint. The preceptor must recognize that a different approach must be taken when supervising each skill.

- **Direct** when the EMT-B is highly motivated but has no experience.
- **Coach** when students have motivation or confidence problems. Coaching provides support and encouragement at a crucial time.
- **Support** those who are unmotivated but who have good skills and experience. This approach is often useful when students have reached a plateau in learning.
- **Delegate** when EMT-Bs are self-motivated and have developed a high level of experience and proficiency.

It is easy to imagine what could happen when an EMT-B who lacks confidence or motivation is designated to a task for which he or she is not ready. Remember, a person is *not* a failure because he or she lacks confidence and motivation. Confidence and motivation are qualities that must be cultivated by organizations and individuals. If you direct, coach, support, and delegate in the appropriate situations, the end result will be a high-quality, life-long EMS provider.

Feedback is essential to any EMS provider; it leads to growth. Provide feedback frequently. You will most likely have to disperse both positive and negative feedback. Remember to "praise in public; reprimand in private."

If you recall an EMT who made a positive impression on you, pass that positive message along to a newcomer. Also recall the traits of people who have negatively influenced you and discard them.

Finally, participate in training or instructor workshops offered in your area. Your role as a teacher, mentor, and preceptor is valuable in and out of the classroom.

■ QUALITY IMPROVEMENT AND MEDICAL DIRECTION

Quality Improvement (QI)

The 1994 DOT curriculum defines quality improvement (QI) as "a system of internal and external reviews and audits of all aspects of an EMS system so as to identify those aspects needing improvement to assure that the public receives the highest quality prehospital care."

Most EMS systems have some type of quality improvement program in place. In some systems it may be called QA (quality assurance) or be a part of a TQM (total quality management) program. The end result is basically the same.

A group of people is usually assigned the function of quality improvement. A quality improvement review session may proceed this way: The group decides to review traumatic cardiac arrest calls for a given period. The run reports will be pulled for all calls meeting that criterion in the set time period. The calls will be reviewed for specific, objective criteria such as scene time, spinal immobilization, other skills, and documentation. If calls are found in which the crew did not appear to meet the standards set by the organization, those crews are notified of the results, and a plan of action is taken to assure that the standards are met in the future.

If calls are found to be exceptional in meeting the standards set by an organization, commendations or letters may be issued documenting the excellent work done by crews who have provided superior patient care and have met or exceeded the desired standards. Quality improvement is not a once-a-month proposition. As an EMT-B you must strive to provide quality care at all times. Your agency's Medical Director must be actively involved in the QI process. (Medical direction will be

[1] Adapted from *Leadership and the One-Minute Manager* by Kenneth H. Blanchard. William R. Morrow, 1985.

discussed later in the chapter.) There are several ways that you can work toward quality patient care and quality improvement every day.

- *Documentation.* Since committees that review prior calls rely on your documentation, this is a critical aspect of the QI process. If a report is incomplete or improperly completed, a QI committee would be forced to assume that substandard care was given. Furthermore, incomplete documentation may result in, or worsen, lawsuits filed against you and your organization. A run report should "tell the story" of your patient so that others reading the report can get a clear picture of the patient's condition, your assessment, and treatment given.

- *Review and Audit Run Reports.* As an EMT-B, you may volunteer to be a member of your agency's QI committee. Even when not functioning as part of a committee, review your run reports before submission to be sure they are complete. Have another person on your crew review your reports for accuracy and completeness.

- *Gathering Feedback from Patients and Hospital Staff.* If you never receive feedback or comments on your patient-care procedures or techniques, you may never improve. Many people can offer comments that will help improve your patient care. Questionnaires sent to patients after a call may be returned with valuable information that can help you improve.

- *Conduct Preventive Maintenance.* Extremes in temperature, the weight of repeated patients, and the nature of emergency scenes take a great toll on your equipment, including your emergency vehicle. Preventive maintenance (PM) and regular equipment checks will extend the life of your equipment and ensure that it will be in good working order for use with the next patient.

- *Continuing Education.* If not used every day, the knowledge and skills you learned in your original EMT class may be forgotten. Also, new techniques and procedures have undoubtedly come about since your certification. Continuing education is an important part of quality improvement. Reading journals, attending seminars or classes, and completing other continuing education endeavors is a necessary part of EMS quality today.

- *Maintain Skills.* Skills that are not practiced frequently usually deteriorate. If you have not performed a traction-splint application in some time, you may require additional practice *before* you perform on a patient. To provide quality patient care, you must maintain proficiency in all skills.

A true quality improvement program transcends agency politics and personalities and focuses on the true issue: *quality.* Members of any profession must continually strive for quality to gain community and peer respect.

Medical Direction

A **Medical Director** is a physician who is responsible for the clinical and patient-care aspects of an EMS system. All ambulance services and rescue squads must have a medical director. The medical director will be actively involved with the QI committee. Many agencies included a physician Medical Director before implementation of the new curriculum, but with the new interventions, such as administering medication and applying automated external defibrillation, use of medical direction becomes even more important.

Medical direction can be **on-line** or **off-line.** *On-line medical direction* (Figure 1–3) was demonstrated in the scenario that opened the chapter. An EMT-B found that a patient had been prescribed nitroglycerin and called medical direction on the patient's phone to obtain permission to assist the patient in taking the medication. The physician that the EMT-B talked to might not have been his agency's Medical Director. Physicians authorized by regional or local agencies may provide medical direction on a call-by-call basis. On-line medical direction may be contacted by telephone, cellular phone, or radio. A brief report on the patient is presented, followed by "orders" from the on-line physician.

Off-line medical direction is done through **standing orders,** or **protocols.** These are orders issued by the medical director that can be used any time a certain situation is encountered. Using the nitroglycerin example from the scenario, if this was a standing order and a strict series of circumstances existed, an EMT-B could assist the patient in administering the nitroglycerin without first calling the physician. The standing order may be issued as shown in Figure 1–4. Your system may have standing orders such as this. Other drugs such as oral glucose, activated charcoal, and prescribed inhalers may have similar orders. **Always follow local protocols.**

The true practice of medicine and the ability to prescribe and administer drugs is primarily given to physicians. If you, as an EMT-B, administer a medication it is generally considered an extension

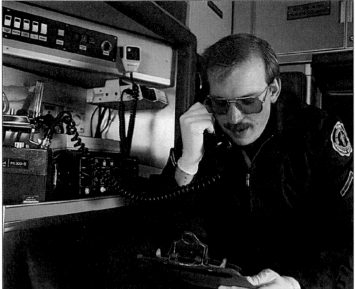

FIGURE 1–3 Communicating with Medical Director.

An EMT-B is authorized to assist the patient in administering nitroglycerin tablets or spray if the following circumstances exist:

1. The nitroglycerin medication has been prescribed to the patient. No other person's nitro may be administered in this situation.

2. The patient must have suspected cardiac chest pain, which may include substernal pain with radiation to the neck, arm, or jaw; or a patient must have a previous cardiac history and be experiencing pain similar to a prior cardiac event.

3. At no point will more than two nitroglycerin tablets be administered in the field without contacting on-line medical direction. The doses are to be administered 5 minutes apart with an evaluation of chest pain and vital signs prior to each dose being administered. This 5-minute wait between administrations includes nitro that may have been taken by the patient before your arrival.

4. Nitroglycerin will be administered only to patients with a systolic blood pressure above 110 mmHg.

5. EMT-Bs will follow directions on the prescription for administration of the drug.

6. Nitroglycerin is a potentially beneficial drug for patients with chest pain. It is a *drug*, however, and must be treated with respect. Monitor the patient carefully before and after administration of this or any drug. **If you have any doubts or questions, contact your on-line physician immediately!**

FIGURE 1–4 A sample protocol.

of the medical director's authority or license. When you carry out an on-line or off-line order, you are the **designated agent** of the physician. This is a tremendous responsibility. You would not be able to perform these tasks without your Medical Director. *Performing advanced skills and medication administration without approval from a Medical Director is the equivalent of practicing medicine without a license.*

Most states have enacted legislation that creates and authorizes the EMS systems in your area. Authority may be given to state, regional, or local agencies to set policies and procedures that affect you as an EMT-B. Become familiar with the regulations that affect you and the agencies that set them.

PEDIATRIC HIGHLIGHT

Medical direction may be valuable when treating pediatric patients. While you receive training in calls involving infants and children, these calls may be infrequent. Remember to take advantage of the guidance that medical direction can provide in general issues, medications, and other problems that you encounter when treating pediatric patients. ■

Minimum Data Set

In order to improve the way EMS cares for patients, research is ongoing. This research includes EMS response, care, and other responsibilities. In order

TABLE 1-1 The Minimum Data Set

Patient information (Gathered at the time of the EMT-B's initial contact with patient on arrival at scene, following all interventions, and on arrival at facility)
• Chief complaint
• Level of consciousness (AVPU)—mental status
• Systolic blood pressure for patients greater than 3 years old
• Skin perfusion (capillary refill) for patients less than 6 years old
• Skin color and temperature
• Pulse rate
• Respiratory rate and effort

Administrative information
• Time of incident report
• Time unit notified
• Time of arrival at patient
• Time unit left scene
• Time of arrival at destination
• Time of transfer of care

for this research to be effective and accurate, researchers must be able to collect similar data from many different systems. If each system's data differed from the next, the data, and, most importantly, the research would be meaningless.

For example, if a study were to focus on survival from cardiac arrest in order to determine how long it took from the time the call was received at a 911 center until the time the EMT-Bs arrived, the researchers may find that there was a problem with the times received from certain systems. One system may use the time the ambulance arrived "on the scene." This may or may not reflect the time that the EMT-Bs reached the patient. In some high-rise buildings it may take another five minutes to reach the patient, once the EMT-Bs arrive at the scene.

A **minimum data set** was developed to standardize arrival time at patient location and other pieces of information (Table 1–1). This data set means that all the data elements should be present in each Prehospital Care Report (PCR) and the definition of each data element should be standardized from region to region and state to state. Note that there are two types of information: patient information and administrative information.

■ MEDICAL/LEGAL AND ETHICAL ISSUES

This section reviews common medical/legal and moral issues. These terms and concepts are largely unchanged from your original training and are presented for the purpose of helping you prepare for certification exams.

Scope of Practice

Simply stated, the scope of practice defines medical/legal boundaries and expectations for the care you provide as an EMT-B. The scope of practice for any medical professional is usually defined by state legislation. Just as physicians, nurses, technicians, and others have definitions of what they are allowed to do, EMT-Bs are also bound by legislative guidelines. The scope of practice of an EMT-B may be enhanced by medical direction through the use of standing orders and protocols.

Consent

Do Not Resuscitate (DNR) Orders

In general, mentally competent patients have the right to refuse care, including resuscitative efforts. This situation is most commonly encountered in a patient with a terminal disease. In most states, refusal of care requires a written order from a physician (a Do Not Resuscitate [DNR] order) before care may be withheld (Figure 1–5). A DNR order is called an "advance directive" because it is signed in advance by the patient. Be sure to review your protocols regarding DNR orders *before* you must make these decisions. A scene in which the patient or family do not want care for a critical illness is not the time to read the manual!

Expressed Consent

In order to provide care for any patient, you must obtain consent. To be able to give consent, a patient must be of legal age, be able to make a rational decision, be mentally competent, and be informed about the care that will be given, the procedures involved, and all related risks. *Consent must be obtained from every conscious, mentally competent adult before rendering treatment.*

Department of Health

Nonhospital Order Not to Resuscitate (DNR order)

Person's Name (Print) _____

Date of Birth ___/___/___

Do not resuscitate the person named above.

Person's Signature _____

Date ___/___/___

Physician's Signature _____

Print Name _____

License Number _____

Date ___/___/___

It is the responsibility of the physician to determine, at least every 90 days, whether this order continues to be appropriate, and to indicate this by a note in the person's medical chart. The issuance of a new form is **NOT** required, and under the law this order should be considered valid unless it is known that it has been revoked. This order remains valid and must be followed, even if it has not been reviewed within the 90 day period.

FIGURE 1–5 A Do Not Resuscitate (DNR) order.

Implied Consent

If a patient is unconscious and therefore unable to give consent, it is assumed or implied that the patient, if he were conscious, would consent to your care. If an unconscious patient regains consciousness and is able to make a rational decision, you must obtain consent to continue care.

Consent of Minors

Minors, because of their age, are unable to give consent. This also applies to individuals who are mentally incompetent. Consent for care of these patients must be obtained from a parent or legal guardian. Each state has its own laws that determine the age at which a minor can legally give consent. The ages for consent may vary depending on whether the child is emancipated (living on his or her own) or married. If a child is critically ill or injured and a parent or guardian is not present, begin care based on implied consent.

Patient Refusal

A patient who is competent and of legal age may refuse your care and/or transportation. The patient may withdraw consent at any time. Most agencies have a "release" form that the patient signs to indicate refusal of care (Figure 1–6). This form should also be witnessed. The purpose of this form is to release the EMT-B and ambulance service from liability should the patient suffer ill effects from the refusal.

A patient must be fully informed of the risks involved with refusing care and/or transportation. A patient who refuses care and whose condition then deteriorates can be a significant source of liability for EMT-Bs, even though the patient signed the "waiver" or release. *Always make every effort to convince the patient to accept your care and transportation.* In the event the patient still refuses, always tell the patient that you can be called again at any time. Furthermore, attempt to convince the patient to call a doctor for follow-up care. Having a family member or other concerned person stay with the patient may also be helpful should problems develop after you leave. Carefully document attempts you have made to convince the patient to accept your care and the provisions you made for the patient when care was refused.

Consent is not always clear cut. It is not always easy to determine if a patient is rational and capable of making informed decisions. In your experience as an EMT-B, you may have responded to calls in which a patient was intoxicated, suf-

fered from head injury, or incurred another medical problem which may have clouded his or her judgment. If patients such as these are allowed to "sign off" and refuse care, you could be held responsible if they suffer a worsening of their condition as a result of not being transported.

There are several steps that can be taken to provide quality care while still respecting the patient's rights. If you question whether a patient is competent to refuse, or if you feel that not caring for the patient may result in a worsening of the patient's condition, you must take action. Consider the following steps:

- *Contact medical direction for advice.* The medical control physician may be able to provide advice and input on the patient's condition and ways to convince the patient to accept your care and transportation.
- *Utilize family members to help the patient accept your care.* Often family members can help convince the patient that care is actually needed. Family members can also provide insight into the patient's reasoning for refusing care (denial, fear of hospitals, etc.).
- *Notify the police if necessary.* In many states, police have the authority to order a patient to be transported against their will. If you have a supervisor, notify him or her as well.

Remember to document all your actions. It is usually considered best to err on the side of caution and seek input from medical control, the police, or other appropriate parties than simply let the patient refuse.

Abandonment

Terminating care of a patient without assuring that the patient is in the hands of a provider at the same or higher level of training is considered abandonment.

Negligence

Negligence is deviation from the accepted standard of care that results in injury to a patient. There are four components to a successful negligence action or lawsuit:

1. The EMT-B had a **duty to act.** This means that the EMT-B was in a situation through employment, position in a volunteer squad, or other

EMS PATIENT REFUSAL CHECKLIST

PATIENT NAME:_____ AGE: _____

LOCATION OF CALL:_____ DATE: _____

AGENCY INCIDENT #:_____ AGENCY CODE: _____

NAME OF PERSON FILLING OUT FORM: _____

I.   ASSESSMENT OF PATIENT (Circle appropriate response for each item)

    1.   Oriented to: Person?   Yes   No
                              Place?   Yes   No
                              Time?   Yes   No
                              Situation?   Yes   No

    2.   Altered level of consciousness?   Yes   No

    3.   Head injury?   Yes   No

    4.   Alcohol or drug ingestion by exam or history?   Yes   No

II.   PATIENT INFORMED (Circle appropriate response for each item)

    Yes   No   Medical treatment/evaluation needed

    Yes   No   Ambulance transport needed

    Yes   No   Further harm could result without medical treatment/
                   evaluation

    Yes   No   Transport by means other than ambulance could be
                   hazardous in light of patient's illness/injury

    Yes   No   Patient provided with Refusal Information Sheet

    Yes   No   Patient accepted Refusal Information Sheet

III. DISPOSITION

    _____   Refused all EMS services

    _____   Refused field treatment, but accepted transport

    _____   Refused transport, but accepted field treatment

    _____   Refused transport to recommended facility

    _____   Patient transported by private vehicle to _____

    _____   Released in care or custody of self

    _____   Released in care or custody of relative or friend

           Name: _____   Relationship: _____

    _____   Released in custody of law enforcement agency

           Agency: _____   Officer: _____

    _____   Released in custody of other agency

           Agency: _____   Officer: _____

IV.   COMMENTS: _____

    _____

    _____

FIGURE 1–6 A sample patient refusal checklist.

position in which the EMT-B is required to provide care *and*

2. The EMT-B breached, or failed to perform, that duty.

3. Injuries or damages were inflicted (may be physical or psychological) *and*

4. The actions (or omissions, lack of action) caused the injury or damage.

Preceptor Pearl

When someone new to the profession is completing a pre-hospital care report (PCR), remember your role as an experienced provider. Coach the new EMT-B to "paint a word picture" of the patient. Someone who has never seen the patient should be able to clearly "picture" the patient by reading the PCR. Remind the newcomer that when it comes to interventions: "If it's not written down, it wasn't performed." Proper documentation is important for liability prevention. ✤

Battery

If a patient who is legally able to refuse care is treated anyway, the patient has grounds for criminal or civil charges against the EMT-B for battery. Battery is subjecting a person to contact against his or her will.

Duty to Act

EMT-Bs, in some situations, have a duty to act. In some cases, this duty is very clear—such as when you are riding an ambulance dispatched to a call. Other times—such as when you are off-duty in another ambulance district—you may not have a legal duty to act, but you may be morally obligated to provide care or take action until EMS arrives. In most cases, for both legal and moral reasons, it is better to provide care than not to.

Confidentiality

When you treat a patient, the details of your assessment and care are confidential—they cannot be told to others. The information may be given to other health care providers who need the information to provide care, under judicial subpoena, when law requires (child abuse, etc.), and for some insurance purposes. Releasing information for other reasons requires a signed release form from the patient.

Organ Retrieval/Organ Donor

There are many people who are waiting to receive donated organs to save or prolong their life. While the EMS care we give to organ donor patients *must* not differ from that for other patients, there are some things that may be done to assist in the harvesting of organs from a donor. If you find yourself caring for a patient who is an organ donor and that patient is in cardiac arrest, continue to treat the patient as you would any other. Advise medical direction that the patient may be an organ donor. The physician may direct you to continue CPR when it normally would be stopped in order to maintain organs in a viable condition. You may confront this situation in a trauma incident in which a patient has mortal wounds. Mortal head injuries are the most common scenario for organ donations. CPR may be initiated solely for the purpose of organ harvesting.

■ EMS AT CRIME SCENES

Crime scenes are very dynamic situations (Figure 1–7). Providing EMS at crime scenes can be very challenging. Your safety is always the most important concern. Crime scenes should always be secured by the police before you enter and begin care. Even then, the perpetrator(s) may return or even be well hidden at the scene.

Once your safety is reasonably assured, there are still some very major issues: patient care, preservation of evidence, and working with the police. This section will give an overview of EMS actions at the crime scene. Just as there are many types of patients, there are many types of crime

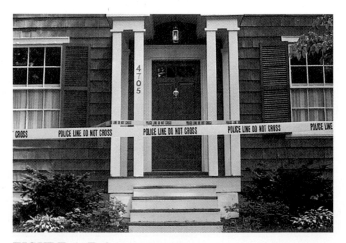

FIGURE 1–7 A crime scene.

scenes and evidence. Use your local resources to set up additional training in conjunction with police agencies in your area.

Scene Safety

Obviously, scene safety is the most important part of any call. Danger at a crime scene may come from things other than human beings. While physical violence is perhaps the most thought-of danger, remember that downed wires, hazardous materials, controlled substances, booby traps, and other materials may pose a danger to you. Even if the danger is not directed at you as an EMS provider, you may still be affected by it.

The police have the training, authority, and responsibility to secure the scene for violent or potentially violent persons. Failing to let police perform this task, or unreasonably attempting it yourself, may cause you to fall victim to the same violence that harmed your patient. Fight the urge to rush in without doing a thorough scene survey. Remember that scenes change rapidly. A scene that was not violent initially may become violent when the perpetrator returns or emerges from hiding. Patients themselves can become violent. You can never be too careful.

Cooperating with the Police

While some may feel that public service agencies automatically cooperate, as an experienced provider you will realize that this is not always the case. Agencies and personnel may fail to cooperate—not out of malicious actions but because emergency scenes are very stressful.

There is one fundamental difference between the responsibilities of police and EMS: EMS must get a trauma patient off the scene in ten minutes or less; the police may have hours to examine a crime scene carefully.

Even the most experienced and well-meaning EMT-B can disturb a crime scene. It is inevitable. One fundamental disturbance is caused by taking the patient to the hospital. This action removes a key piece of evidence (the patient) from the scene.

The combination of the stress felt by members of both agencies plus their conflicting roles is often the cause of less than ideal EMS/police interaction. The following steps may help prevent these negative interactions:

- *Learn to identify and preserve evidence.* While you must always put patient care first (after your own safety) at any scene, learn how to recognize evidence and preserve it. Knowledge of types of evidence can help you carry out your patient-care tasks and help you to preserve valuable evidence.

- *Be observant.* Small things may be the key to a criminal case. Remembering the condition of the area when you arrive is very important. Whether the door was unlocked, whether the lights were on or off, and statements made by the patient can be extremely important.

- *Remember what you touch.* Remembering what you touch is very important at a crime scene. You may find it necessary to move a patient from a couch to the floor to provide treatments such as CPR. You may also need to move furniture to perform this task. Remembering these actions and reporting them to the police is very important. If you do not, a police officer at the scene may see furniture moved and blood in two locations. The officer may improperly conclude that a struggle took place because of changes you made.

- *Minimize your impact on the scene.* While you may have to move items at the scene, do so carefully and minimally. A good rule of thumb would be to do what you must to provide proper patient care and no more. Remember what changes have been made and report them to the police.

- *Communication and training* It may not be possible to provide a thorough report to the police and still keep your time at the scene to an acceptable level. Many police agencies will request a statement about your actions and observations at the crime scene. Do this according to your agency's policies. There is a good chance that you will be required to testify about the conditions at the crime scene and the actions you took while there and en route to the hospital. When the call is over, critique the scene from a patient-care as well as an evidence-preservation standpoint. Invite police officers to speak at your training sessions to learn more about crime scenes.

You may also be sent to calls that appear to be routine medical or trauma calls which later are determined to be crime scenes. Many experienced EMT-Bs have received calls days, weeks, or months later from a police officer indicating that a call they had been to some time ago was actually a crime. EMT-Bs may also uncover situations that are suspicious and be the first to alert the police to a crime. In either case, being observant will help you to remain safe, to uncover the mechanism of injury or medical history, and to document important facts about the patient.

Crime scenes are challenging situations. Your first priority is always patient care, with attention to aspects of the crime scene that may be pre-served as you go. Remember that you are under a certain amount of stress at a crime scene. So are the police. Any interpersonal relationship will suffer when stress is added; crime scenes are no different. Understanding, training, and cooperation will make the next crime scene you respond to successful for both yourself and the police.

CHAPTER REVIEW

■ SUMMARY

The new curriculum emphasizes assessment-based thinking rather than diagnosis. In addition, it allows the EMT-B to assist patients with some medications, which enhances the relationship between the EMT-B and medical direction.

The EMS system has been developed to provide prehospital as well as hospital emergency care. It includes the 911 or other emergency access system, dispatchers, First Responders, EMTs, the hospital emergency department, physicians, nurses, physicians' assistants, and other health professionals.

The EMT-B's responsibilities include safety; patient assessment and care; lifting, moving, and transporting patients; transfer of care; and patient advocacy. An EMT-B must have certain personal and physical traits to assure the ability to do the job. In addition, the seasoned EMT-B is asked to take on the role of preceptor, coaching less-experienced EMT-Bs.

Education (including refresher training and continuing education), quality improvement procedures, and medical direction are all essential to maintaining high standards of EMS care.

■ REVIEW QUESTIONS

1. List the components of the Emergency Medical Services (EMS) system.
2. List the roles and responsibilities of the EMT-B.
3. Define quality improvement (QI). Describe the quality improvement program in place in your EMS system.
4. Describe the difference between on-line and off-line medical direction. Give an example of each.

5. Define the following terms:
   scope of practice   Do Not Resuscitate
   expressed consent   (DNR) order
   negligence   implied consent
                              duty to act

6. List several ways to identify and preserve evidence at a crime scene.

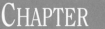
The Well-Being of the EMT-Basic

- *Emotions and Stress*
- *Scene Safety*

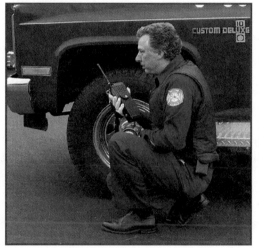

■ *Learning how to safeguard your well-being as an EMT-Basic is critical. During your EMS service you will be exposed to all kinds of stress, including that which accompanies death and dying. You will also sometimes be exposed to dangerous situations. It is important to learn strategies to help you stay emotionally well and physically safe.*

Scene safety is perhaps the most important part of any call. Without assuring your safety and the safety of others at the scene, the remainder of the call is destined to fail. This chapter *deals with the concept of scene size-up, with a primary emphasis on scene safety. Texts that are designed for EMT-Bs taking their original class cover some scene-safety issues, but in less detail. As a practicing EMT-B, you have experience in emergency scenes, patient assessment, management, and other aspects of the EMS call. With this experience, you will find it easier to integrate scene-safety methods. You have experienced unsafe or potentially unsafe scenes and recognize the value of scene safety for every call.*

MAKING THE TRANSITION

- Scene size-up is a formal part of the patient assessment process.
- Size-up is performed before the initial assessment and includes determining BSI needed, scene safety, mechanism of injury/nature of illness, and the number of patients.

OBJECTIVES

Numbered objectives below are from the United States Department of Transportation 1994 EMT-Basic National Standard Curriculum.

■ KNOWLEDGE AND ATTITUDE

At the completion of this chapter, you should be able to:

Well-Being of the EMT-Basic

1. List the possible emotional reactions that the EMT-Basic may experience when faced with trauma, illness, death, and dying. (pp. 21–23)
2. Discuss the possible reactions that a family member may exhibit when confronted with death and dying. (p. 23)
3. State the steps in the EMT-Basic's approach to the family confronted with death and dying. (p. 23)
4. State the possible reactions that the family of the EMT-Basic may exhibit due to their outside involvement in EMS. (p. 21)
5. Recognize the signs and symptoms of critical incident stress. (p. 21)
6. State possible steps that the EMT-Basic may take to help reduce/alleviate stress. (pp. 22–23)

7. Explain the need to determine scene safety. (pp. 23-24)

Scene Size-Up

1. Recognize hazards/potential hazards. (pp. 23–24)
2. Describe common hazards found at the scene of a trauma and a medical patient. (pp. 24–27)
3. Determine if the scene is safe to enter. (p. 24)
4. Discuss common mechanisms of injury/ nature of illness. (pp. 24–26)
5. Discuss the reason for identifying the total number of patients at the scene. (pp. 24–25)
6. Explain the reason for identifying the need for additional help or assistance. (pp. 24–25)
7. Explain the rationale for crew members to evaluate scene safety prior to entering. (pp. 26–29)
8. Serve as a model for others explaining how patient situations affect your evaluation of mechanism of injury or illness. (pp. 24–26)

■ SKILLS

1. Observe various scenarios and identify potential hazards.

Your EMS unit receives a call for an unknown problem at 1243 E. Magnolia Street. The Emergency Medical Dispatcher tells you that the caller "hung up" before further information could be obtained.

You arrive in the area of the residence and begin the size-up even before leaving the rig. You note that there is no activity outside the residence. You carefully approach the residence and begin to get a "funny feeling" about the call.

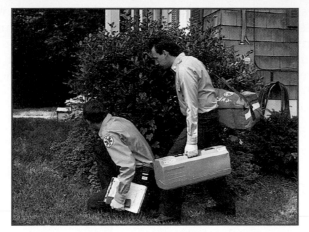

Your partner moves to ring the doorbell, but you stop him. "It's too quiet," you say. "The house is dark. Let's get back and listen for a second." You only need to listen for about two seconds when you hear glass breaking and the beginning of shouting.

One of the individuals in the residence who is shouting sounds intoxicated and is making threats to the other. You wisely decide to return to the ambulance and move to a safe place until the police arrive. You inform the dispatcher of your observations and wait for word from the police that the scene is secure.

Once you are called back to the scene, you are briefed by the police. You maintain a higher level of observation since violence can always reoccur. The call was an injury as a result of a family fight. Your scene-safety skills prevented you from walking into the middle of a dispute and possibly being injured. ■

One of your most important jobs is to stay emotionally well and physically safe. Remember: If the EMT-B becomes a victim, he is of little or no use to a patient and may put other rescuers in jeopardy. Ways to safeguard your well-being include understanding and dealing with the stress that normally accompanies critical incidents, ensuring scene safety, and taking body substance isolation (BSI) precautions before treating a patient.

■ EMOTION AND STRESS

Causes of Stress

Emergencies are stressful. That is their nature. While most emergencies are considered "routine," some calls seem to have a higher potential for causing excess stress on EMS providers. They include the following.

- *Multiple-casualty incident (MCI)*—a single incident in which there are multiple patients.

- *Calls involving infants and children*—these calls are known to be particularly stressful to all health-care providers.
- *Severe injuries*—calls involving injuries that cause major trauma or distortion to the human body.
- *Abuse and neglect of children, adults, and the elderly*
- *Death of a coworker*

Stress may be caused by a single event or it may be the cumulative result of several incidents. Remember that any incident may affect you and coworkers differently. Two EMT-Bs on the same call may have opposite responses. Try never to make negative judgments about another person's reaction.

Stress may also stem from a combination of factors, including problems in your personal life. One common cause of stress is people who "just don't understand" the job. For example, your EMS organization may require you to work on weekends and holidays. Time spent on call may be frustrating to friends and family members. They may not understand why you can't participate in certain

CHAPTER 2 The Well-Being of the EMT-Basic—Emotions and Stress, Scene Safety **21** social activities or why you can't leave a certain area. You might get frustrated, too, because you can't plan around the unpredictable nature of emergencies. Then, after a very trying or exciting call, for instance, you may wish to share your feelings with a friend or someone you love. You find instead that the person does not understand your emotions. This can lead to feelings of separation and rejection, which are highly stressful.

Signs and Symptoms of Stress

The signs and symptoms of stress include irritability with family, friends, and coworkers; inability to concentrate; changes in daily activities, such as difficulty sleeping or nightmares, loss of appetite, and loss of interest in sexual activity; anxiety; indecisiveness; guilt; isolation; and loss of interest in work.

Dealing with Stress

Life-Style Changes

There are several ways to deal with stress. They are called "life-style changes," and they include the following.

- *Develop more healthful and positive dietary habits.* Avoid fatty foods and increase your carbohydrate intake. Also reduce your consumption of alcohol and caffeine, which can have negative effects including an increase in stress and anxiety and disturbance of sleep patterns.
- *Exercise.* When performed safely and properly, this life-style change helps to "burn off" stress. It also helps you deal with the physical aspects of your responsibilities, such as carrying equipment and performing physically demanding emergency procedures.
- *Devote time to relaxing.* Try relaxation techniques, too. These techniques, which include deep-breathing exercises and meditation, are valuable stress reducers.

In addition to the changes you can make in your personal life to help reduce and prevent stress, there are also changes you can make in your professional life. If you are in an organization with varied shifts and locations, consider requesting a change to a different location that offers a lighter call volume or different types of calls. You

may also want to change your shift to one that allows more time with family and friends.

There are many types of help available for EMT-Bs and others who are experiencing stress. Seek them out. It is not a sign of weakness. There are many professionals who can help you deal with the stress you feel, and much of the care may be covered by health insurance policies.

Critical Incident Stress Debriefing (CISD)

A **critical incident stress debriefing (CISD)** is a process in which a team of trained peer counselors and mental health professionals meet with rescuers and health care providers who have been involved in a major incident. The meetings are generally held within 24 to 72 hours after the incident. The goal is to assist emergency care workers in dealing with the stress related to that incident.

The CISD is an open discussion of the feelings experienced during and after the call. Participants are encouraged to talk about any fears or reactions they have had. It is critical that the CISD does not become a method of investigation of the events of the call. Everything discussed at the meetings is confidential and all participants are asked not to disclose information once the meeting is over. Any breech in the confidentiality of the discussion prevents others from sharing information that can help them. After the open discussion, the CISD team offers suggestions on how to deal with and overcome the stress. It is important once again to state that stress after a major incident is normal and should be expected. The CISD process can help to accelerate the recovery process.

Sometimes a "defusing session is held within the first few hours after a critical incident. While CISD includes all personnel involved in the incident, a defusing session is usually limited to a small group, often the people who were most directly involved with the most stressful aspects of the incident. It provides them an opportunity to vent their feelings and receive information about the stress they may feel before the larger group meets.

After a CISD, follow-up is essential. A member of the peer team should contact all CISD attendees within 24 hours to offer support and referrals. No two emergency care workers will perceive, experience, or recover from critical incident stress in the same way. The process of overcoming the stress will be different from person to person. Resources must be available immediately as well as long after the incident, including "anniversary dates"—anniversaries of stressful events.

Comprehensive critical stress management goes beyond the CISD session to include pre-incident stress education, on-scene peer support, one-on-one support, disaster support services, spouse and family support, community outreach programs, and other health and welfare programs such as wellness programs. Remember, stress is a normal and perhaps an inevitable response to a critical incident. Learn to recognize the signs and symptoms, and find out where to turn for help in your area.

Understanding Reactions to Death and Dying

As an EMT-B, you will undoubtedly be called to patients who are in various stages of a terminal illness. Understanding what the families and the patients go through can help you deal with the stress they feel as well as your own.

When a patient finds out that he is dying, he goes through emotional stages, each varying in duration and magnitude, sometimes overlapping, and all affecting both the patient and the family.

- *Denial or "not me."* The patient denies that he is dying. This puts off dealing with the inevitable end of the process.
- *Anger or "why me?"* The patient becomes angry at his situation. This anger is commonly vented upon family members and EMS personnel.
- *Bargaining or "okay, but first let me..."* In the mind of the patient bargaining seems to postpone death, even for a short time.
- *Depression or "okay, but I haven't..."* The patient is sad, depressed, and despairing, often mourning things not accomplished, dreams that won't come true. He retreats into a world of his own, unwilling to communicate with others.
- *Acceptance or "okay, I'm not afraid."* The patient may come to accept death, although he does not welcome it. Often, the patient may come to accept the situation before family members do. At this stage, the family may need more support than the patient.

The patient and family are on an emotional roller coaster after a terminal condition has been diagnosed, and their reactions may not be the same. People may actually seem to be in more than one stage at the same time, or their attitudes may reflect thoughts that do not fit easily into any of the stages. However, a general understanding of the process can help you to communicate with them effectively.

As an EMT-B, you will encounter sudden, unexpected death, for example as a result of a motor vehicle collision. In cases of sudden death, family members are likely to react with a wide range of emotion.

There are several steps or approaches that you can take in dealing with the patient and family members confronted with death or dying.

- *Recognize the patient's needs.* Treat the patient with respect and do everything you can to preserve the patient's dignity and sense of control. For example, talk directly to the patient. Avoid talking about the patient to family members in the patient's presence as if the patient were incompetent or no longer a living person. Be sensitive to how the patient seems to want to handle the situation. For example, allow or encourage the patient to share feelings and needs, rather than cutting off such communications because of your own embarrassment or discomfort. Respect the patient's privacy if he does not want to communicate personal feelings.
- *Be tolerant of angry reactions from the patient or family members.* There may be feelings of helpless rage about the death or prospect of death. The anger is not personal. It would be directed at anyone in your position.
- *Listen empathetically.* You can't "fix" the situation, but just listening with understanding and patience will be very helpful.
- *Do not falsely reassure.* Avoid saying things like "Everything will be all right," which you, the patient, and the family all know is not true. Offering false reassurance will only be irritating or convey the impression that you don't really understand.
- *Offer as much comfort as you realistically can.* Comfort both the patient and the family. Let them know that you will do everything you can to help or to get them whatever help is available from other sources. Use a gentle tone of voice and a reassuring touch, if appropriate.

■ SCENE SAFETY

Depending on when you began your EMT training, you may remember that scene safety was not always considered a top priority. Assessment began with the patient's airway. Times have changed. EMT-Bs now realize that there are dangers, not only from violence, but from environmental and chemical factors, pets, and more. Although the text you studied in your original EMT-B classes covered scene safety, it most likely

TABLE 2-1 Components of the Scene Size-Up

Size-Up Component	Actions
Scene Safety	Make sure that the scene is safe from all potential hazards (violence, hazmat, fire, explosion, unstable vehicles or surfaces, etc.).
BSI Review	Make sure your BSI precautions are adequate for the patient and situation.
Mechanism of Injury (trauma) Nature of Illness (medical)	Determine whether the call is trauma or medical in nature. Observe for physical forces in injury.
Number of Patients and Needed Resources	Determine number of patients and if resources will be needed. Call for additional help before beginning patient care.

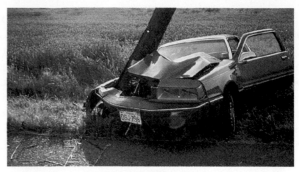

A. Motor vehicle accident.

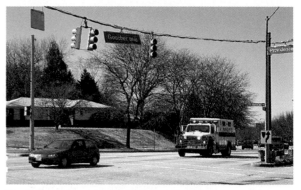

B. Emergency vehicle operation.

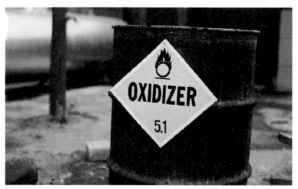

C. Hazardous materials.

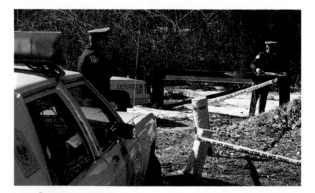

D. Crime scene.

FIGURE 2-1 Always be alert to potential hazards as you approach a scene.

was not detailed since it is difficult to present such material to students who have never been on calls or who have minimal experience in responding to calls. Furthermore, in your initial training, you were learning all parts of the patient assessment process and probably had minimal time to spend on learning all the principles of scene safety. This chapter reviews the concept of scene size-up, with concentration on scene-safety techniques.

The scene size-up is the first step of the patient assessment process and it begins the assessment with a logical theme: It will not be possible to act as an EMT-B if you are injured. The size-up also focuses on several other factors that must be determined early on, such as the mechanism of injury (MOI) and the resources needed to adequately handle the call (Table 2–1). The parts of the size-up include:

- *Scene Safety.* The first and foremost part of the size-up is safety. This process begins before you approach the scene or exit the ambulance (Figure 2–1). Observe the scene as you drive up and before you exit the vehicle. The process continues throughout the call since hazards can change and violence can escalate at any time.

- *Body Substance Isolation Review.* One of the initial determinations that must be made during the size-up is the amount of body substance isolation equipment that will be required for the call (Figure 2–2). Make this determination as soon as possible. Getting to the patient

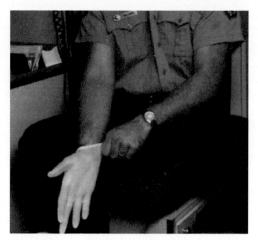

FIGURE 2-2 During scene size-up make the determination about what body substance isolation equipment you will require.

without appropriate equipment can be awkward and potentially dangerous.

- *Mechanism of Injury/Nature of Illness.* Even before you touch the patient, you should have some idea about the patient's complaint. Before care can begin, determine the mechanism of injury/nature of illness.

Some physical force (mechanism of injury) causes a traumatic injury. For example, in the case of a motor vehicle accident, there are three obvious impacts (Figure 2-3). It is your responsibility to determine this force, how it applies to a patient's condition, and the care you will provide. The most obvious examples are whether cervical spine stabilization is required and whether there is a potential for hidden injuries.

Specific types of motor vehicle collisions have specific injury patterns (Table 2-2). The amount of deformity in the passenger compartment is also significant in determining MOI. Injury from falls depends on the height, the surface landed on, and the part of the body that struck the ground. Penetrating injuries always have a high index of suspicion since the path of damage under the skin cannot be seen.

A person with a medical problem will have a nature of illness. Once trauma is ruled out, it is necessary to determine what type of medical problem the patient is experiencing.

- *Determine the Number of Patients.* Determine the number of patients early in the call, since you are less likely to call for help once you become involved with patient care. This may

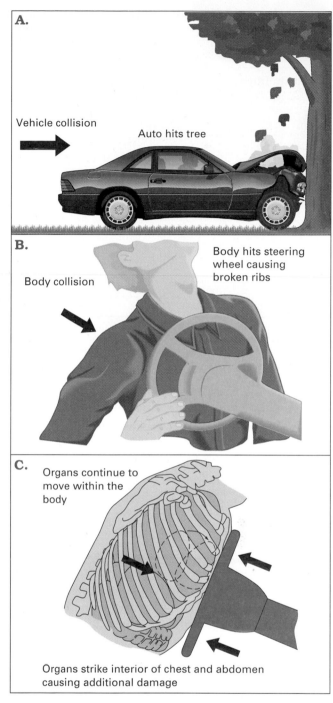

FIGURE 2-3 A. A vehicle strikes an object. **B.** The occupant continues to move forward and collides with steering wheel. **C.** The organs continue to move forward and collide with the inside of the chest and other organs.

range from simply calling for an additional ambulance in smaller incidents to activation of a multiple-casualty incident (MCI) plan. Don't forget to request any special resources that you may need (hazmat, power company, etc.).

TABLE 2-2 Mechanisms of Injury—Motor Vehicle Accidents

Type of Collision	Possible Injury Patterns
Head-On Impact	**Up-and-Over Pathway:** The body may be thrown over the steering wheel. The head and neck may sustain injuries from the windshield while the chest and abdomen may strike the steering wheel.
	Down-and-Under Pathway: The body slides under the steering wheel. There may be chest and abdominal injuries with pelvis, femur, knee, and lower leg injuries.
Rear Impact	Injuries to the cervical spine—especially when a head rest is not used. Other injury types are possible.
Side Impact	The patient on the side of the collision absorbs more energy than a person on the opposite side. The body and head may be pushed in opposite directions laterally. Suspect all injury patterns, especially if patients may have struck door post, etc. Determine the extent (in inches) of intrusion into passenger compartment.
Rotational Impact	A **rotational impact** occurs when a vehicle is struck, then spins. This often results in collisions with other vehicles or objects and results in multiple injury patterns.
Rollover	As with rotational impacts, **rollovers** cause multiple injury patterns. Items inside the vehicles become projectiles causing further injury.

Note: Attempt to determine if occupant restraints (safety belts) were in use at the time of the collision and what type was used (lap belt, lap and shoulder belt, etc.). Also determine if an airbag was deployed and "lift and look" under the airbag after the patient has been removed since the driver may have hit the steering wheel after the bag was deployed.

There are various sections in this text that deal with specific components of the scene size-up. Chapter 3 deals with body substance isolation. Chapter 18 covers hazardous material incidents. MCI procedures are covered in Chapter 17.

Scene-Safety Techniques

Observation

The best way to avoid danger is to prevent it. To prevent danger, you must observe it early. The On the Scene for this chapter described an alert EMT-B who recognized a dangerous situation. Had the EMT-B knocked on the door not observing the danger, he would have been exposed to the violence. It was a combination of factors, including the fact that the caller hung up, the house was dark, and the unusual silence at the scene that made the EMT-B suspicious. Since emergency calls are usually very active, these factors added together were cause for suspicion.

While "gut feelings" are usually correct, it is also important to develop concrete information about a call. Always check for these indicators of danger at a scene:

• *Fighting or Loud Voices.* Fighting is a relatively obvious sign of trouble, but one that is often ignored. Loud voices, posturing, or other signs of imminent fighting are also indicators. While you might not be the one who is involved in the fight, you can still be injured. Since you may appear as a symbol of authority, you could be attacked. Fighting may take place on the street or in the home. Domestic violence is alarmingly common and a source of many EMS calls.

• *Intoxicants or Illegal Drugs.* When people abuse alcohol or other drugs, their behavior becomes unpredictable. Many of us have seen intoxicated persons acting anywhere from sleepy to combative. When drugs are abused or they are observed on the scene, it is likely that the criminal element associated with the drugs is close by.

• *Weapons.* Weapons are a clear indicator of potential danger. When weapons are visible or in use, or their use is threatened, retreat! Remember that almost anything may be used as a weapon. It takes careful observation of the people and surroundings at a scene to prevent the use of a weapon against you.

• *Crime Scenes.* These scenes can cause dangers when the crime is in progress—as well as after the crime has been committed. It is not unusual for the perpetrators to be in hiding at the scene. They may also return to the scene during your time there. There have been calls where the "victim" assaults police and EMT-Bs! Even if the police have secured the crime scene, consider it potentially dangerous at all times.

- *Pets.* Almost any dog can be dangerous if it or its owners are threatened. There are many breeds of dogs that are trained to protect and attack. Exotic animals may also pose a threat to the EMT-B.

Use of Your Senses

Use your senses to observe and prevent danger. While it is sometimes difficult to remember to constantly observe, practicing observational techniques daily will make this task second nature.

When it comes to safety, some senses are obviously better applied than others. Sight is the sense most EMT-Bs think of when it comes to safety; you are able to see a weapon, unstable vehicle, or hazmat situation and respond appropriately. But do not underestimate the remaining senses. Hearing, as shown in the On the Scene, is vital for detecting scene dangers. The sense of hearing is beneficial because one does not need to see the danger directly in order to detect it. You can listen from other rooms, from behind doors, or from some distance away. Smell is valuable for identifying dangerous chemicals, leaking gasoline, and other situations that may pose a hazard. The senses of touch and taste are not practical to use since they brings you too close to the danger.

Some people claim to have a "sixth sense." If you do, heed it. Your gut feeling may not require immediate action, but may simply create a reason for you to react more slowly and to observe carefully until you can gain more information.

Many crime victims have told police that they "had a feeling" that something was about to happen but that they ignored that feeling. Act cautiously until the feeling is resolved, but avoid overreacting.

Response to Danger

When you observe danger, these tactics can help keep you safe until the police or other appropriate agencies arrive to secure the scene:

- *Use cover and concealment* (Figure 2–4). No doubt you have heard of the term "take cover." **Cover** is taking a position behind some sturdy barricade that will hide your body and offer ballistic protection. Examples of cover include brick walls, the engine of your ambulance, and large trees. Surprisingly, some common items offer little coverage. The box of an ambulance offers little or no protection. Most doors and walls are also poor cover.

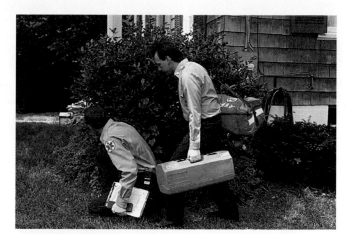

A.

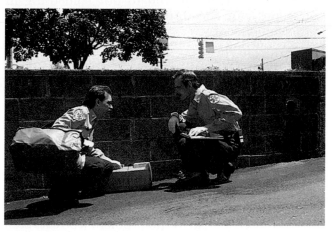

B.

FIGURE 2–4 A. Concealing yourself is placing your body behind an object that can hide you from view. **B.** Taking cover is finding a position that both hides you and protects your body from projectiles.

Concealment is hiding your body, but it does not offer protection from projectiles and should be used only when solid cover cannot be found safely. Doors, walls, smaller trees, and shrubs can be used for concealment.

- *Retreat.* If danger is observed, the most appropriate action is immediately moving a safe distance away. Retreat when you confront hazardous materials, unstable vehicles and terrain, and violence. When you are retreating from danger, a common mistake is not getting far enough away. It is best to have a clear idea exactly how far is far enough *before* a potentially life-threatening situation.

Move to a position where there are two major obstacles between you and the violence. If a dangerous person is able to get through one of the obstacles, one remains there as a buffer. One or both of the obstacles should be *cover.* One of the obstacles can be distance, as in moving several hundred yards away. However, distance alone will not provide protection from projectiles.

Ideally, you should be able to get away from the danger *and* find a position of cover. This way, if someone tries to move toward you, you have time to retreat further and find another position of cover. When possible, return to the rescue vehicle and drive away. However, this should be done only when it is safe to go to your vehicle.

- *Use distractions if necessary.* If you must retreat, it may help you to put something in the path of the danger. If you are fleeing through a doorway, wedging the stretcher there will slow down a potential aggressor. Throwing a medical kit at someone's feet will have a similar effect.

- *Carry a portable radio.* If you do confront danger, it must be reported. Carry a portable radio, especially if you are unable to return to the ambulance. When you report the danger, provide as much information as possible, such as:
  - The location of the problem
  - The nature of the problem (fighting, gunshots, dangerous drugs)
  - Your response to the problem (retreat, etc.)
  - Details about the incident

In the On the Scene example, the EMT-B was able to determine that there were two participants involved in the dispute. Advise the dispatcher of the number and gender of the people involved, their location in the residence, and whether alcohol is involved.

Many EMT-Bs are concerned about preventing liability when retreating from a scene. The key to any liability prevention is adequate, objective documentation. Document all the indicators of potential danger and your response to them. When you retreat from the scene, do not return to service. Stand by until the scene is safe—when care can be performed safely. Document the time you left and returned to the scene. Notify a supervisor if necessary.

Carrying weapons can be cause for liability—and danger. Carrying a weapon may give you a false sense of security. You may enter scenes from which you would normally retreat. It is also dangerous to carry any weapon you are not trained to use: You wouldn't think of using advanced life support equipment unless you were an AEMT. Also remember that weapons may be taken from you and used against you or your partners. The use of a weapon may also result in considerable liability. Observation and proper response before the danger strikes are much safer and more practical methods of dealing with danger than is the use of weapons.

Planning for Safety

It is always best to plan for safety. Planning begins with having a base of safety knowledge, such as the information presented earlier in this chapter. To be safe, these are certain things that can be done in advance:

- *Work together.* The sum of a team's efforts is greater than its individual parts. This is especially true when it comes to safety. Crews can work together to observe and can use predetermined signals to communicate dangers to other members of the crew.

  Split up the carrying of equipment between crew members so no one person is bogged down. Having a hand free helps you to hold railings, open doors, stabilize yourself on uneven surfaces, and retreat more easily.

- *Make your equipment work for you.* Make sure your equipment is easily carried and not burdensome. Carry the equipment that you will realistically need in kits of a reasonable size and shape.

- *Dress for safety.* Wear clothing or protective equipment that is appropriate for the task you are performing. Hazardous material incidents and rescue scenes require specific safety equipment (see Chapters 17 and 18). Everyday EMS work requires safe shoes and outerwear that is reflective and appropriate for the weather.

- *Use body armor, if necessary.* Some EMT-Bs wear body armor, also known as bulletproof vests (Figure 2–5). Many metropolitan EMS agencies are providing body armor for employees or contributing a sum toward its purchase. Even if body armor isn't for you at this time, the following information can help you make an informed decision about its purchase and possible use.
  - Body armor isn't totally bulletproof. It will stop most handgun bullets, but not rifle

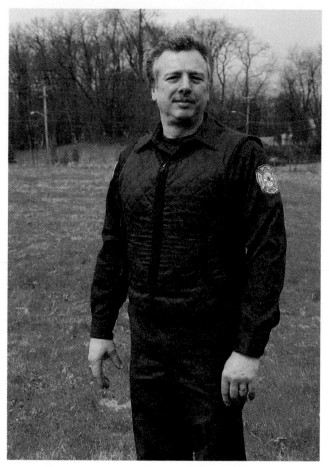

FIGURE 2–5 Body armor, or bulletproof vest.

bullets. Body armor isn't a guarantee; it is an added safety measure that you may choose to take.

- Body armor may stop knife penetration and prevent trauma from steering wheel impact in motor vehicle accidents.

- To be effective, equipment must be worn! Choose comfortable body armor and a practical way to wear it. A quilted cover designed for outerwear will be very hot in the summer. A vest will not afford any protection when it is in your locker or behind the seat of the ambulance.

- Body armor is flexible. It is not truly "armor." The panels are made of soft Kevlar™ or other fibers that are woven together to give ballistic protection.

Scene safety techniques are not designed to instill paranoia. In our chosen career as EMT-Bs, it would be unrealistic to believe that we will never face danger. Emergencies are dynamic events at which emotions run high. If we accept that the skill of observation is necessary, then that skill will be part of our activities on every call, just as are patient assessment or splinting skills.

CHAPTER REVIEW

■ SUMMARY

The scene size-up is the first part of any call. It requires initial as well as continual attention to scene safety throughout the call. Be alert for hazardous materials, unstable vehicles or surfaces, violence, and other dangers.

During the size-up, make a determination of what body substance isolation precautions are necessary. It is essential to be prepared before reaching the patient. Once you reach the patient it is very important that you determine the mechanism of injury/nature of illness in order to provide proper patient care. Finally, it is important to determine the number of patients that are at the

scene. If there are more than the current resources can handle, call for help *before* beginning care. You are less likely to call for help after being immersed in patient care. Call in advance for additional resources such as the fire department, hazmat teams, and utility companies.

The best way to remain safe is to be observant and spot danger before it strikes. This involves the use of your senses and a careful survey of the scene. When you do observe danger, you should retreat and attain a position of cover or concealment. Working with others on your crew will help you to remain safe.

■ REVIEW QUESTIONS

1. List the five types of calls that have a higher potential for causing stress in EMS providers.

2. Describe the purpose and process of a critical incident stress debriefing (CISD).

3. Explain the stages of emotion that are experienced by a patient or the family of a patient who is dying.

4. Describe ways an EMT-B should deal with the emotions experienced by a patient or the family of a patient who is dying.

5. List the four components of the scene size-up.

6. What is the difference between mechanism of injury and nature of illness? How is each determined?

7. Why is it important to make an early determination of the number of patients?

8. List four indicators of a potentially violent scene.

9. If you encounter danger and must retreat, how far away should you retreat? Why?

10. What is body armor? Describe its uses and pitfalls.

CHAPTER 3

Infection Control

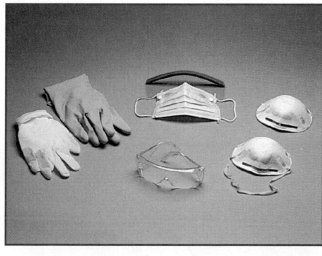

■ As an experienced EMT-B, you now know the importance of ensuring your safety from exposure to potentially infectious blood or other body fluids through body substance isolation (BSI) both before, during, and after patient care activities. The use of hand washing and of personal protective equipment (PPE) has become a crucial part of every EMS provider's practice. As you are aware, attitudes and practices have changed over the past several years regarding exposure to blood and other body fluids in order to minimize contracting a potentially infectious disease.

This increased awareness has also extended beyond the EMS providers' well-being to our patients as well. Decontamination and cleaning or disposing of equipment that has been soiled or used during patient care activities has also changed over the years. An EMT-B must be acutely aware of the cleanliness of patient care equipment to decrease any potential for passing on an infectious disease from patient to patient.

This chapter outlines the OSHA requirements 29 CFR Part 1910.1030 of an exposure control plan for annual refresher training regarding bloodborne pathogens, reviews the Ryan White CARE Act reporting requirements, and reviews the body substance isolation considerations for EMT-Bs during an ambulance call as well as decontamination procedures for emergency equipment and vehicles.

MAKING THE TRANSITION

■ EMT-Bs' requirements under OSHA 1910.1030 and the Ryan White CARE Act are explained.

■ Proper BSI and PPE required during all phases of an ambulance call are considered.

■ Changes in EMT-Bs' attitudes regarding blood and other potentially infectious materials are emphasized.

OBJECTIVES

The numbered objectives below are from the United States Department of Transportation 1994 EMT-Basic National Standard Curriculum.

■ KNOWLEDGE AND ATTITUDE

At the completion of this chapter, you should be able to:

1. Discuss the importance of body substance isolation. (pp. 33–34, 38–44)

2. Describe the steps the EMT-B should take for personal protection from airborne and bloodborne pathogens. (pp. 33–34)

3. List the personal protective equipment necessary during exposure to airborne and bloodborne pathogens. (pp. 35, 37–38)

4. Explain the rationale for serving as an advocate for the use of appropriate protective equipment. (pp. 31, 34, 35–36)

5. Summarize the importance of preparing the unit for the next call. (pp. 38–44)

6. Distinguish among the terms cleaning, disinfection, high-level disinfection, and sterilization. (p. 41)

7. Describe how to clean or disinfect items following patient care. (pp. 38–44)

■ SKILLS

1. Given a scenario with a potential infectious exposure, the EMT-B will use appropriate personal protective equipment. At the completion of the scenario, the EMT-B will properly remove and discard the protective equipment.

2. Given the above scenario, the EMT-B will complete cleaning and disinfection of all equipment used during patient care.

ON THE SCENE

You and your partner have just completed the morning checklist for your vehicle. You have restocked the necessary equipment and supplies. You know that you, your partner, and the vehicle are ready to respond to any call. Just as you settle in to study for the upcoming EMT-Intermediate pre-test, the alert tone goes off, and dispatch sends you to an emergency call for a 58-year-old man who is "vomiting blood."

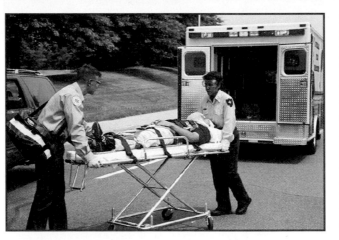

En route the dispatcher reports that the patient is conscious, alert, and breathing, but he does have a history of alcohol abuse. As part of your **scene size-up**, you don your gloves, mask, and eye protection since there is a likelihood that blood or body fluid will be splashed with the vomitus. As you arrive on scene, you note there do not appear to be any hazards for you or your partner at this single family residence. As your partner gathers the jump kit and you grab the clipboard, a woman comes to the front door and tells you the patient is in the bathroom. As you enter the house, you smell a distinct odor of feces and blood. Although you have only one patient, you consider the need for ALS backup because of the patient's potential for blood loss.

You enter the bathroom to find the man slumped against the bathtub. You introduce yourself, and he tells you his name is William Verrill. He asks that you call him "Billy." You begin your **initial assessment** by noting his general appearance, which is not good. Billy tells you he is a recovering alcoholic, has been vomiting blood for the past thirty minutes, and has blood in his stools. There are large blood clots in the toilet bowl. He is conscious and alert, with a patent airway and rapid breathing. His radial pulse is weak and rapid. Since you know Billy could have severe internal bleeding, you consider him a high-priority patient. You have your partner request from the dispatcher an ALS back-up to your location. Since Billy's vomiting has stopped, you decide to place him on high-flow oxygen via a non-rebreather mask.

You have your partner get the ambulance stretcher as you continue with the **focused history and physical–medical patient**. Billy tells you that he was outside working in the garden when he felt sick to his stomach. He came into the bathroom and began to vomit dark red blood that turned to bright red after a few episodes. He did not have any pain prior to vomiting but now complains his stomach hurts from the vomiting. Billy points out that he was a heavy drinker for about twenty years but that he has been "dry" for the last year. He has had some problems with his liver in the past, but for the last year he has been fairly healthy. He is not allergic to anything and does not take any medications. He last ate at breakfast three hours ago. Your physical exam does not reveal any other signs or symptoms other than pain when his stomach is palpated. His vital signs are blood pressure 102/60, pulse 110, respirations 22, and his skin is pale, cool, and

clammy. He tells you that the blood pressure you've obtained is low for him.

You and partner load Billy on to the stretcher to move him to the ambulance. Your partner tells you that ALS is not readily available, so you begin transport to the receiving hospital. Since Billy has started to vomit again, you decide to put on a gown to protect your clothes and skin from contact with the blood and emesis.

While en route to the hospital, you perform an **ongoing assessment**. You again check Billy's overall general appearance, mental status, and ABCs. His vital signs remain the same, the oxygen is still flowing, and there seems to be a slight improvement in skin color. Billy's last vomiting episode has subsided, although not all the blood and emesis were caught by the basin. You know this will have to be cleaned up at the hospital.

At the hospital you transfer care to the emergency department staff and give a report to the triage nurse on duty. You place Billy on the cardiac trauma room stretcher and leave him in the hands of the emergency department staff. You strip the linen from the ambulance stretcher and put it in the dirty linen hamper. You note that there is some blood on the side of the stretcher and tell your partner about it. You discard your gown, gloves, mask, and eye protection into the biohazard trash can and begin your patient care report. Your partner dons heavy-duty rubber gloves to clean the stretcher and the patient compartment of the ambulance. ■

■ THE EXPOSURE CONTROL PLAN

Purpose

The Occupational Safety and Health Administration (OSHA) has developed and enforces standards for EMT-Bs to use when dealing with bloodborne pathogens, called Title 29 CFR 1910.1030. This standard will be reviewed in this section and may be used by EMT-Bs as a basis for their annual refresher training requirements.

The OSHA standard requires an EMS service or employer to establish an **exposure control plan**. The exposure control plan must include:

• General hazards associated with exposures to blood or body fluids

• Specific tasks considered to present a potential exposure to these hazards
• Job classifications or descriptions of the employees/personnel expected to perform the above tasks
• Personal protective equipment (PPE) and safe work practices designed to prevent exposures
• Vaccination (hepatitis B) requirements
• Training requirements under the exposure control plan
• Exposure determination and follow-up medical care including record keeping

As you know, bacteria and viruses are organisms or pathogens that may cause infections or diseases. The spread of pathogens may be through contact with blood or other body fluids or through the air. Direct contact with blood or other body fluids through an open wound or break in the skin, mucous membrane of the mouth, nose or eyes, or parenteral contact (stick by a needle or other sharp object) increases the risk for contracting a bloodborne disease such as human immunodeficiency virus (HIV) or hepatitis B (HBV). Airborne pathogens are spread through tiny droplets released by breathing, sneezing, or coughing. These pathogens may be absorbed through the EMT-B's eyes or inhaled into the respiratory system. Airborne pathogens will be covered in more detail under the Ryan White Act.

Occupational Exposure

Since it is impossible to determine which body fluids are infectious, *ALL* blood and other body fluids must be considered infectious, and appropriate safeguards must be taken whenever these fluids are present. When an EMT-B has contact with blood or other body fluid through a break in the skin, eyes, mucous membranes, or parenteral contact resulting from the performance of his or her duties, this is referred to as **occupational exposure**. Duties in which EMS providers are considered "at risk" include CPR, airway management maneuvers, emergency medical care such as bleeding control for trauma victims, other medical emergencies such as childbirth, and cleaning/decontamination of equipment used during patient-care activities.

Universal Precautions and Body Substance Isolation

Exposure control plans outline procedures to use when the potential for contact with blood or other body fluids exists. **Universal precautions**, or **body substance isolation (BSI)**, are infection-control procedures designed to reduce the risk for exposure to potentially infectious blood or other body fluids. Because each situation you encounter is slightly different, it is important that you take the appropriate BSI for the specific situation you are faced with.

Both the employer and the employee are responsible for ensuring that proper BSI techniques are followed. The employer is responsible for implementing the exposure control plan, as well as providing appropriate training, immunizations, and the proper **personal protective equipment (PPE)**. The employee has the responsibility

to take the training, use the proper PPE, and follow the exposure control plan. The employee is to use the proper PPE except in the most extraordinary circumstances, such as when an off-duty EMT-B encounters a patient who must be given CPR. Extraordinary situations are reserved for those instances when, in the EMT-B's professional judgment, the specific PPE will prevent the delivery of appropriate emergency medical care or will pose an increased hazard to the safety of the employee(s). Documentation of these extraordinary situations is required and must be followed up by the employer.

Engineering Controls

The exposure control plan must also include **engineering controls** that outline specific procedures to follow in dealing with blood or other body fluid specimens, contaminated equipment, contaminated needles, sharps containers, and disposal of contaminated disposable items. Blood or other body fluid specimens should be labeled with the appropriate "biohazard" identification and placed in a leak-proof container (Figure 3–1).

Non-disposable equipment that is contaminated with blood or other body fluids should be immediately examined for any contaminants and cleaned with disinfectant prior to returning it to service. If equipment cannot be adequately decontaminated, then it must be labeled with a "biohazard" identification.

Contaminated needles or other "sharps" should not be recapped, bent, or otherwise altered and should be placed immediately into a puncture- and leak-proof container appropriately labeled with a "biohazard" identification. Such containers should not be allowed to overflow and should be replaced routinely and disposed of properly.

Following a call, contaminated disposable items such as dressings, bandages, and gloves,

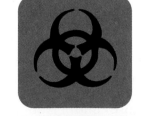

FIGURE 3–1 This biohazard symbol must be included on the labels of containers used for disposal of contaminated items.

should be disposed of immediately in an appropriately marked "biohazard" waste container. This action usually takes place while you are at the receiving facility but in some cases may occur at the ambulance station or base. Detailed procedures for cleaning and disinfecting equipment are presented later in this chapter.

Work Practice Controls

Work practice controls are the part of the exposure control plan used to complement the engineering controls. This section of the plan includes promotion of hand washing, usually the best defense against contracting an infectious disease. It also outlines procedures for dealing with contaminated needles or other sharps, procedures for personnel to follow regarding eating, drinking, or applying cosmetics in the patient compartment of the vehicle, and procedures to minimize the splashing or spattering of blood and other body fluids.

Personal Protective Equipment

The OSHA standards require that personal protective equipment (PPE) must be used any time there is a potential for contact with blood or other body fluids to prevent the transmission of any diseases. Always follow BSI guidelines and wear appropriate PPE on every call. Personal protective equipment is considered "appropriate" only if it prevents blood or other body fluids from passing through the skin or reaching the eyes, mouth, or other mucous membranes. Personal protective equipment includes:

- Disposable latex gloves
- Impervious gowns
- Eye shields or protection
- Surgical masks
- Resuscitation bags such as BVM
- Pocket masks with one-way valves

All PPE used during patient care should be disposed of or cleaned according to procedures outlined in the exposure control plan. Protective gloves may be either latex, vinyl, or other similar synthetic material and should be worn if there is the possibility of contact with blood or other body fluids that may occur during bleeding control, suctioning, CPR, or any situation in which han-

dling or touching contaminated items or surfaces is anticipated. Gloves should not be washed but should be replaced between patients or if punctured, ripped, or torn.

When there is anticipated blood or other body fluid splash or spatter, eye protection and masks should be worn because the mucous membranes of the eyes are capable of absorbing fluids. Protective eyewear should provide protection from the front and the sides. EMS services should provide goggles or nonprescription eyewear for employees to use; in the case of prescription glasses, protective clip-on barriers should be available.

Impervious gowns should be worn to protect clothing from spilled or splashed blood or other body fluids that occur during childbirth or other bleeding. In cases of suspected tuberculosis (TB), a high-efficiency particulate air (HEPA) respirator is required.

Housekeeping Procedures

Housekeeping procedures are outlined in an exposure control plan to establish and maintain sanitary conditions of the workplace and vehicle. All employees are responsible for ensuring that vehicles and work areas are kept clean and sanitary. This portion of an exposure control plan also establishes a schedule for cleaning as well as methods of decontaminating work areas and vehicles. These procedures are presented later in this chapter.

Vaccinations

All employers are required to make available to all identified employees the hepatitis B virus (HBV) vaccination series free of charge. Hepatitis B is an infection of the liver caused by the hepatitis B virus and is one of several types of infections that can affect the liver. HBV infections can occur in two forms—the acute phase and the chronic phase. The acute phase occurs just after a person becomes infected and lasts from a few weeks to several months. Most people will recover after the acute phase and no longer be infectious. However, some people are infected for the remainder of their lives and are chronic carriers of the HBV.

Acute hepatitis B begins with symptoms such as loss of appetite, generalized weakness, nausea, vomiting, a jaundice or yellow appearance, and dark-colored urine. However, over half the people infected with HBV never become sick or ill. HBV is passed by blood or other body fluids through direct contact with nonintact skin, mucous membranes, unprotected sexual intercourse, or parenteral contact (needle stick).

As an EMS provider, you are at risk for exposure to blood or other body fluids. For this reason, if possible, you should be immunized with the HBV vaccine. The vaccinations are given in three shots: the first shot within 10 days of the initial job functions, the second shot one month after the first, and the third shot five months after the second.

An EMS employee may elect to decline the series of shots but will then need to sign a hepatitis vaccination declination form. The signing of the form, however, does not preclude the employee from deciding that he or she wishes to be vaccinated at a later date. In this case, the employer is still required to make the vaccination available. All vaccination records should be stored in the medical records of the employee's personnel files.

Post-Exposure Procedures

By definition, an exposure is any occurrence of blood or other body fluids coming in contact with non-intact skin, the eyes, other mucous membranes, or parenteral contact, e.g., needle stick. In general, post-exposure procedures require immediate washing of the affected area with soap and water, medical evaluation, and follow-up reporting to document the circumstances surrounding the exposure. If feasible and applicable to state law, the source individual's and employee's blood should be tested for the presence of HBV and HIV. The exposed employee may also be required to attend post-exposure counseling. All information obtained through post-exposure follow-up is confidential and becomes part of the employee's medical record.

Preceptor Pearl

Since an exposure incident can be anxiety provoking to new EMT-Bs, discuss with them your state laws and local policies regarding post-exposure procedures. ❖

Other Plan Requirements

Other parts of the exposure control plan include hazard requirements, training requirements, and record keeping. The "biohazard" label is required

to be affixed to all containers used to store, transport, or ship blood or other body fluids. Also, EMT-Bs must be provided with training that includes information about the employer's exposure control plan, general disease transmission, uses and limitations of PPE, workplace practices that reduce or prevent exposures, exposure incident procedures, and labeling requirements. OSHA also requires that records be kept for medical and training purposes. Medical records are confidential and kept for the duration of employment plus thirty years. Training records are kept for three years.

■ RYAN WHITE CARE ACT

In 1994, the Centers for Disease Control (CDC) issued the final notice for the Ryan White Comprehensive AIDS Resources Emergency (CARE) Act. This federal mandate applies to all 50 states and establishes procedures by which all emergency response employees (EREs) can determine if they have been exposed to a potentially infectious disease while providing patient care. EREs includes all EMS, firefighting, and police personnel who provide emergency medical care. The Ryan White Act identifies a list of potentially life-threatening, infectious, and communicable diseases to which EREs may be exposed. This list includes infectious pulmonary tuberculosis, HIV/AIDS, hepatitis B, hemorrhagic fevers, plague, diphtheria, meningococcal disease, and rabies.

The Ryan White Act requires that "every State public health officer must designate an official of every employer of EREs in the State who will be responsible for notifying EREs of exposure." This person, called the **Designated Officer**, or D.O., is responsible for gathering all information regarding an exposure to an airborne or bloodborne infectious disease and reporting to the receiving medical facility to request a determination of exposure. There are two separate notification procedures—one for airborne exposures, another for bloodborne exposures as shown in Figure 3–2.

The reason for the two distinct reporting requirements is that exposure to airborne diseases, such as infectious pulmonary tuberculosis, may not be evident until well after the patient is transferred to the medical facility. Tuberculosis is usually diagnosed during hospitalization. However, you will know immediately if you had significant contact with blood or other body fluids and can request immediate follow-up.

FIGURE 3–2
Under the Ryan White CARE Act, there is a procedure for finding out and following up if you have been exposed to a life-threatening infectious disease.

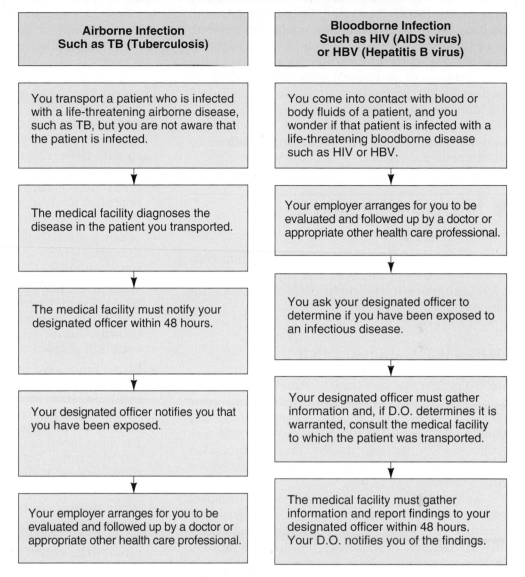

INFECTIOUS DISEASE EXPOSURE PROCEDURE

Airborne Infection Such as TB (Tuberculosis)

You transport a patient who is infected with a life-threatening airborne disease, such as TB, but you are not aware that the patient is infected.

↓

The medical facility diagnoses the disease in the patient you transported.

↓

The medical facility must notify your designated officer within 48 hours.

↓

Your designated officer notifies you that you have been exposed.

↓

Your employer arranges for you to be evaluated and followed up by a doctor or appropriate other health care professional.

Bloodborne Infection Such as HIV (AIDS virus) or HBV (Hepatitis B virus)

You come into contact with blood or body fluids of a patient, and you wonder if that patient is infected with a life-threatening bloodborne disease such as HIV or HBV.

↓

Your employer arranges for you to be evaluated and followed up by a doctor or appropriate other health care professional.

↓

You ask your designated officer to determine if you have been exposed to an infectious disease.

↓

Your designated officer must gather information and, if D.O. determines it is warranted, consult the medical facility to which the patient was transported.

↓

The medical facility must gather information and report findings to your designated officer within 48 hours. Your D.O. notifies you of the findings.

Several states have laws regarding patient testing after an exposure that are not covered under the Ryan White Act. Review all applicable laws in your area regarding your rights to request patient testing after an exposure incident.

■ TUBERCULOSIS REQUIREMENTS

In 1993, OSHA, based upon the 1990 Centers for Disease Control (CDC) recommendations, issued policies and procedures for providing care for patients with suspected or confirmed TB called "Guidelines for Preventing the Transmission in Health Care Settings with Special Focus on HIV-Related Issues." These guidelines outline those situations in which there is a risk for contracting and transmitting TB, procedures for prevention of transmission, and the training required for use of personal protective equipment such as a high-efficiency particulate air (HEPA) respirator.

As an EMT-B, you should suspect TB in patients who have a suppressed immune system such as occurs in HIV/AIDS, in prison populations and in nursing homes. Patients may have a productive cough of either sputum or blood, night sweats, loss of appetite, weight loss, lethargy or weakness, and fever. Always consider any patient who is coughing as potentially infectious.

In cases of potential exposure to exhaled air of a patient with potential or confirmed TB, OSHA requires that a HEPA respirator that is approved by the National Institute for Occupational Safety and Health (NIOSH) be used. You are required to be "fit tested" and medically evaluated prior to wearing any HEPA mask. An employer is required to provide a written procedure for training in the use of the mask and how it should be cleaned, as well as a plan for medical surveillance, including TB Mantoux skin tests.

Always review your state, local, and employer policies and procedures regarding airborne or bloodborne pathogens.

■ BSI AND AMBULANCE CALL PHASES

Various BSI techniques and other infection control procedures outlined in the exposure control plan take place in the three phases of an ambulance call.

Before the Ambulance Call

Before performing any duties as an EMS provider, make sure you review and understand your employer's specific exposure control plan. You should also have all of the necessary vaccinations, such as HBV, as well as the TB Mantoux skin test or purified protein derivative (PPD) test for tuberculosis.

As you begin each shift, you should inspect your vehicle for cleanliness as you complete other equipment checklists. All equipment, especially airway, oxygen, and suction equipment, should be in good working order and free of any blood or other body fluids from previous patient-care activities. If any equipment is found to be contaminated, it should be immediately cleaned and checked for proper functioning. Some EMS services have a daily or weekly infection-control cleaning schedule that should be followed. In general, however, all surfaces should be checked and cleaned of any blood or body fluids. Any contaminated items in waste receptacles should be emptied, and the receptacles should be cleaned. Sharps containers should be checked to ensure they are not overflowing or leaking. Never attempt to empty sharps containers; when full, they should be sealed and disposed of properly. Check to make sure you have adequate supplies of infection-control equipment such as gloves, masks, eye protection, biohazard waste bags, and intermediate- and low-level disinfectants for cleaning up

spills of blood or other body fluids. Also remember to wash your hands after cleaning or disinfecting any equipment or vehicle surfaces and prior to going on any calls.

During the Ambulance Call

Most exposure control plans require the use of PPE based upon the degree of risk associated with each call. General guidelines to follow are:

- Wear disposable gloves anytime there is a potential for contact with blood or other body fluids. Always change gloves between patients.
- Wash your hands with soap and water after removing gloves and before each time you eat or use cosmetics.
- Wear protective eyewear when there is a risk for blood or other body fluid spatter—for example childbirth, endotracheal intubation, or major trauma. Adapt removable side shields to prescription glasses.
- Wear protective gowns when there are large splash areas of blood or other body fluids—for example when dealing with emergency childbirth or major trauma victims. The gowns should be designed to provide a barrier that prevents blood or other body fluids from reaching your inner clothing or skin. If your clothing does become contaminated, have a change of uniform readily available.
- Wear a surgical-type mask or face shield in cases where there is anticipated blood or other body fluid spatter—for example emergency childbirth, endotracheal intubation, or major trauma. In cases of potential infectious respiratory tuberculosis, a high-efficiency particulate air (HEPA) respirator is required.

In addition to PPE, use other protective/barrier equipment such as face shields and/or pocket masks with one-way valves to decrease the possibility of any disease transmission. Always try to minimize your exposure to any blood or body fluids to decrease the risk of an exposure to an infectious disease.

Termination of the Ambulance Call

Even after you have transferred care of the patient to the receiving facility, your call has not ended. As an EMT-B, you are responsible for preparing for the next call by decontaminating and cleaning any equipment used for patient-care activities and the ambulance.

Always wash your hands after transferring care at the receiving facility. The practice of good hand-washing techniques is the best defense against the transmission of infectious or potentially infectious blood or body fluids. Wash your hands with soap and water or other disinfectant as soon as possible upon removing gloves after patient contact.

Follow engineering controls and housekeeping procedures to ready yourself, your crew, and the ambulance for the next response. While still at the receiving facility, take the following steps (Skill Summary 1):

1. *Prepare the ambulance for service.* While wearing heavy duty, rubber, dishwashing-style gloves, quickly clean the patient compartment. Follow biohazard disposal procedures according to your agency's exposure control plan. Clean up blood, vomitus, and other body fluids that may have soiled the floor and wipe down any equipment that has been splashed. Place disposable towels used to clean up blood or body fluids directly in a red bag. Remove and dispose of trash such as bandage wrappings and opened but unused dressings. Sweep away caked dirt that may have been tracked into the patient compartment. Sponge up water and mud from the floor that may have been tracked in due to inclement weather. Bag dirty linens or blankets to be appropriately laundered and use a deodorizer to neutralize odors of vomit, urine, and feces.

2. *Prepare respiratory equipment for service.* Clean and disinfect nondisposable, used BVMs and other reusable parts of respiratory-assist devices that were used during the call. This will keep them from becoming reservoirs of infectious agents that can easily contaminate the next patient. Disinfect the suction unit and place used disposable items in a plastic bag and seal it. Replace the items with the spare ones carried in the ambulance.

3. *Replace expendable items.* If you have a supply replacement agreement with the hospital, replace expendable items from the hospital storerooms on a one-for-one basis. However, do not abuse this exchange program. Keep in mind that the constant abuse of a supplies replacement program usually leads to its discontinuation.

4. *Exchange equipment according to your local policy.* Exchange items such as splints and spine boards. Several benefits are associated with an equipment exchange program: there is no need to subject patients to injury-aggravating movements just to recover equipment, crews are not delayed at the hospital, and ambulances can return to quarters fully equipped for the next response. When equipment is available for exchange, quickly inspect it for completeness and operability. Parts are sometimes lost or broken when an immobilizing device is removed from a patient. If you do find that a piece of equipment is broken or incomplete, notify someone in authority so the device can be repaired or replaced.

5. *Make up the ambulance stretcher.* Each service has its own favorite way to make up the stretcher. It is a good practice to clean the mattress and flip it over prior to making the stretcher. Learn the procedure for your service and always make up the stretcher so it is neat and clean.

Preceptor Pearl

Remember if patients see stained sheets or other examples of failure to prepare a vehicle, they may also question the quality of care they will receive! Remind new EMT-Bs that they can make a good first impression on their patients and the patients' families by making the stretcher presentation a matter of personal and professional pride! ❖

Specific cleaning and decontamination solutions used will vary according to local procedures. Three levels of disinfectants are used: a high-level disinfectant (strong enough to destroy mycobacterium tuberculosis), an intermediate-level disinfectant such as 1:100 solution of bleach (1 part bleach to 100 parts water), and a low-level disinfectant such as Lysol®. Sterilization, another process used to clean and disinfect equipment, is generally used in a hospital and is not practical in the out-of-hospital setting (Skill Summary 2).

You may elect to wait until back in quarters to disinfect and clean equipment (Skill Summary 3). However, always remember to bag this equipment properly to isolate and separate it from clean equipment while returning to quarters. This prevents the possibility that you will use "dirty" equipment if you receive a call prior to disinfecting and cleaning. If the floor, cots, or walls of the vehicle are blood-covered, then the ambulance may need to be placed out of service until cleaning can occur. At the station, place all contaminated equipment in the proper solution for disinfection and cleaning. Clean and dry equipment as needed. Check the ambulance for any surfaces that may have come in

Actions That Can Be Taken at the Hospital

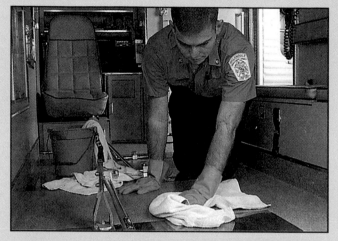

1. Clean the ambulance interior as required.

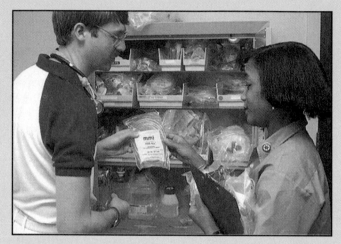

2. Replace respiratory equipment as required.

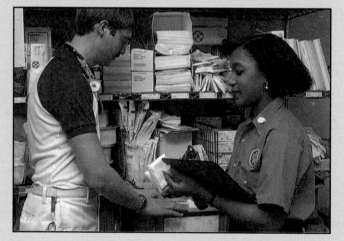

3. Replace expendable items per local policies.

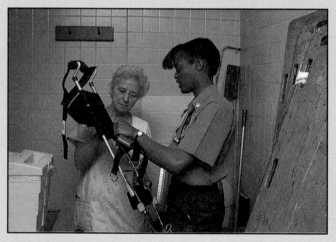

4. Exchange equipment per local policies.

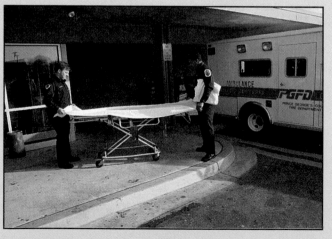

5. Make up the wheeled stretcher.

Cleaning and Disinfecting Equipment

There are four levels of cleaning and disinfecting.

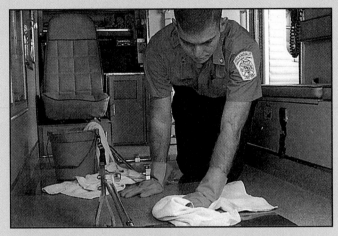

1. A **low-level disinfectant** approved by the U. S. Environmental Protection Agency, for example a commercial product such as Lysol, will clean and kill germs on ambulance floors and walls.

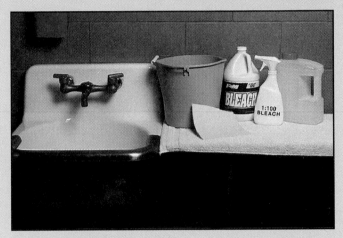

2. An **intermediate-level disinfectant**, such as a mixture of 1:100 bleach-to-water, can be used to clean and kill germs on equipment surfaces.

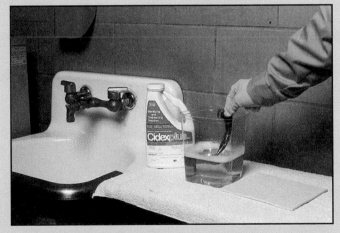

3. A **high-level disinfectant**, such as Cidex Plus, will destroy all forms of microbial life except high numbers of bacterial spores.

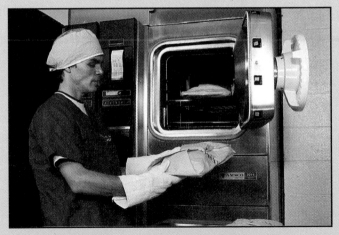

4. Sterilization is required to destroy all possible sources of infection on equipment that will be used invasively.

Termination of Activities in Quarters

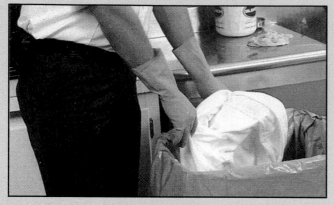

1. Place contaminated linens in a biohazard container, noncontaminated linens in a regular hamper.

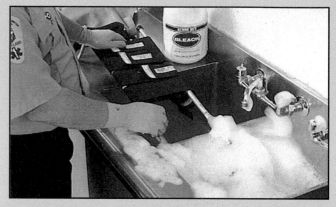

2. Remove and clean patient-care equipment as required.

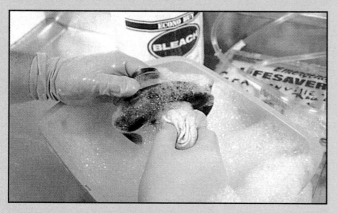

3. Clean and sanitize respiratory equipment as required.

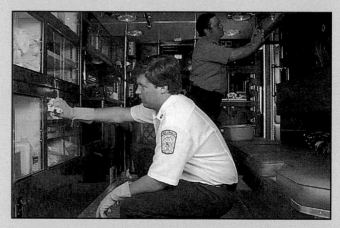

4. Clean and sanitize the ambulance interior as required. Any devices or surfaces that have come into contact with a patient's blood or other body fluids must be cleaned with germicide.

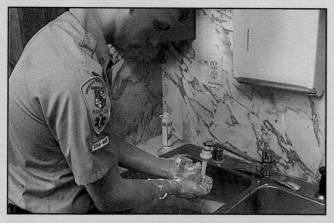

5. Wash thoroughly. Change soiled clothing. If exposed to a communicable disease, you should do this first.

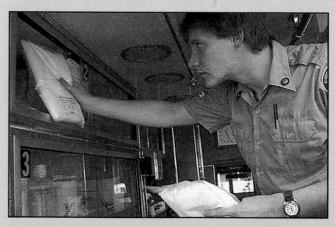

6. Replace expendable items as required.

Skill Summary 3–3 (continued)

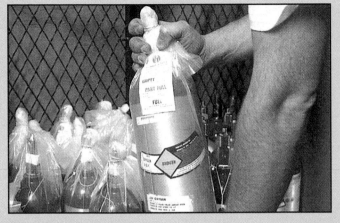

7. Always replace oxygen cylinders as necessary.

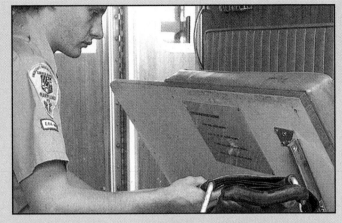

8. Replace patient-care equipment as needed.

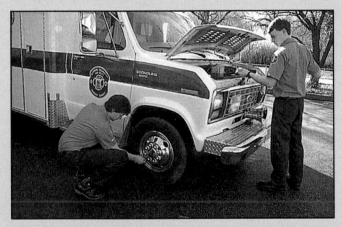

9. Maintain the ambulance as required. Report problems that will take the vehicle out of service.

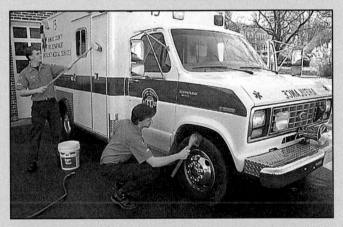

10. Clean the ambulance exterior as needed.

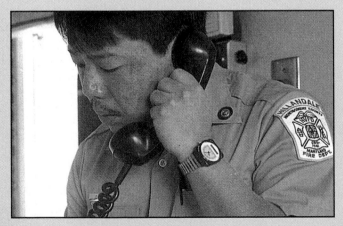

11. Report the unit ready for service.

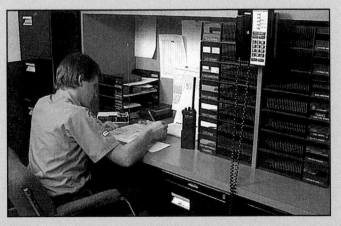

12. Complete any unfinished report forms as soon as possible.

contact with blood or other body fluids. After the equipment and vehicle have been cleaned, wash your hands thoroughly and check to see if your uniform has become soiled with blood or other body fluids. Prepare yourself for service by washing your hands and changing your uniform if it was soiled with a body substance on the call; replace expendable items with items from the unit's storeroom; refill oxygen cylinders even if only a small volume of gas was used; replace patient care equipment; check vehicle fluid levels, tire pressures, warning devices, and lights; clean the vehicle (a clean exterior lends a professional appearance to an ambulance); check the vehicle for broken lights, glass and body damage, door operation, and other parts that may need repair or replacement, complete any unfinished report forms and report the unit ready for service.

CHAPTER REVIEW

■ SUMMARY

The Occupational Safety and Health Administration (OSHA) has developed and enforces standards for EMT-Bs to use when dealing with bloodborne pathogens. The OSHA standard requires an EMS service or employer to establish an exposure control plan that identifies hazards associated with exposure to blood or other body fluids, identifies job classifications that are at risk for exposure, establishes procedures for using PPE, provides HBV vaccinations and training, determines exposure, and provides follow-up.

The Ryan White Comprehensive AIDS Resources Emergency (CARE) Act mandates and establishes procedures by which all emergency response employees (EREs)—including all EMS, firefighters, and police personnel who provide emergency medical care—can find out if they have been exposed to a potentially infectious disease such as infectious pulmonary tuberculosis, HIV/AIDS, hepatitis B, hemorrhagic fevers, plague, diphtheria, meningococcal disease, and rabies. A Designated Officer (D.O.) is assigned for each ERE employer who is responsible for exposure investigation and notification. There are two separate notification procedures, one for airborne exposures and another for bloodborne exposures.

Body substance isolation should be used in all phases of an ambulance call. Before any ambulance call you should ensure that you and your crew are aware of the local policies and procedures, that equipment is clean, and that the vehicle is free from any blood or body fluid contamination.

All employees are responsible to ensure that the vehicles and work areas are maintained in a clean and sanitary condition. Housekeeping procedures are outlined in an exposure control plan to establish and maintain sanitary conditions of the workplace and vehicle. Cleaning schedules and decontamination procedures should be established by each employer and used after each contact with blood or body fluids.

■ REVIEW QUESTIONS

1. Explain how airborne and bloodborne pathogens enter the body.
2. What is the purpose of OSHA's standard 29 CFR 1910.1030?
3. List and give a brief statement about the purpose of each component of an exposure control plan.
4. Why and when should you wear a HEPA respirator?
5. Explain the purpose of the Ryan White CARE Act.
6. List the BSI techniques and other infection-control procedures that take place during the three phases of an ambulance call.

CHAPTER 4

Airway

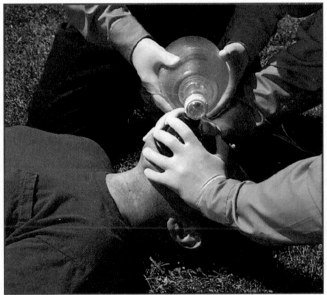

■ As an EMT-B you have heard it over and over again, "Open the airway, clear the airway, assure a patent airway!" Often, the most basic techniques prove to be the most effective life-saving techniques we can provide for our patients. After assuring that the scene is safe for yourself and your crew, the first priority of all patient care is to open the airway. If you do not master the skills of airway care, all other treatments are likely to be futile.

This chapter reviews airway anatomy, how to examine a patient for adequate and inadequate breathing, how to open the airway for the medical and the trauma patient, how to insert oral and nasal airways, suctioning, ventilation with the pocket mask and BVM, and oxygen administration. Your patients will rely on your ability to "expertly" know why, when, and how to use the airway maintenance, ventilation, and oxygenation skills covered in this chapter. For some of us that means constant practice with ventilation equipment that is not used on a daily basis. After all, their long-term survival depends on your quick actions in the field.

MAKING THE TRANSITION

- Importance of BSI is emphasized.
- Use of the two-person bag-valve-mask technique is encouraged.
- Use of a flow-restricted, oxygen-powered ventilation device (FROPVD) is explained.
- Assisting with endotracheal tube placement is recommended.
- Simplified approach to oxygen therapy is included.

OBJECTIVES

The numbered objectives below are from the United States Department of Transportation 1994 EMT-Basic National Standard Curriculum. Objectives with colored bullets that follow in italics are from the EMT-Basic Transitional Program.

■ KNOWLEDGE AND ATTITUDE

At the end of this chapter, you should be able to:

1. Name and label the major structures of the respiratory system on a diagram. (pp. 48, 49)
2. List the signs of adequate breathing. (p. 49)
3. List the signs of inadequate breathing. (pp. 49–50)
4. Describe the steps in performing the head-tilt, chin-lift. (pp. 50–51)
5. Relate mechanism of injury to opening the airway. (pp. 50, 51)
6. Describe the steps in performing the jaw thrust. (pp. 51, 52)
7. State the importance of having a suction unit ready for immediate use when providing emergency care. (pp. 52, 55)
8. Describe the techniques of suctioning. (p. 57)
9. Describe how to artificially ventilate a patient with a pocket mask. (pp. 57, 58)
10. Describe the steps in performing the skill of artificially ventilating a patient with a bag-valve mask while using the jaw thrust. (pp. 57, 60)
11. List the parts of a bag-valve-mask system. (pp. 58–59)
12. Describe the steps in performing the skill of artificially ventilating a patient with a bag-valve mask for one and two rescuers. (pp. 57, 58–61)
13. Describe the signs of adequate artificial ventilation using the bag-valve mask. (pp. 59, 60)
14. Describe the signs of inadequate artificial ventilation using the bag-valve mask. (p. 61)
15. Describe the steps in artificially ventilating a patient with a flow-restricted, oxygen-powered ventilation device. (p. 61)
16. List the steps in performing the actions taken when providing mouth-to-mouth and mouth-to-stoma artificial ventilation. (pp. 58, 61)
17. Describe how to measure and insert an oropharyngeal (oral) airway. (pp. 52–54)
18. Describe how to measure and insert a nasopharyngeal (nasal) airway. (pp. 54–55)
19. Define the components of an oxygen delivery system. (pp. 64–65)
20. Identify a nonrebreather face mask and state the oxygen flow requirements needed for its use. (p. 66)
21. Describe the indications for using a nasal cannula versus a nonrebreather face mask. (p. 66)
22. Identify a nasal cannula and state the flow requirements needed for its use. (p. 66)
23. Explain the rationale for basic life support artificial ventilation and airway protective skills taking priority over most other basic life support skills. (p. 45, 50)
24. Explain the rationale for providing adequate oxygen through high-inspired oxygen concentrations to patients who, in the past, may have received low concentrations. (p. 66)
- *Discuss the changed philosophy of oxygenation and ventilation interventions. (pp. 45, 57)*
- *State the order of preference for the various methods of ventilating a patient. (p. 57)*
- *Value the rationale for the modified methods of oxygen delivery and ventilation techniques. (pp. 57–66)*

■ SKILLS

1. Demonstrate the steps in performing the head-tilt, chin-lift.
2. Demonstrate the steps in performing the jaw thrust.
3. Demonstrate the techniques of suctioning.
4. Demonstrate the steps in providing mouth-to-mouth artificial ventilation with body substance isolation (barrier shields).
5. Demonstrate how to use a pocket mask to artificially ventilate a patient.
6. Demonstrate the assembly of a bag-valve-mask unit.
7. Demonstrate the steps in performing the skill of artificially ventilating a patient with a bag-valve mask for one and two rescuers.

8. Demonstrate the steps in performing the skill of artificially ventilating a patient with a bag-valve mask while using the jaw thrust.

9. Demonstrate artificial ventilation of a patient with a flow-restricted, oxygen-powered ventilation device.

10. Demonstrate how to artificially ventilate a patient with a stoma.

11. Demonstrate how to insert an oropharyngeal (oral) airway.

12. Demonstrate how to insert a nasopharyngeal (nasal) airway.

13. Demonstrate the correct operation of oxygen tanks and regulators.

14. Demonstrate the use of a nonrebreather face mask and state the oxygen flow requirements needed for its use.

15. Demonstrate the use of the nasal cannula and state the flow requirements for its use.

16. Demonstrate how to artificially ventilate the infant and child patient.

17. Demonstrate oxygen administration for the infant and child patient.

- *Demonstrate the use of the bag-valve mask utilizing two rescuers without missing any critical criteria listed on the skill sheets in the 1994 EMT-Basic Transitional Program.*

- *Demonstrate the use of the oxygen-powered ventilation device.*

- *Given various scenarios, be able to adequately demonstrate techniques of ventilations using mouth-to-mask, two-person BVM, flow-restricted, oxygen-powered ventilation device and one-person BVM.*

ON THE SCENE

One evening, fifty-five-year-old Marie Wishard is watching TV with her son, Tony, when she begins to experience shortness of breath. At first she ignores it, but as it continues, Tony can tell something is wrong and calls 911. Upon your arrival, your **scene size-up** reveals no hazards inside this suburban home. Tony leads you to his mother and introduces her to you. You ask Mrs. Wishard if you may help her and she agrees.

You quickly conduct your **initial assessment**, gaining a general impression of an alert middle-aged woman who is sitting at the edge of her chair concentrating on her breathing. You discover no immediate life threats with her airway,

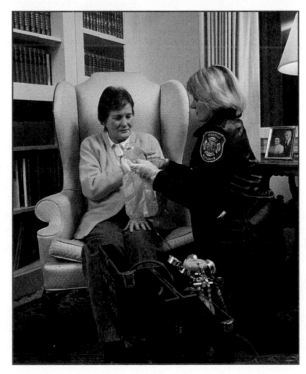

breathing, or circulation. You begin the **focused history and physical exam**. As your partner gets a set of vitals, you begin to take Mrs. Wishard's history by asking about her breathing difficulty.

You: Mrs. Wishard, could you tell me about your breathing?
Mrs. Wishard: I cannot catch my breath. (She answers in a short, choppy sentence.)
You: On a scale of 1 to 10, with 10 being the worst breathing difficulty you ever had, how would you rate the difficulty?
Mrs. Wishard: About a 6. (At this point, her son volunteers that she is an asthmatic.)
You: I am going to put this oxygen mask (nonrebreather) on you. It will help you breathe.

Did you take any medications to help you breathe?
Mrs. Wishard: I took two puffs on my inhaler, but it didn't help. Should I take another puff?
You: Well let me ask you a few more questions, and then I'll contact the doctor in the emergency department to see if he wants me to assist you with your inhaler.

As you prepare for transport, you notice Mrs. Wishard is no longer struggling to breathe. You have also asked the **OPQRST** questions as well as the **SAMPLE history**, which revealed that Mrs. Wishard has a history of a recent upper respiratory infection and asthma. She also states she has been smoking two packs of cigarettes a day for 37 years. She has a productive cough with white sputum.

You: Has the oxygen helped your breathing?
Mrs. Wishard: Oh yes, it seems to be getting better.

En route to the hospital, you perform **ongoing assessment**, checking Mrs. Wishard's vital signs, fit of the oxygen mask, and the liter flow rate into the mask. You also give a radio report to the emergency department. When you call **medical direction**, the physician asks you to assist Mrs. Wishard with administering her bronchodilator, since she is still experiencing some shortness of breath (dyspnea), although her pulse rate is normal. The physician also suggests that you continue the oxygen therapy, since it seems to be helping the patient's condition. ■

■ AIRWAY ANATOMY AND PHYSIOLOGY REVIEW

Another word for breathing is **respiration**. The body system that allows breathing to occur is the respiratory system. As an EMT-B, you should be able to label the following major structures on a diagram (Figure 4–1A).

- **Nose**—allows air entry, warms inhaled air, and filters out impurities with the help of nose hairs and mucus
- **Mouth**—one of the openings to the airway and respiratory system that allow the taking in of air
- **Oropharynx**—inside of the mouth posterior to the tongue leading to the throat
- **Nasopharynx**—area between the nasal passages and the oropharynx
- **Epiglottis**—flap of tissue that covers the glottic opening of the trachea when swallowing or gagging takes place
- **Trachea**—tube in the front of the throat that carries air to the lungs; windpipe
- **Cricoid cartilage**—tissue covering the front of the larynx
- **Larynx**—voice box that holds the vocal cords and the glottic opening to the trachea
- **Bronchi**—right and left mainstem tubes leading into the lungs
- **Lungs**—organs where oxygen is exchanged for carbon dioxide

- **Alveoli**—grapelike sacs within the lungs that are surrounded by capillaries whose red blood cells pick up inhaled oxygen and drop off carbon dioxide to be exhaled
- **Diaphragm**—large primary muscle of breathing which separates the thorax from the abdomen

The respiratory system enables the body to inhale oxygen, which is used by all the cells and organs in the body, and to exhale carbon dioxide, the major waste product of respiration. If anything obstructs or disrupts the breathing process, the patient is likely to develop the sensation of shortness of breath (**dyspnea**) and be at risk for respiratory failure.

When the diaphragm contracts, it moves downward as the intercostal muscles pull the ribs up and out to create a larger cavity into which air can rush. This is called **inhalation**. The lungs are wrapped in two membranes, the *visceral pleura* directly around the lung tissue and the *parietal pleura* directly around the inside of the ribs. These membranes have a small amount of fluid between them that causes them to stick together like a drop of water between two glass slides under a microscope. Due to this "surface tension," when the intercostal muscles move the rib cage, the lungs also enlarge in size.

When the diaphragm relaxes, it moves upward as the intercostal muscles allow the ribs to fall back in and down. This action decreases the space inside the chest cavity and forces out air in the lungs (Figure 4–1B). This process is referred to as **exhalation**.

Patient Assessment **Adequate Breathing**

When examining a patient for **adequate breathing**:

- Look for adequate and equal expansion of both sides of the chest with inhalation.
- Listen for air entering and leaving the nose, mouth, and chest. The breath sounds should be present and equal on both sides of the chest. Any sounds heard from the mouth should be free of gurgling, gasping, crowing, and wheezing. Feel for air moving out of the nose or mouth.
- Check for typical skin coloration. There should be no blue or gray discolorations.
- Take note of the rate, rhythm, quality, and depth of breathing typical for a person at rest. ◼

Adequate breathing consists of a normal rate of 12 to 20 per minute for an adult, 15 to 30 for a child, and 25 to 50 for an infant. A patient with adequate breathing should exhibit equal and present breath sounds and have visible and symmetric chest expansion with minimal effort.

Patient Assessment **Inadequate Breathing**

When evaluating patients with **inadequate breathing**, you may observe any of the following signs:

- Chest movements are absent, minimal, or uneven.
- Movements associated with breathing are limited to the abdomen (diaphragmatic or abdominal breathing).
- Breath sounds are diminished or absent.
- Noises such as wheezing, snoring, gurgling, or gasping are heard during breathing.
- The rate of breathing is too rapid or too slow compared to the norms given above.
- Breathing is very shallow, is very deep, or appears labored.
- The patient's skin, lips, tongue, ear lobes, or nail beds are blue (cyanotic) or gray.
- Inspirations are prolonged, indicating a possible upper airway obstruction.

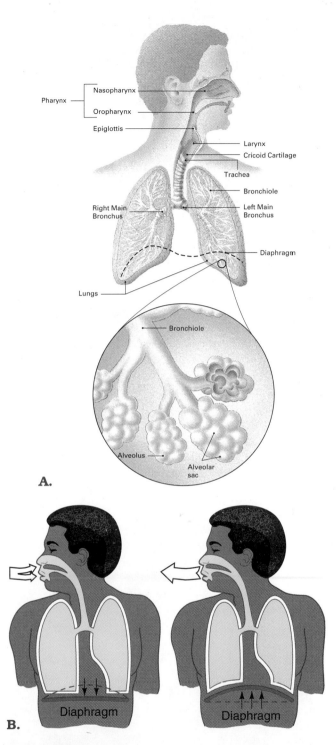

A.

B.

FIGURE 4–1 A. The respiratory system. **B.** The lungs and diaphragm.

- Expirations are prolonged, indicating a possible lower airway obstruction.
- The patient is unable to speak or cannot speak in full sentences due to shortness of breath.

- In children, there may be retractions, or pulling in, of the muscles above the sternum and clavicles and between and below the ribs.
- Nasal flaring or widening of the nostrils may be present, especially in infants and children. ■

■ OPENING THE AIRWAY—MEDICAL AND TRAUMA PATIENTS

The **airway** is the passageway by which air enters or leaves the body. The structures of the upper airway include the nose, mouth, pharynx, and larynx. The larynx contains the epiglottis, which separates the upper airway from the lower airway. The lower airway contains the trachea, lungs, bronchi, and alveoli.

Airway assessment is usually done on a patient in the supine position (Figure 4–2). If a patient is found in a sitting position or slumped over the wheel of a car, carefully move him to assess his airway status.

Moving a trauma patient before immobilizing the head and spine could cause serious injury. If you suspect injury to the spine, protect the patient's head and neck as you position him. As you know, airway and breathing have priority over spine protection and must be assured as quickly as possible. If the trauma patient must be moved in order to open the airway or to provide ventilations, you will probably not have time to provide immobilization with a cervical collar, head immobilizer, and long spine board. In this case, manually stabilize the head and spine while a partner or two help you reposition the patient into a supine position. Then you can stabilize the patient's head and do a jaw-thrust maneuver to open the airway.

You will need to open and maintain the airway in any patient who cannot do so for himself. This includes patients without a gag reflex, patients with an altered level of consciousness, or patients in respiratory or cardiac arrest. Most airway obstructions are anatomical obstructions caused by the tongue flopping back into the patient's airway when the head is flexed. When a patient is unconscious, the tongue frequently loses muscle tone and muscles of the lower jaw relax. Since the tongue is attached to the lower jaw (mandible), the risk of airway obstruction is even greater during unconsciousness.

Preceptor Pearl

A common sign of a partial airway obstruction is a snoring noise. As an experiment, if you can do so without waking up a snoring person, simply hyperextend the person's neck and listen as the snoring noise disappears! ✦

Head-Tilt, Chin-Lift Maneuver

The basic procedure for opening the airway to correct the position of the tongue is called the **head-tilt, chin-lift**. As you can see in Figure 4–3, when the jaw is pulled or lifted, the tongue moves away from the back of the throat. This procedure provides the maximum opening of the airway.

- Once the patient is in the supine position, place one hand on the forehead and place the fingertips of the other hand under the bony area at the center of the patient's lower jaw.
- Use your fingertips to lift the chin and to support the lower jaw. Move the jaw forward to a point where the lower teeth are almost touching the upper teeth (Figure 4–4).
- If a patient has no gag reflex, use an oral airway to keep the tongue from occluding his airway. In some situations it may be helpful to use the thumb of the hand supporting the chin to pull back the patient's lower lip. To avoid being bitten, do not insert your thumb into the patient's mouth.

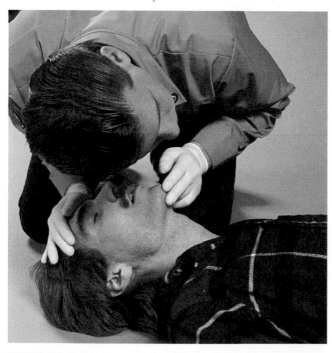

FIGURE 4–2 Positioning the patient for airway evaluation and care.

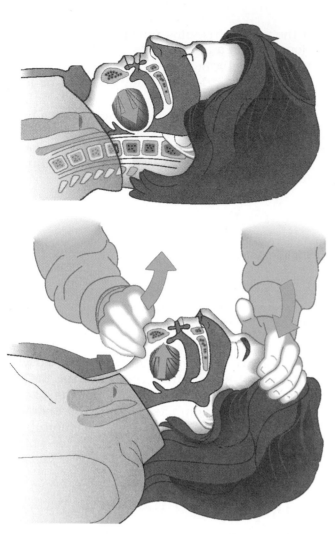

FIGURE 4–3 Procedures for opening the airway to help position the tongue.

PEDIATRIC HIGHLIGHT

When performing the head-tilt, chin-lift on a child, be careful not to push in on the fleshy tissue under the chin as it may actually cause the tongue to partially occlude the airway. Hold by the chin bone only. Also, do not hyperextend the infant's neck; simply place it into an extended position. Hyperextension could occlude the soft trachea and larynx. ■

Jaw-Thrust Maneuver

If you suspect that the patient may have a possible spinal injury, the head-tilt, chin-lift is not indicated since it can harm the patient with a neck/cervical injury. The **jaw-thrust** maneuver is

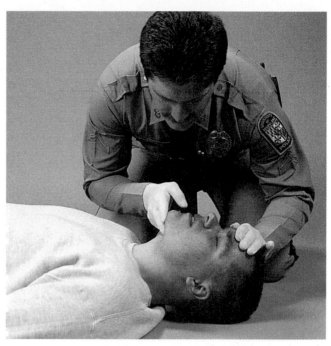

FIGURE 4–4 The head-tilt, chin-lift maneuver.

the only recommended procedure for use on conscious or unconscious patients when trauma is suspected.

- Keep the patient's head, neck, and spine aligned, moving him as a unit as you place him in the supine position. It will take more than one EMT-B to move the patient into this position, and the person holding the neck should direct all movement of the patient.
- Kneel at the top of the patient's head, resting your elbows on the same surface on which the patient is lying.
- Carefully reach forward and place one hand on each side of the patient's lower jaw, at the angle of the jaw below the ears (Figure 4–5).
- Stabilize the patient's head with your forearms while using your index fingers to "jut the jaw" by pushing the patient's lower jaw forward. It is essential that you have your fingers behind the angle of the jaw, not just on the bottom; otherwise you will just shut the patient's mouth. You may need to retract the patient's lower lip with your thumb to keep the mouth open. *Do not* tilt or rotate the patient's head since any movement may cause an injury to the cervical spine.

Preceptor Pearl

There is no such thing as a one-handed jaw thrust! If a trauma victim's airway is being held open with only one hand, it is unlikely that he is being adequately ventilated. ✜

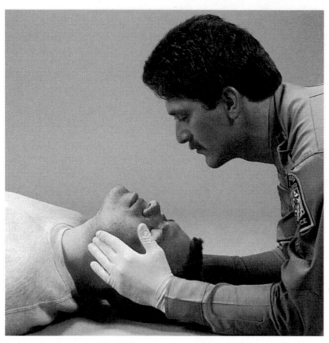

FIGURE 4–5 The jaw-thrust maneuver.

■ USING AIRWAY ADJUNCTS

Devices that aid in maintaining an open airway are referred to as **airway adjuncts**. In addition to performing either the head-tilt, chin-lift, or jaw-thrust maneuver in a trauma patient, two common airway adjuncts are used: the **oropharyngeal airway (OPA)** and the **nasopharyngeal airway (NPA)**. *Oro* refers to the mouth, *naso* the nose, and *pharyngeal* the throat.

Use these general guidelines for OPAs and NPAs:

- Always take body substance isolation precautions when working in or around a patient's airway. This includes gloves, mask, and an eyeshield.
- Use OPAs only on patients who do not have a gag reflex. The **gag reflex** causes vomiting or retching when something is placed in the back of the throat. When a patient is unconscious, the gag reflex usually disappears but may reappear as he begins to regain consciousness. A patient with a gag reflex may tolerate the NPA because it does not go as deeply into the pharynx.
- Open the patient's airway manually before using an airway adjunct.
- *Do not* continue to insert the OPA if the patient starts to gag. Continue manual maneuvers and,

if the patient remains unconscious, try insertion again in a few minutes.
- While the OPA or NPA is in place, continue to provide either the head-tilt, chin-lift, or jaw-thrust maneuver.
- While the OPA or NPA is in place, always have a rigid-tipped suction device readily available.
- If the patient regains consciousness or develops a gag reflex, remove the airway adjunct immediately.

Preceptor Pearl

When a patient has no gag reflex, it is your primary responsibility to protect his airway from occlusion or aspiration (sucking in) of foreign material because the patient can no longer safeguard himself. While you could initially "save the patient," if he was allowed to aspirate during the time of your airway care, he could die from aspiration pneumonia over the next days or weeks. ❖

There are a number of advanced airway adjuncts that are elective sections of the EMT-B curriculum. Chapter 19 introduces the use of advanced airway adjuncts such as the endotracheal tube, EOA, EGTA, PtL®, and Combitube®. The state and local Medical Directors decide which, if any, of these devices are taught in your region.

The Oropharyngeal Airway (OPA)

Since you are an experienced prehospital provider, you have most likely used an OPA frequently. Let's review how to measure and insert an OPA. The OPA cannot be used effectively unless you select the correct airway size for the patient. Always measure the proper size first before using an OPA. If the wrong size is used, you could actually occlude the patient's airway. The proper size will extend either from the center of the patient's mouth to the angle of the jaw OR from the corner of the mouth to the ear lobe (Figure 4–6). Use these guidelines for inserting an OPA:

- Take body substance isolation precautions.
- First place the patient on his back and open the airway using either the head-tilt, chin-lift OR jaw-thrust maneuver if you suspect trauma.
- Open the patient's jaws using the **cross-fingered technique** (Figure 4–7). Cross the thumb and forefinger of one hand and place them on the patient's upper and lower teeth at the corner of the mouth. Then spread your fingers apart.

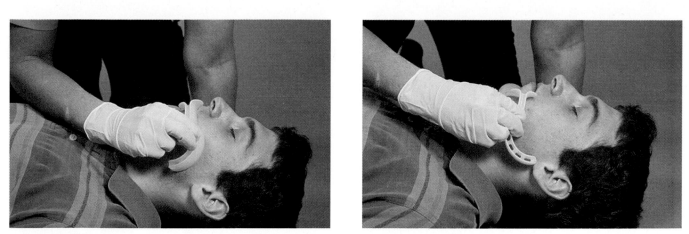

FIGURE 4–6 The oropharyngeal airway is chosen and checked for size.

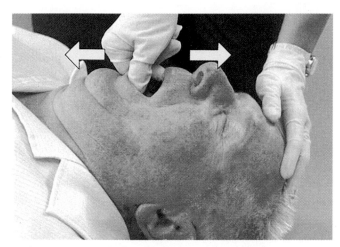

FIGURE 4–7 Cross-fingered technique.

- Position the correct size airway so that its tip is pointing toward the roof of the patient's mouth. Insert the airway by sliding it along the roof of the patient's mouth (Figure 4–8), past the soft tissue hanging down from the back (the uvula), or until you meet resistance against the soft palate. Be certain not to push the patient's tongue back into the throat.
- Now flip the airway 180 degrees over the tongue (Figure 4–9) so the tip is pointing down into the patient's throat. This prevents pushing the tongue back.
- Once the OPA has been inserted, place the non-trauma patient in a maximum head-tilt position (hyperextension). Check to see that the airway flange is against the patient's lips. If the airway is too long or short, replace it with the proper size.

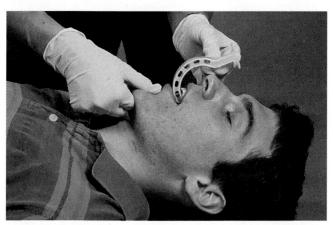

A.

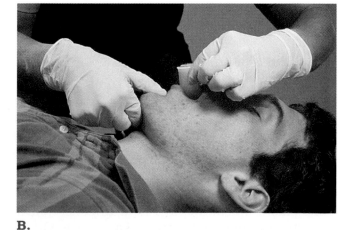

B.

FIGURE 4–8 A. The airway may be inserted with the tip pointing to the roof of the mouth and then ... **B.** the airway is rotated into position.

Airway insertion

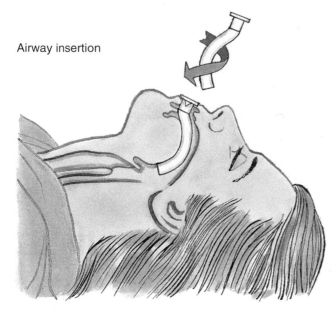

FIGURE 4–9 Note that when the airway is properly positioned, the flange rests against the patient's lips.

An alternative insertion method for adults is to place the airway tip already pointing "down" towards the patient's throat, using a tongue depressor to press the tongue down and forward to avoid obstructing the airway.

PEDIATRIC HIGHLIGHT

The preferred method for inserting an airway in infants and children is to use a tongue depressor and insert the airway straight in. This method prevents damage of the soft palate or uvula. ■

The Nasopharyngeal Airway (NPA)

NPAs are not as widely used as OPAs, but those who use them often prefer them because they do not stimulate a gag reflex. They are useful on patients with clenched teeth or oral injuries. When a patient has clenched teeth and the airway is filled with secretions, the NPA and a suction catheter provide access to the secretions without ever opening the patient's mouth. Because the hard plastic nasal airways tend to cause nasal bleeding, soft flexible latex nasal airways are used in the field. The sizes used for adults range from 28, 30, 32, to 34 "French." A small adult female would take a 28 and a large male would take a 34.

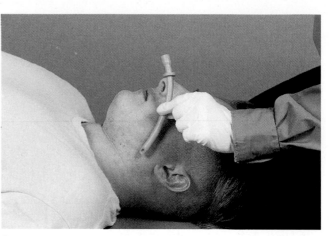

A.

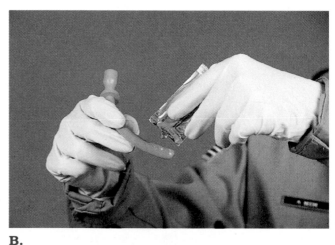

B.

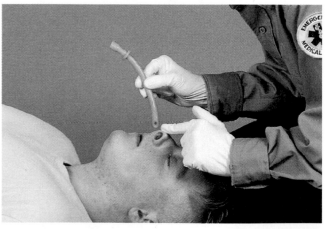

C.

FIGURE 4–10 A. Measuring, **B.** lubricating, and **C.** inserting a nasopharyngeal airway.

There are two ways to size these adjuncts: use an NPA that is the diameter of the patient's smallest finger or use one that extends from the tip of the patient's nose to the ear lobe (Figure 4–10A).

Your goal is to insert the largest diameter that will fit into the nostril!

To insert an NPA:

- Take body substance isolation precautions.
- Lubricate the NPA with a water-based lubricant such as KY jelly®, Lubifax®, or Surgilube® (Figure 4–10B). *Do not* use an oil-based lubricant such as Vaseline®, which can damage the tissue lining the nasal cavity and, if aspirated, can cause pneumonia.
- Gently push the tip of the nose upward while keeping the patient's head in a neutral position (Figure 4–10C). Most NPAs are designed to be placed in the right nostril. The beveled, or angled, portion at the tip of the airway should face toward the nasal septum, the wall that separates the nostrils.
- Insert the airway into the nostril, advancing until the flange rests firmly against the patient's nostril. Never force an NPA. If you experience any difficulty advancing the airway, pull it out, rotate 180 degrees, and try to insert it in the other nostril.

Do not attempt to use an NPA if there is evidence of clear (cerebrospinal) fluid coming from the nose or ears. This may indicate a skull fracture in the base of the cranium, which could potentially create an opening for the NPA to enter the brain.

■ WHY SUCTION PATIENTS?

As you know, keeping the patient's airway clear of vomitus, secretions, blood, and foreign materials is an important job. If a patient aspirates foreign material into the lungs, complications ranging from severe pneumonia to complete airway obstruction could occur.

The esophagus and stomach are lined with a tough coating that can tolerate anything from spicy sauces to peanuts and beer. In fact, the stomach contains hydrochloric acid, which helps break down food in the stomach. The trachea and lungs, however, are made up of very delicate tissue that is easily damaged. When a patient is unconscious and regurgitates or vomits stomach contents into the pharynx, there is a danger that some of this "toxic" material may be aspirated into the lower airway. It only takes about an ounce of stomach acid to cause a potentially lethal pneumonia. So make clearing the patient's airway your first priority!

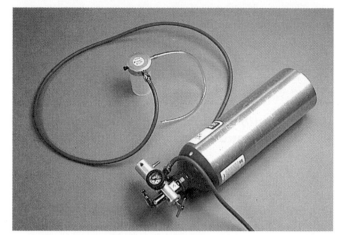

A.

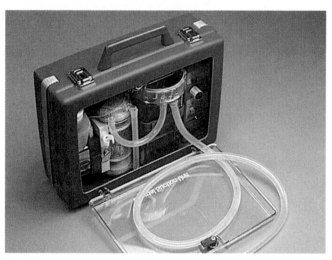

B.

FIGURE 4–11 A. An oxygen-powered portable suction unit. **B.** An electric battery-powered portable suction unit.

Suction Devices

There are basically three types of suction units: electric-, oxygen-, or gas-powered; the third type is manual (Figure 4–11). There are "on-board" or portable versions of each. Typical on-board units are mounted near the head end of the stretcher and are powered by the suction vacuum produced by the engine's manifold or the vehicle's battery. To be effective, a suction unit should furnish an air intake of at least 30 liters per minute at the open end of the collection tube. This will occur if the system can generate a vacuum of no less than 300 mmHg when the collecting tube is clamped.

Since patients can vomit or have fluid in their airways at any time, *always* carry a portable suction unit to the patient's side. Some EMT-Bs carry a "turkey baster" as a manual unit until the larger unit is at the patient's side.

PEDIATRIC HIGHLIGHT

Carry a bulb syringe in your pediatric kit to use as a manual suction unit for infants and toddlers. ■

There are pros and cons to each type of portable suction unit; use a unit that works best for your service area. Things to consider when choosing a portable suction unit include:

- *How easy is it to clean?* Material in the suction unit tubing and reservoir is a biohazard. Many units now have self-contained disposable parts that limit your potential exposure to the infectious materials you collect.
- *Does it deplete too much oxygen?* If you rely on an oxygen-powered suction unit, you may find that it runs down smaller tanks of oxygen quickly, consuming oxygen that should be administered to the patient.
- *Is the collection container large enough?* If you will be away from the ambulance for a long time and there is a great amount of suctioning to be done, you may have a problem if the collection container is too small.
- *How reliable is the unit?* Manual units work well when there is someone to pump them. Many EMT-Bs carry a manual hand-operated suction unit such as the V-Vack™ in their first-in bag to cover them until they return to the ambulance. Electric units work well, but the batteries should be checked every shift.

In addition to the suction unit, you need tubing, tips, and catheters. The tubing should be thick-walled, nonkinking, and wide-bored. It must allow "chunks" of suctioned material to pass through it. A tube that kinks or collapses decreases the amount of suction. The tubing must also be long enough to reach from the wall of the ambulance to the patient's head when the patient is on the stretcher. If it is necessary to suction a large volume of thick material, the tubing can be used without a tip as long as the steps for suctioning are followed.

PEDIATRIC HIGHLIGHT

If you immobilize a toddler on a long spine board, make sure the child is affixed to the head end, not placed in the center of the board.

This will guarantee that the suction tubing, as well as the oxygen tubing, will reach from the wall of the ambulance to the patient's face. ■

The most popular type of **suction tip** is the rigid pharyngeal tip, also called a "**Yankauer**," "tonsil sucker," or "tonsil-tip." Basically it is a disposable straight version of the suction tip a dentist places in the corner of your mouth. The Yankauer offers excellent control over the distal end of the device as you suction a patient's mouth and throat. It also has a larger bore than a catheter. However, be sure the Yankauer has a port to use as an on-off control. This way, with one hand you can open the mouth using the cross-fingered technique, while the other hand controls the Yankauer as well as the on-off control.

If the patient has a gag reflex, be careful not to cause gagging or to stimulate the vagus nerve by tickling the back of the throat. The vagus nerve, when stimulated, will cause the heart rate to slow down—a dangerous occurrence in critical situations. Always suction a few seconds at a time with a maximum of 15 seconds before oxygenating a patient. Always keep the end of the tip in sight to avoid damaging any soft tissue.

Suction **catheters** are flexible plastic tubes that come in various sizes identified by a number French. The larger the number, the larger the catheter. A "14 French" catheter is larger than an "8 French." Actually, catheters are designed to be passed down a tube such as an endotracheal tube or a nasal airway. Some catheters have an on-off control port. For those that do not, it is necessary to kink the tubing to turn the suction on and off. When using a suction catheter, use the largest diameter that fits. Measure the catheter from the center of the mouth to the angle of the jaw OR the corner of the mouth to the ear lobe. The length measured should be the maximum placed into the mouth at one time. Three hands are needed to properly position a catheter that is not being placed down a tube. One hand is used to open the mouth, another is used to control movement of the catheter tip, and the "third hand" is needed to turn the vacuum on and off.

Preceptor Pearl

No suction unit is designed to clear the airway of large chunks of meat or a linguini dinner the patient ate prior to having a cardiac arrest! Make sure you open the airway and sweep out such large food particles with a gloved finger before suctioning. ✢

Techniques of Suctioning

Use these steps for suctioning:

- *Always use body substance isolation precautions.* Most EMT-Bs routinely wear gloves when suctioning, but fail to wear masks and eyeshields. Yet, the potential for being sprayed with oral secretions or other infectious material is greatest when suctioning a patient. Use eyewear that you feel comfortable wearing and wear a mask or a combination mask and eyeshield.

- *Position yourself at the patient's head and turn the patient to the side, if patient is not at risk of a cervical injury.* Positioning the patient in this way allows secretions to drain from the mouth. If the patient has a potential cervical spine injury, one EMT-B should maintain manual stabilization of the patient's neck while another quickly suctions. If you are unable to adequately suction the patient in the supine position, it will be necessary for at least two rescuers to carefully log roll the patient. Remember that the airway is the highest treatment priority. If the patient is immobilized on a long spine board, then the entire spine board should be rolled on its side.

- *Measure the catheter.* It is not necessary to measure a rigid-tip catheter as long as you do not lose sight of the tip. If using a flexible catheter, measure the same way you measure for an OPA.

- *Open the mouth using the cross-fingered technique.* Clear the mouth of large pieces of material by using a finger sweep as necessary. If the patient has an OPA inserted, remove it while you are suctioning.

- *Place the Yankauer so that the convex (bulging-out) side is against the roof of the patient's mouth. Insert the tip to the base of the tongue.* Follow the pharyngeal curvature (Figure 4–12). *Do not* push the tip down into the throat or into the larynx.

- *Apply suction only after the Yankauer or catheter tip is in place.* Suction on the way out, moving the catheter from side to side for a maximum of 15 seconds. Then reoxygenate the patient. Remember that as long as the suction unit is on, it is removing oxygen from the patient's respiratory system.

Preceptor Pearl

Rather than counting out fifteen seconds as the maximum amount of time for suctioning, just take a breath and hold it before beginning to suction. When you need a breath, so does the patient. So stop suctioning and allow the patient to breathe. ✣

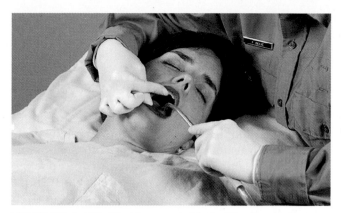

FIGURE 4–12 Placing a rigid tip Yankauer.

■ VENTILATION MANAGEMENT AND ASSISTANCE

If you determine that either a patient is not breathing or his respiratory effort is inadequate, it is necessary to immediately provide artificial ventilation. Artificial ventilation is the forcing of air, or oxygen, into the lungs when a patient has either stopped breathing or has inadequate breathing. After years of researching various artificial ventilation techniques, in 1992 the American Heart Association recommended that the technique used for ventilation be done in the following order of preference:

- *Mouth-to-mask with high-flow supplemental oxygen at 15 liters, or more, per minute* This procedure allows for delivery of a large volume of oxygen and provides an excellent mask seal that is created by the use of both hands on the mask.

- *Two-person bag-valve mask with high-flow supplemental oxygen at 15 liters, or more, per minute* When using the BVM, one rescuer uses two hands to seal the mask with the "double OK hand position," as the second rescuer squeezes the bag. This also gives the EMT-B a good sense of the patient's lung compliance.

- *Flow restricted, oxygen-powered ventilation device* This procedure provides excellent volume. In fact, you need to watch closely to prevent overinflation, which would fill the patient's stomach with gas. In the field, this device is not recommended for use on infants and children.

- *One-person bag-valve mask with supplemental oxygen at 15 liters, or more, per minute* The one-handed mask seal is difficult to maintain over a long time period.

If the patient has been endotracheal intubated by a paramedic or a specially trained EMT-B, the first choice would be the one-person bag to ET technique discussed later in this chapter.

Mouth-to-Mask Ventilation

Mouth-to-mask ventilation is performed using a pocket face mask. The pocket face mask, or barrier protection device, is made of soft, collapsible material that can be easily carried in your pocket, jacket, glove compartment, or purse (Figure 4–13). Most EMT-Bs carry a pocket mask in their first-in bag.

Face masks and barrier protectors have an important infection-control purpose. To prevent direct contact with the patient's mouth, ventilations are given into a valve in the mask. Most pocket masks have one-way valves that allow ventilations to enter but prevent the patient's exhaled air from exiting through the ventilation port into the rescuer. The pocket mask must be made of see-through plastic so you can observe the color of the patient's face and immediately respond if the patient begins to regurgitate.

Use these steps when applying the pocket mask:

1. Take body substance isolation precautions. Wear gloves and an eyeshield. You will be unable to wear a disposable mask.

2. Position yourself at the patient's head and open the airway. It may be necessary to quickly suction and clear obstructions in the patient's mouth. If available, insert an OPA to help keep the patient's airway open.

3. Connect oxygen to the inlet on the face mask. Run oxygen at 15 liters or more per minute.

4. Position the mask on the patient's face so that the apex is over the bridge of the nose and the

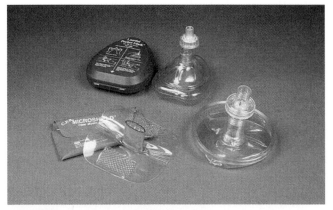

FIGURE 4–13 Barrier devices.

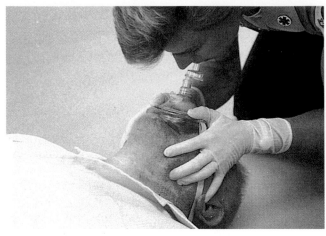

FIGURE 4–14 Mouth-to-mask ventilation.

base is between the lower lip and prominence of the chin.

5. Hold the mask firmly in place while maintaining the proper head tilt (Figure 4–14). To lift the jaw forward, place both thumbs on the sides of the mask and the index, third, and fourth fingers on each side of the patient's face between the angle of the jaw and the ear lobe. Jut the jaw up to the mask; avoid squeezing the mask down onto the face since this squeezing closes the mouth and airway.

6. Take a deep breath and exhale into the mask's one-way valve at the top of the mask port. Each ventilation should be delivered over 1½ to 2 seconds in adults and 1 to 1½ seconds in infants and children. Watch closely for the patient's chest to rise—this is your primary goal.

7. Remove your mouth from the port and allow for passive exhalation. Continue the procedure for ventilating following the rescue breathing or CPR guidelines.

Preceptor Pearl

Begin mouth-to-mask ventilations immediately if oxygen is not available. ❖

Bag-Valve-Mask Ventilation

The bag-valve mask is a hand-held ventilation device which may be referred to as a bag-valve-mask unit, system, or device; resuscitator; Ambu-bag™; or BVM. It is used to ventilate a non-breathing patient as well as to assist the respirations of a patient who is not adequately ventilating on his own. The parts of the BVM include the clear face mask with air cushion, the nonrebreather valve, the squeezable bag, the oxygen reservoir, and the oxygen inlet. When you are ventilating a patient, the BVM provides an excellent barrier to infection but must be properly disposed of or sterilized after its use.

BVMs come in various sizes. Ambulances should carry the adult, pediatric, and neonatal, or newborn, sizes. The bag must be a self-refilling shell. The system must have a nonjam valve that allows an oxygen inlet flow of 15 liters or more per minute. The valve should be nonrebreathing to prevent the patient from rebreathing his own exhalation and not subject to freezing in the cold temperatures experienced in the field. Most systems have the standard 15/22 mm respiratory fitting to ensure a proper fit with other respiratory equipment, face masks, and endotracheal tubes.

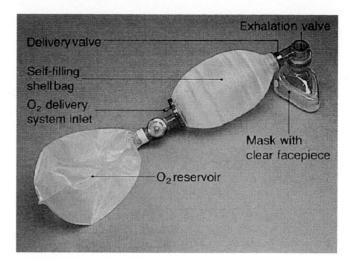

FIGURE 4–15 The typical bag-valve-mask with a closed reservoir system.

Preceptor Pearl

If the BVM you are using has a pop-off valve, discard it and order a new one without a pop-off valve. Often rescuers who thought they were ventilating patients using a BVM with a pop-off valve discovered that they were blowing out the entire oxygen volume through the pop-off valve. The AHA recommendations clearly state that BVMs with pop-off valves should not be used, even on pediatric patients. ✣

Preceptor Pearl

In the field, never use a BVM without the reservoir. Without a reservoir, the BVM would produce only about 50% oxygen if attached to an oxygen source, or 21% if not attached to an oxygen source. When resuscitating a patient with a BVM, your goal is to deliver 90% to 100% oxygen. ✣

The BVM's squeezable bag is designed to hold anywhere from 1,000 to 1,600 milliliters of air, depending on the brand. According to the AHA guidelines, at least 800 milliliters of air must be delivered to the patient with each squeeze of the bag. The BVM should always be used with an oxygen reservoir system attached. To operate the BVM, the oxygen should flow at 15 liters or more per minute.

There are two types of reservoir systems—open and closed. In the **open system,** the BVM usually has a long open tube, or elephant's trunk, which backfills with oxygen between ventilations. When the bag is squeezed, the oxygen in it goes into the patient; then the bag immediately fills with the oxygen that has collected in the reservoir. Since the end of the tube is open to the outside environment, there is a possibility that some room air will mix with the oxygen in the bag. Therefore, oxygen concentration is usually expressed as 90% oxygen.

In the **closed system,** a collapsible bag acts as the reservoir (Figure 4–15). Since this bag is not open to the outside environment, it contains 100% oxygen. The closed system operates the same way as the open system, but since there is no outside air mixed with the contents of the reservoir, the patient receives 100% oxygen.

Two-Person Bag-Valve-Mask Ventilations

The most difficult part of delivering BVM ventilations is obtaining an adequate mask seal so that air does not leak in or out around the mask's edges. It is difficult to maintain the seal with one hand while squeezing the bag with the other. For this reason, the one-person bag-valve mask technique is often inadequate. It is strongly recommended that BVM ventilation be performed by two rescuers. This technique can be used when no trauma is suspected or it can be modified by using a jaw-thrust maneuver if potential spinal trauma is suspected.

To perform BVM ventilation when *no trauma* is suspected (Figure 4–16A):

1. Take body substance isolation precautions.
2. Open the patient's airway using the head-tilt, chin-lift technique. Suction as needed and insert an OPA or NPA.
3. Select the proper size BVM for the patient (infant, child, or adult).
4. Kneel at the patient's head. Position thumbs over the top half of the mask, index and middle fingers over the bottom half.
5. Place the apex of the triangular mask over the bridge of the patient's nose; then lower the mask over the mouth and upper chin.

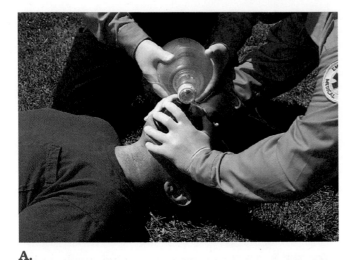

A.

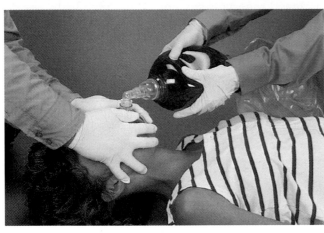

B.

FIGURE 4–16 A. Providing bag-valve-mask ventilations when there is no suspected trauma. **B.** Providing bag-valve-mask ventilations when trauma is suspected.

6. Use the ring and little fingers (the middle fingers may also be used) to bring the patient's jaw up to the mask and maintain the head-tilt, chin-lift.

7. The second rescuer should kneel at the patient's side and connect the bag to mask, if this has not already been done. While you maintain the mask seal, the second rescuer should squeeze the bag with two hands until the patient's chest rises. The rate should be once every 5 seconds for an adult or once every 3 seconds for infants and children.

To use the BVM on a patient that you suspect has *spinal trauma* (Figure 4–16B):

1. Take body substance isolation precautions.

2. Open the patient's airway using the jaw-thrust maneuver. Suction as needed and insert an OPA or NPA.

3. Select the proper size BVM for the patient (infant, child, or adult).

4. Kneel at the patient's head. Place the apex of the triangular mask over the bridge of the patient's nose, then lower the mask over the mouth and upper chin.

5. Place thumbs over the nose portion of the mask and place your index and middle fingers over the portion of the mask that covers the mouth, reaching to grasp the angle of the jaw.

6. Use the ring and little fingers to jut the patient's jaw, bringing the jaw up to the mask without tilting the head or neck.

7. The second rescuer should kneel at the patient's side and ventilate as described above for the nontrauma patient.

Preceptor Pearl

It is impossible to do a one-handed jaw thrust; therefore, it is impossible to use a BVM on an unconscious trauma patient unless the patient has an endotracheal tube inserted or a second rescuer can assist you. ❖

One-Person Bag-Valve-Mask Ventilations

As noted above, the one-person BVM procedure is the last choice for artificial ventilation. If it must be performed because of the lack of helpers or the lack of an available flow-restricted, oxygen-powered ventilation device or a pocket mask, then follow these steps:

1. Take body substance isolation precautions.

2. Position yourself at the patient's head about 12 to 18 inches above the supine patient. Establish an open airway using the head-tilt, chin-lift technique. Suction and insert an OPA or NPA.

3. Select the correct size mask for the patient. Position the mask on the patient's face as described above.

4. Use the "OK hand position" by forming a "C" with the thumb and index finger around the ventilation port. Use the middle, ring, and little fingers under the patient's jaw to pull it up to the mask.

5. With the other hand, squeeze the bag against the side of the patient's face once every 5 seconds. The squeeze should be a full one, causing the patient's chest to rise.

6. Release pressure on the bag and let the patient exhale passively. While this takes place, the bag refills with oxygen from the reservoir.

Preceptor Pearl

If you hear any leaks during BVM ventilation, immediately reopen the airway and reposition the mask seal to correct the mask leak. If the chest does not rise and fall, check for airway obstruction or obstruction in the BVM system. Consider inserting an OPA if one is not yet in place. If these steps are unsuccessful, do not continue to ventilate the patient inadequately. If corrections prove unsuccessful, quickly switch to the two-person BVM technique, pocket-mask technique, or flow-restricted, oxygen-powered ventilation device. ✤

The BVM can be used to artificially ventilate patients with a stoma who are found to be in severe respiratory distress or respiratory arrest. These patients often have thick secretions blocking the stoma that will first need to be suctioned with a catheter. Use this procedure:

1. Take body substance isolation precautions.

2. Clear any mucus plugs or secretions from the stoma.

3. Keep the patient's head and neck in the neutral position. It is unnecessary to position a stoma breather's airway prior to ventilating.

4. Use a pediatric-sized mask to establish a seal around the stoma.

5. Ventilate at the appropriate rate for the seal around the stoma.

6. If unable to ventilate through the stoma, consider sealing the stoma and attempting artificial ventilations through the mouth and nose. (This technique may work if the patient is a partial neck breather. It will not work in a patient whose trachea has been permanently connected to the neck opening, since there is no remaining connection to the mouth, nose, or pharynx.)

The Flow-Restricted, Oxygen-Powered Ventilation Device (FROPVD)

A flow-restricted, oxygen-powered ventilation device uses pressurized oxygen delivered through a mask to provide artificial ventilation. This device is similar to the traditional positive-pressure ventilator, multifunction regulator, or "demand-valve resuscitator" but includes a redesigned valve that

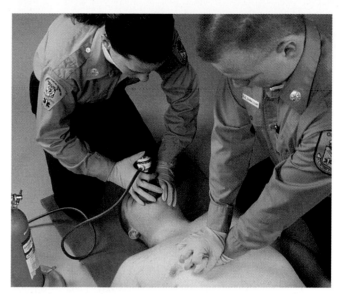

FIGURE 14–17 Providing ventilations with a flow-restricted, oxygen-powered ventilation device.

optimizes ventilations and safeguards the patient (Figure 4–17). In the past, the FROPVD was referred to as MTV (manual transport ventilator). A ventilator called ATV (automatic transport ventilator) is commonly used by ALS providers for inter-facility transport (see Chapter 19).

PEDIATRIC HIGHLIGHT

The flow-restricted, oxygen-powered device is designed to be used only on adults unless members of your service have been specially trained in its use for children and a very sophisticated unit in which the ventilation volume can be adjusted is available. ■

The procedure for mask seal using the FROPVD is the same as the one-person or two-person BVM. When purchasing a FROPVD, look for these features:

• Peak flow rate of 100% oxygen at up to 40 liters per minute

• Inspired pressure relief valve that opens at approximately 60 cm of water pressure

• Audible alarm when the relief valve is activated

• Rugged design and construction

• Trigger that enables the EMT-B to use both hands to maintain a mask seal while triggering the device

• Satisfactory operation in both normal and extreme environmental conditions

ASSISTING WITH ENDOTRACHEAL TUBE PLACEMENT

The "gold standard" for airway care is the endotracheal tube. All other airway devices are, at best, secondary. This is because the endotracheal tube is directly inserted into the trachea, forming an open pathway for air, oxygen, or medications to be blown into the lungs. In addition, adult sizes have an inflatable cuff that seals off the trachea to minimize the risk of aspiration.

In some areas, EMT-Bs are trained to perform endotracheal intubation. This skill is taught as an elective (see Chapter 19: Advanced Airway Management). In other areas, only paramedics are trained to perform endotracheal intubation.

When assisting in intubation, you may be asked to hyperventilate the patient with the BVM for about a minute or so before the paramedic inserts the ET tube. This can be accomplished by ventilating once every two seconds. The paramedic then places the nontraumatic patient in the sniffing position (neck elevated approximately two inches, chin and nose thrust forward, and head tilted back) to align the mouth, throat, and trachea. The paramedic then removes the OPA and passes the ET tube through the mouth (sometimes the nose), into the throat past the vocal cords, and into the trachea. This procedure usually requires a laryngoscope to illuminate the airway and to move the tongue and other obstructions out of the way.

In order to maneuver the tube past the vocal cords correctly, the paramedic needs to see them. You may be asked to push the vocal cords into view by gently and carefully pressing your thumb and index finger just to either side of the medial throat over the cricoid cartilage. This procedure is known as cricoid pressure or Sellick's maneuver.

Once the tube is properly placed, the cuff is inflated with air from a 10 cc syringe. To assure proper placement of the ET tube, the paramedic, while holding the tube, uses a stethoscope to listen for lung sounds on both sides and over the epigastrium (the area of the upper abdomen just under the xiphoid process). If the tube is incorrectly placed, the paramedic immediately repositions or removes the tube, asks you to reoxygenate the patient, and repeats the intubation procedure.

The correctly positioned tube is anchored in place with tape. The entire procedure, including the last ventilation, passing the tube, and the next ventilation, should take less than 30 seconds.

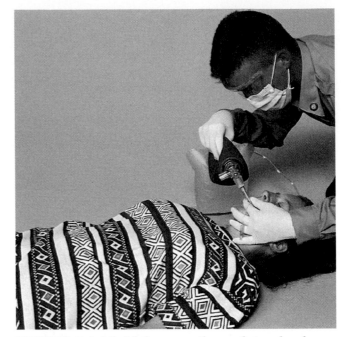

FIGURE 14–18 Make sure the endotracheal tube does not move. Hold it with two fingers against the patient's teeth.

Complications

When asked to ventilate the intubated, or "tubed," patient, keep in mind that it takes very little movement to displace the ET tube. Look at the graduations on the side of the tube. In the typical adult male, for example, the 22 cm mark will be at the teeth when the tube is properly placed. If the tube moves, report this to the paramedic immediately.

Be especially careful not to disturb the ET tube. If the tube is pushed in, it will most likely enter the right mainstem bronchus, preventing oxygen from entering the patient's left lung. If the tube is pulled out, it can easily slip into the esophagus and send ventilations directly to the stomach. This is a fatal complication if it goes unnoticed. When holding the tube, place two fingers of one hand against the patient's teeth (Figure 4–18).

If you are ventilating a breathing patient, be sure to time your breaths with the respiratory efforts of the patient. You want to enlarge the patient's breaths, not fight them. Pay close attention to how the ventilations feel. Report any change in resistance, since increased resistance when ventilating with the BVM is one of the first signs of air escaping through a hole in the lungs and filling the space around the lungs (pneumothorax). A change in resistance can also indicate that the tube has slipped into the esophagus.

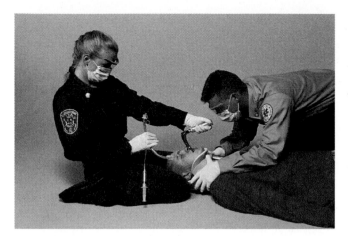

FIGURE 14–19 To assist in the intubation of a patient with suspected cervical-spine injury, maintain manual stabilization throughout the procedure.

Whenever a patient is to be defibrillated, carefully remove the bag from the tube, because the weight of the unsupported bag may accidentally dislodge the tube. Watch for any changes in the patient's mental status. As the patient becomes more alert, he or she may need to be restrained from pulling the tube out.

Assisting with a Trauma Intubation

Occasionally you will be asked to assist in the endotracheal intubation of a patient with a suspected cervical-spine injury. Since using the sniffing position increases the risk of neck injury, you may be required to provide manual in-line stabilization during the entire procedure.

To accomplish this, the paramedic holds manual stabilization while you apply a rigid cervical collar. (In some systems the patient may be intubated without the collar.) Since the paramedic must stay at the patient's head, it is necessary for you to stabilize the head and neck from the patient's side (Figure 4–19). Once you are in position, the paramedic leans back and uses the laryngoscope to bring the patient's vocal cords into view in order to tube him.

After intubation, you hold the tube against the patient's teeth until placement is confirmed and the tube is anchored. At that time, you can change your position to a more comfortable one. However, until the patient is immobilized on a long backboard, it is necessary to assign another rescuer to maintain manual stabilization while you ventilate the patient.

Preceptor Pearl

Never assume that a collar alone provides adequate immobilization. In addition to a collar, manual stabilization must be used until the patient's head is taped in place on the backboard. ✜

■ OXYGEN ADMINISTRATION

One of the most beneficial treatments an EMT-B can provide is oxygen. **Hypoxia** is an insufficient supply of oxygen to the body's tissues. If a patient develops hypoxia while breathing atmospheric air (which contains only 21% oxygen), it is essential that the patient receive aggressive oxygen therapy. Clinically, the hypoxic patient may present with cyanosis or with restlessness and confusion if the brain is not receiving adequate oxygen.

Indications

Indications for oxygen include:

- Shock or hypoperfusion
- Respiratory distress or arrest
- Cardiac abnormality or arrest
- Patients with chronic lung disorders who present in respiratory distress
- Smoke or toxic fume inhalation
- Poisoning or drug overdose causing ventilations that are too shallow or too slow
- Multiple system trauma patients
- Head trauma resulting in brain tissue swelling and hypoxia
- Stroke, seizure, or diabetic emergency

Hazards

The use of oxygen can involve nonmedical and medical hazards.

Nonmedical hazards:

- If a pressurized oxygen cylinder is dropped and the valve breaks off, the cylinder can become a missile injuring everything and everyone in its path.
- Oxygen supports combustion, causing fire to burn more rapidly.
- Oxygen under pressure and oil do not mix. When they come in contact, an explosion can occur. Never lubricate an oxygen cylinder.

Medical hazards:

- Oxygen toxicity or air sac collapse can occur in an environment where high-concentration oxygen has been administered to a patient for an extended time period, such as in hospitals and long-term care facilities.

- If premature infants are given too much oxygen, eye damage may occur. Excessive oxygen, along with other factors, can cause scar tissue to develop on the eyes' retinas. However, in the field, if you suspect that an infant or premature infant is in respiratory distress, never withhold oxygen for fear of injuring the patient's eyes.

- Patients with chronic lung diseases such as asbestosis, black lung, emphysema, and chronic bronchitis, as well as elderly asthmatics, may be in the last stage of these diseases. In cases such as these, administering high-concentration oxygen could cause breathing stoppage. Although such breathing stoppage is rare, always evaluate the patient's oxygen needs. If a patient is in respiratory distress, administer high-concentration oxygen. If a patient has a minor problem, such as a twisted ankle, and normally is on a twenty-foot nasal cannula at home, then continue the liter flow and device the patient has been using at home.

The normal stimulus to breathe is the level of carbon dioxide in the blood. In chronic lung diseases, gas, mostly carbon dioxide, is trapped in the lungs due to chronic lower airway obstruction. When this occurs, the chronic obstructed pulmonary disease (COPD) patient switches over to a secondary stimulus to breathe—a low level of oxygen in the blood. This condition is called "hypoxic drive." A patient who is in hypoxic drive and who is administered high-concentration oxygen would stop breathing because his blood level of oxygen would be so high that the brain thinks no more oxygen is needed.

Preceptor Pearl

In the field, you may never see oxygen toxicity or other adverse conditions that result from oxygen administration since the time required for such conditions to develop is lengthy. Therefore, if the patient requires oxygen and is adequately ventilating himself, use a nonrebreather mask at 15 liters per minute; otherwise ventilate the patient. The bottom line: Never withhold high-concentration oxygen from a patient who needs it! ❖

Oxygen Delivery Systems

Oxygen equipment used in the field must be safe, lightweight, portable, and dependable.

Oxygen Cylinder

The standard source of oxygen is the oxygen cylinder, which is made of seamless steel or alloy, and is filled with oxygen under pressure, usually 2,000 to 2,200 psi when full. A tank is ¾ full when it reads 1,500 psi, ½ full when it reads 1,000 psi, and ¼ full at 500 psi. Change the tank when it is at 500 or less, but never allow it to empty completely since this can damage the inside of the tank. Cylinders come in various sizes. The higher the letter in the alphabet, the larger the cylinder. For example, a "D" tank holds 350 liters of oxygen, and an "E" tank holds 625 liters. The larger tanks, such as a "G" tank, which holds 5,300 liters, or an "H" tank, which holds 6,900 liters, are used on board the ambulance.

The United States Pharmacopoeia has assigned a color code to distinguish compressed gases. Green and white cylinders have been assigned to all grades of oxygen. Also, unpainted stainless steel or aluminum cylinders are frequently used for oxygen.

Safety is a prime concern when working with oxygen cylinders.

When using an oxygen tank, *ALWAYS:*

- Use pressure gauges, regulators, and tubing that are intended for use with oxygen.

- Use nonferrous metal oxygen wrenches for changing gauges and regulators or for adjusting flow rates to avoid sparks.

- Ensure that valve seal inserts and gaskets are in good condition to prevent dangerous leaks.

- Use medical grade oxygen. Industrial oxygen contains impurities. The cylinders should be labeled "OXYGEN U.S.P." and should not be more than five years old.

- Open the valve of an oxygen cylinder fully, then close it half a turn. This prevents someone else from thinking the valve is closed and attempting to force it open. Remember: "Right is Tight and Left is Loose."

- Store reserve oxygen cylinders in a cool, vented room, properly secured in place.

- Have oxygen cylinders hydrostatically tested every five years. Some tanks only need testing every ten years, if they have a star after the date of test (e.g., 4M92*). The date a cylinder was last tested is stamped on the cylinder.

When using an oxygen tank, *NEVER:*

- Drop a tank or let it fall against any object. When transporting a patient with an oxygen cylinder, make sure the oxygen cylinder is strapped or secured to the stretcher.

- Leave an oxygen tank standing in an upright position without being secured.

- Allow smoking around oxygen equipment in use. Clearly mark the area of use with signs that read "OXYGEN—NO SMOKING."

- Use grease, oil, or fat-based soaps on devices that will be attached to an oxygen supply cylinder. *Do not* handle these devices when your hands are greasy. Use greaseless tools when making connections.

- Use adhesive tape to protect an oxygen tank outlet or to mark or label any oxygen tank or delivery apparatus. The oxygen can react with the adhesive and debris and cause a fire.

- Try to move an oxygen cylinder by dragging it or rolling it on its side or bottom.

Regulators

A pressure regulator must be attached to the oxygen cylinder to measure the amount of pressure in the tank and the liters you wish to flow. Regulators are either screw-in types for the larger tanks or pin-yoke assembly types. The pin system is designed to assure that the regulator is used only on an oxygen tank. The procedure for changing the regulator on a tank is as follows:

1. Select desired cylinder. Check the label for Oxygen U.S.P.
2. Place the cylinder in an upright position and stand to one side.
3. Remove the plastic wrapper or cap protecting the cylinder outlet.
4. Keep the plastic washer and change if necessary.
5. "Crack" the main valve for a second.
6. Select the correct pressure regulator and flowmeter (either pin yoke or threaded).
7. Place cylinder valve gasket on regulator oxygen port.
8. Make certain that the pressure regulator is closed.
9. Align pins or thread by hand.
10. Tighten the T-screw for the pin yoke by hand or tighten the threaded outlet with a wrench.
11. Attach tubing and appropriate oxygen delivery device.

Flowmeters

The flowmeter allows control of the flow of oxygen in liters per minute. It is connected to the regulator but may be a separate unit as in the on-board oxygen system. The three types of flowmeters commonly used in the field are:

- Bourdon Gauge Flowmeter™ This flowmeter operates at most any angle and is fairly rugged, but the gauge is inaccurate. When the tubing is kinked, the flowmeter doesn't compensate for the back pressure, and the gauge will give a false high reading.

- Pressure-Compensated Flowmeter (Thorpe™ tube-type) This unit is gravity dependent so it must be in an upright position. It has a ball float in an upright glass tube and indicates very accurately the flow at all times. It is often used in the on-board system.

- Constant Flow Selector Valve This type of flowmeter is gaining popularity for use with portable tanks. It allows for adjustment in stepped increments (2, 4, 6, 8, ... 15 liters per minute).

Humidifiers

A humidifier can be connected to the flowmeter to provide moisture to the dry oxygen coming from the supply cylinder. Dry oxygen can dehydrate the mucous membranes of a patient's airway and lungs. When used for a short time, oxygen dryness is not a problem. However certain patients (infants, children, and those with COPD or respiratory burns) are better off if offered humidified oxygen, especially on long ambulance trips. Sterile, single-use humidifiers are also available and should be considered, rather than changing a humidifier's water with every shift as is often done.

Preceptor Pearl

Some EMT-Bs like to keep Betadyne® in their on-board suction container to keep it clean. However, putting Betadyne® in the humidifier could kill an asthmatic patient. Never use any substance other than sterile water in the humidifier unless directed by a physician! ✚

Delivering Oxygen to the Breathing Patient

Two devices are used in the field to treat patients who are breathing and have adequate ventilation—the nonrebreather mask and the nasal cannula. If patients need oxygen, give them a high flow of 15 liters per minute with a **nonrebreather mask**, which produces an oxygen concentration of 80 to 90%.

Excluding the BVM with a reservoir or a flow-restricted, oxygen-powered ventilation device, the nonrebreather mask is the best way for an EMT-B to deliver high concentrations of oxygen. The mask must be properly placed on the patient's face to provide the necessary seal, which ensures that a high concentration is delivered. The reservoir bag must be inflated before the mask is placed on the patient's face. To inflate the reservoir bag, use your finger to cover the exhaust port or the connection between the mask and the reservoir. The reservoir must always contain enough oxygen so that it does not deflate by more than one third when the patient takes his deepest inspiration. Oxygen supply can be maintained by flowing at least 15 liters per minute. Air exhaled by the patient does not return to the reservoir; instead it escapes through a flutter valve in the face piece.

New design features allow for one emergency port in the mask so that the patient can still receive atmospheric air should the oxygen supply fail. This feature keeps the mask from delivering 100% oxygen but is a necessary safety feature. Nonrebreather masks come in infant, child, and adult sizes.

Some patients will not tolerate a mask-type delivery device because they feel "suffocated" by the mask. If they need the higher concentration of oxygen, try to convince them to use the nonrebreather mask. For the patient who refuses to wear a nonrebreather mask, the **nasal cannula** is better than no oxygen at all. A nasal cannula provides low oxygen concentrations between 24 and 44%. Oxygen is delivered to the patient by the two prongs that rest in the patient's nostrils. The device is usually held to the patient's face by placing the tubing over the patient's ears and securing the slip-loop under the patient's chin.

When a cannula is used, deliver no more than 6 liters of oxygen per minute. At higher flow rates, the cannula begins to feel like a windstorm in the nose and dries out the nasal mucous membranes.

CHAPTER REVIEW

■ SUMMARY

The first priority of all patient care is to open the airway. As practicing EMT-Bs, you have used airway maintenance, ventilation, and oxygenation skills over and over. Through continuing education, you become aware of revisions in the curriculum that lead to improvement of patient care.

For example, in this chapter you learned that the new curriculum emphasizes use of the bag-valve mask as a two-rescuer skill. In addition, the curriculum encourages EMT-Bs to use the FROPVD, to assist with endotracheal intubation, and to implement simplified oxygen therapy.

■ REVIEW QUESTIONS

1. Describe how you can tell if a patient is breathing adequately.
2. Describe how you can tell if a patient is breathing inadequately.
3. Explain the differences between opening the airway of a medical patient and opening that of a trauma patient.
4. Demonstrate how to measure and insert an OPA.
5. Demonstrate how to insert an NPA and explain why water-soluble jelly is used.

6. Discuss the procedure of suctioning and explain the benefits of using a rigid tip.
7. Explain why a BVM should be used with two rescuers rather than one.
8. List the hazards of using oxygen.
9. Explain how to safely handle an oxygen cylinder.
10. Explain why all patients are given oxygen by a nonrebreather mask unless they cannot tolerate it.

Patient Assessment— Medical Patient

■ For years, EMT-Bs have assessed medical and trauma patients in different ways. The U.S. DOT Revised 1994 EMT-B National Standard Curriculum recognizes this and encourages EMT-Bs to assess each patient in the appropriate manner. This chapter describes the assessment of a medical patient—a patient who is not injured. Most of the assessment consists of gathering a history of the present illness, a past medical history, and a set of vital signs.

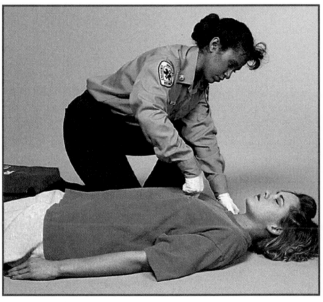

Assessing a responsive medical patient is very different from assessing an unresponsive medical patient. The curriculum recognizes this, too, and describes how to evaluate each of those patients.

The EMT-B will be able to administer medications to some patients and to assist others in taking their own medications. In these cases, there are specific questions to ask that will determine whether the medication is the appropriate intervention. Since many things can be going on at the same time with any particular patient, the obvious treatment may not always be the best or only treatment. Determining this accurately depends on an appropriate assessment that is done well.

MAKING THE TRANSITION

■ The initial step in detecting and treating immediate threats to life is now called the initial assessment instead of the primary survey.

■ The next steps in the assessment depend on the category into which a patient falls: medical or trauma; responsive or unresponsive; significant mechanism of injury or no significant mechanism of injury; adult, child, or infant.

■ Re-evaluate stable patients every 15 minutes, unstable patients every 5 minutes.

OBJECTIVES

The numbered objectives below are from the United States Department of Transportation 1994 EMT-Basic National Standard Curriculum. Objectives with colored bullets that follow in italics are from the EMT-Basic Transitional Program.

■ KNOWLEDGE AND ATTITUDE

At the completion of this chapter, you should be able to:

Initial Assessment

1. Summarize the reasons for forming a general impression of the patient. (p. 74)
2. Discuss methods of assessing altered mental status. (pp. 74, 75, 77)
3. Differentiate between assessing the altered mental status in the adult, child, and infant patient. (pp. 74, 75, 77)
4. Discuss methods of assessing the airway in the adult, child, and infant patient. (pp. 74, 77)
5. Describe methods used for assessing if a patient is breathing. (pp. 74, 77)
6. State what care should be provided to the adult, child, and infant patient with adequate breathing. (pp. 74, 77)
7. State what care should be provided to the adult, child, and infant patient without adequate breathing. (pp. 74, 77, 81, 82)
8. Differentiate between a patient with adequate and inadequate breathing. (pp. 74, 77, 81, 82)
9. Distinguish between methods of assessing breathing in the adult, child, and infant patient. (pp. 81–82)
10. Compare the methods of providing airway care to the adult, child, and infant patient. (p. 77)
11. Describe the methods used to obtain a pulse. (pp. 74–75)
12. Differentiate between obtaining a pulse in an adult, child, and infant patient. (pp. 74–75)
13. Discuss the need for assessing the patient for external bleeding. (p. 75)
14. Describe normal and abnormal findings when assessing skin color. (p. 75)
15. Describe normal and abnormal findings when assessing skin temperature. (p. 75)
16. Describe normal and abnormal findings when assessing skin condition. (p. 75)
17. Describe normal and abnormal findings when assessing skin capillary refill in the infant and child patient. (pp. 75–76)
18. Explain the reason for prioritizing a patient for care and transport. (p. 76)
19. Explain the importance of forming a general impression of the patient. (p. 74)
20. Explain the value of performing an initial assessment. (pp. 71, 74)

Focused History and Physical Exam—Medical

1. Describe the unique needs for assessing an individual with a specific chief complaint with no known prior history. (pp. 76, 80)
2. Differentiate between the history and physical exam that is performed for responsive patients with no known prior history and responsive patients with a known prior history. (pp. 76–83)
3. Describe the unique needs for assessing an individual who is unresponsive or has an altered mental status. (p. 87)
4. Differentiate between the assessment that is performed for a patient who is unresponsive or has an altered mental status and other medical patients requiring assessment. (pp. 71–90)
5. Attend to the feelings that these patients might be experiencing. (pp. 77, 80)

Vital Signs and SAMPLE History

1. Identify the components of vital signs. (pp. 80–84)
2. Describe the methods used to obtain a breathing rate. (pp. 81–82)
3. Identify the attributes that should be obtained when assessing breathing. (pp. 81–82)
4. Differentiate between shallow, labored, and noisy breathing. (p. 81)
5. Describe the methods used to obtain a pulse rate. (p. 82)
6. Identify the information obtained when assessing a patient's pulse. (p. 82)
7. Differentiate between a strong, weak, regular, and irregular pulse. (p. 82)

8. Describe the methods used to assess the skin color, temperature, condition (capillary refill in infants and children). (pp. 82, 83)

9. Identify the normal and abnormal skin colors. (p. 83)

10. Differentiate between pale, blue, red, and yellow skin color. (p. 83)

11. Identify the normal and abnormal skin temperature. (p. 83)

12. Differentiate between hot, cool, and cold skin temperature. (p. 83)

13. Identify normal and abnormal skin conditions. (p. 83)

14. Identify normal and abnormal capillary refill in infants and children. (pp. 73, 75–76)

15. Describe the methods used to assess the pupils. (pp. 82–83)

16. Identify normal and abnormal pupil size. (pp. 82–83)

17. Differentiate between dilated (big) and constricted (small) pupil size. (pp. 82–83)

18. Differentiate between reactive and nonreactive pupils and equal and unequal pupils. (pp. 82–83)

19. Describe the methods used to assess blood pressure. (pp. 83–84)

20. Define systolic pressure. (p. 83)

21. Define diastolic pressure. (p. 83)

22. Explain the difference between auscultation and palpation for obtaining a blood pressure. (p. 83)

23. Identify the components of the SAMPLE history. (pp. 78, 80, 90)

24. Differentiate between a sign and a symptom. (p. 80)

25. State the importance of accurately reporting and recording the baseline vital signs. (p. 80)

26. Discuss the need to search for additional medical identification. (p. 80)

27. Explain the value of performing the baseline vital signs. (p. 80)

28. Recognize and respond to the feelings patients experience during assessment. (pp. 77–78)

29. Defend the need for obtaining and recording an accurate set of vital signs. (p. 80)

30. Explain the rationale for recording additional sets of vital signs. (p. 80)

31. Explain the importance of obtaining a SAMPLE history. (p. 80, 90)

Ongoing Assessment

1. Discuss the reasons for repeating the initial assessment as part of the ongoing assessment. (pp. 84–86, 90)

2. Describe the components of the ongoing assessment. (pp. 84–85)

3. Describe trending of assessment components. (p. 80)

4. Explain the value of performing an ongoing assessment. (pp. 84–86, 90)

5. Recognize and respect the feelings that patients might experience during assessment. (pp. 79–80)

6. Explain the value of trending assessment components to other health professionals who assume care of the patient. (p. 80)

● *Establish the relationship between assessment and intervention. (pp. 71, 74)*

● *Explain the six components of the patient assessment. (pp. 71–76)*

● *Recognize and advocate the rationale for the EMT-Basic to perform assessment-based patient care. (pp. 67, 71)*

■ SKILLS

Initial Assessment

1. Demonstrate the techniques for assessing mental status.

2. Demonstrate the techniques for assessing the airway.

3. Demonstrate the techniques for assessing if the patient is breathing.

4. Demonstrate the techniques for assessing if the patient has a pulse.

5. Demonstrate the techniques for assessing the patient for external bleeding.)

6. Demonstrate the techniques for assessing the patient's skin color, temperature, condition, and capillary refill (infants and children only).

7. Demonstrate the ability to prioritize patients.

Focused History and Physical Exam—Medical

1. Demonstrate the patient care skills that should be used to assist with a patient who is responsive with no known history.
2. Demonstrate the patient care skills that should be used to assist with a patient who is unresponsive or has an altered mental status.

Vital Signs and SAMPLE History

1. Demonstrate the skills involved in assessment of breathing.
2. Demonstrate the skills associated with obtaining a pulse.
3. Demonstrate the skills associated with assessing the skin color, temperature, and condition, and capillary refill in infants and children.
4. Demonstrate the skills associated with assessing the pupils.

5. Demonstrate the skills associated with obtaining blood pressure.
6. Demonstrate the skills that should be used to obtain information from the patient, family, or bystanders at the scene.

Ongoing Assessment

1. Demonstrate the skills involved in performing the ongoing assessment.

● *Perform the six components of assessment without missing any critical criteria listed on the skill sheets in the 1994 EMT-Basic Transitional Program.*

● *Given various medical and trauma scenarios, adequately evaluate patients and state the interventions that would be provided without missing any critical criteria listed on the skill sheets in the 1994 EMT-Basic Transitional Program.*

ON THE SCENE

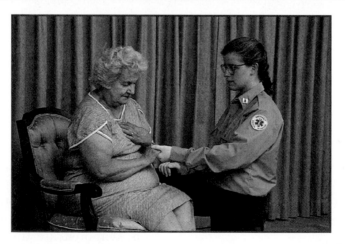

Early one Monday morning, you respond to a call for a woman with chest pain. As your vehicle approaches the scene, you do a **scene size-up.** There is nothing in front of the building that indicates any danger, but you continue to be observant as you put on your gloves and start walking to the front door. A worried, elderly man answers the door and shows you to his wife, Mrs. Holmes.

You get a **general impression** of an alert but anxious woman sitting in a living room chair. She appears approximately 70 years old. You do not see any reason to believe the patient has sustained an injury. As you introduce yourself, you observe her breathing and note

that it may be a little faster than usual, but there is no apparent difficulty breathing. Her chest is rising and falling without any audible abnormal sounds. As you confirm the patient's chief complaint and begin your history gathering, you feel her radial pulse. It is full and a little rapid. At the same time, you notice that Mrs. Holmes' skin is pale, cool, and sweaty. You look for external bleeding, but see none.

At the end of the **initial assessment,** you know that the patient's name is Karen Holmes and you conclude that for now the patient has a patent airway and her breathing and circulation are adequate. Although the patient does not have any "red flags" that would cause you to transport her immediately, the patient's chief complaint of chest pain makes you reluctant to spend any more time than necessary at the scene.

Since there is no reason to suspect trauma, you proceed with the **focused history and physical exam—medical patient.** You gather a history of the present illness and discover that the patient's pain started about three hours ago when she was at rest. It started out as a mild feeling of pressure and progressed over the course of an hour to a crushing pain in the middle of her chest. It radiates to the left shoulder. She tells you that this is the worst pain she's ever experienced in her life.

Your partner places a nonrebreather mask on the patient.

As part of gathering a SAMPLE history, you ask the patient whether she has any other complaints. You learn that she feels a little short of breath and sick to her stomach. She has no allergies to any medications. She takes Hydrodiuril for high blood pressure, but has no other health problems. The last thing she had to eat or drink was a breakfast of coffee and a muffin an hour ago. She has been in good health until this morning.

As you interview the patient, your partner gets a complete set of vital signs. Mrs. Holmes has a pulse of 92 and full, respirations of 24 and unlabored, a blood pressure of 156/90, and skin that is pale, cool, and sweaty. ■

When you assess a medical patient, you get most of your information from the history and vital signs. You can usually get this information only from an individual who is able to communicate with you. For the purpose of learning to assess a medical patient, this patient is referred to as responsive.

Since the individual who cannot communicate with you cannot give you a history, assessing this patient will necessarily be different. The assessment of the unresponsive medical patient is described in the second part of this chapter.

■ THE RESPONSIVE PATIENT

Scene Size-Up

EMTs are accustomed to evaluating a trauma scene for threats. A medical scene can also be a source of danger. Household animals, distraught family members, and unsafe buildings all present hazards that the EMT-B must be alert for. Chapter 2 described the importance of scene size-up and how to improve your skills in performing it.

Another very important function of scene size-up is determining whether you are dealing with a trauma patient, a medical patient, or a patient who is both. This chapter focuses only on the medical patient—a patient who has not sustained trauma.

Initial Assessment

Early in the development of EMS, experts in emergency care realized the importance of quickly finding and correcting immediate threats to life. This step in the assessment process was called the primary survey. It started out rather simply as a mental status check followed by evaluation of the airway, breathing, and circulation (ABCs). As time went on, varying authorities, groups, and textbooks expanded on the primary survey. Additional steps were incorporated so that in some areas ABC became ADCD (D for Disability) or even ADCDE (E for Expose). In a few places, the primary survey was complete only if the EMT took a complete set of vital signs.

The purpose of the primary survey, to quickly find and correct immediate threats to life, had been lost in these improvements. The primary survey was no longer quick and was being used to find problems that were not immediate threats to life. Largely for this reason, the 1994 EMT-B National Standard Curriculum abandoned the use of the term "primary survey." Instead, a new term, "initial assessment," is now used to describe the rapid series of steps that can be used to quickly find and control immediate threats to life.

There are six elements of the initial assessment: general impression, mental status, airway, breathing, circulation, and identification of priority patients (Skill Summary 5–1). In performing an initial assessment, you also discover information

Initial Assessment

> **Note:** *A trauma patient has been used to summarize the steps in the initial assessment.*

FIRST take body substance isolation precautions.

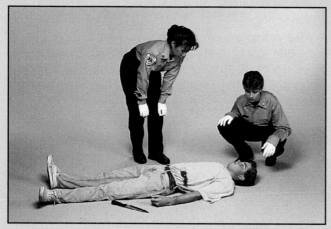

1. Form a general impression of patient and patient's environment.

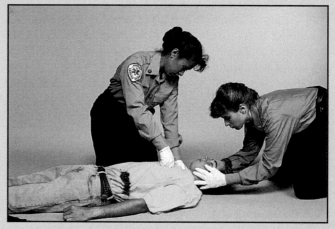

2. Assess patient's mental status using AVPU.

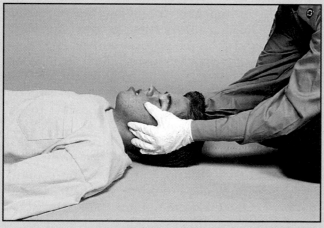

3. Assess airway. (Intervention: Perform appropriate maneuver to open and maintain airway. If necessary, suction, insert oro- or nasopharyngeal airway.)

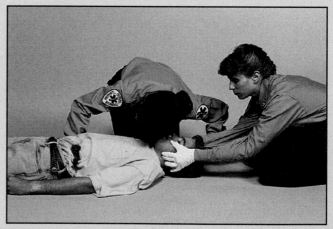

4. Assess breathing. (Interventions: If respiratory arrest or inadequate breathing, ventilate with 100% oxygen. If breathing above 24/min, give high-concentration oxygen.)

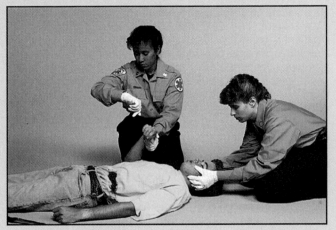

5. Evaluate circulation by taking the patient's pulse and evaluating skin color, temperature, and condition, and ...

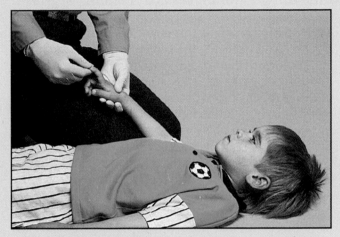

... in infants and children also assess circulation by testing capillary refill. (Interventions: For indications of poor circulation, treat for shock.)

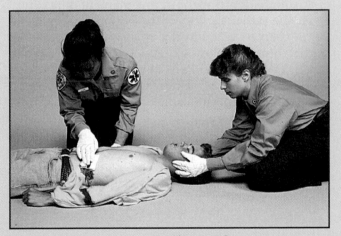

Assess and control severe bleeding.

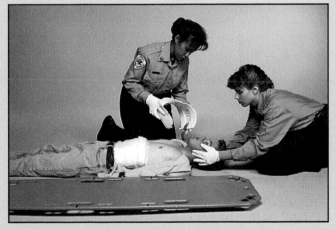

6. Make a decision about patient's priority for further assessment, interventions, or immediate transport.

that determines the kind and extent of assessment you will perform next, e.g., responsive or unresponsive.

General Impression

After you finished your EMT course and gained some experience, you probably developed a "sixth sense" that alerted you when there was something wrong with a patient. There is now a name for this: the general impression. Forming a general impression allows you to determine, at least initially, the priority of care. You do this by evaluating the environment, the patient's appearance, and the patient's chief complaint, among other things. As part of your general impression, you should also determine the patient's age and gender. In addition, you determine whether the patient is injured or ill or both. If the patient has sustained an injury, you should look for the mechanism of injury (MOI). If the patient is ill, you should determine the nature of illness. Additionally, you may see an immediate threat to life before you can even perform an initial assessment, such as a heavily bleeding wound. It is appropriate to treat an immediate threat to life before proceeding further.

Mental Status

You begin your evaluation of mental status as you approach the patient and introduce yourself. You should tell the patient your name, that you are an emergency medical technician, and that you are there to help.

The response you get will vary. Most of the time, the patient is awake, with eyes open, and is able to answer questions. At other times, a patient's eyes may be closed, but he will respond to the sound of your voice. Another possibility is that the patient does not respond to voice, but moves or speaks only after you apply a painful stimulus. The most serious possibility is that the patient does not respond to either your voice or a painful stimulus. This is the AVPU system of assessing mental status (Figure 5–1). An appropriate painful stimulus may include rubbing your knuckles on the patient's sternum, squeezing the trapezius muscle (although not in a patient who may have a cervical spine injury), or pinching the muscle between the thumb and index finger. This last method has the advantage of allowing you to compare the response to a painful stimulus on each side of the body.

Although a true mental status check includes more than just applying a verbal or painful stimulus, during the initial assessment you do not need any more information than this to determine your next steps. There is usually time later to gather more detailed information on the patient's mental status.

Preceptor Pearl

Many EMT-Bs, especially at the beginning of their careers, are reluctant to apply a painful stimulus. Instead, perhaps out of a sense of shyness or a reluctance to harm the patient, they apply only a mild stimulus that is not sufficient to rouse the patient. The EMT then notifies the hospital that the patient is unresponsive to verbal and painful stimuli; but on arrival at the emergency department, the staff is easily able to elicit a response with a brisk sternal rub or a pinch of the trapezius. Watch for this tendency with new or inexperienced EMT-Bs and give them the benefit of your experience. ❖

Airway and Breathing

In the responsive patient, there is rarely difficulty in confirming that the patient's airway is patent. You can determine this by the absence of any trauma to the airway, the patient's alertness, the lack of blood or other fluid in the mouth, and the ability to speak without difficulty. You can also note that the respiratory rate appears to be in the normal range (although you do not stop to count respirations during the initial assessment) and that breathing is of adequate depth without any signs of difficulty.

If the patient's respiratory rate appears to be faster than 24 per minute, you should administer high-concentration oxygen by nonrebreather mask. You may also wish to apply oxygen early to patients with respirations in the normal range, based on the patient's chief complaint, e.g., chest pain or shortness of breath. If the patient's breathing is inadequate, you should ventilate with oxygen. Although responsive patients sometimes do have inadequate breathing, it is much more likely that you will find this condition in unresponsive patients.

Circulation

Evaluating circulation involves checking three things simultaneously: pulse, bleeding, and perfusion.

When assessing a responsive patient, the easiest and least intrusive way of checking the pulse is to feel the radial pulse on the thumb side of the anterior wrist. If you don't feel a radial pulse, palpate a carotid pulse. In children less than a year old, the brachial pulse inside the upper arm is more reliable.

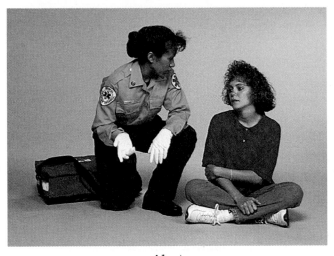

Alert

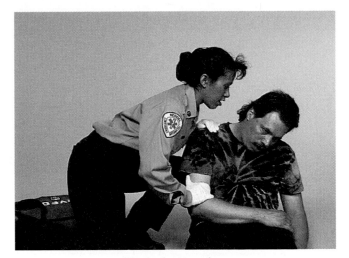

Verbal stimulus

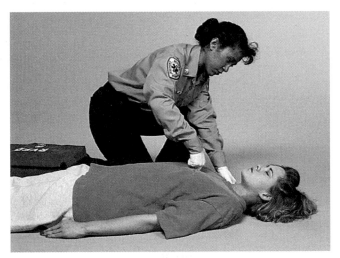

Painful stimulus

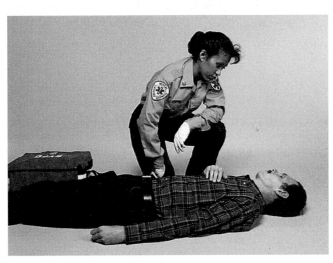

Unresponsive

FIGURE 5-1 The AVPU system of mental status assessment.

Palpating the pulse provides valuable information about the status of the patient's circulation. A rapid, weak pulse leads you to suspect shock (hypoperfusion). A slow pulse in a child or infant may be an indication of the need for you to ventilate the patient with oxygen. The most common finding on checking the pulse is a full (neither weak nor bounding) pulse in the normal range for the age of the patient (Table 5–1).

At the same time that you are palpating the pulse, look around the patient for blood and any continuing bleeding. If you see bleeding, control it now to minimize blood loss. To evaluate perfusion, check skin color, temperature, and condition. Under normal conditions, most people have skin that is pink, warm, and dry. In dark-pigmented individuals, the nailbeds, lips, and inner surface of the eyelids may be a better source of

information than the skin. Abnormal skin conditions include pallor (pale skin from blood loss, shock, fright), cyanosis (blue or blue-gray color from hypoxia), flushed (redness from exertion or exposure to heat), and jaundice (yellowish cast from liver disease).

When you feel the patient's skin temperature, you will frequently find it to be warm—the way it should be. It can also be hot (from fever or exposure to heat), cool (from hypoperfusion), or cold (from exposure to cold temperature).

Skin condition refers to the amount of moisture on the skin. Normally, skin is dry. You may also find it moist or wet. If the skin is both cool and moist, it is called clammy, a condition that can result from hypoperfusion.

In children under six years, also evaluate capillary refill by pressing on the end of the nail, the

CHAPTER 5 Patient Assessment—Medical Patient

TABLE 5–1 Pulse, Normal Ranges

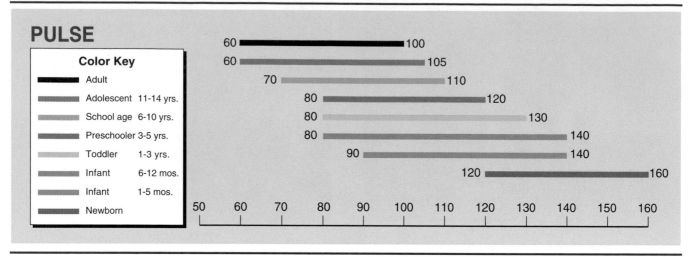

Concept for Table 5–1 by Christine M. Yuhas, practicing EMT, State of New Jersey.

back of the hand, or the top of the foot. After you release the pressure of your finger, the color should change from white to pink. If it takes more than two seconds for this to happen, this is abnormal and may be a sign of shock (hypoperfusion) or exposure to cold.

(See Table 5–2 for a summary of assessment steps for mental status and the ABCs for adults, children, and infants.)

Identification of Priority Patients

The "sixth sense" you may have developed with experience probably alerts you that particular patients need to be transported promptly. This is indeed the case in certain circumstances. Some patients need additional treatment and stabilization that can only be provided in an emergency department or operating room. Table 5–3 lists some conditions that fit in this category.

Focused History and Physical Exam— Medical

Once immediate threats to life have been detected and corrected, you can proceed to gather information that will determine the interventions you need to provide and that will assist the emergency department staff in their preparation for the patient's arrival. The traditional medical model of assessment includes a history and physical exam. EMT-Bs also gather a history and perform a physical exam, but one that is tailored to provide the information necessary for decision making in the field.

The four elements of the focused history and physical exam for a responsive medical patient are the OPQRST history, SAMPLE history, physical exam, and baseline vital signs (Skill Summary 5–2).

OPQRST History

The history of the present illness you learned about in your EMT course is also known as the OPQRST history because this acronym serves as a reminder of the information that must be obtained. The OPQRST history allows you to describe the chief complaint in some detail.

Onset	What were you doing when the episode started?
Provokes	Did anything bring on this episode?
Quality	What kind of pain are you having?
Radiation	Does the pain spread anywhere?
Severity	How bad is the pain? How does it compare to previous episodes?
Time	When did the episode start? Has the pain changed since it started?

OPQRST is very useful for conditions characterized by pain, but, as you may have discovered, needs to be modified when a patient's chief complaint does not involve pain. For example, when interviewing a patient with shortness of breath, it

TABLE 5–2 Initial Assessment of Adults, Children, and Infants

	Adults	Children 1–6 yrs.	Infants to 1 yr.
Mental Status	AVPU: Is patient alert? responsive to verbal stimulus? responsive to painful stimulus? unresponsive? If alert, is patient oriented to person, place, and time?	As for adults	If not alert, shout as a verbal stimulus, flick feet as a painful stimulus. (Crying would be infant's response.)
Airway	Trauma: jaw thrust Medical: head-tilt, chin-lift. Consider oro- or nasopharyngeal airway, suctioning.	As for adults, but see Chapter 4 for special child airway techniques. If performing head-tilt, chin-lift, do so without hyperextending (stretching) the neck.	As for children, but see Chapter 4 for special infant airway techniques.
Breathing	If respiratory arrest, perform rescue breathing. If depressed mental status and inadequate breathing (slower than 8 per minute), ventilate with bag-valve mask and 100% oxygen. If alert and respirations are more than 24 per minute, give 100% oxygen by nonrebreather mask.	As for adults, but normal rates for children are faster than for adults. (See Table 5–4 for normal child respiration rates.) Parent may have to hold oxygen mask to reduce child's fear of mask.	As for children, but normal rates for infants are faster than for children and adults. (See Table 5–4 for normal infant respiration rates.)
Circulation	Assess skin, radial pulse, bleeding. If cardiac arrest, perform CPR. See Chapter 12 on how to treat for bleeding and shock.	Assess skin, radial pulse, bleeding, capillary refill. See Table 5–1 for normal child pulse rates (faster than for adults). If cardiac arrest, perform CPR. See Chapter 12 on how to treat for bleeding and shock.	Assess skin, brachial pulse, bleeding, capillary refill. See Table 5–1 for normal infant pulse rates (faster than for children and adults). If cardiac arrest, perform CPR. See Chapter 12 on how to treat for bleeding and shock.

TABLE 5–3 High Priority Conditions

Poor general impression
Unresponsive
Responsive, but not following commands
Difficulty breathing
Shock
Complicated childbirth
Chest pain with systolic blood pressure less than 100
Uncontrolled bleeding
Severe pain anywhere

does not make sense to ask the patient whether the shortness of breath radiates anywhere.

Important principles to remember when interviewing a patient include:

- *Position yourself properly.* You should be close to the patient and at about the same height without being so close that the patient feels "closed in."

- *Introduce yourself in a calm, confident, and reassuring manner.* Although emergencies may be routine to you, chances are this is not the case for the patient. Reassuring the patient and behaving in a calm, professional manner does wonders in establishing a rapport.

- *Ask how the patient would like to be addressed.* Treat patients with respect by asking them how they would like you to address them. Many of

Focused History and Physical Exam—Medical Patient—Responsive

First take body substance isolation precautions.

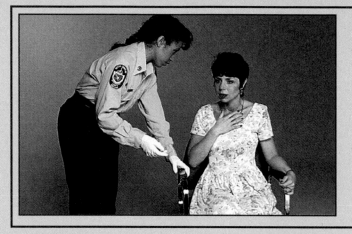

HISTORY OF PRESENT ILLNESS

Ask the "OPQRST" questions:
Onset
Provokes
Quality
Radiation
Severity
Time

SAMPLE HISTORY

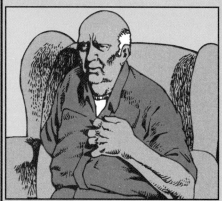

Signs and symptoms

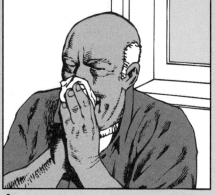

Allergies

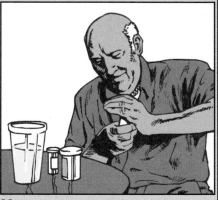

Medicines

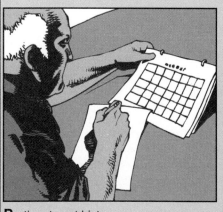

Pertinent past history

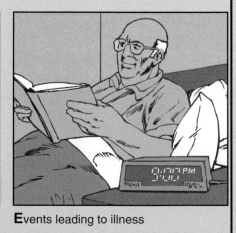

Last oral intake

Events leading to illness

Skill Summary 5–2 (continued)

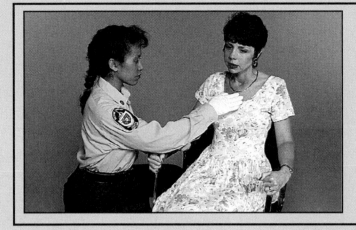

FOCUSED PHYSICAL EXAM

Quick exam of affected body part or system

Assess as needed:
- Head
- Neck
- Chest
- Abdomen
- Pelvis
- Extremities
- Posterior

VITAL SIGNS

Assess the patient's vital signs.
- Respirations
- Pulse
- Skin color, temperature, condition (capillary refill in infants and children)
- Pupils
- Blood pressure

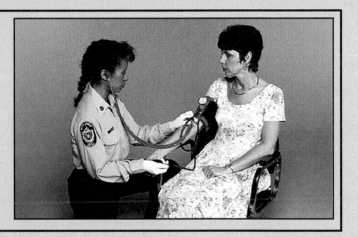

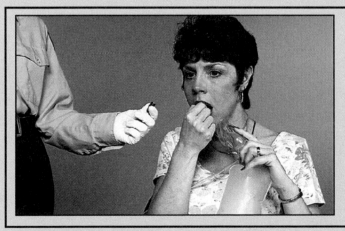

INTERVENTIONS AND TRANSPORT

Contact on-line medical direction as needed.
Perform interventions as needed.
Transport patient.

your patients will be older than you, some considerably so. Many elderly patients feel comfortable being on a first-name basis with EMT-Bs, but some prefer being addressed as "Mrs." or "Ms." or "Mr."

- *Ask open-ended questions.* Avoid questions that the patient can answer "yes" or "no." By asking questions like "Where is the pain?" instead of "Is the pain in the center of your chest?" you avoid leading the patient into saying what you want or expect to hear.

SAMPLE History

The SAMPLE history is not exactly the same as the past medical history, but the two have a lot in common. The "S" for signs and symptoms really acts as a bridge between the history of the present illness (OPQRST) and the past medical history (AMPLE). This information may be very useful to the emergency department staff in determining the proper treatment. In the unresponsive patient, you may be able to gather some of this history from a medical ID tag or from family members.

<u>S</u>igns/ Symptoms	What's wrong? Be sure to ask about associated symptoms; for example, in the patient with a chief complaint of chest pain, you should ask whether the patient is having any difficulty breathing or shortness of breath.
<u>A</u>llergies	Is the patient allergic to any medications, foods or environmental substances?
<u>M</u>edications	What medications (both prescription and over-the-counter) does the patient take?
<u>P</u>ertinent past history	What medical illnesses has the patient had in the past or is the patient receiving treatment for now? If the patient is injured, has this area been injured before?
<u>L</u>ast oral intake	What did the patient last eat or drink? This information can help you prepare for potential airway problems, especially in the patient who is nauseated.
<u>E</u>vents leading to the injury or illness	What, if anything, happened that led to today's problem?

Physical Exam

In the responsive medical patient, there is typically little useful information an EMT-B can gain through physical examination of the patient. To a certain extent, this is not unique to EMS but is also true in other areas of health care for the medical patient. The history frequently determines what interventions you should provide. There are times, though, when it may be appropriate to examine certain areas based on the patient's chief complaint. For example, if your patient is complaining of abdominal pain, you should gently palpate the four quadrants of the abdomen, looking for tenderness, rigidity, and pulsations. Chapter 6 describes physical examination of the trauma patient, but some of the techniques described for trauma patient assessment also apply to medical patient assessment.

If your patient has chest pain or shortness of breath, you may wish (or local protocols may direct you) to assess for neck vein distention, ankle edema, and abnormal breath sounds. The EMT-B curriculum includes evaluation of equality of breath sounds, but not the recognition of abnormal breath sounds. If your local protocols direct you to describe abnormal breath sounds, you should have received training in this technique and you should review it frequently.

Evaluation of neck veins, ankles, and breath sounds will not change any of the treatment you can administer as an EMT-B, but some systems may wish EMT-Bs to obtain such evaluation for other reasons, such as whether to request ALS backup. Follow your local protocols.

As appropriate, assess these areas in responsive medical patients: head, neck, chest, abdomen, pelvis, extremities, and posterior aspect of the patient.

Baseline Vital Signs

The importance of accurate vital signs should not be underestimated. Many treatment decisions are a direct result of the vital signs. An EMT-Basic must be able to accurately assess and record a patient's vital signs. This is important not only for the first assessment (baseline vital signs), but also for repeated assessments when trends in a patient's condition may be detected. A trend in a patient's vital signs may alert the emergency department staff to the need to prepare certain equipment or a particular area of the emergency department.

There are five vital signs that must be measured: respirations, pulse, skin, pupils, and blood

TABLE 5-4 Respirations—Rates and Sounds

Normal Respiration Rates (breaths per minute, at rest)	
Adults	12 to 20 Above 24: Serious Below 8: Serious
Infants and Children	
Adolescent 11–14 years	12 to 20
School age 6–10 years	15 to 30
Preschooler 3–5 years	20 to 30
Toddler 1–3 years	20 to 30
Infant 6–12 months	20 to 30
Infant 0–5 months	25 to 40
Newborn	30 to 50

Respiratory Sounds	Possible Causes/Interventions
Snoring	Airway blocked/Open patient's airway; Prompt transport
Wheezing	Medical problem such as asthma/Assist patient in taking prescribed medications; Prompt transport
Gurgling	Fluids in airway/Suction airway; Prompt transport
Crowing (harsh sound when inhaling)	Medical problem that cannot be treated on the scene/Prompt transport

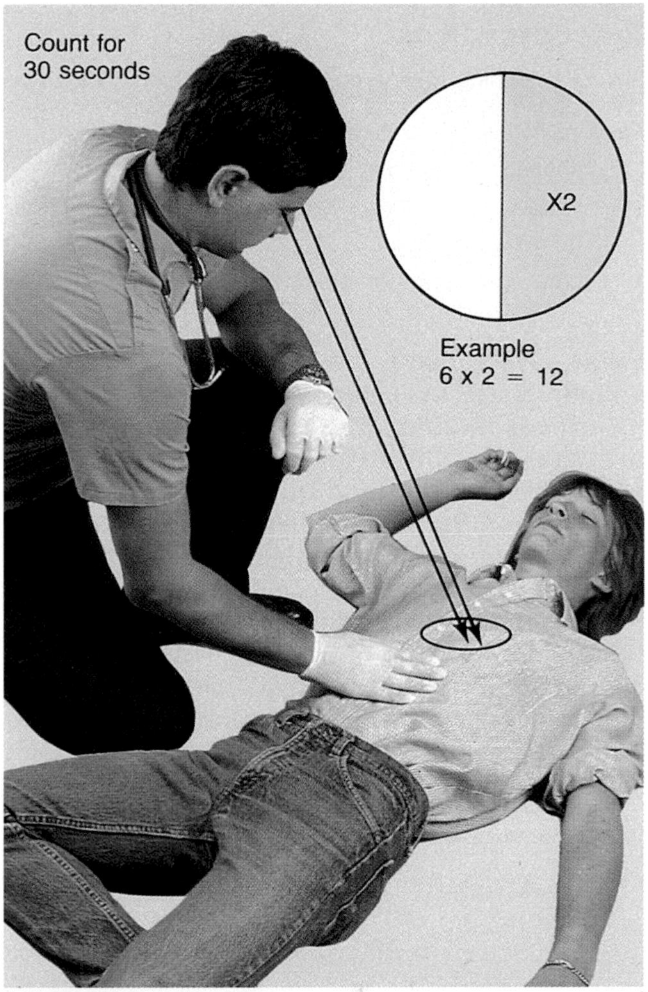

Count for 30 seconds

X2

Example
6 x 2 = 12

FIGURE 5-2 Respiration rate and quality are vital signs.

pressure. In the hospital, temperature is another vital sign that is frequently obtained, but in the field it has little value under ordinary circumstances and can be difficult to obtain accurately.

Respirations Respirations, one of the most frequently forgotten vital signs, are easily assessed by observing the patient's chest rise and fall. You determine the rate by counting the number of breaths in a 30-second period and multiplying by two (Figure 5–2).

Preceptor Pearl

New EMT-Bs, in their desire to explain to the patient everything that is going on, may say something like, "I'm going to count your breathing right now, so just relax." Of course, the patient who knows someone is counting his breathing rate will think about it and probably breathe either faster or slower as a result. If you hear new EMT-Bs using this approach, remind them that counting a respiratory rate should be done without bringing the patient's attention to it. ❖

The quality of respirations is easy to determine while assessing the rate. Quality falls into one of four categories—normal, shallow, labored, or noisy.

A patient with *normal* respirations shows average chest wall motion and does not use accessory muscles to breathe. *Shallow* respirations show only slight chest or abdominal wall motion. *Labored breathing* is usually easy to recognize by an increase in the effort of breathing, grunting, and stridor; the use of accessory muscles; and sometimes outright gasping. In children, you may also see nasal flaring and retractions in the supraclavicular (above the clavicles) and intercostal (between the ribs) areas. The fourth category of breathing is *noisy*. Noisy respirations are just that—easy to hear because of the noise they make (Table 5–4).

Noisy breathing means obstructed breathing. When you hear these noises, administer high-concentration oxygen and institute these treatments:

snoring	open the airway
wheezing	ask the patient if he has a prescribed inhaler
gurgling	suction
crowing	transport promptly ✤

Pulse The radial pulse is the pulse you should initially assess in all patients one year or older. In infants less than one year old, assess the brachial pulse instead. When assessing the pulse, feel for rate and quality. Determine the rate by counting the number of beats you feel in thirty seconds and multiplying that number by two (Figure 5–3).

The quality of the pulse is classified as strong or weak and regular or irregular (Table 5–5). Use only gentle pressure when palpating the pulse. This is especially true if you cannot feel a radial pulse and try the carotid pulse instead. Too much pressure can actually "shut off" the pulse by not allowing any blood to pass through the artery past where you are pressing. When palpating a carotid pulse, especially in elderly patients, you may also

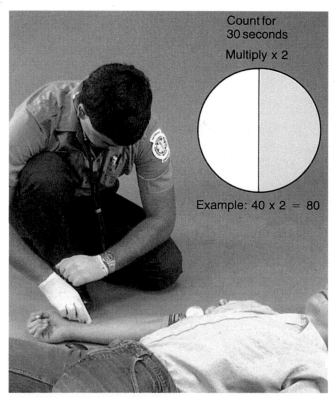

FIGURE 5–3 Assessing pulse rate and quality.

Count for 30 seconds
Multiply x 2
Example: 40 x 2 = 80

TABLE 5–5 Pulse

Normal Pulse Rates (beats per minute, at rest)	
Adults	60 to 100
Infants and Children	
Adolescent 11–14 years	60 to 105
School age 6–10 years	70 to 110
Preschooler 3–5 years	80 to 120
Toddler 1–3 years	80 to 130
Infant 6–12 months	80 to 140
Infant 0–5 months	90 to 140
Newborn	120 to 160

Pulse	Significance/Possible Causes
Rapid, regular, and full	Exertion, fright, fever, high blood pressure, first stage of blood loss
Rapid, regular, and thready	Shock, later stages of blood loss
Slow	Head injury, drugs, some poisons, some heart problems
No pulse	Cardiac arrest (clinical death)

Infants and Children: A high pulse in an infant or child is not as great a concern as a slow pulse. A slow pulse (heart rate) may indicate imminent cardiac arrest.

slow the pulse by inadvertently putting pressure on an area called the carotid sinus. Naturally, you should refrain from assessing carotid pulses on both sides of a patient at one time.

Skin The steps in evaluation of the skin are the same as the steps performed in the initial assessment. Evaluate the color, temperature, and condition of the skin, looking for abnormalities like cyanosis or clammy skin (Table 5–6).

Pupils The pupils have been called the windows to the brain, and for good reason. They can give a very quick indication of serious problems in the brain, such as hypoxia or swelling inside the skull.

Assess the pupils by briefly shining a light into the patient's eyes one at a time. When you do this, cover the eye that you are not assessing. This will prevent light in that eye from affecting the size of the pupil in the other one. When you assess pupils, look for size, reactivity, and equality (Table 5–7). Dilated pupils are very big, so big that it is difficult to tell what color eyes the patient has. Constricted pupils are very small. Normal pupils are in between these two extremes. A normal pupil constricts when you shine a light

TABLE 5-6 Skin Color, Temperature, and Condition.

Skin Color	Significance/Possible Causes
Pink	Normal in light-skinned patients or at inner eyelids, lips, nail beds of dark-skinned patients
Pale	Constricted blood vessels possibly resulting from blood loss, shock, heart attack, emotional distress
Cyanotic (blue)	Lack of oxygen in blood cells and tissues resulting from inadequate breathing or heart function
Flushed (red)	Exposure to heat, high blood pressure, emotional excitement
Jaundiced (yellow)	Liver abnormalities
Mottling (blotchiness)	Occasionally in patients with shock

Skin Temperature/Condition	Significance/Possible Causes
Cool, clammy	Usual sign of shock, anxiety
Cold, moist	Body is losing heat
Cold, dry	Exposure to cold
Hot, dry	High fever, heat exposure
Hot, moist	High fever, heat exposure
"Goose pimples" accompanied by shivering, chattering teeth, blue lips, and pale skin	Chills, communicable disease, exposure to cold, pain, or fear

into it and returns to its normal size after you remove the light. Normal pupils also are the same size when you first look at them and each constrict at about the same rate when you shine a light into them.

Blood Pressure The arterial blood pressure obtained with a BP cuff (or sphygmomanometer) is actually two pressures, the systolic and diastolic. These are the pressures against the walls of the arteries when the heart is contracting and relaxing.

The **systolic blood pressure** is the first distinct sound of blood flowing through the artery as the pressure in the blood pressure cuff is released. This is a measurement of the pressure exerted

TABLE 5-7 Pupils

Pupil Appearance	Significance/Possible Causes
Dilated (larger than normal)	Fright, blood loss, drugs, treatment with eye drops
Unequal	Stroke, head injury, eye injury, artificial eye
Lack of reactivity	Drugs, lack of oxygen to brain

against the walls of the arteries during contraction of the heart. There are two methods of obtaining a blood pressure, **auscultation** and **palpation**. To auscultate the blood pressure, place a cuff of the appropriate size on the upper arm of the sitting or supine patient. The cuff should fit snugly. Find the location of the brachial artery by palpating just medial to the center of the crease of the elbow. Put a stethoscope in your ears so that the ear pieces face forward, and place the diaphragm over the brachial artery. Inflate the cuff until you can no longer hear the pulse. Slowly deflate the cuff until you hear the first return of the sound of the artery. This is the systolic pressure. Continue to deflate slowly until you no longer hear the sound. This is the **diastolic pressure.** Allow the cuff to deflate the rest of the way quickly. When listening for the diastolic pressure, be careful not to put any more pressure than necessary on the diaphragm. Too much pressure will give you a falsely low diastolic pressure.

To palpate the blood pressure, position the cuff in the same way as before. Instead of putting the stethoscope diaphragm over the brachial artery, palpate the radial pulse. Inflate the cuff until you can no longer feel the pulse. Slowly deflate the cuff until you feel the return of the

TABLE 5–8 Blood Pressure

Blood Pressure Normal Ranges		
	Systolic	*Diastolic*
Adults	90 to 150	60 to 90
Infants and Children	Approx. 80 plus (2 × age)	Approx. 2/3 Systolic
Adolescent 11–14 years	average 115 (94 to 140)	average 59
School age 6–10 years	average 105 (80 to 122)	average 57
Preschooler 3–5 years	average 99 (78 to 116)	average 65

Blood Pressure	*Significance/Possible Causes*
High blood pressure	Medical condition, exertion, fright, emotional distress or excitement
Low blood pressure	Athlete or other person with normally low blood pressure; blood loss; late sign of shock

Note: The systolic blood pressure usually parallels the pulse rate; that is, when the pulse (heart) rate increases, the systolic blood pressure increases, too.

Infants and Children: Blood pressure is usually not taken on a child under 3 years. In cases of blood loss or shock, a child's blood pressure will remain within normal limits until near the end, then fall swiftly.

pulse. This is the systolic pressure. Allow the cuff to deflate the rest of the way, since there is no way to get an accurate diastolic pressure by palpation.

When obtaining a blood pressure, be sure to use the proper size cuff. A cuff that is the right width should take up about two-thirds of the distance between the shoulder and the elbow. It should also have a bladder that does not overlap when the cuff is wrapped around the arm. The center of the bladder should be over the brachial artery when it is positioned properly.

Hypertension (high blood pressure) has many definitions, but most authorities would agree that it is present when the diastolic is greater than 90 millimeters of mercury (mm Hg) (Table 5–8). Hypertension is important because it indicates that the heart is working harder than it should to pump blood to the body. When the heart pumps, no blood leaves the left ventricle until the ventricle generates a pressure greater than the diastolic pressure (the diastolic is the lowest pressure in the arteries). If the diastolic pressure is higher than it should be, then the heart has to pump extra hard in order to do its job. Left untreated, this additional workload on the heart has the effect of weakening the heart and worsening other cardiovascular diseases such as angina.

Hypertension is rarely something to be concerned about in the short term. However, document it and bring it to the attention of the hospital staff.

PEDIATRIC HIGHLIGHT

Cuff size is especially important when assessing children. You should determine a blood pressure in all patients older than three years. Below this age, the blood pressure is difficult to obtain and has very limited value. Instead, the general appearance of the patient, e.g., weak, in respiratory distress, or unresponsive, is more valuable than the numbers obtained from a blood pressure measurement. ■

You should reassess the patient's vital signs as part of your ongoing assessment and also after each medical intervention.

Ongoing Assessment

Your job of assessing the patient does not stop after you have finished your assessment at the scene and performed appropriate interventions. Keeping a close eye on the patient is an important part of your continuing care of a patient.

There are five parts of the ongoing assessment: repeating the initial assessment, re-establishing patient priority, reassessing and recording vital signs, repeating a focused assessment regarding the patient's complaint or injuries, and checking interventions you have administered (Skill Summary 5–3).

Ongoing Assessment

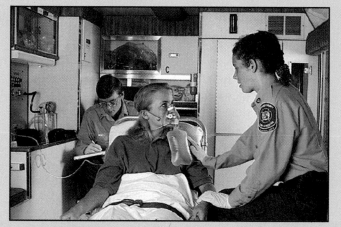

1. Repeat the initial assessment. At this time, evaluate patient priority.

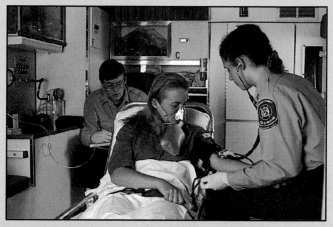

2. Reassess and record vital signs.

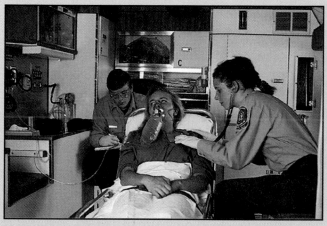

3. Repeat focused assessment.

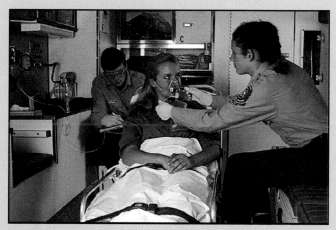

4. Check interventions.

You should perform ongoing assessment at least every fifteen minutes for stable patients, and every five minutes for unstable patients. You should record the results of your ongoing assessment as soon as possible so that you have an accurate record of changes in the patient's condition that allow you to detect trends.

Repeating the initial assessment means reassessing the patient's mental status, maintaining an open airway, monitoring breathing for rate and quality, reassessing the pulse for rate and quality, and monitoring skin color and temperature. After gathering this information, you can determine whether the patient's condition has changed in a way that should alter the priority of the patient.

Repeating vital signs can also give you valuable information about whether you need to alter your treatment of the patient. In addition, you should also reassess the patient's complaint. For example, if the patient is having chest pain, ask how the pain is and whether it has changed.

Finally, you should check the interventions you have performed. Make sure that if you have started oxygen, it is still flowing. If the bag on the nonrebreather mask is not filling adequately, make sure the tubing is still attached, the flowmeter is set at the appropriate rate, e.g., 15 liters per minute, and there is still oxygen in the tank.

Whenever you check the interventions that you have performed for a patient, you should try to take a fresh look at the patient. Attempt to see the patient as though you had never seen him before. This may help you to more objectively evaluate the adequacy of your interventions and adjust them as necessary.

ON THE SCENE

You receive a call to respond to the scene of an unconscious but breathing elderly woman. As you approach the scene, you size it up for any dangers. Seeing nothing that appears to be dangerous, you put on disposable gloves and enter the house. A concerned middle-aged man brings you to a room in the back of the house where his mother, Mrs. Schell, is lying in bed. As you get closer to

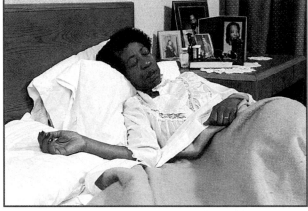

the patient, you get a **general impression** of an approximately seventy-year-old woman who appears to be asleep or unconscious. You bend over next to the bed and shake her shoulder as you say loudly into her ear, "Mrs. Schell! Mrs. Schell! Can you hear me?" She doesn't respond, so you pinch her shoulder. She moans a little bit. Next, you open her airway with the head-tilt, chin-lift maneuver and evaluate her breathing. Respirations appear to be about twenty per minute and adequate in depth. As your partner holds Mrs. Schell's chin up, you feel her radial pulse. You estimate it to be about seventy or eighty per minute and full. You see no bleeding. Her skin is warm and dry. You decide this is a high-priority patient because of her unconsciousness and threatened airway. Your system

does not have paramedics, but if it did, you would call for them now.

Since the patient cannot give you any history, you perform a rapid physical exam. You find nothing abnormal. You look for a medical identification tag, but find none. At the same time, your partner, who has inserted a nasal airway and started oxygen by nonrebreather mask, gets a set of vital signs. The patient has a pulse of 84, regular and full, respirations of 22 and adequate, blood pressure of 184/90, skin that is warm, pink, and dry, and pupils that are equal but sluggish to react. Before your partner leaves to get the stretcher, the two of you turn the patient onto her side to protect her airway. The patient's son is able to tell you that his mother complained of a headache before lying down for a nap. She is allergic to sulfa drugs. She takes no medications and has no history of illnesses. The last time she ate or drank anything was lunch about two hours ago.

Your partner arrives with the stretcher and you transport Mrs. Schell on her side while still administering high-concentration oxygen. Reassessment en route reveals no changes. ■

■ THE UNRESPONSIVE PATIENT

Evaluating an unresponsive patient can be much more challenging than evaluating a patient who is able to communicate with you. Since the history gives much more information than the physical exam on medical patients, you are able to get valuable information from the responsive patient. But for the unresponsive patient, you must gather all of the useful information you can find in other ways. This means performing a rapid physical exam and getting as much history as possible from family members or bystanders (Skill Summary 5–4).

Initial Assessment

The initial assessment of an unresponsive medical patient has the same goals as in the responsive patient: find and detect immediate threats to life and guide further assessment and treatment. In this case, though, completing the initial assessment will frequently take longer because of the additional steps you need to take to secure and maintain an airway.

General Impression

As before, look at the environment and the patient, noting whether the patient is ill or injured, and determining the patient's gender and approximate age.

Mental Status

When dealing with an unresponsive patient, you will not find one who gets an "A" on the AVPU scale. At best, the patient may respond to verbal stimuli. When describing the mental status of a patient like this, it is important to describe both the stimulus and the patient's response to it. For example, the patient might moan in response to a painful stimulus.

Airway

Managing the airway of an unresponsive patient requires considerably more work than when the patient is responsive. Since this is a medical patient and trauma has been ruled out, open the airway with the head-tilt, chin-lift maneuver. This should relieve any snoring that is the result of the tongue partially obstructing the airway. Also insert an oral or nasal airway.

Breathing

In Chapter 4, you reviewed how to determine whether a patient's breathing is adequate. This is a skill that is very important in the initial assessment of an unresponsive patient. After seeing a number of patients over the years, an EMT-B can easily be lulled into a false sense of security. Most unresponsive patients you see will be breathing adequately, but you must quickly find the ones who are not and begin ventilating them quickly.

Circulation

Evaluating circulation in the unresponsive patient is no different from evaluating circulation in the responsive patient. Check the radial pulse (brachial in infants under one year of age) for rate and quality. Look for and correct external hemorrhage. Check the patient's skin color, temperature, and condition.

Identification of Priority Patients

A patient who is unresponsive is automatically a high-priority patient. The patient's airway is at risk and there are many possible causes of altered mental status, some of which can be life threatening.

Focused History and Physical Exam— Medical

Since the patient cannot give you a history, get information in other ways. The best sources are a physical exam of the patient and a history from a family member or friend.

Rapid Physical Exam

Examine the patient by inspecting (looking) and palpating (pressing or touching) these areas: the head, neck, chest, abdomen, pelvis, extremities, and the posterior aspect of the body. Remove any clothing covering the area so that you can get a good look at it, then replace clothing after you have finished examining that area.

Baseline Vital Signs

With so little history available, vital signs become even more important than usual. Be sure to assess the pulse, respirations, blood pressure, skin, and pupils. Before going any further in your assessment, position the patient to protect his

Focused History and Physical Exam—Medical Patient—Unresponsive

First take body substance isolation precautions.

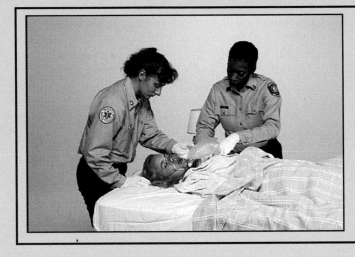

RAPID PHYSICAL EXAM

Rapid exam of entire body

Rapidly assess:
- Head
- Neck
- Chest
- Abdomen
- Pelvis
- Extremities
- Posterior

VITAL SIGNS

Assess the patient's vital signs.
- Respiration
- Pulse
- Skin color, temperature, condition (capillary refill in infants and children)
- Pupils
- Blood pressure

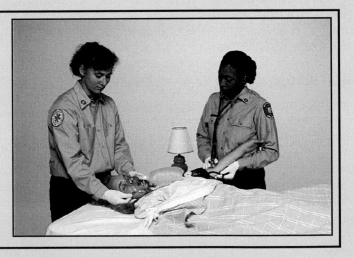

Skill Summary 5–4 *(continued)*

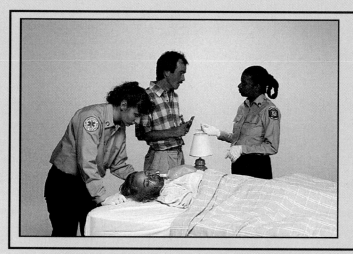

SAMPLE HISTORY

Interview family and bystanders to get as much information as possible about the patient's problem. Ask about:

Signs and symptoms (Ask the "OPQRST" questions regarding **O**nset, **P**rovocation, **Q**uality, **R**adiation, **S**everity, and **T**ime)

Allergies

Medicines

Pertinent past history

Last oral intake

Events leading to problem

INTERVENTIONS AND TRANSPORT

Contact on-line medical direction as needed.
Perform interventions as needed.
Transport patient.

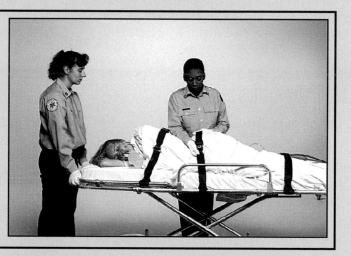

airway. Turn him on his side so that secretions drain out of his mouth and he is in a good position to avoid aspiration if he vomits.

Obtain SAMPLE History

Since the patient is unable to tell what history he has, interview family members, bystanders, or friends before you leave the scene. They may have information that is valuable to the emer-gency department staff and which they will be unable to obtain.

Ongoing Assessment

Check the same things in the ongoing assessment of the unresponsive patient as you did for the responsive patient. Pay special attention to the airway in this case.

CHAPTER REVIEW

■ SUMMARY

The assessment of a medical patient—a patient who is not injured—consists of gathering a history of the present illness, a past medical history, and a set of vital signs. However, the assessment of a responsive medical patient differs from the assessment of an unresponsive medical patient. When assessing a responsive medical patient you can usually get most of your information from the history the patient gives you and from the vital signs taken. However, evaluating an unresponsive medical patient can be much more challenging since you must gather all of the useful information you can find in other ways. This means performing a rapid physical exam and getting as much history as possible from family members, friends, or bystanders.

Your job of assessing the patient does not stop after you have finished your assessment at the scene and performed appropriate interventions. You must also continue your care of the patient by performing ongoing assessment, which includes repeating the initial assessment, reestablishing patient priority, reassessing and recording vital signs, repeating a focused assessment regarding the patient's complaint or injuries, and checking interventions you have administered.

■ REVIEW QUESTIONS

1. List the six elements of the initial assessment.

2. Explain the purpose of forming a general impression.

3. Describe the AVPU system of assessing mental status.

4. When evaluating circulation, what three things must be checked simultaneously?

5. Explain the acronyms OPQRST and SAMPLE.

6. Name the five vital signs and explain how they are measured.

7. Explain the steps in the ongoing assessment and tell how often it should be performed.

8. Describe how the evaluation of a responsive medical patient differs from the evaluation of an unresponsive medical patient.

Patient Assessment—
Trauma Patient

■ *Trauma patients make up only a small portion of EMS patients, but they are one of the most visible reasons for the existence of EMS systems. Although medical patients receive a great deal of attention today, it was the unnecessary deaths of patients on the highways in the 1960s that led to the American system of delivering EMS.*

Today, the death rate from trauma on the highways is decreasing because of successful prevention measures, organized systems of trauma care, attention to the airway, control of bleeding, and prompt transport. Although EMT-Bs can and do participate in all of these components of trauma care, the last

three are critical EMT-B interventions if patients are to survive potentially fatal injuries.

Trauma patients with significant internal injuries usually require interventions that are not available in the field. Rarely, if ever, can out-of-hospital providers stabilize a critical trauma patient. Such patients require interventions that are available only in an emergency department or an operating room.

Most trauma patients do not have critical injuries. Distinguishing between critical and non-critical patients can be difficult, but a systematic, efficient approach to assessment will make this process much easier.

MAKING THE TRANSITION

■ The trauma patient with a significant mechanism of injury should receive a limited physical exam (the rapid trauma assessment) at the scene and prompt transport.

■ During the physical exam, you should search for DCAP-BTLS (deformities, contusions, abrasions, punctures/penetrations, burns, tenderness, lacerations, and swelling).

■ If a trauma patient is complaining of pain in the pelvis, do not compress it. You will cause the patient a great deal of pain without gathering any additional useful information.

OBJECTIVES

The numbered objectives below are from the United States Department of Transportation 1994 EMT-Basic National Standard Curriculum. Objectives with colored bullets that follow in italics are from the EMT-Basic Transitional Program.

Note: Many of the objectives in Chapter 5 also pertain to the material in this chapter. The objectives on assessment in the EMT-B curriculum have been separated so that only those describing assessment of trauma patients are included in this chapter. The transition course objectives for assessment are included in Chapter 5 and are repeated here.

■ KNOWLEDGE AND ATTITUDE

At the completion of this chapter, you should be able to:

Initial Assessment

1. State reasons for management of the cervical spine once the patient has been determined to be a trauma patient. (pp. 95, 96, 97, 100–101)

Focused History and Physical Exam—Trauma

1. Discuss the reasons for reconsideration concerning the mechanism of injury. (p. 94)

2. State the reasons for performing a rapid trauma assessment. (pp. 96–97)

3. Recite examples and explain why patients should receive a rapid trauma assessment. (pp. 96–97)

4. Describe the areas included in the rapid trauma assessment and discuss what should be evaluated. (pp. 96, 97–98)

5. Differentiate when the rapid assessment may be altered in order to provide patient care. (p. 97)

6. Discuss the reason for performing a focused history and physical exam. (pp. 96, 98)

7. Recognize and respect the feelings that patients might experience during assessment. (p. 93)

Detailed Physical Exam

1. Discuss the components of the detailed physical exam. (pp. 104–105)

2. State the areas of the body that are evaluated during the detailed physical exam. (pp. 104–105)

3. Explain what additional care should be provided while performing the detailed physical exam. (pp. 104–105)

4. Distinguish between the detailed physical exam that is performed on a trauma patient and that of the medical patient. (p. 104)

5. Explain the rationale for the feelings that these patients might be experiencing. (p. 93)

● *Establish the relationship between assessment and intervention. (p. 94)*

● *Explain the six components of the patient assessment. (pp. 94–96)*

● *Recognize and advocate the rationale for the EMT-Basic to perform assessment-based patient care. (p. 93)*

■ SKILLS

Focused History and Physical Exam—Trauma

1. Demonstrate the rapid trauma assessment that should be used to treat a patient based on mechanism of injury.

Detailed Physical Exam

1. Demonstrate the skills involved in performing the detailed physical exam.

● *Perform the six components of assessment without missing any critical criteria listed on the skill sheets in the 1994 EMT-Basic Transitional Program.*

● *Given various medical and trauma scenarios, adequately evaluate patients and state the interventions that would be provided without missing any critical criteria listed on the skill sheets in the 1994 EMT-Basic Transitional Program.*

You receive a call for a motor-vehicle collision just a half mile away. As your partner drives the ambulance to the scene, you review the potential hazards that such a call can present. You see nothing that appears dangerous as you pull up. Upon getting out of the ambulance, you take BSI precautions; then you sniff the air, but detect no gasoline or other odors that would make you suspicious. You start your **initial assessment** when you

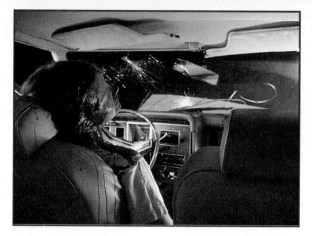

see the patient. She is an approximately twenty-year-old female who appears unconscious, with her head back against the headrest. The vehicle, a medium-size car, has sustained significant damage. Your partner begins manual immobilization of the patient's head and cervical spine as you assess the patient's mental status. The patient moans in response to verbal stimuli, but does not say anything intelligible. Your partner opens her airway with a jaw thrust and evaluates her breathing by looking, listening, and feeling. You hear no abnormal sounds from her airway and see that her breathing is approximately twenty per minute and adequate in depth. Her radial pulse is weak and rapid (at a rate of 120). A quick but careful look around reveals some blood on the patient's face, but no continued external bleeding. Her skin is pale, cool, and sweaty. You determine that this is a high-priority patient; she has an altered mental status and signs of shock (hypoperfusion). If the ALS crew was available, you would call

them, but you know that they are working a cardiac arrest on the other side of town.

Because of the need to transport the patient promptly, you and your partner decide to perform a rapid extrication. As a police officer and fire-fighter get your stretcher, long spine board, and other equipment, you perform a **rapid physical exam**. You find a scalp laceration that is oozing blood slowly, an abrasion on the front of the chest where it might have hit the steering wheel, equal breath sounds, and a tender abdomen. The patient's pulse is now 132 and weaker; blood pressure is 110/80; respirations are 22; the skin is pale, cool, and sweaty; and pupils are equal and reactive.

After you size and apply a cervical collar, you quickly but carefully move the patient to the long spine board, where you immobilize her. Less than ten minutes after you arrived, you have left the scene. Once in the ambulance, you repeat the **initial assessment** to ensure that no life-threatening conditions are present. Next, you perform a **detailed physical exam**, which reveals no additional injuries. **Ongoing assessment** is cut short by your arrival at the hospital.

As you bring the patient into the trauma room, you describe to the doctor and nurses what you found and what you did for the patient. They are grateful for your description of the car and are not surprised that you were unable to get a SAMPLE history on the patient. ■

When examining a patient, tell the patient what you are going to do. In particular, let the patient know when there may be pain or discomfort. Stress the importance of the examination and work to build the patient's confidence.

Some trauma patients require significant interventions from the EMS system if they are to survive and do well. Most of the things an EMT-B can do that will make the difference between life and death are included in the initial assessment. Sometimes a rapid trauma exam will also reveal serious conditions that the EMT-B must manage. Mastering a systematic, efficient way to detect

these conditions is an essential part of being an EMT-B.

■ SCENE SIZE-UP

Sizing up the scene is a critical part of any assessment. A trauma scene in particular can present a confusing array of information that the EMT-B must quickly evaluate and use to make decisions. For example, scene size-up is more than just looking for downed power lines as you approach. It includes taking body substance isolation (BSI) precautions, evaluating the scene for actual and potential dangers, examining the mechanism of injury, and determining whether to institute mass-casualty procedures (see Chapter 17). You reviewed the principles of BSI and scene safety in Chapter 2. This chapter will concentrate on mechanism of injury.

The first step is to anticipate, based on dispatch information, what you might encounter when you arrive at the scene. This can help you to begin a plan of action. For example, if you receive a call for a motor-vehicle collision, you should anticipate blunt trauma with possibly the need for extrication. On the other hand, a patient with a stab wound will have a penetrating injury, with very little need for extrication under ordinary circumstances. Beware, though, of depending too much on dispatch information. As you have no doubt discovered, the scene you arrive at sometimes bears little resemblance to the scene your dispatcher described. The patient in the motor vehicle may have gone off the road because he lost consciousness from hypoglycemia. The patient with the stab wounds may also have fallen (or been pushed) down a flight of stairs. Use dispatch information to start a plan, but be prepared to change your plan based on additional information at the scene.

The goals of your assessment are always the same—to detect and correct conditions you can treat, to gather information for other members of the health care team, and to identify and respond to trends in the patient's condition. How you accomplish these goals in the trauma patient will depend to a great extent on the mechanism of injury. In all trauma patients, you begin with the initial assessment, followed by a focused history and physical exam. En route to the hospital, you will conduct an ongoing assessment.

In the patient with a significant mechanism of injury, after you perform the initial assessment, you will conduct a focused history and physical exam by doing a rapid physical exam, getting baseline vital signs, and gathering a SAMPLE history. En route to the hospital, if time allows, you will perform a detailed physical exam and ongoing assessment, re-evaluating the patient for changes and trends.

In the patient without a significant mechanism of injury, after you perform the initial assessment, you will examine areas the patient tells you are injured, in addition to areas you suspect may have been injured based on your evaluation of the mechanism of injury. You will also get baseline vital signs and gather a SAMPLE history. En route, you will perform ongoing assessment.

■ SIGNIFICANT MECHANISM OF INJURY

Experience has shown that certain mechanisms carry with them a greater risk of serious or life-threatening injury. Some are quite apparent, such as a gunshot to the chest. Others are not as obvious, e.g., how far can someone fall before it is likely that he or she will sustain serious injury? Trauma specialists and researchers have examined thousands of cases and drawn up a list of some of the more dangerous mechanisms of injuries (Table 6–1). This is only a partial list, though. It is important that the EMT-B have a high index of suspicion. When in doubt, assume that the patient has a significant mechanism of injury and treat him or her as such.

Initial Assessment

The components of the initial assessment are the same in medical and trauma patients, but they

TABLE 6–1 Significant Mechanisms of Injury

Significant Mechanisms of Injury
Ejection from vehicle
Death in same passenger compartment
Falls of more than 15 feet or 3 times patient's height
Roll-over of vehicle
High-speed vehicle collision
Vehicle-pedestrian collision
Motorcycle crash
Unresponsive or altered mental status
Penetrations of the head, chest, or abdomen, e.g., stab and gunshot wounds
Additional Significant Mechanisms of Injury for a Child
Falls from more than 10 feet
Bicycle collision
Vehicle in medium speed collision

can take very different forms. This is because of the potential for spinal cord injury in trauma patients. You should suspect potential spine injury in any patient who has sustained significant force to the upper part of the body or when there is a wound to the head, face, or neck. As you assess and treat a patient you suspect has a potential spine injury, avoid, as much as possible, moving the neck and head. Even a slight movement in the wrong direction can turn a potential spine injury into an actual injury to the spinal cord that can be devastating or even life threatening.

There are six parts of the initial assessment:

- Forming a general impression
- Assessing mental status
- Assessing the airway
- Assessing breathing
- Assessing circulation
- Determining the priority of the patient

Forming a General Impression

As with the medical patient, you form your general impression by looking at the patient and getting an idea of the severity of the patient's condition. You also gather information such as the patient's sex and approximate age. It is at this point that you start to determine whether the patient is injured or ill or both. If you see an immediate threat to life in the initial assessment, it is appropriate to treat it at this time.

Assessing Mental Status

The AVPU system of determining mental status gives you a good way of describing the type of stimulus you used and the patient's response to it. For example, a patient may moan in response to verbal stimuli or may withdraw both hands from a painful stimulus. When applying a painful stimulus, be sure not to cause or worsen an injury. To avoid this, it is wise to avoid pinching the trapezius muscle near the neck in trauma patients. At the same time that you assess mental status, your partner should apply manual immobilization of the head and neck (Figure 6–1).

Assessing the Airway

If the patient is not talking (crying for children and infants), assume that the airway is not open and take steps to establish an open airway. When assessing the airway of a patient with a potential

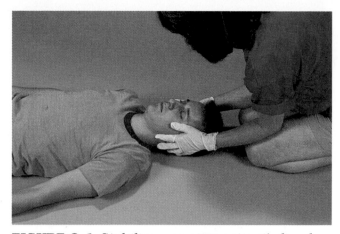

FIGURE 6–1 Stabilize a supine patient's head from the top.

spine injury, you must take care not to move the patient's head or neck any more than necessary. The jaw thrust is the preferred way to open the airway of the patient who cannot keep his airway open alone. Suction the mouth and oropharynx to remove blood and other fluids as necessary.

Assessing Breathing

If the patient is unresponsive, put your ear near his mouth and look toward his chest. Look, listen, and feel for air movement. If the patient is responsive, look at the chest as you approach him. Estimate the rate and depth of the patient's breaths. If he is unresponsive and his breathing is less than eight per minute, ventilate with high-concentration oxygen. This is also appropriate if the patient's breathing is faster than eight per minute, but inadequate in depth.

If the depth of the patient's breathing is sufficient but the rate is faster than twenty-four per minute, give him high-concentration oxygen by nonrebreather mask.

Assessing Circulation

To determine how adequate the patient's circulation is, check pulse, bleeding, and perfusion. The radial pulse is easy to find and allows you not only to check the rate and strength, but also to gauge how good the circulation is in the extremities. If the radial pulse is difficult to find, palpate the carotid pulse.

Significant external bleeding is uncommon, but important to identify and correct. Direct pressure on a heavily bleeding wound will stop or slow hemorrhage from all but the most serious of wounds (see Chapter 12).

TABLE 6–2 High-Priority Conditions

Poor general impression
Unresponsive
Responsive, but not following commands
Difficulty breathing
Shock (hypoperfusion)
Complicated childbirth
Chest pain with systolic blood pressure less than 100
Uncontrolled bleeding
Severe pain anywhere

It is easy to determine the adequacy of perfusion by checking skin color, temperature, and condition.

PEDIATRIC HIGHLIGHT

In children and infants, capillary refill gives additional information about perfusion. A capillary refill time greater than two seconds indicates reduced perfusion from either shock or exposure to cold temperatures. ■

Determining the Priority of the Patient

Table 6–2 lists a number of high-priority conditions. Your local protocols may describe others. Some systems have very clearly defined conditions that require scene time to be kept to a minimum. In addition, this is the time to decide whether advanced life support (ALS) backup is needed. You will also, based on the information gathered so far, decide the next steps in the assessment.

Focused History and Physical Exam—Trauma

When you are treating a patient who has a significant mechanism of injury, you should spend as little time at the scene as possible. Rather than doing a complete physical exam at the scene, you should perform a rapid trauma assessment and perform a detailed physical exam en route. This is why you should reconsider the mechanism of injury at this point in the assessment.

Rapid Physical Exam

The rapid physical exam, or rapid trauma assessment, is a quick assessment that allows you to find major problems that need to be identified and treated quickly. The rapid trauma assessment consists of inspecting, palpating, and auscultating particular areas of the body: the head, neck, chest, abdomen, pelvis, extremities, and posterior. When you assess these areas, search for DCAP-BTLS: deformities, contusions, abrasions, punctures/penetrations, burns, tenderness, lacerations, and swelling. The steps of the rapid trauma assessment are shown in Skill Summary 6–1.

A part of the rapid trauma assessment is not assessment at all: It is application of a cervical collar to limit motion of the head and neck. Even after the collar is in place, the person applying manual immobilization must continue to hold the head and neck still. No collar limits motion enough for you to depend on it alone. Skill Summary 6–2 describes the proper sizing and application of a cervical collar.

Baseline Vital Signs

A complete set of baseline vital signs is essential in both determining the patient's condition now and detecting changes in the patient's condition later. Be sure to determine the patient's respirations; pulse; blood pressure; and skin color, temperature, and condition. As appropriate, assess the pupils.

SAMPLE History

Although a trauma patient has an injury and not an illness, there is still important information you can gain when gathering a SAMPLE history. Remember to determine **S**igns/symptoms, **A**llergies, **M**edications, **P**ertinent past history, **L**ast oral intake, and **E**vents leading to the injury. The patient may have a medical condition that affects the way you or the emergency department staff manage the patient.

You should also find out more about how the patient was injured. If the patient was in a motor vehicle, some questions to ask include:

- Was the patient wearing a lap belt, a shoulder belt, or both?
- Was there any loss of consciousness?
- Did the patient strike the inside of the vehicle?

Focused History and Physical Exam— Trauma Patient

First take body substance isolation precautions.

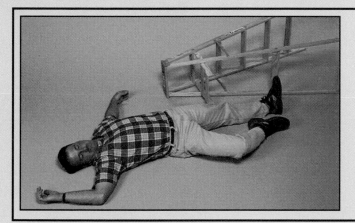

MECHANISM OF INJURY

Reassess mechanism of injury.

If there is no significant mechanism of injury (e.g., patient has a cut finger), focus the physical exam only on the injured part.

If the mechanism of injury is significant:
- Continue spine stabilization
- Consider requesting ALS personnel
- Reconsider transport decision
- Reassess mental status and ABCs
- Perform rapid trauma assessment

RAPID TRAUMA ASSESSMENT

Rapidly assess each part of the body for the following problems (say "Dee-cap - B-T-L-S" as a memory prompt):

Deformities	Burns
Contusions	Tenderness
Abrasions	Lacerations
Punctures and Penetrations	Swelling

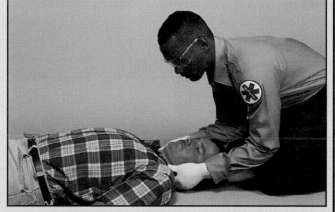

Head: DCAP-BTLS plus crepitation

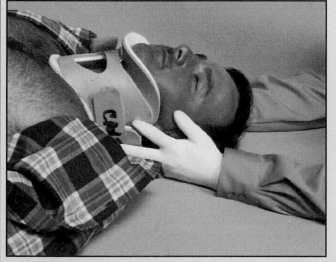

Neck: DCAP-BTLS plus jugular vein distention and crepitation (then place cervical collar)

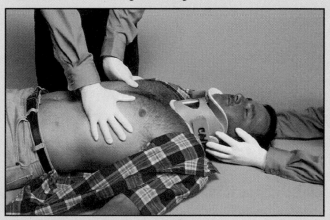

Chest: DCAP-BTLS plus crepitation and breath sounds (absent/present, equal)

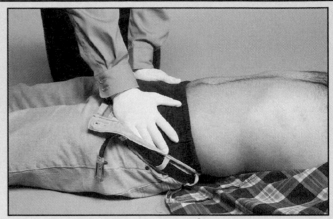

Abdomen: DCAP-BTLS plus firm, soft, distended

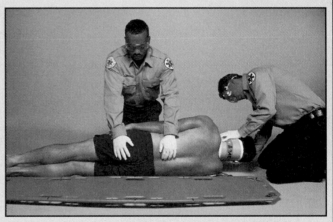

Pelvis: DCAP-BTLS. Gentle compression for tenderness

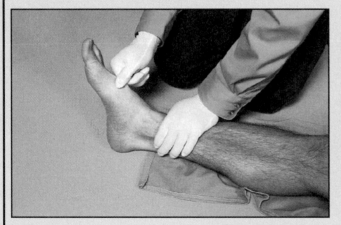

Extremities: DCAP-BTLS plus distal pulse, sensation, motor function

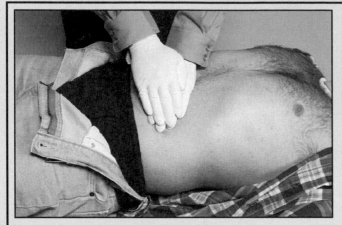

Posterior: DCAP-BTLS (To examine posterior, roll patient using spinal precautions.)

VITAL SIGNS

Assess the patient's vital signs:
- Respiration
- Pulse
- Skin color, temperature, condition, plus capillary refill in infants and children
- Pupils
- Blood pressure

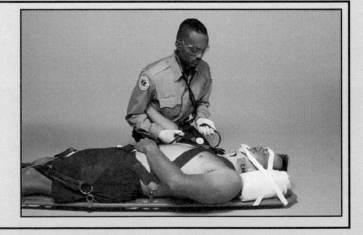

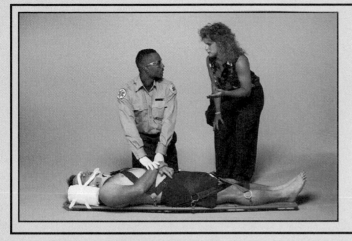

SAMPLE HISTORY

Interview patient, or if patient is unresponsive, interview family and bystanders to get as much information as possible about the patient's problem. Ask about:

<u>S</u>igns and symptoms
<u>A</u>llergies
<u>M</u>edicines
<u>P</u>ertinent past history
<u>L</u>ast oral intake
<u>E</u>vents leading to problem

INTERVENTIONS AND TRANSPORT

Contact on-line medical direction as needed. Perform interventions as needed.

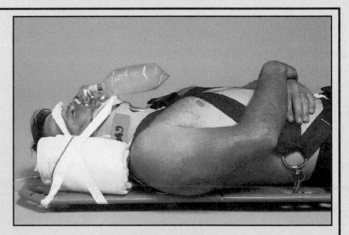

Package and transport patient.

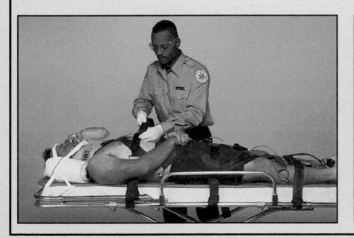

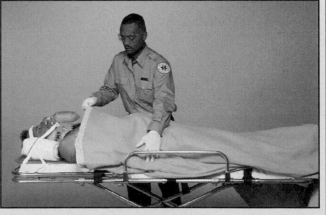

Cervical Collars

Rigid cervical collars are applied to protect the cervical spine. **Do not** apply a soft collar.

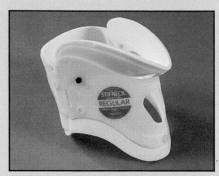

STIFNECK™—Rigid extrication

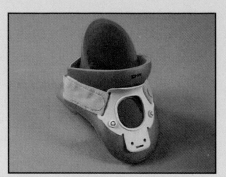

PHILADELPHIA CERVICAL COLLAR™

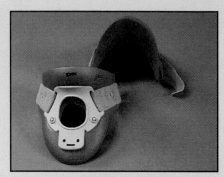

PHILADELPHIA CERVICAL COLLAR™—Opened

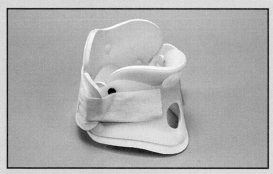

NEC-LOC™—Rigid extrication

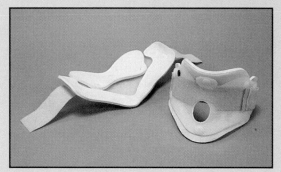

NEC-LOC™—Opened

Sizing a Rigid Cervical Collar

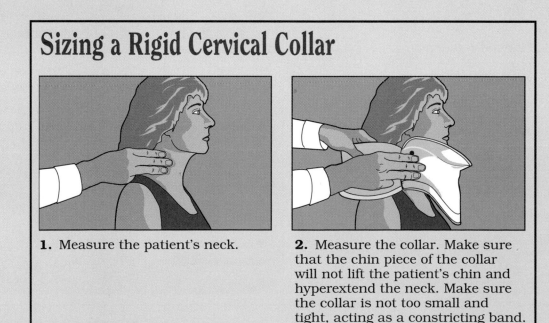

1. Measure the patient's neck.

2. Measure the collar. Make sure that the chin piece of the collar will not lift the patient's chin and hyperextend the neck. Make sure the collar is not too small and tight, acting as a constricting band.

Stifneck™ Collar—Seated Patient

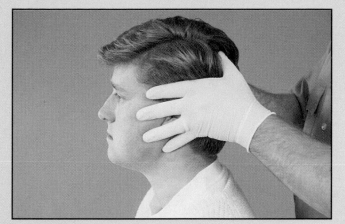

1. Stabilize the head and neck from the rear.

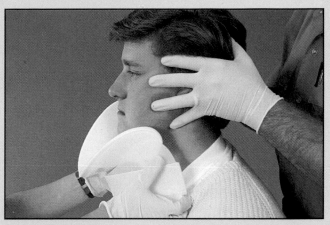

2. Properly angle the collar for placement.

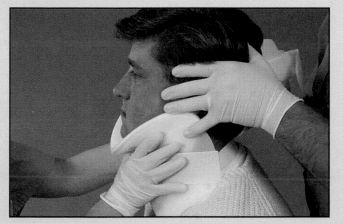

3. Position the collar bottom.

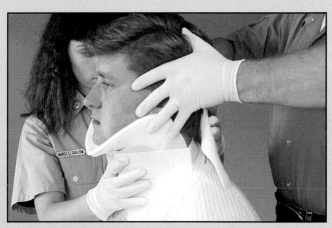

4. Set collar in place around neck.

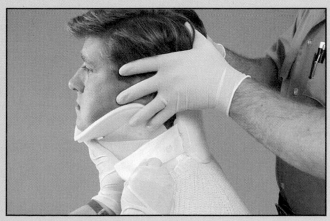

5. Secure the collar.

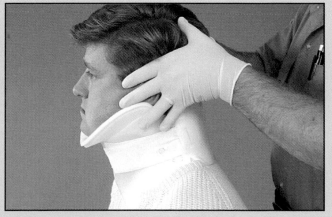

6. Spread fingers and maintain support.

Stifneck™ Collar—Supine Patient

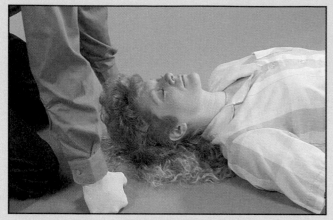

1. Kneel at patient's head.

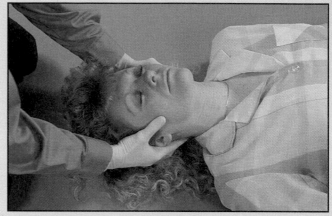

2. Stabilize the head and neck.

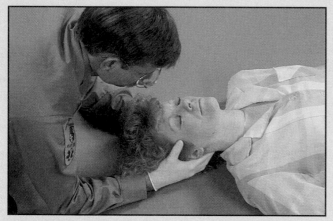

3. Maintain stabilization.

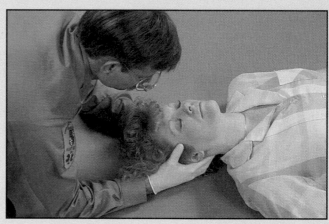

4. Set collar in place.

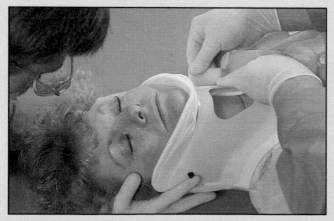

5. Secure the collar.

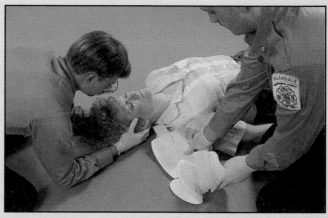

6. Continue to stabilize.

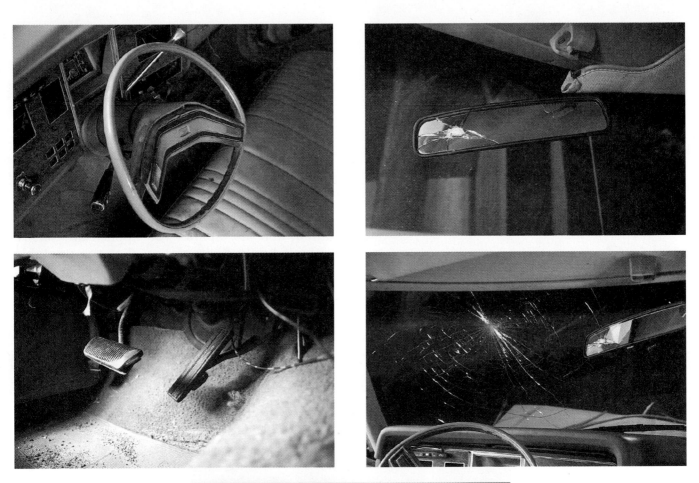

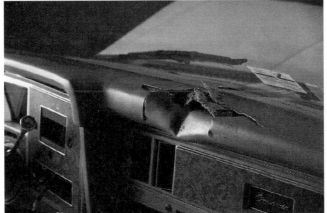

FIGURE 6–2 Deformities to the interior of a vehicle may show where a person has struck the surface, revealing a mechanism of injury.

Examination of the vehicle (Figure 6–2) will lead to answers to the following questions:

- Is there deformity of the steering wheel?
- Is there deformity of the pedals, mirror, gearshift, or other items inside the vehicle?
- Is the windshield cracked or spiderwebbed?

If the patient was on a motorcycle, bicycle, or all-terrain vehicle, find out:

- Was the patient wearing a helmet?
- If there is a helmet but it is not on the patient when you arrive, who removed it?

Detailed Physical Exam

The best place to perform the detailed physical exam is generally en route to a hospital.

There are two other ways in which the detailed physical exam differs from the rapid trauma exam. First, the detailed physical exam includes examination not only of the areas you assessed in the rapid trauma exam, but also the face, ears, eyes, nose, and mouth (Skill Summary 6–3). Second, it is done more slowly, allowing you more time to be thorough and to locate injuries.

Ongoing Assessment

There are five steps in the ongoing assessment:

- Repeat the initial assessment.
- Re-establish the priority of the patient.
- Reassess and record vital signs.
- Reassess injuries found previously.
- Check the interventions you have instituted.

For the trauma patient with a significant mechanism of injury, an intervention check might include verifying that oxygen continues to flow into the nonrebreather mask, the straps on the backboard are snug without compromising respiration, and any splints you applied are secure without limiting circulation. For the unstable patient, ongoing assessment should be repeated every five minutes.

ON THE SCENE

You receive a call for a man with a "cut arm bleeding badly." You and your partner encounter no hazards responding to the scene. When you arrive, you see a middle-aged man near the side of the house. He is holding a bloody towel on his left wrist. Next to him is a storm window with shattered glass. As you get out of the ambulance, you put on disposable gloves. Your **initial assessment** takes only a few seconds—he is alert, with a patent airway and no breathing difficulty. The radial pulse on his uninjured wrist is rapid and strong. Although the towel appears quite bloody, there does not seem to be any more bleeding. His skin is pink, warm, and dry.

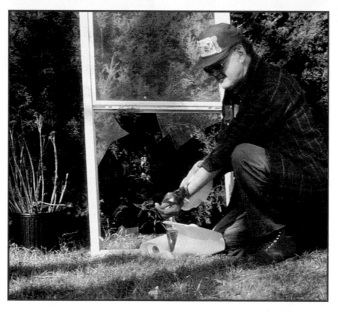

You focus your exam on the injury to the wrist. The patient confirms that he was not injured anywhere else. Examination of the area reveals a 3-centimeter laceration that is not bleeding. You look for glass in the wound, but find none. Your partner gets a set of vital signs as you dress and bandage the wound and gather a SAMPLE history.

En route to the hospital, you repeat the **initial assessment**, reassess the wound for bleeding, and check the circulation distal to the bandage. When you arrive at the hospital, you turn the patient over to the emergency department staff. ■

■ NO SIGNIFICANT MECHANISM OF INJURY

Most trauma patients are not critically injured. In these cases, you have a little more time to assess and treat them. However, it is important to keep a high index of suspicion. When in doubt, treat the patient as though he or she has a significant mechanism of injury.

Examining the Head During the Detailed Physical Exam

The detailed physical exam includes reexamination of the head, neck, chest, abdomen, pelvis, extremities, and posterior body, as was done during the rapid trauma assessment (review Skill Summary 6–1). During the detailed physical examination of the head, however, the face, ears, eyes, nose, and mouth are given particular attention, as shown below.

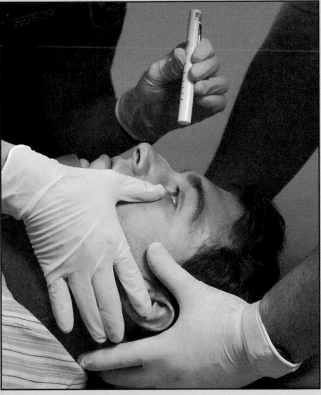

1. Examine the scalp, cranium, and face.

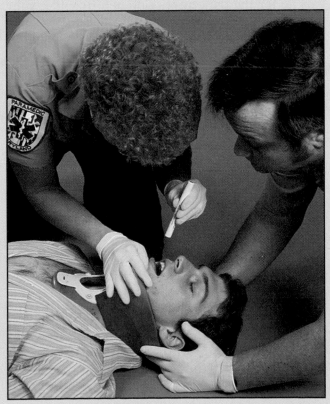

2. Examine the ears.

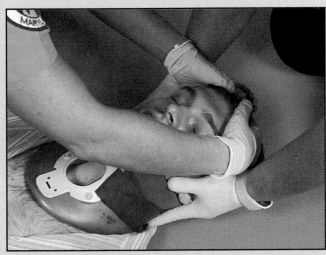

3. Examine the eyes.

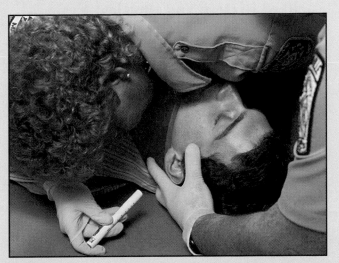

4. Examine the nose and mouth.

Initial Assessment

The initial assessment consists of the same six steps as before: general impression, mental status, airway, breathing, circulation, and patient priority identification. Although most patients without a significant mechanism of injury will not display any life-threatening problems, do not be lulled into a false sense of security. Evaluate every patient for threats to life as soon as you can.

Focused History and Physical Exam— Trauma

In situations where there is no significant mechanism of injury, your history and physical exam are truly focused. You assess the areas the patient has injured and also areas you believe may have been injured based on your evaluation of the mechanism of injury. Search for the same wounds and signs that you looked for in the physical exam of the patient with a significant mechanism of injury (DCAP-BTLS). As part of your focused history and physical exam, you should also assess baseline vital signs and gather a SAMPLE history.

Ongoing Assessment

If the patient does not have a significant mechanism of injury and is stable, you should reassess at least every fifteen minutes. This includes repeating the initial assessment, re-establishing the priority of the patient, reassessing and recording vital signs, reassessing injuries, and checking the interventions you have instituted.

CHAPTER REVIEW

■ SUMMARY

In one moment, trauma can change a perfectly healthy person into a patient with life-threatening injuries. Although there are limits to what you can do for the patient outside of a hospital, your actions can sometimes literally mean the difference between life and death. In order to help the patient with critical injuries, you must quickly find and treat threats to life. By following a systematic approach to assessment, you will find the conditions that you can treat and that will make a difference in the patient's outcome.

Scene size-up is always the first step, followed quickly by the initial assessment. If the patient has no significant mechanism of injury, you assess the areas the patient tells you are injured, in addition to areas where you suspect injury because of the mechanism of injury. Just as you do for every patient, you take vital signs and gather a SAMPLE history. En route, you perform ongoing assessment.

If the patient has a significant mechanism of injury, after you perform the initial assessment, you perform a rapid trauma exam, take vital signs, and gather a SAMPLE history. You immobilize the patient's spine and transport promptly. En route, as time allows, you perform a detailed physical exam and ongoing assessment. By following this systematic approach, you will provide the trauma patient with the best chance for survival and return to a normal life.

■ REVIEW QUESTIONS

1. List the mechanisms of injury that should lead you to the decision to perform a rapid trauma exam.

2. Describe how the initial assessment for trauma patients is different from the initial assessment for medical patients.

3. What areas do you assess in the detailed physical exam that you do not evaluate in the rapid trauma exam?

4. What should you listen for when auscultating the chest of a trauma patient?

5. What signs should you look for in the neck before applying a cervical collar?

6. Besides DCAP-BTLS, what signs do you search for when performing the rapid trauma exam?

7. Describe the ongoing assessment of a trauma patient with a significant mechanism of injury.

CHAPTER 7

Communications and Documentation

There are many different ways in which an EMT-B communicates on a call. Understanding and speaking to patients, family members, and bystanders all require excellent interpersonal communication skills.

Communication with the hospital requires special communications skills. As you know, assessing a patient thoroughly and delivering quality care are two major tasks of the EMT-B. However, excellent prehospital care will not be continued in the hospital if the emergency department is unprepared for the patient's arrival. Therefore, by providing information in an orderly, efficient manner, the EMT-B can help ensure that the patient

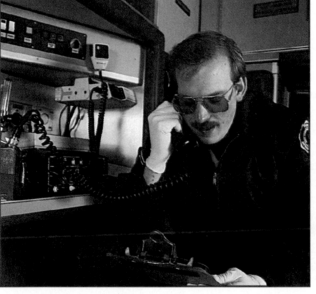

will continue to receive quality care.

Radio transmissions help to inform other members of the health care team about a patient while you are taking care of him, but what happens after you transfer patient care? After the patient is transferred to a floor or critical care unit, the staff require critical information about what happened to the patient before he arrived. However, they can learn this information only if you document your assessment findings and treatment in an organized, comprehensive manner. The prehospital care report you complete is an important link in the chain of communication for your patient.

MAKING THE TRANSITION

- The 1994 curriculum describes the information you should transmit in a radio report and the order in which you should transmit it.
- A minimum data set describes the minimum information each EMS system should collect.
- Special situations require alterations in the usual manner of documenting incidents.

OBJECTIVES

The numbered objectives below are from the United States Department of Transportation 1994 EMT-Basic National Standard Curriculum.

■ KNOWLEDGE AND ATTITUDE

At the completion of this chapter, you should be able to:

Communications

1. List the proper methods of initiating and terminating a radio call. (pp. 110–112)
2. State the proper sequence for delivery of patient information. (p. 112)
3. Explain the importance of effective communication of patient information in the verbal report. (pp. 111–112)
4. Identify the essential components of the verbal report. (p. 112)
5. Describe the attributes for increasing effectiveness and efficiency of verbal communications. (pp. 110–111)
6. State legal aspects to consider in verbal communication. (p. 111)
7. Discuss the communication skills that should be used to interact with the patient. (pp. 109–110)
8. Discuss the communication skills that should be used to interact with the family, bystanders, and individuals from other agencies while providing patient care, as well as the difference between skills used to interact with the patient and those used to interact with others. (pp. 109–110)
9. List the correct radio procedures in the following phases of a typical call: (pp. 110–112)
   - To the scene
   - At the scene
   - To the facility
   - At the facility
   - To the station
   - At the station

10. Explain the rationale for providing efficient and effective radio communications and patient reports. (p. 109)

Documentation

1. Explain the components of the written report and list the information that should be included in the written report. (pp. 112–116)
2. Identify the various sections of the written report. (pp. 112–115)
3. Describe what information is required in each section of the prehospital care report and how it should be entered. (pp. 112–115)
4. Define the special considerations concerning patient refusal. (pp. 116–118)
5. Describe the legal implications associated with the written report. (pp. 112, 116, 117)
6. Discuss all state and/or local record and reporting requirements. (pp. 113, 118, 119)
7. Explain the rationale for patient care documentation. (pp. 112–113)
8. Explain the rationale for the EMS system gathering data. (pp. 112–113)
9. Explain the rationale for using medical terminology correctly. (p. 113)
10. Explain the rationale for using an accurate and synchronous clock so that information can be used in trending. (p. 113)

■ SKILLS

Communications

1. Perform a simulated, organized, concise radio transmission.
2. Perform an organized, concise patient report that would be given to the staff at a receiving facility.
3. Perform a brief, organized report that would be given to an ALS provider arriving at an incident scene at which the EMT-B was already providing care.

Documentation

1. Practice completing a prehospital care report.

You are the preceptor for Karen, a student in an EMT-B course. Karen has ridden on one shift during which she observed several calls. She is curious about radio communications and documentation. You show her the regional protocol for radio communications as well as several prehospital care reports.

You explain that the radio communication protocol lists the pieces of information that an EMT-B should transmit to the hospital. To help teach Karen how to organize this kind of information, you ask her to create an imaginary patient or to think of one she has observed on your shift and to give a simulated radio report. She is hesitant, but with some encouragement from you, she is able to start:

"Good Samaritan, this is Manchester. We are eight minutes out with a 76-year-old male complaining of abdominal pain that started three hours ago. He describes

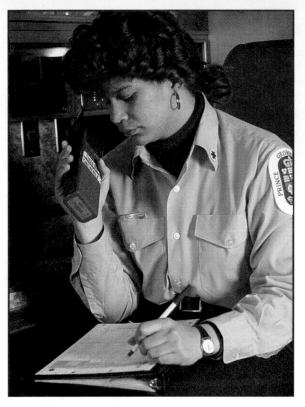

the pain as burning in nature and is also complaining of nausea. He has no medical history. He is alert and oriented. He appears to be in minimal distress. Pulse is 84; BP is 160 over 90; skin is pale, cool, and dry. We are giving him oxygen at 12 liters per minute by nonrebreather. There has been no change in his condition."

You compliment Karen on her report, but remind her to include the patient's respiratory rate and the physical examination of the patient's abdomen. She takes the constructive criticism well.

Next, you review with Karen some prehospital care reports from the last few shifts. Karen is impressed with the completeness and organization of the reports. Before you can ask her to practice writing one, you get a call. You tell Karen that you will complete the report for this call, but that she will soon have an opportunity to practice her documentation skills. ■

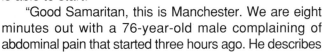

When members of the health care team are able to give and receive information about a patient in a clear, concise manner, this communication leads to improved patient care. Such vital communication starts in the dispatch phase and continues throughout the call, ending only after completion of transport. As an EMT-B and member of the patient's health care team, you must have excellent verbal and written communication skills to assure that the appropriate individuals receive the information they need to treat the patient. In fact, this continuum of patient care is dependent upon effective and efficient communication skills.

■ COMMUNICATIONS

General Principles of Communication

There are many ways human beings communicate. This chapter focuses on the verbal and written forms. There are other nonverbal methods of communication, though, that you must keep in mind when dealing with a patient, family member, friend, bystander, public safety officer, or fellow EMS provider. Particularly when dealing with patients, keep these simple principles in mind:

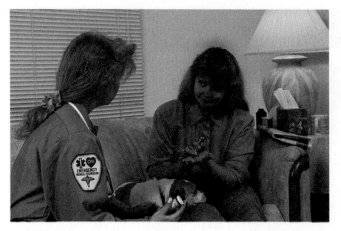

FIGURE 7–1 If possible, position yourself at or below the patient's eye level to be less intimidating and to aid communication.

- *Make and keep eye contact with the patient.* Remember that some cultures discourage eye contact. If there are ethnic enclaves in your community, find out more about these cultures to ensure that you can appropriately communicate with them.

- *When practical, position yourself at a level lower than the patient.* Do this only when the scene is safe (Figure 7–1).

- *Be honest with the patient.* If a patient asks you a direct question, give the best answer you can.

- *Use language the patient can understand.* Asking a patient whether he has ever had an MI is not likely to be as effective as asking if he has ever had a heart attack or heart problem.

- *Be aware of your own body language.* Taking a defensive stance can sometimes make you appear to be unapproachable.

- *Speak clearly, slowly, and distinctly.*

- *Use the patient's proper name,* either first or last, depending on the circumstances. Ask the patient what he or she wishes to be called.

- *If a patient has difficulty hearing, speak clearly with your lips visible.*

- *Allow the patient enough time to answer a question before asking the next one.* When you are trying to move quickly and spend as little time on the scene as possible, it is easy to appear rushed. This can fluster patients, making it even harder for them to describe their chief complaints. It can also antagonize an already anxious patient.

- *Act and speak in a calm, confident manner.* Even if you don't feel confident, look and act that way. A patient wants to feel that you know what you are doing. If you appear unsure, the patient may avoid talking to you, waiting instead to talk to the doctor at the hospital.

Preceptor Pearl

Not every patient you see is lucky enough to have good hearing. You may need to use an interpreter or other means of communicating with these patients. This can be time consuming, so phrase your questions carefully and clearly, with the intent of getting as much useful information as possible from each question. Similarly, when dealing with a patient who does not speak English, you may have to wait for an interpreter to repeat what you said. When an interpreter is not available, you may find that a pocket medical guide for non-English speaking patients can be useful. ✣

PEDIATRIC HIGHLIGHT

Children can also be a communication challenge. It is especially important that you speak to a child at the child's level. Kneel, if necessary, to make eye contact and use words the child will understand. You should be extremely careful to be honest with children. They sense falsehoods more quickly than do many adults. ■

Radio Use

Although the information in this section is intended to describe use of radios, much of it also applies to the use of cellular telephones. Your system should have guidelines on what equipment to use under different circumstances (Table 7–1).

The dispatcher plays a pivotal role in EMS. The dispatcher gets essential information from the caller about the nature and location of the call, as well as keeps track of certain events. To accomplish this, the dispatcher must be kept informed. In particular, you need to notify the dispatcher:

- that you received the call
- when your unit is en route
- when you arrive at the scene
- when you leave the scene
- when you arrive at the hospital
- when you leave the hospital
- when you are back at quarters

In many rural areas, EMS notifies the local hospital when responding to a call. This allows the limited staff to make contingency plans so that they are not overwhelmed.

TABLE 7-1   Principles of Radio Communication

Follow these principles when using the EMS radio system.

- Make sure that your radio is on and the volume is adjusted properly.
- Reduce background noise by closing the vehicle window when possible.
- Listen to the frequency and ensure that it is clear before beginning a transmission.
- Press the "press to talk" (PTT) button on the radio, then wait one second before speaking. This prevents cutting off the first few words of your transmission.
- Speak with your lips about two to three inches from the microphone.
- When calling another unit or base station, use their unit number or name, followed by yours. "Dispatcher, this is Ambulance 2."
- The unit being called will signal that the transmission should start by saying "go ahead" or another regionally accepted term: "Ambulance 2, this is the dispatcher. Go ahead." If the unit you are calling tells you to "stand by," wait until they tell you they are ready to take your transmission.
- Speak slowly and clearly.
- Keep transmissions brief. If a transmission takes longer than 30 seconds, stop at that point and pause for a few seconds so that emergency traffic can use the frequency if necessary.
- Use plain English. Avoid codes.
- Do not use phrases like "be advised." These are implied and serve no purpose.
- Courtesy is assumed, so there is no need to say "please," "thank you," and "you're welcome."
- When transmitting a number that might be unclear (15 may sound like 16 or 50), give the number, then repeat the individual digits. Say "15, one-five."
- Anything said over the radio can be heard by the public on a scanner. Do not use the patient's name over the radio. For the same reason, do not use profanities or statements that tend to slander any person. Use objective, impartial statements.
- Use "we" instead of "I." As an EMT-B you will rarely be acting alone.
- "Affirmative" and "negative" are preferred over "yes" and "no" because the latter are difficult to hear.
- Give assessment information about your patient, but avoid offering a diagnosis of the patient's problem. For example, say "Patient complains of chest pain," but not "Probably having a heart attack."
- After transmitting, say "Over." Wait for acknowledgment that the person to whom you were speaking heard your message.
- Avoid codes, slang, or abbreviations that are not authorized.
- Use EMS frequencies only for authorized EMS communication.

In some systems, EMT-Bs receive medical direction through the receiving hospital. In others, medical direction is at a separate site. In either case, EMT-Bs need to contact medical direction to get orders for administering certain medications and occasionally to obtain additional advice about patient care. When communicating with medical direction, the EMT-B needs to make these radio transmissions organized, concise, and pertinent. Since the physician will base the decision on whether to order medications and additional procedures on the information you provide, you must make sure this information is accurate.

When you receive an order for a medication or procedure (or denial of such a request), repeat the order back word for word. This ensures that the order you are about to implement is the one the physician intended. If you receive an order that is unclear or that appears to be inappropriate, ask the physician to repeat the order again. If it is still unclear, discuss it with the physician until it is clear and you feel comfortable. At times like this, the telephone may be the preferred method of communicating. It allows you to speak more comfortably and to say certain things that are not appropriate over the airwaves or are confidential (e.g., the patient's name). Moreover, an ordinary telephone is superior to a cellular phone if you are going to discuss confidential information since cellular phone transmissions are not confidential.

The information you provide about a patient allows the receiving hospital to prepare for the patient's arrival, which includes selecting the right room, equipment, and personnel. Your report should include this information, in this order (unless local protocol dictates otherwise):

- ID and level of certification of provider
- Estimated time of arrival
- Patient's age and sex
- Chief complaint
- Brief, pertinent history of the present illness
- Major past illnesses
- Mental status
- Baseline vital signs
- General impression
- Pertinent findings of the physical exam
- Emergency medical care given
- Response to emergency medical care

As part of your ongoing assessment, you will re-evaluate the patient frequently. In accordance with local protocol, advise the hospital of updated vital signs. If the patient's condition takes a turn for the worse, you must notify the hospital so that the patient will get the appropriate care upon arrival.

Reporting to the Hospital Staff

After you arrive at the hospital, you should give a verbal report to the staff. Oftentimes, the nurse who receives the patient has not obtained all of the information you gave in your radio report. When done properly, your verbal report shows the emergency department staff that you did a good assessment and gave quality care. Start by introducing the patient by name. Summarize the information you gave over the radio. Then describe information that was not appropriate or necessary for a radio transmission: additional history, additional vital signs, and any other treatments you have given the patient.

■ DOCUMENTATION

Prehospital Care Report (PCR)

As an experienced EMT-B, you have had considerable experience in preparing prehospital care reports. You are also aware that these reports vary from system to system. As you learned in Chapter 1, the U.S. Department of Transportation has developed a minimum data set—the elements that are recommended for inclusion on a prehospital care report (see Chapter 1, Table 1–1). Each system is encouraged to collect at least this much information so that system evaluation and quality improvement can occur.

Functions

The prehospital care report has many functions.

- *Continuity of Care* It is easy for EMT-Bs to feel that no one in the hospital reads the prehospital care report because it is often not read immediately in the emergency department. However, at a later time a nurse or physician may read it more carefully. If the patient is admitted, staff on the floor or in a critical care unit may depend on your PCR to gain information about the scene and the patient's initial condition. This is information that was available only to you and, if not documented, may be lost to the hospital staff forever.
- *Legal Document* Many EMT-Bs consider this function of the PCR to be the most important one because the form may be used in court proceedings. The form does not go to court alone, though; the person who completed it must ordinarily also appear in court. The best way to avoid legal problems with the PCR is to do a good job completing it.

  A clear, comprehensive, and well-written report documents the condition of the patient upon EMS arrival, the emergency medical care the patient received, any changes in the patient's condition, and the status of the patient on arrival at the hospital. The report should include both objective and subjective information. An example of objective information is a description of the patient's appearance. Subjective information could include the patient's SAMPLE history. The PCR should avoid the EMT-B's opinions on nonmedical findings; for example, derogatory comments about the patient's appearance or hygiene.
- *Educational* PCRs can demonstrate not only proper documentation techniques, but also how to handle unusual and uncommon cases.
- *Administrative* Agencies that bill for their services need accurate information in order to get reimbursement. Many services also compile statistics that help them to determine the best locations for their vehicles and to provide adequate staff and equipment.

- *Research* Advancing the quality of EMS is virtually impossible without adequate information. If a service or region enters data into a computerized database, it becomes much easier to determine where promising areas of research lie.
- *Evaluation and Continuous Quality Improvement* These areas are closely related to research and just as dependent on data. Without a system to identify problems, an EMS system is not fulfilling all of its responsibilities. Progressive systems go further and try to prevent problems from occurring by carefully evaluating all of the information at their disposal.

Principles of Completion

Most EMS agencies use the traditional paper form for recording information about a call (Figures 7–2, 7–3). A few services use a computerized run form. This usually takes the form of an "electronic clipboard" (Figure 7–4). With computer technology advancing rapidly, it is difficult to determine what the clipboard of the future will look like.

Regardless of the way information is collected, there are certain characteristics all of these approaches have in common. There are two sections of the form, one for run data and one for patient data. The run data section includes the date, times, service, unit, and names of crew members. It is important that clocks used to record times be accurate and synchronous. If your dispatcher's clock is five minutes different from your wristwatch, then administrative times (call received, arrival at scene, etc.) and patient times (e.g., vital signs) may conflict.

The patient data section includes

- Patient name, address, date of birth, sex, and age
- Insurance information
- Nature of call
- Mechanism of injury
- Location of patient
- Treatment administered prior to arrival of EMT-B
- Signs and symptoms
- Baseline vital signs
- SAMPLE history
- Care administered
- Changes in patient condition

There are usually two ways you can complete this information, check boxes and open-ended narrative. Check boxes are not only quick and easy to complete, they also make gathering statistics easier. But patients don't always fit easily into the categories that are set up on any one form. On the other hand, the narrative section allows you to explain things and to go into more detail. When filling in check boxes, be sure to fill in the box completely and avoid stray marks if your form is scanned into a computer.

If your form has a narrative section, there are a number of important principles to keep in mind.

- Describe, don't conclude.
- Include pertinent negatives (for example, a patient with chest pains denies difficulty breathing).
- Record important observations about the scene (suicide note, weapon, etc.).
- Avoid radio codes.
- Use abbreviations only if they are standard.
- When information of a sensitive nature is documented, note the source of that information, (for example, certain communicable diseases).
- Be sure to spell words correctly, especially medical words. If you do not know how to spell a word, find out or use a different one.
- Every time you reassess the patient, record the time and your findings.
- Be sure to fulfill other state and local requirements.

Confidentiality is a vital issue in documentation. Although the form itself is considered confidential, it is important to remember that the information on the form is also considered confidential.

After you complete the PCR, you will need to distribute different copies of the form to different individuals or agencies. Generally, the service retains the original copy and one copy is inserted in the patient's hospital medical record. In some areas, another copy is used for data collection and one goes to the medical director or quality improvement coordinator. Be familiar with local protocol and procedures that describe where the different copies of the form should be distributed.

Falsification

An **error of omission** is the failure to do something for the patient, in either assessment or treatment. An **error of commission** is doing something for or to the patient, but doing it poorly or in a manner that is harmful to the patient. When either of these

MAINE EMS

PRESS DOWN, YOU ARE MAKING THREE COPIES

RUN REPORT #	Mo.	Day	Year	M T W Th F S Sun	SERVICE NAME	SERVICE NO.	VEHICLE NO.	ALS ☐ Performed ☐ Back-up Called	SERVICE RUN NO.
746118									

NAME

STREET OR R.F.D.

CITY/TOWN | STATE | ZIP

AGE / DATE OF BIRTH | ☐ Male ☐ Female | PHONE

INCIDENT LOCATION: ADDRESS | CITY/TOWN

TRANSPORTED TO: | TREATING / FAMILY PHYSICIAN

TRANSPORTATION / COMMUNICATIONS PROBLEMS

BILLING INFORMATION

CREW LICENSE NUMBERS

☐ Medical
- ☐ Cardiac
- ☐ Poisoning/OD
- ☐ Respiratory
- ☐ Behavioral
- ☐ Diabetic
- ☐ Seizure
- ☐ CVA
- ☐ OB/Gyn
- ☐ Other ______

☐ Trauma
- ☐ Multi-Systems Trauma
- ☐ Head
- ☐ Spinal
- ☐ Burn
- ☐ Soft Tissue Injury
- ☐ Fractures
- ☐ Other ______

☐ Code 99

R	L	LUNG SOUNDS
☐	☐	CLEAR
☐	☐	ABSENT
☐	☐	DECREASED
☐	☐	RALES
☐	☐	WHEEZE
☐	☐	STRIDOR

TYPE OF RUN
- ☐ Emergency Transport
- ☐ Routine Transfer
- ☐ Emergency Transfer
- ☐ No Transport
- ☐ Refused Transport

TIME	CODE		ODOMETER
		Call Received	
		Enroute	
		At Scene	
		From Scene	
		At Destination	
		In Service	

☐ MEDICATIONS ☐ ALLERGIES

CHIEF COMPLAINT:

TIME	PULSE	RESP	BP	PUPILLARY RESPONSE	SKIN	VERBAL RESPONSE	MOTOR RESPONSE	EYE OPENING RESPONSE	CAPILLARY REFILL
			/			5 4 3 2 1	6 5 4 3 2 1	4 3 2 1	☐ Normal ☐ Delayed ☐ None
			/			5 4 3 2 1	6 5 4 3 2 1	4 3 2 1	☐ Normal ☐ Delayed ☐ None
			/			5 4 3 2 1	6 5 4 3 2 1	4 3 2 1	☐ Normal ☐ Delayed ☐ None

☐ MVA ☐ Concern AOB/ETOH SEAT BELTS: ☐ Used ☐ Not Used ☐ N/A ☐ Helmet Used

MUTUAL AID: Assisted/Assisted by Service # ______ Time Called: ______

PATIENT'S SUSPECTED PROBLEM:

746118

	Cleared Airway		Extrication
	Artificial Respiration/BVM		Cervical Immobilization
	Oropharyngeal Airway		KED/Short Board
	Nasopharyngeal Airway		Long Board
	CPR—Time:		Restraints
	Bystander CPR		Traction Splinting
	AED		General Splinting
	Suction		Cold Application
	Oxygen—LPMin___ ☐ Nasal ☐ Mask		MAST Inflated
	Pulse Oximetry		
	Autovent		

☐ Medication Administered ☐ Defib Lic #______

☐ Monitor ☐ Chest Decomp

☐ Pacing ☐ Cpricothyrotomy

MEDICAL CONTROL ☐ Written Order/Protocol ☐ Verbal Order/Protocol

IV — Total Attempts
☐ SUC LIC.# ______ ___
☐ UNSUC LIC.# ______ ___

EOA — Total Attempts
☐ SUC LIC.# ______ ___
☐ UNSUC LIC.# ______ ___

ET — Total Attempts
☐ SUC LIC.# ______ ___
☐ UNSUC LIC.# ______ ___

LIC #	EKG RHYTHM	TIME	MEDS / DEFIB / C-VERT	DOSE W/S	ROUTE

NAME OF E.D. TREATING PHYSICIAN SIGNATURE OF CREW MEMBER IN CHARGE

COPY 1 HOSPITAL

FIGURE 7–2 The Maine prehospital care report has fill-in boxes and narrative spaces.

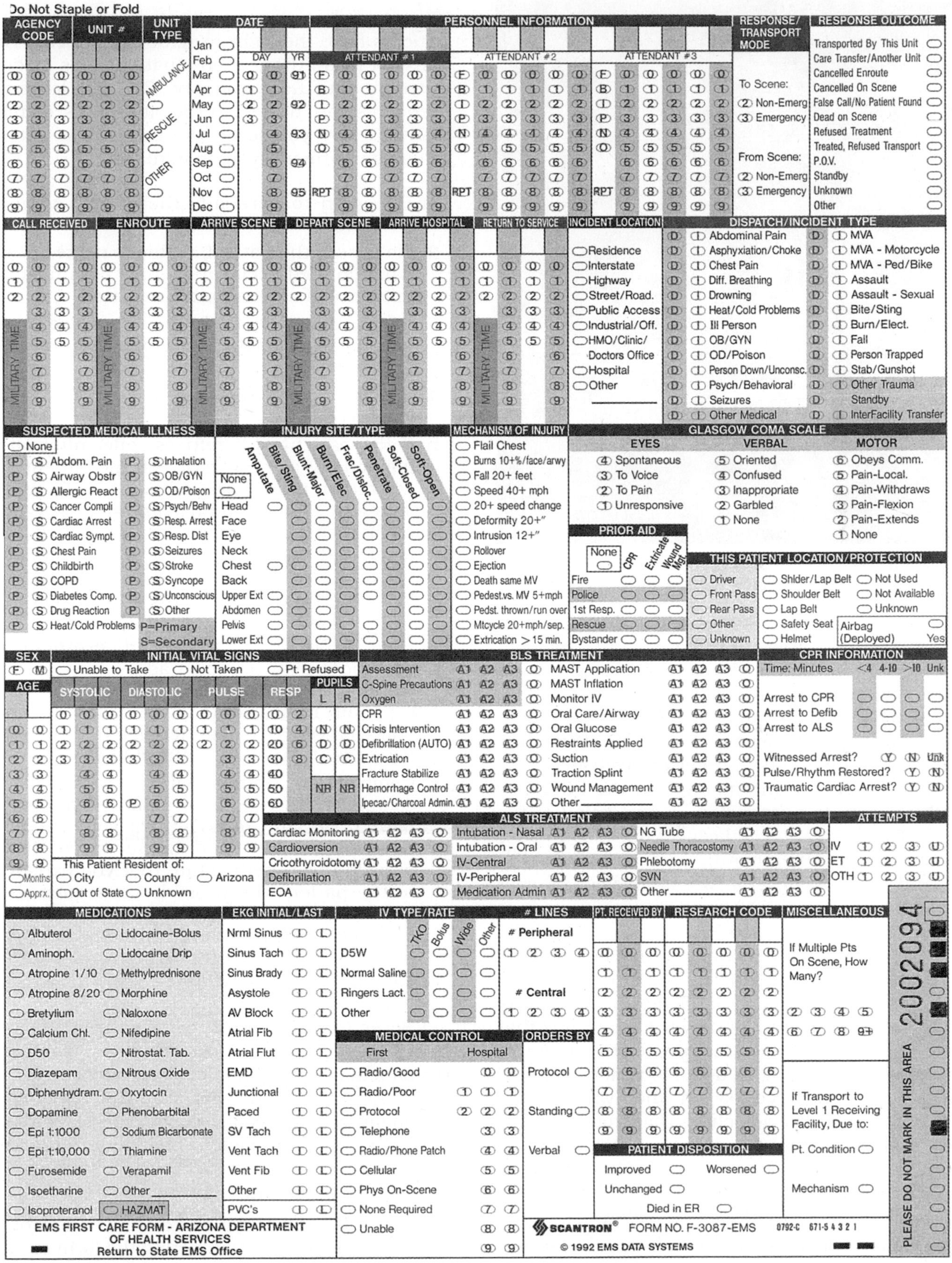

Do Not Staple or Fold

AGENCY CODE | UNIT # | UNIT TYPE: AMBULANCE, RESCUE, OTHER | DATE: Jan, Feb, Mar, Apr, May, Jun, Jul, Aug, Sep, Oct, Nov, Dec; DAY; YR: 91, 92, 93, 94, 95

PERSONNEL INFORMATION: ATTENDANT #1, ATTENDANT #2, ATTENDANT #3 (F, B, D, P, N, O, RPT)

RESPONSE/TRANSPORT MODE: To Scene: Non-Emerg, Emergency; From Scene: Non-Emerg, Emergency

RESPONSE OUTCOME: Transported By This Unit; Care Transfer/Another Unit; Cancelled Enroute; Cancelled On Scene; False Call/No Patient Found; Dead on Scene; Refused Treatment; Treated, Refused Transport; P.O.V.; Standby; Unknown; Other

CALL RECEIVED | ENROUTE | ARRIVE SCENE | DEPART SCENE | ARRIVE HOSPITAL | RETURN TO SERVICE (MILITARY TIME)

INCIDENT LOCATION: Residence; Interstate; Highway; Street/Road.; Public Access; Industrial/Off.; HMO/Clinic/Doctors Office; Hospital; Other ______

DISPATCH/INCIDENT TYPE: Abdominal Pain; Asphyxiation/Choke; Chest Pain; Diff. Breathing; Drowning; Heat/Cold Problems; Ill Person; OB/GYN; OD/Poison; Person Down/Unconsc.; Psych/Behavioral; Seizures; Other Medical; MVA; MVA - Motorcycle; MVA - Ped/Bike; Assault; Assault - Sexual; Bite/Sting; Burn/Elect.; Fall; Person Trapped; Stab/Gunshot; Other Trauma; Standby; InterFacility Transfer

SUSPECTED MEDICAL ILLNESS: None; Abdom. Pain; Airway Obstr; Allergic React; Cancer Compli; Cardiac Arrest; Cardiac Sympt.; Chest Pain; Childbirth; COPD; Diabetes Comp.; Drug Reaction; Heat/Cold Problems; Inhalation; OB/GYN; OD/Poison; Psych/Behv; Resp. Arrest; Resp. Dist; Seizures; Stroke; Syncope; Unconscious; Other. P=Primary S=Secondary

INJURY SITE/TYPE: None; Amputate; Bite/Sting; Blunt-Major; Burn/Elec; Frac/Disloc.; Penetrate; Soft-Closed; Soft-Open. Head; Face; Eye; Neck; Chest; Back; Upper Ext; Abdomen; Pelvis; Lower Ext

MECHANISM OF INJURY: Flail Chest; Burns 10+%/face/arwy; Fall 20+ feet; Speed 40+ mph; 20+ speed change; Deformity 20+"; Intrusion 12+"; Rollover; Ejection; Death same MV; Pedest.vs. MV 5+mph; Pedst. thrown/run over; Mtcycle 20+mph/sep.; Extrication > 15 min.

GLASGOW COMA SCALE: EYES: (4) Spontaneous; (3) To Voice; (2) To Pain; (1) Unresponsive. VERBAL: (5) Oriented; (4) Confused; (3) Inappropriate; (2) Garbled; (1) None. MOTOR: (6) Obeys Comm.; (5) Pain-Local.; (4) Pain-Withdraws; (3) Pain-Flexion; (2) Pain-Extends; (1) None

PRIOR AID: None; CPR; Extricate; Wound Mgt. Fire; Police; 1st Resp.; Rescue; Bystander

THIS PATIENT LOCATION/PROTECTION: Driver; Front Pass; Rear Pass; Other; Unknown; Shlder/Lap Belt; Shoulder Belt; Lap Belt; Safety Seat; Helmet; Not Used; Not Available; Unknown; Airbag (Deployed) Yes

SEX: F M. AGE. Months; Apprx.

INITIAL VITAL SIGNS: Unable to Take; Not Taken; Pt. Refused. SYSTOLIC; DIASTOLIC; PULSE; RESP; PUPILS L R (N, D, C, NR)

This Patient Resident of: City; County; Arizona; Out of State; Unknown

BLS TREATMENT (A1 A2 A3 O): Assessment; C-Spine Precautions; Oxygen; CPR; Crisis Intervention; Defibrillation (AUTO); Extrication; Fracture Stabilize; Hemorrhage Control; Ipecac/Charcoal Admin.; MAST Application; MAST Inflation; Monitor IV; Oral Care/Airway; Oral Glucose; Restraints Applied; Suction; Traction Splint; Wound Management; Other______

CPR INFORMATION: Time; Minutes <4 4-10 >10 Unk. Arrest to CPR; Arrest to Defib; Arrest to ALS. Witnessed Arrest? Y N Unk; Pulse/Rhythm Restored? Y N; Traumatic Cardiac Arrest? Y N

ALS TREATMENT (A1 A2 A3 O): Cardiac Monitoring; Cardioversion; Cricothyroidotomy; Defibrillation; EOA; Intubation - Nasal; Intubation - Oral; IV-Central; IV-Peripheral; Medication Admin; NG Tube; Needle Thoracostomy; Phlebotomy; SVN; Other______

ATTEMPTS: IV; ET; OTH (1 2 3 U)

MEDICATIONS: Albuterol; Aminoph.; Atropine 1/10; Atropine 8/20; Bretylium; Calcium Chl.; D50; Diazepam; Diphenhydram.; Dopamine; Epi 1:1000; Epi 1:10,000; Furosemide; Isoetharine; Isoproterenol; Lidocaine-Bolus; Lidocaine Drip; Methylprednisone; Morphine; Naloxone; Nifedipine; Nitrostat. Tab.; Nitrous Oxide; Oxytocin; Phenobarbital; Sodium Bicarbonate; Thiamine; Verapamil; Other______; HAZMAT

EKG INITIAL/LAST: Nrml Sinus; Sinus Tach; Sinus Brady; Asystole; AV Block; Atrial Fib; Atrial Flut; EMD; Junctional; Paced; SV Tach; Vent Tach; Vent Fib; Other; PVC's

IV TYPE/RATE: TKO; Bolus; Wide; Other. D5W; Normal Saline; Ringers Lact.; Other

LINES: # Peripheral; # Central

MEDICAL CONTROL: First; Hospital. Radio/Good; Radio/Poor; Protocol; Telephone; Radio/Phone Patch; Cellular; Phys On-Scene; None Required; Unable

ORDERS BY: Protocol; Standing; Verbal

PT. RECEIVED BY | RESEARCH CODE

PATIENT DISPOSITION: Improved; Worsened; Unchanged; Died in ER

MISCELLANEOUS: If Multiple Pts On Scene, How Many? 2 3 4 5 6 7 8 9+. If Transport to Level 1 Receiving Facility, Due to: Pt. Condition; Mechanism

PLEASE DO NOT MARK IN THIS AREA 2002094

EMS FIRST CARE FORM - ARIZONA DEPARTMENT OF HEALTH SERVICES Return to State EMS Office

SCANTRON® FORM NO. F-3087-EMS 0792-C 671-5 4 3 2 1 © 1992 EMS DATA SYSTEMS

FIGURE 7–3 The Arizona prehospital care report has a scannable segment that can be read by a computer.

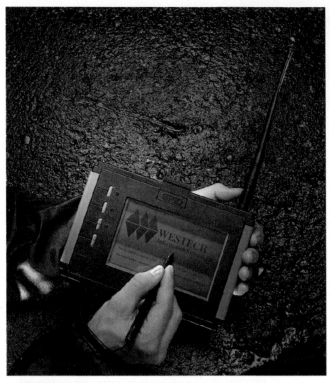

FIGURE 7–4 A pen-based computer can read handwriting and convert it to computer text.

errors occurs, never try to cover it up. Instead, document what did or did not happen and what steps you took (if any) to correct the situation. You are not expected to be perfect; attempting to cover up a mistake usually makes the situation a lot worse than admitting an error occurred.

Falsification of information on the PCR may lead not only to suspension or revocation of the EMT-B's certification or license, but also to poor patient care. Other health care providers who depend on the form get a false impression of what findings were discovered in patient assessment or what treatment was given.

One of the areas in which it may be tempting to "make up" information is in the recording of the patient's vital signs. It is essential to quality patient care to document only the vital signs that were actually taken. In the area of treatment, it can also be tempting to document, for example, that you administered oxygen when you actually forgot to do it. Do not chart that you gave the patient a treatment unless you actually did.

Patient Refusal

As you learned in Chapter 1 and from your field experience, some patients refuse treatment and transportation. This is very frustrating, but it is important to remember that competent adult patients have the right to refuse treatment. This does not mean that, when a patient says he does not want your help, you say "OK" and leave the scene. Instead, approach the situation systematically. Before you leave the scene of a patient refusing treatment, you should:

1. Try again to persuade the patient to go to a hospital.
2. Make sure the patient is able to make a rational, informed decision—e.g., is not under the influence of alcohol or other drugs.
3. Inform the patient why he should go to the hospital and what may happen to him if he does not.
4. Consult medical direction as your local protocol directs.
5. If the patient still refuses, offer alternative methods of gaining care, tell the patient you will return if he changes his mind, document your assessment findings and the emergency medical care given, then have the patient sign a refusal form (Figure 7–5). Every EMS agency should have a refusal form that has been reviewed by both the medical director and an attorney.
6. Have a family member, police officer, or bystander sign the form as a witness. If the patient refuses to sign the refusal form, it is especially important to have a family member, police officer, or bystander sign the form verifying that the patient refused to sign.
7. Complete the prehospital care report just as completely as you do for a patient you transported. Be sure to document your complete patient assessment and the care you wished to provide the patient. State that you explained to the patient the possible consequences of failure to accept care. Document that you offered the patient alternative methods of gaining care and that you offered to return if the patient changed his mind.

Never tell a patient not to call EMS again. Doing so will open you to significant liability if the patient's condition takes a turn for the worse. If you have a patient who calls EMS frequently and inappropriately, consult your medical director about the best approach to handle the situation.

Correction of Errors

There are two times you can discover an error on a PCR: while you are completing the form or after you distributed the copies of the form. For example,

REFUSAL INFORMATION SHEET

PLEASE READ AND KEEP THIS FORM!

This form has been given to you because you have refused treatment and/or transport by Emergency Medical Services (EMS). Your health and safety are our primary concern, so even though you have decided not to accept our advice, please remember the following:

1) The evaluation and/or treatment provided to you by the EMS providers is not a substitute for medical evaluation and treatment by a doctor. We advise you to get medical evaluation and treatment.

2) Your condition may not seem as bad to you as it actually is. Without treatment, your condition or problem could become worse. If you are planning to get medical treatment, a decision to refuse treatment or transport by EMS may result in a delay which could make your condition or problem worse.

3) Medical evaluation and/or treatment may be obtained by calling your doctor, if you have one, or by going to any hospital Emergency Department in this area, all of which are staffed 24 hours a day by Emergency Physicians. You may be seen at these Emergency Departments without an appointment.

4) If you change your mind or your condition becomes worse and you decide to accept treatment and transport by Emergency Medical Services, please do not hesitate to call us back. We will do our best to help you.

5) DON'T WAIT! When medical treatment is needed, it is usually better to get it right away.

I have received a copy of this information sheet.

PATIENT SIGNATURE: _____ DATE: _____

WITNESS SIGNATURE: _____ DATE: _____

AGENCY INCIDENT #: _____ AGENCY CODE: _____

NAME OF PERSON FILLING OUT FORM: _____

G 11A

FIGURE 7–5 A refusal information sheet from Spokane County Emergency Medical Services, Washington State.

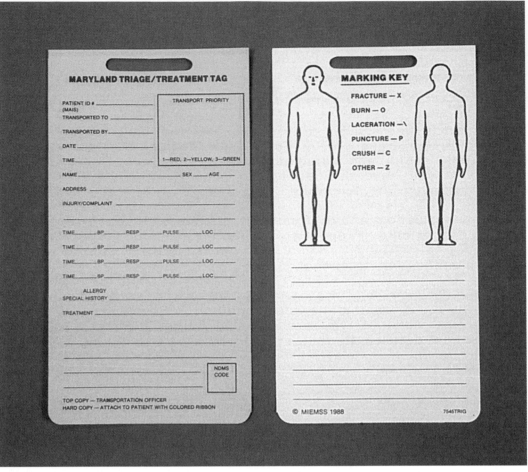

FIGURE 7–6 During a multiple-casualty incident, triage tags are used to document information for each patient.

you thought you were writing "albuterol," but someone was talking about nitroglycerin as you began writing. When you check the form, you discover you wrote the wrong medication name. To correct this, draw a single horizontal line through the error, initial it, and write the correct information beside it. Do not try to obliterate the error: This may be interpreted as an attempt to cover up a mistake. If you discover an error after you submit the report form, the procedure is a little different. Draw a single line through the error (preferably in a different color ink), initial and date it, and add a note with the correct information. If you neglected to include some important information, add a note with the correct information, the date, and your initials.

Special Situations

There are several instances where the usual principles of documentation don't meet the needs of the situation. These can include charting patient care at multiple-casualty incidents and documenting unusual incidents.

Multiple-Casualty Incidents (MCI) There are days when your service is very busy and you do not have time to complete a form immediately after each call. Although everyone would like to avoid these situations, they are sometimes inevitable in EMS. When you don't have enough time to complete the form before the next call, keep your notes and fill out the report later.

Multiple-casualty incidents (MCIs) are a special case. The very nature of an MCI prevents you from completing the form immediately after you have transported a patient. Fortunately, good local MCI plans include some means of recording important medical information temporarily (like a triage tag) that can be used later to complete the form (Figure 7–6). The standard for documentation in an MCI is not the same as for a typical call. Your local plan should have guidelines.

Special Situation Reports Unusual events occur from time to time that do not fit into the usual system of documenting patient care. When an EMS provider is stuck by a contaminated needle, for example, special care must be taken to document this, preferably on a form made for this purpose. Other types of injury to crew members also need to be documented. There are other events that you may need to report to local authorities, and occasionally you may need to explain an unusual event on a call.

Whatever the nature of the incident, you should submit any required report in a timely manner to the authority described by local protocol. The report should be accurate and objective, with careful attention to the facts of the case. Be very careful about speculation. It is prudent for you to keep a copy of the report for your own records.

CHAPTER REVIEW

■ SUMMARY

One of the things that intimidates many new EMT-Bs is talking on the radio. Just knowing that what you say is being broadcast to potentially thousands of listeners is enough to make even superb providers hesitate and lose their confidence. However, knowing exactly what you need to say and knowing the order in which you are going to say it makes all the difference. By performing an excellent assessment and following your local communication protocol, you will be able to provide important information to other members of the health care team.

Another skill that is not on a typical EMT-B's list of favorite activities is completing the PCR. Generally, this is because of the narrative section of the form. Again, knowing what you need to write and having a system to organize it increases confidence. By performing both of these skills well, you will forge an essential link in the chain that continues the patient's care.

■ REVIEW QUESTIONS

1. Describe three general principles of communication.

2. Describe how communicating with children can differ from communicating with adults.

3. What is the order in which patient information should be transmitted over the radio?

4. How should you deal with an order from medical direction that you feel is inappropriate?

5. List three principles to use in completing the PCR.

6. Describe how to correct an error while you are writing the PCR.

7. How should you handle a patient who is refusing transport?

CHAPTER 8

General Pharmacology

■ As an EMT-B, you carry several medications on your EMS unit that you can give a patient under specific conditions. There are additional medications that, when they have been prescribed, you are permitted to assist the patient in taking with medical direction's approval.

Being able to give the proper medication in an emergency can prove lifesaving for your patient.

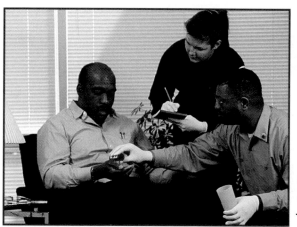

This chapter provides basic information on what you need to know in order to assist a patient with his prescribed medications, provided your medical director agrees that this is the most appropriate course of action.

The chapter concludes with the six common categories of medications that patients often take that you find in the field and that are relevant to patient care.

MAKING THE TRANSITION

- ■ Medications carried on the ambulance are explained.
- ■ Medications the EMT-B may assist the patient in taking with medical direction's approval are discussed.

OBJECTIVES

The numbered objectives below are from the United States Department of Transportation 1994 EMT-Basic National Standard Curriculum.

■ KNOWLEDGE AND ATTITUDE

At the completion of this chapter, you should be able to:

1. Identify which medications will be carried on the unit. (p. 123)
2. State the medications carried on the unit by the generic names. (p. 123)
3. Identify the medications which the EMT-B may assist the patient with administering. (pp. 124–125)
4. State the medications the EMT-B can assist the patient with by the generic names. (pp. 124–125)
5. Discuss the forms in which the medications may be found. (p. 126)
6. Explain the rationale for the administration of medications. (p. 121)

■ SKILLS

1. Demonstrate general steps for assisting patient with self-administration of medications.
2. Read the labels and inspect each type of medication.

ON THE SCENE

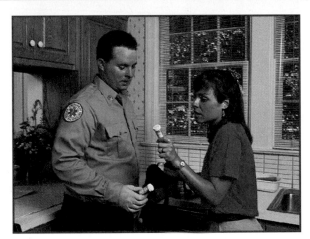

On a bright fall morning, Peggy Martin dropped by her mother's apartment. She finds her mother unconscious in bed and dials 911. You pull on gloves as you arrive at the scene. You ring the doorbell and introduce yourself to Peggy when she answers. She leads you to a bedroom, nervously saying, "Mom's in here. I can't wake her up." Her mother's name, Peggy tells you, is Laura Foster.

Your **scene size-up** reveals a safe scene and no apparent mechanism of injury. During your **initial assessment,** you find that Mrs. Foster is unresponsive but she is breathing and has a pulse. Because of her depressed mental status, you remove the pillow from behind her head, open her airway using the head-tilt, chin-lift, suction secretions from her mouth, and give her oxygen by nonrebreather mask. She is a high priority for rapid transport. You should call for paramedic back-up immediately.

You begin your **focused history and physical exam** and gather as much of a SAMPLE history as possible from the daughter. She tells you that she found her mother unconscious in bed about 15 minutes ago but does not know how long she had been that way. Mrs. Foster has no allergies that her daughter knows of.

"What medicines has your mother been taking?" you ask. "I don't know, but I'll get her purse," Peggy replies. She produces several containers of prescription medicines. You write down the information from the labels and tell Peggy you want to bring the containers along with her mother to the emergency department. You complete your on-scene assessment and place Mrs. Foster in the ambulance. En route to the hospital, you include the information about the medicines in your **radio report** and **documentation.** You perform an **ongoing assessment** every five minutes until you arrive at the ED. When you transfer Mrs. Foster to the ED staff, you also hand over the medicine containers.

In Mrs. Foster's case, the information provided by the medicine containers was critical. Although Peggy knew that her mother had been feeling "upset" lately, she did not know what medications her mother had been taking. The medications turned out to be tranquilizers, and Mrs. Foster may have accidentally overdosed—a clue that allowed the ED staff to treat Mrs. Foster quickly and effectively. ■

The study of drugs—their sources, characteristics, and effects—is called **pharmacology**. In the On the Scene scenario, recall that you did not ask Mrs. Foster's daughter, "Is your mother on *drugs?*" Rather you used the term "medications," because the general public often associates the word *drugs* with illegal or abused substances. Among themselves, EMS personnel usually use the terms *medications* and *drugs* interchangeably.

This chapter discusses the medications carried by EMT-Bs on the ambulance, as well as the medications that you may assist the patient in taking with approval from medical direction. The forms of medications, the names of common types of medications, and why they are used are also covered.

■ MEDICATIONS AN EMT-B CAN ADMINISTER

There are six medications that an EMT-B can administer: *activated charcoal, oral glucose, oxygen, prescribed inhalers, nitroglycerin,* and *epinephrine*. The information below is a brief introduction to each of them.

Medications Carried on the Ambulance

As an EMT-B, you carry activated charcoal, oral glucose, and oxygen on the ambulance. The specific circumstances in which these drugs are used are discussed in the appropriate chapter of this text.

Activated Charcoal

Activated charcoal is a powder prepared from charred wood, usually pre-mixed with water (Figure 8–1). It is used to treat a poisoning or overdose where a substance was ingested and is in the patient's digestive tract. Activated charcoal absorbs poisons and prevents them from being absorbed by the body. (The procedure for administering activated charcoal is included in Chapter 11.)

Oral Glucose

Glucose is a kind of sugar. **Oral glucose** is a form of glucose that is taken by mouth to treat a patient with an altered mental status and a history of diabetes. The brain is very sensitive to low blood sugar, often caused by poorly managed diabetes, and this can cause an altered mental status. Oral glucose usually comes in a tube of gel (Figure 8–2) that you can apply to a tongue depressor and

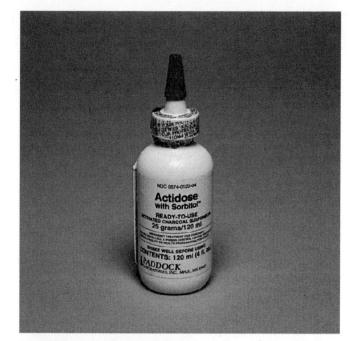

FIGURE 8–1 Activated charcoal is often used in poisoning cases.

place between the patient's cheek and gum. This area is very vascular, and the glucose is easily absorbed into the bloodstream and carried to the brain. This may begin to reverse the patient's life-threatening condition. (The procedure for administering oral glucose is included in Chapter 11.)

Oxygen

Oxygen is a gas commonly found in the atmosphere. Pure oxygen is used as a drug to treat any patient whose medical or traumatic condition causes him or her to be, or potentially be, hypoxic (Figure 8–3). Throughout your EMS training you have learned many situations in which oxygen

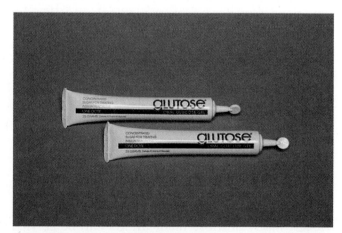

FIGURE 8–2 Oral glucose may help a diabetic.

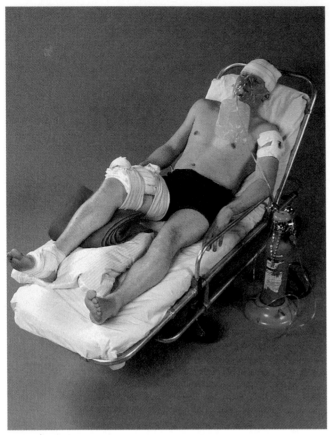

FIGURE 8–3 Oxygen is a powerful drug.

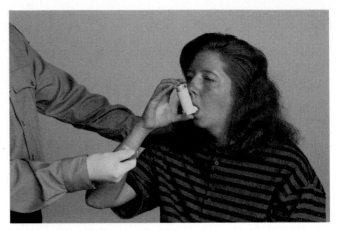

FIGURE 8–4 A prescribed inhaler may help a patient with respiratory problems.

should be administered. (The procedure for administering oxygen therapy is included in Chapter 4.)

Prescribed Medications

Three medications—prescribed inhalers, nitroglycerin, and epinephrine—are drugs that an EMT-B may assist the patient in taking. If the medications are prescribed for the patient by a physician, you need permission from medical direction by phone or radio, or there may be a standing medical order that permits you to assist a patient with these kinds of medication. *Always comply with the protocols of your EMS system.*

Prescribed Inhalers

There are various medications that patients may carry to help them through a period of breathing difficulty. Most often COPD patients (history of emphysema or chronic bronchitis) or asthmatics carry a "bronchodilator," a drug designed to dilate the constricted bronchial tubes to make breathing easier. Many of these medications can be carried in an **inhaler,** which contains an aerosol form of a

drug in a spray device with a mouthpiece so the patient can spray the medication directly into the airway (Figure 8–4).

Since many bronchodilators also have some effect on the heart, an increased heart rate or patient jitteriness are common side effects of treatment.

You need permission from medical direction to help a patient self-administer a prescribed inhaler. Be sure to determine that the inhaler is actually the patient's and not that of a family member or bystander. (The procedures for assisting a patient with an inhaler are included in Chapter 10.)

Nitroglycerin

Many patients with problems such as recurrent chest pain, or who have had a heart attack, carry **nitroglycerin** pills or spray. Nitroglycerin (Figure 8–5) is a drug that helps to dilate the coronary

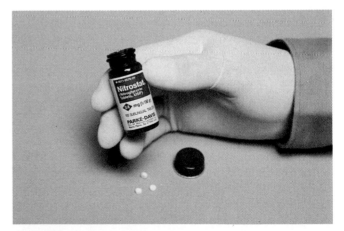

FIGURE 8–5 Nitroglycerin is often prescribed for chest pain.

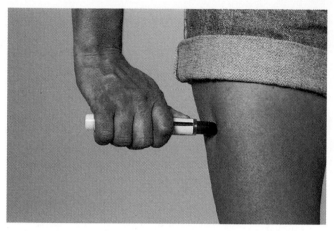

FIGURE 8–6 The Epi-Pen® is an epinephrine auto-injector.

vessels that supply the heart muscle with blood. It is often called "nitro." This drug is taken by the patient when he begins to have chest pain he believes to be cardiac in origin. It is not uncommon for EMT-Bs to treat patients who have already taken a nitro pill or who are carrying a bottle of nitroglycerin and have not thought to try one of their pills. You need permission from medical direction to help the patient self-administer his nitroglycerin. Be sure to determine that the nitroglycerin is actually the patient's and not that of a family member or bystander.

Since nitro causes a dilation of blood vessels, a drop in blood pressure is a potential side effect of administration. If this occurs, lay the patient flat and re-contact medical direction. (The procedures for assisting a patient with nitro are covered in Chapter 9.)

Epinephrine Auto-Injectors

When a patient is highly allergic to substances like shellfish or penicillin, or to a bee sting or a snake bite, he may have a very severe reaction. This reaction may cause airway obstruction and/ or cardiovascular collapse. This **anaphylactic reaction** can be reversed by using a drug called **epinephrine.** Epinephrine is a medication that will help to constrict the blood vessels, correct heart rhythm problems, and relax airway passages. Because severe allergic reactions are almost immediately life-threatening, epinephrine must be administered quickly. Many patients who are prone to severe allergic reactions carry an epinephrine auto-injector (Figure 8-6). This is a syringe with a spring-loaded needle that will release and inject epinephrine into the muscle when the auto-injector is pushed against the

thigh. If you need to assist a patient with the use of his epinephrine auto-injector, be sure to determine that the auto-injector is actually the patient's and not that of someone else.

Since epinephrine has a potent effect on the heart and vascular system, increased heart rate and blood pressure commonly occur after epinephrine administration. (The procedures for assisting a patient with epinephrine are covered in Chapter 10.)

■ GENERAL INFORMATION ABOUT MEDICATIONS

Drug Names

Each drug is found in *U.S. Pharmacopoeia* (USP), a comprehensive government publication, listed by its generic name (a general name that is not the brand name of any manufacturer). Actually, each drug has at least three names: the chemical name, the generic name, and one or more trade (brand) names given the drug by various manufacturers. For example, *epinephrine* is a generic drug name. Its chemical name is B-(e,4 dihydroxyphenyl)-a-methylaminoethanol. (Chemical names are technical formulas used only by scientists or manufacturers.) Epi-Pen® is the trade name of an epinephrine auto-injector.

What You Need to Know to Give a Medication

Every drug has **indications,** or specific circumstances, when it is appropriate to administer the drug to a patient. For example, nitro is indicated when a patient has squeezing, dull pressure chest pain.

Each drug also has **contraindications,** or specific circumstances when it is *not* appropriate, and may be harmful, to administer to a patient. For example, nitro is contraindicated if the patient has low blood pressure, because nitro, in dilating the coronary arteries, causes a slight drop in the systolic BP.

As discussed above, a **side effect** is any action of a drug other than the desired actions. Some side effects are predictable, like the drop in BP from nitro. If you were not aware of this side effect and gave the drug to a patient who started out with low BP, the results could be devastating. The patient's BP might "bottom out," which is definitely not a desirable effect for a cardiac patient.

Forms of Medications

Medications come in different forms. A few examples are:

- Compressed powders or tablets, such as nitro pills
- Liquids for injection, such as the epinephrine in an auto-injector
- Gels, such as the paste in a tube of oral glucose
- Suspensions, such as the thick slurry of activated charcoal in water
- Fine powder for inhalation, such as that in a prescribed inhaler
- Gases for inhalation, such as oxygen
- Sublingual (under-the-tongue) sprays such as a nitro spray
- Liquid that is vaporized, such as a fixed-dose nebulizer

Medication Administration Rights

Before administering a drug to any patient, you must confirm the order, write it down, and then check the "four rights" by asking yourself the following questions as you select the drug and confirm that it is not expired.

- Do I have the *right patient?*
- Is this the *right medication?*
- Is this the *right dose?* (Generally a dose is given in milligrams.) and,
- Am I giving this drug by the *right route* of administration?

The route of drug administration affects the rate the drug enters the bloodstream and arrives at its target organ to achieve its desired effect. Methods of administration include:

- Oral, or swallowed
- Intravenous, or injected into a vein
- Intramuscular, or injected into a muscle
- Sublingual, or dissolved under the tongue
- Subcutaneous, or injected into the deep skin
- Endotracheal, sprayed into the ET tube and absorbed by the lungs
- Inhaled, or breathed into the lungs in tiny aerosol particles from an inhaler or mask

After any drug is given to a patient, it is important that you reassess the patient to see how the drug has affected him. Obtain another set of vitals and compare them to the baseline vitals you took before administering the drug. The ongoing assessment should include an evaluation of the changes in the patient's condition and vital signs after administration of medicine. Be sure to always document the patient's response to each drug intervention. For example, "The respiratory distress decreased after five minutes of oxygen by nonrebreather mask."

Medications Patients Often Take

It would be impossible to memorize all the types of medications your patients may be taking. Mrs. Foster in the On the Scene scenario was taking tranquilizers. She might also have been taking or misusing other drugs, causing her altered mental status. Perhaps she was taking insulin for diabetes, or Dilantin® to control seizures, or morphine for pain, or Inderal® for a heart rhythm disorder. The drugs a patient is taking are often a clue to a preexisting medical condition or, if improperly used, may be a cause of his or her current problem.

It is a good idea to have a resource from which you can find out additional information about a patient's medications en route to the hospital. Many ambulances carry a *Physician's Desk Reference,* or *PDR,* for this purpose. Most EMT-Bs carry, or have available to them, a pocket guide that contains information such as generally used abbreviations. These guides list commonly prescribed medications along with the general category of that drug to help you understand what it is used for.

Preceptor Pearl

Remember that your main purpose in finding out what medications the patient is taking is *not* to make a diagnosis but to report this information to the ED staff. ❖

The list below gives the six common categories of drugs you find in the field that are relevant to patient care, with a few examples of drugs in each category. (The trade names are capitalized; the generic names are not.) There are many other categories in addition to those listed here.

- *Analgesics*—drugs prescribed for pain relief. Examples: Darvon (propoxyphene), morphine,

Nubain (nalbuphine),Tylenol (acetaminophen), Advil (ibuprofen), aspirin, codeine, and methadone.

- *Antiarrhythmics*—drugs prescribed for heart rhythm disorders. Examples: Lanoxin (digoxin), Inderal (propranolol), and Pronestyl (procainamide).

- *Anticonvulsants*—drugs prescribed for prevention and control of seizures. Examples: Dilantin (phenytoin), Mysoline (primidone), phenobarbital, Zarnotin (ethosuximide), and Tegretol (carbamazepine).

- *Antihypertensives*—drugs prescribed to reduce high blood pressure. They may act by controlling the sympathetic nervous system to relax the arterioles. They may also increase salt and water elimination. Examples: Capoten (captopril), Tenormin (atenolol), Lasix (furosemide), Esidrix (hydrochlorothiazide), and Aldomet (methyldopa).

- *Bronchodilators*—drugs that relax the smooth muscles of the bronchial tubes. These medications provide relief of bronchial asthma and other allergies affecting the respiratory system. Examples: Alupent (metaproterenol), Bronkosol (isoetharine), Slo-bid (theophylline), Brethaire (terbutaline), and Ventolin or Proventil (albuterol).

- *Antidiabetic agents*—drugs prescribed to control a hyperglycemic patient's sugar level and to provide insulin. Examples: Novolin or Humulin (insulin), Orinase (tolbutamide), Glucotrol (glipzide), Diabeta or Micronase (glyburide), and Diabinese (chlorpropamide).

CHAPTER REVIEW

■ SUMMARY

The medications activated charcoal, oral glucose, and oxygen are carried on the ambulance so the EMT-B may administer them to patients under specific conditions. The following medications are those that, if prescribed for the patient, the EMT-B may assist the patient in using or taking: prescribed inhalers, nitroglycerin, and epinephrine auto-injectors. You may need to have permission from medical direction to assist the patient with a prescribed inhaler, nitroglycerin, or an epinephrine auto-injector. Always follow your local protocols.

There are a variety of medications that patients may be taking. You will try to establish this during the SAMPLE history. These drugs may be identified by a variety of generic and trade names. Your main purpose in finding out what drugs the patient is taking is to report this information to the ED staff.

■ REVIEW QUESTIONS

1. Name the drugs that are carried on an ambulance and that may be administered by the EMT-B under certain circumstances without specific orders from medical direction.

2. Name the drugs an EMT-B may assist a patient in taking if they have been prescribed for him and with approval by medical direction.

3. Name five different forms of drugs.

4. Name the "four rights" you must check before administering a drug.

5. Name seven routes by which drugs may be administered.

6. List medications used to control hypertension.

7. Name six categories of medications found in the field.

8. List drugs used to control diabetes.

9. List drugs a patient with a history of COPD may be taking.

10. List drugs a patient with a seizure history may be taking.

CHAPTER 9

Medical Emergencies
■ *Cardiac*

■ *Trauma was the reason modern EMS systems came into being, but cardiac emergencies are what made EMS a household term. Laypeople don't know a joule from a diamond, but they do know that when someone is defibrillated, he jumps off the floor. In fact, the public have seen so much about EMS on television that they have come to expect actions like defibrillation.*

Public awareness about nitroglycerin also runs high.

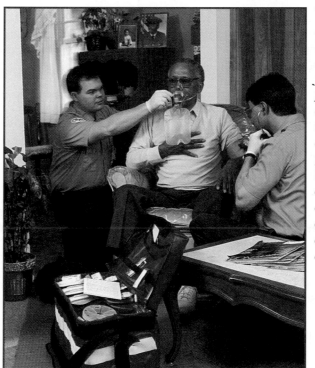

What medical movie doesn't have a character popping at least one nitro? Most people know that nitroglycerin is for chest pain, but they don't pretend to understand it. In addition, there are some things you need to know about nitroglycerin before you help a patient in taking his own. This chapter will go over the management of cardiac problems, with special emphasis on automated defibrillation and nitroglycerin administration.

MAKING THE TRANSITION

- The emphasis in EMT-B courses has changed from distinguishing among the different causes of cardiac problems to management based on the patient's signs and symptoms.
- When your patient has chest pain, an adequate blood pressure, and his own nitroglycerin, you can now assist him in taking it.
- As an EMT-B, you are expected to be able to operate an automated external defibrillator.

OBJECTIVES

The numbered objectives below are from the United States Department of Transportation 1994 EMT-Basic National Standard Curriculum. Objectives with colored bullets that follow in italics are from the EMT-Basic Transitional Program.

■ KNOWLEDGE AND ATTITUDE

At the completion of this lesson, you should be able to:

1. Describe the structure and function of the cardiovascular system. (p. 133)

2. Describe the emergency medical care of the patient experiencing chest pain/discomfort. (pp. 134–137)

3. List the indications for automated external defibrillation (AED). (pp. 139, 141)

4. List the contraindications for automated external defibrillation. (pp. 139, 140)

5. Define the role of the EMT-B in the emergency cardiac care system. (pp. 132–133)

6. Explain the impact of age and weight on defibrillation. (pp. 140, 141)

7. Discuss the position of comfort for patients with various cardiac emergencies. (p. 134)

8. Establish the relationship between airway management and the patient with cardiovascular compromise. (p. 134)

9. Predict the relationship between the patient experiencing cardiovascular compromise and basic life support. (pp. 146–147)

10. Discuss the fundamentals of early defibrillation. (p. 137)

11. Explain the rationale for early defibrillation. (p. 137)

12. Explain that not all chest pain patients result in cardiac arrest and, therefore, do not need to be attached to an automated external defibrillator. (pp. 132–133, 137–138)

13. Explain the importance of prehospital ACLS intervention if it is available. (pp. 137–138)

14. Explain the importance of urgent transport to a facility with Advanced Cardiac Life Support if it is not available in the prehospital setting. (pp. 137, 139, 146)

15. Discuss the various types of automated external defibrillators. (pp. 139–140)

16. Differentiate between the fully automated and the semiautomated defibrillator. (pp. 139–140)

17. Discuss the procedures that must be taken into consideration for standard operations of the various types of automated external defibrillators. (pp. 139–147)

18. State the reasons for assuring that the patient is pulseless and apneic when using the automated external defibrillator. (pp. 139–141)

19. Discuss the circumstances that may result in inappropriate shocks. (pp. 139, 141)

20. Explain the considerations for interruption of CPR, when using the automated external defibrillator. (p. 141)

21. Discuss the advantages and disadvantages of automated external defibrillators. (pp. 145–146)

22. Summarize the speed of operation of automated external defibrillation. (p. 145)

23. Discuss the use of remote defibrillation through adhesive pads. (pp. 145–146)

24. Discuss the special considerations for rhythm monitoring. (pp. 139, 141)

25. List the steps in the operation of the automated external defibrillator. (pp. 141–145)

26. Discuss the standard of care that should be used to provide care to a patient with persistent ventricular fibrillation and no available ACLS. (p. 146)

27. Discuss the standard of care that should be used to provide care to a patient with recurrent ventricular fibrillation and no available ACLS. (p. 147)

28. Differentiate between the single rescuer and multi-rescuer care with an automated external defibrillator. (pp. 146–147)

29. Explain the reason for pulses not being checked between shocks with an automated external defibrillator. (p. 145)

30. Discuss the importance of coordinating ACLS trained providers with personnel using automated external defibrillators. (p. 146)

31. Discuss the importance of post-resuscitation care. (p. 147)

32. List the components of post-resuscitation care. (p. 147)

33. Explain the importance of frequent practice with the automated external defibrillator. (p. 147)

34. Discuss the need to complete the Automated Defibrillator: Operator's Shift Checklist. (pp. 147, 148)

35. Discuss the role of the American Heart Association (AHA) in the use of automated external defibrillation. (pp. 137, 138)

36. Explain the role medical direction plays in the use of automated external defibrillation. (p. 147)

37. State the reasons why a case review should be completed following the use of the automated external defibrillator. (p. 147)

38. Discuss the components that should be included in a case review. (p. 147)

39. Discuss the goal of quality improvement in automated external defibrillation. (p. 147)

40. Recognize the need for medical direction of protocols to assist in the emergency medical care of the patient with chest pain. (pp. 135, 137, 138)

41. List the indications for the use of nitroglycerin. (pp. 134, 137, 138)

42. State the contraindications and side effects for the use of nitroglycerin. (pp. 134, 138)

43. Define the function of all controls on an automated external defibrillator, and describe event documentation and battery defibrillator maintenance. (pp. 141–145, 147)

44. Defend the reasons for obtaining initial training in automated external defibrillation and the importance of continuing education. (p. 147)

45. Defend the reason for maintenance of automated external defibrillators. (p. 147)

46. Explain the rationale for administering nitroglycerin to a patient with chest pain or discomfort. (pp. 132, 134)

● *Describe the relationship between assessment findings and medical interventions for cardiac emergencies. (pp. 132–133)*

● *Defend the rationale for the EMT-Basic to carry and assist with medications. (pp. 132, 134)*

■ SKILLS

1. Demonstrate the assessment and emergency medical care of a patient experiencing chest pain/discomfort.

2. Demonstrate the application and operation of the automated external defibrillator.

3. Demonstrate the maintenance of an automated external defibrillator.

4. Demonstrate the assessment and documentation of patient response to the automated external defibrillator.

5. Demonstrate the skills necessary to complete the Automated Defibrillator: Operator's Shift Checklist.

6. Perform the steps in facilitating the use of nitroglycerin for chest pain or discomfort.

7. Demonstrate the assessment and documentation of patient response to nitroglycerin.

8. Practice completing a prehospital care report for patients with cardiac emergencies.

● *Given medical scenarios, demonstrate the ability to properly assess the patient and demonstrate the ability to properly utilize the intervention of nitroglycerin.*

● *Given a cardiac arrest scenario, demonstrate the use of the AED without missing any critical criteria listed on the skill sheets in the 1994 EMT-Basic Transitional Program.*

You receive a call for a man who has collapsed at work. The caller tells your dispatcher that the patient is unconscious and someone has started CPR. You arrive four minutes after receiving the call. You find an approximately 60-year-old man lying on the floor with a secretary doing CPR on him. As she sees you come in the door, she says, "Thank goodness you're here!" and stops CPR.

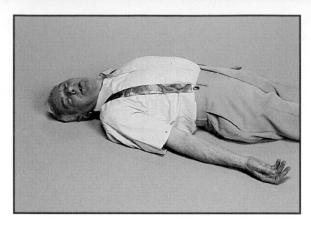

Your partner immediately moves to the patient's head as you position yourself and your automated external defibrillator next to the patient's chest. As your partner confirms that the patient is unresponsive, not breathing, and pulseless, you open up the automated external defibrillator and begin your report to the tape recorder.

You apply the monitoring/defibrillation pads to the patient's chest. When the machine signals that it is ready, you say, "Stop CPR and clear the patient." You look to be sure no one is touching the patient and press the analyze button. The AED begins to charge up and in about 7 or 8 seconds indicates that you should deliver a shock. You say "Clear!" in a loud voice, look to be sure no one is touching the patient, and press the shock button. The patient jumps a little bit. You press the analyze button again and repeat the steps to deliver a second shock. You press the analyze button a third time, but this time the AED gives you a "No shock" message.

Your partner checks the patient's carotid and reports that she finds a slow pulse. When she checks for breathing, she finds none, so she begins ventilating the patient with a flow-restricted, oxygen-powered ventilation device. You call for ALS, but no one is available right now. With help from a police officer, you get the patient onto a spine board and the stretcher, being sure to monitor the patient's pulse frequently and not interfere with your partner's ventilations.

En route to the hospital, the patient begins to breathe on his own. You continue to ventilate him until his breathing is adequate and then switch him over to a nonrebreather mask at 15 liters of oxygen per minute. By the time you arrive at the emergency department, the patient is starting to wake up.

You follow up a few days later with a doctor in the emergency department and discover that the patient is doing well after suffering a myocardial infarction. He is scheduled to be discharged after some more tests and rehabilitation. ■

More than a half million people die from cardiovascular disease in the United States every year. Many of these deaths occur before the patient reaches a hospital. However, defibrillation, if performed early enough, can prevent some of them. Rapid defibrillation is the single most important factor in increasing survival from cardiac arrest caused by ventricular fibrillation.

For patients who are not in cardiac arrest but who are experiencing cardiac-related chest pain, EMT-Bs can now, in addition to oxygen administration, assist them in taking their own nitroglycerin. This can sometimes relieve pain and the anxiety that accompanies it. When patients meet certain conditions, it should be safe for the EMT-B to assist them in taking this medication.

■ CARDIAC COMPROMISE

In your EMT-A course, your instructor probably described a number of cardiac conditions, including myocardial infarction, angina pectoris, congestive heart failure, and pulmonary edema. If you had no health care experience, these descriptions probably didn't mean much to you. Imagining what a living, breathing patient looks like based on a list of signs and symptoms is very difficult if you don't have any firsthand experience with sick people. Now that you have had some experience, you may feel comfortable making a tentative "diagnosis" or conclusion about what the cause of the patient's condition may be. But at the same time, you start treating the patient without letting the time-consuming process of determining the cause delay your care. After all, even physicians sometimes have difficulty reaching the correct diagnosis in these cases.

Because it is so difficult to determine with certainty a cardiac patient's diagnosis, it is important to have a high index of suspicion and to overtreat when in doubt. At the EMT-B level, the risk of overtreatment is extremely low and the potential benefit is very high. Rather than spend time determining whether a patient is having a myocardial infarction (MI) or an episode of angina, it is more appropriate to begin treatment and prompt transport.

Patient Assessment **Cardiac Compromise**

Your EMT-A book listed different cardiac conditions with their accompanying signs and symptoms. It then described the treatment for each condition. There may have been minor differences, but the essential treatment was the same for all of them. Since these cardiac conditions share the same principles of management, the EMT-B curriculum groups all of these conditions together into one category called **cardiac compromise**.

Signs and Symptoms
Cardiac compromise is characterized by any of a number of signs and symptoms such as:

- pain or a squeezing, dull pressure in the chest, commonly radiating down the arms or up to the jaw
- difficulty breathing
- a feeling of impending doom
- epigastric pain or discomfort
- nausea and vomiting
- sudden onset of sweating.

These signs and symptoms can arise for a number of reasons. When the heart is functioning normally, both the mechanical and electrical aspects function in a coordinated manner. When one of these systems malfunctions, however, the patient can experience any one of a number of conditions that fall into the category of cardiac compromise. ■

However, before we consider these conditions, let's briefly review the anatomy and physiology of the heart. The normal heart has four chambers,

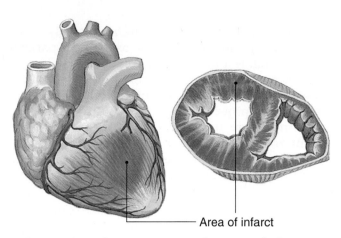

FIGURE 9–1 Cross section of myocardial infarction.

an atrium and a ventricle on both the left and right sides. Blood comes into the atrium, flows into the ventricle, and is then pumped out of the heart. The left side of the heart pumps blood out through the aorta where it then is channeled through arteries, arterioles, and capillaries throughout the body. When the blood gets to the capillaries, it gives oxygen and nutrients to the cells, and picks up carbon dioxide and wastes in exchange. The blood then travels through venules and veins to the right side of the heart. Here it is pumped out through the pulmonary arteries to the capillaries surrounding the alveoli in the lungs. Again, oxygen and carbon dioxide are exchanged and the blood returns via the pulmonary veins to the left side of the heart where it begins the cycle again.

Like any muscle, the heart needs oxygen and nutrients and a way to get rid of carbon dioxide and wastes. This is done through the coronary arteries, a system of blood vessels that come off the aorta immediately after it leaves the heart. If one or more of these arteries become blocked, the patient may (or may not) experience symptoms. If the blockage is sufficient to cut off enough of the blood supply to cause death of heart tissue, the patient has had a **myocardial infarction (MI)** or heart attack (Figure 9–1). Depending on the location and extent of the damage, the patient may sustain a cardiac arrest, or experience chest pain, epigastric distress, sudden onset of weakness and sweating, or nothing at all.

If some of the heart tissue has its blood supply temporarily restricted (but not to the point of causing cell death), the patient has **angina pectoris**. Typically during one of these episodes, the patient experiences chest pain that is relieved by stopping strenuous activity, taking nitroglycerin, or increasing the percentage of oxygen the patient is breathing. Not all cases of angina are typical or respond to these measures, though. Differentiating MI from angina can be difficult at times—even for experienced physicians.

Congestive heart failure (CHF) is another common cardiac problem seen in EMS systems. This condition is characterized by buildup of fluid in the lungs or other areas of the body. It results from an inability of one or both sides of the heart to pump out all the blood that is coming in. If the trouble is on the left side (as often happens), the blood coming into the left side of the heart from the lungs begins to back up. The pressure in the pulmonary veins increases, causing the pressure in the capillaries surrounding the alveoli to increase also. The distance between a capillary and an alveolus is extremely small in order to allow oxygen and carbon dioxide to pass through. When fluid pressure in the capillaries increases significantly, this short distance allows fluid to pass into the alveoli, obstructing the airway. This is why you sometimes see patients with severe CHF or pulmonary edema coughing up pink, frothy sputum.

If the right side of the heart is experiencing difficulty, blood backs up into the systemic circulation. In this case, you may see distended neck veins and edema in the ankles, among other things.

The electrical system of the heart is an integral part of this activity. The heart has specialized fibers that conduct electrical impulses that stimulate the cells in the heart to contract. Ordinarily, the heart's own natural pacemaker in the right atrium, called the **sinoatrial node**, is the starting point for these impulses, which simultaneously travel to both the atria and the ventricles. The atria immediately contract and squeeze blood into the ventricles, providing them with about 10% to 20% more blood than if the atria did not do this. The impulses to the ventricles don't arrive until about one- to two-tenths of a second later, allowing time for this "priming" of the pump to occur. An abnormality with the conduction system can cause a number of different problems. For example, the patient's heart rate may become extremely fast or extremely slow.

Sometimes, the heart's electrical system loses all ability to regulate these impulses and the cells all fire randomly (**ventricular fibrillation, or VF**). The patient's heart then no longer beats in a coordinated fashion and the patient experiences cardiac arrest.

As you can see, there are many different presentations that patients with cardiac problems can have. However the patient presents, you will still need to perform the following:

- Perform the initial assessment.
- Perform a focused history and physical exam. Inquire about onset, provocation, quality, radiation, severity, and time. Get a SAMPLE history.
- Take baseline vital signs.

■ Patient Care Cardiac Compromise

The mainstay of management of cardiac compromise is oxygen. A commonly administered medication, oxygen can correct the hypoxia that sometimes accompanies cardiac emergencies (Skill Summary 9–1). There is virtually no risk to the patient and the potential benefit is very high. The other medication that may be appropriate is nitroglycerin (NTG). Nitroglycerin is a very powerful drug that dilates blood vessels and reduces the workload of the heart. This reduces the heart's demand for oxygen and can prevent further hypoxic damage to the heart. Because nitroglycerin is so powerful and has significant side effects (like hypotension), it is not for every patient. It should be safe to administer nitroglycerin to a patient who has been evaluated by a physician and received a prescription for it. Even then, it is taken only for specific reasons, e.g., chest pain or discomfort, and can still occasionally produce serious side effects.

Emergency Care Steps
1. Place the patient in a position of comfort, typically sitting up. This is the desirable position for patients with difficulty breathing. Patients who are hypotensive (systolic blood pressure less than 90) will usually feel better lying down. This position allows more blood to flow to the brain. Occasionally, you will see a patient who has both difficulty breathing and hypotension, in which case it may not be easy to find a good position. The best way to determine this is to ask the patient what position will relieve his difficulty breathing without making him weak or lightheaded.
2. Apply high-concentration oxygen through a nonrebreather mask if this has not already been done. If the patient has or develops an altered mental status, you will need to open and maintain his airway. If he is not breathing adequately, you will also need to ventilate him.

Chest Pain Management

FIRST take body substance isolation precautions.

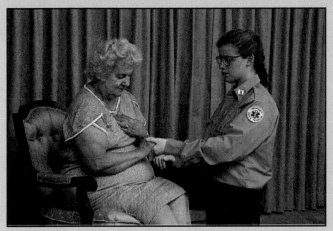

1. Perform the initial assessment.

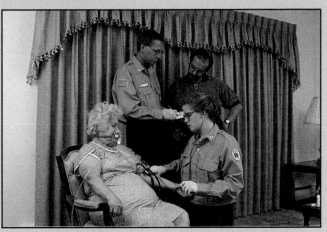

2. Provide high-concentration oxygen by non-rebreather mask. Perform the focused history and physical exam for a medical patient. Document findings.

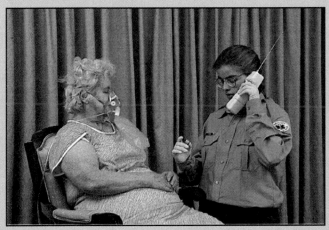

3. If patient meets nitroglycerin criteria and has prescribed nitroglycerin, ask the patient about the last dose taken. Consult medical direction with regard to assisting the patient in taking the medication.

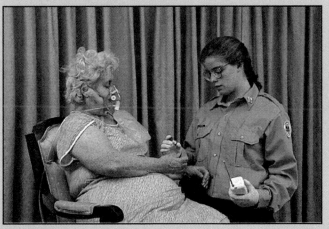

4. Check the four rights: right patient, right drug, right dose, right route. Check the expiration date.

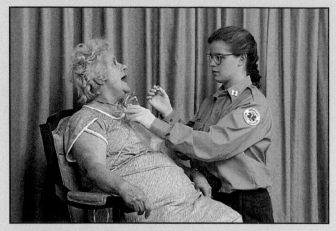

5. Remove oxygen mask. Ask patient to open mouth and lift tongue.

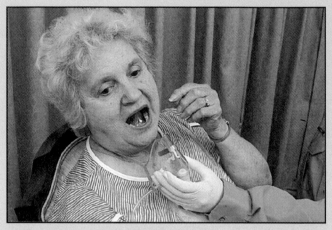

6. Place the nitroglycerin tablet under the tongue, or ...

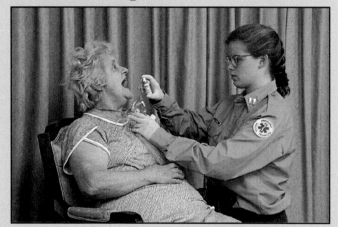

7. ... if the nitroglycerin is in spray form, spray the medication under the tongue according to label directions.

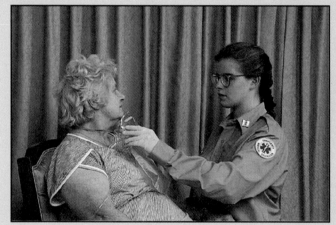

8. Have patient close mouth and hold the nitroglycerin under the tongue. This is an area where the medication will be quickly absorbed.

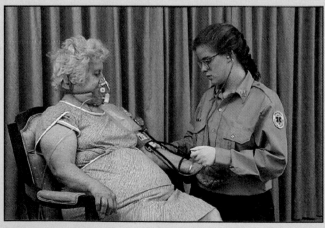

9. Replace oxygen mask. Reassess the patient. Document findings.

Always be prepared for the patient to go into cardiac arrest.

3. Call ALS if available in your system.
4. a. Transport promptly if the patient has any one of these things:
   - no history of cardiac problems, or
   - a history of cardiac problems, but does not have nitroglycerin, or
   - a systolic blood pressure of less than 100.

   b. Give the patient (or help the patient take) nitroglycerin if all of the following conditions are met (Skill Summary 9–2):
   - the patient complains of chest pain
   - the patient has a history of cardiac problems
   - the patient's physician has prescribed nitroglycerin (NTG)
   - the patient has the nitroglycerin with him
   - the systolic blood pressure is greater than 100, and
   - medical direction authorizes administration of the medication.

   c. After giving one dose of the nitroglycerin, repeat another dose in 3 to 5 minutes if all of the following conditions are met:
   - the patient experiences no relief, and
   - the systolic blood pressure remains greater than 100, and
   - medical direction authorizes another dose of the medication.

Administer up to a maximum of three doses of nitroglycerin, reassessing vital signs and chest pain after each dose. If the blood pressure falls below 100 systolic, treat the patient for shock (hypoperfusion). Transport promptly. ■

Preceptor Pearl

The new EMT-B student doesn't have the experience you have. Although giving oxygen may seem second nature to you, the student may still find this a new experience. You may be more interested in what is causing the patient's condition than in the routine aspects of oxygen administration. Before you overwhelm the student with information about cardiac emergencies, find out how much experience the student has, how comfortable he or she is with cardiac emergencies, and how much interest the student has in learning more. With a brand new, inexperienced student, it may be appropriate just to discuss in general terms what may be going on with the patient. If the student has the background and interest, you may be able to cover this information and also give the student the benefit of your additional experience and education by describing the pathophysiology of the patient's condition. However, remember to put the student's need to learn before your desire to teach. ✤

■ CARDIAC ARREST

Only one to two percent of the emergency calls in a typical EMS system are cardiac arrests, but many systems dedicate a significant amount of their resources to handling these cases. This is probably related to both the ancient desire to bring someone back from the dead and the recent advances in technology that sometimes allow us to actually accomplish this.

The Chain of Survival

For the patient in cardiac arrest to have the greatest possible chance of survival, the EMS system must be configured properly and EMS responders must act quickly and efficiently. The American Heart Association has summarized the four major factors that affect the likelihood of recovery from cardiac arrest: early access, early CPR, early defibrillation, and early advanced care. Together, these elements make up the chain of survival (Figure 9–2).

Early access means that someone who sees a patient collapse, or finds the patient already collapsed, notifies EMS quickly. This depends on having a well-educated public, an easy-to-remember phone number (like 9–1–1), and an efficient dispatch system.

Early CPR depends on having either a CPR-trained bystander nearby or being able to send first responders who can perform CPR. This is where the value of training laypeople in CPR becomes apparent.

Early defibrillation means delivering the first defibrillatory shock while it can still do some good. Every minute a heart remains in VF without being defibrillated reduces the patient's chance of survival by 8% to 12%. This is why virtually no one is resuscitated if the response time of the person with the defibrillator is more than 8 minutes. Automated defibrillation keeps to a minimum the time from arrival of the defibrillator to delivery of the first shock.

A few patients arrest after the arrival of EMS. This is why you must always be prepared for the patient to go into cardiac arrest. Most patients you see in cardiac arrest, though, are already pulseless when EMS receives the call.

Early advanced care refers to interventions such as endotracheal intubation and administration of medications. Strengthening the first three elements in the chain of survival can produce

Nitroglycerin

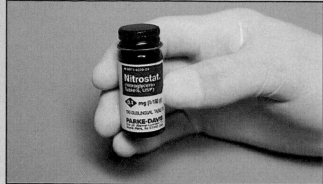

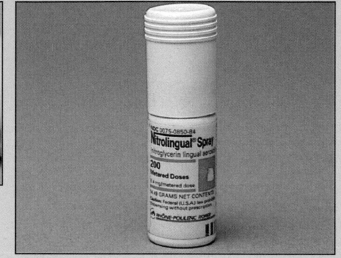

MEDICATION NAME
1. Generic: nitroglycerin
2. Trade: Nitrostat™, Nitrolingual® Spray

INDICATIONS
All of the following conditions must be met:
1. The patient complains of chest pain.
2. The patient has a history of cardiac problems.
3. The patient's physician has prescribed nitroglycerin (NTG).
4. The systolic blood pressure is greater than 100 systolic.
5. Medical direction authorizes administration of the medication.

CONTRAINDICATIONS
1. The patient has hypotension or a systolic blood pressure below 100.
2. The patient has a head injury.
3. The patient is an infant or child.
4. The patient has already taken the maximum prescribed dose.

MEDICATION FORM
Tablet, sublingual (under-the-tongue) spray

DOSAGE
One dose, repeat in 3 to 5 minutes. If no relief, systolic blood pressure remains above 100, and if authorized by medical direction, up to a maximum of three doses.

ADMINISTRATION
1. Perform focused assessment for cardiac patient.
2. Take blood pressure. (Systolic pressure must be above 100.)
3. Contact medical direction if no standing orders.
4. Assure right medication, right patient, right dose, right route. Check expiration date.
5. Assure patient is alert.
6. Question patient on last dose taken and effects. Assure understanding of route of administration.
7. Ask patient to lift tongue and place tablet or spray dose under tongue (while wearing gloves) or have patient place tablet or spray under tongue.
8. Have patient keep mouth closed with tablet under tongue (without swallowing) until dissolved and absorbed.
9. Recheck blood pressure within 2 minutes.
10. Record administration, route, and time.
11. Perform reassessment.

ACTIONS
1. Relaxes blood vessels
2. Decreases workload of heart

SIDE EFFECTS
1. Hypotension (lowers blood pressure)
2. Headache
3. Pulse rate changes

REASSESSMENT STRATEGIES
1. Monitor blood pressure.
2. Ask patient about effect on pain relief.
3. Seek medical direction before readministering.
4. Record assessments.

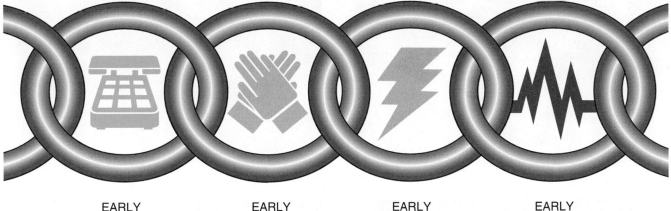

Chain of Survival

EARLY
ACCESS

EARLY
CPR

EARLY
DEFIBRILLATION

EARLY
ADVANCED CARE

FIGURE 9–2 The Chain of Survival (American Heart Association).

significant improvements. Strengthening the fourth element may improve the survival rate even further.

As an EMT-B, your responsibilities at a cardiac arrest include not only performing one- and two-rescuer CPR, but also

- using an automated external defibrillator
- requesting ALS backup (when appropriate)
- ventilating with a bag-valve-mask or flow-restricted, oxygen-powered ventilation device
- lifting and moving the patient
- suctioning, using airway adjuncts
- interviewing family members and bystanders to obtain information related to the arrest.

Types of Automated External Defibrillators

Defibrillators are either manual or automated. A manual defibrillator is the kind typically found in an emergency department. The operator interprets the electrocardiographic (ECG) rhythm and makes the decision whether to shock. An automated defibrillator, on the other hand, has a micro-processor that interprets the rhythm and deter-

mines whether it is appropriate to deliver a shock. A fully automated defibrillator operates without the need for any action by the operator except to turn on the power and attach the monitoring/defibrillation pads to the patient. A semi-automatic defibrillator, after analyzing the rhythm, advises the EMT-B to deliver a shock, if appropriate. Semi-automatic defibrillators are sometimes called shock advisory defibrillators (Figure 9–3).

Automated defibrillators have been extremely accurate in discriminating between patients who do and do not need shocks. The most common reason for an incorrect decision by an automated defibrillator is improper use by the person operating the machine, e.g., attaching an AED to a patient who has a pulse or not charging the batteries. Occasionally, an AED will make an error that is not the result of operator error. In this case, the machine will almost always fail to deliver a shock rather than deliver an inappropriate shock.

An EMT-B should not attach an AED to a patient who has a pulse because many defibrillators advise shocks for ventricular tachycardia when the rate exceeds a certain value, for example, above 180 beats per minute. You should attach an AED only to an unresponsive, pulseless, nonbreathing patient to avoid delivering inappropriate shocks.

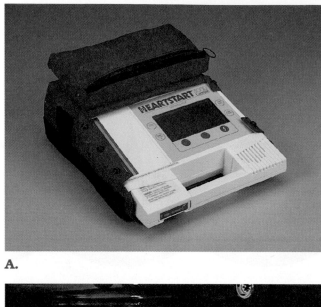

A.

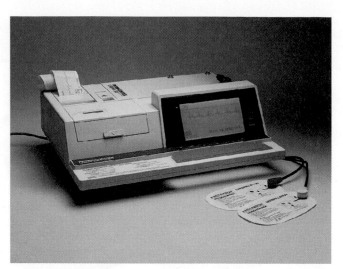

B.

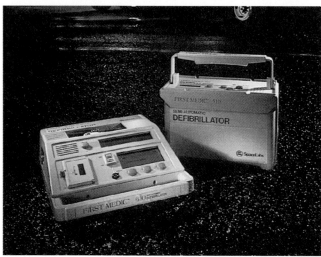

C.

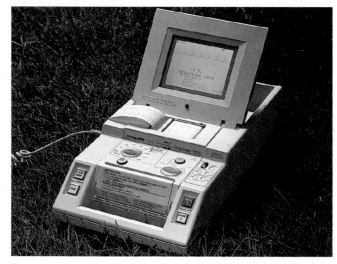

D.

FIGURE 9–3 AEDs from **A.** Laerdal, **B.** PhysioControl, **C.** First Medic, and **D.** Marquette.

PEDIATRIC HIGHLIGHT

Infants and children rarely go into cardiac arrest because of ventricular fibrillation. In adults, cardiac arrest is often the result of a problem with the heart, the most common cause being myocardial infarction. In infants and children, on the other hand, cardiac arrest is typically the end result of a respiratory problem. This causes them to become bradycardic and then asystolic. Rarely do they go into VF.

Since defibrillation is the appropriate treatment for VF, this means a defibrillator has very limited value in the treatment of a pediatric arrest patient. The best treatment for

an infant or child in arrest is CPR, with special attention to the airway and ventilation, along with prompt transport to an appropriate facility. Using an AED on a child will delay transport without any reason to believe that it will help the patient. ◼

◼ Patient Assessment **Cardiac Arrest**

As with all calls, you should protect yourself from infectious diseases by using body substance isolation equipment and procedures. This is especially important in the case of a cardiac arrest, where blood and other body fluids are commonly found.

- Perform the initial assessment. If a bystander is doing CPR when you arrive, have the bystander stop. Verify pulselessness and apnea. Look for external blood loss.

- After you have started or resumed CPR, you should perform a focused history and physical exam. Inquire about onset, trauma, and signs and symptoms that were present before the patient collapsed. Get a SAMPLE history if you can. Do not let history gathering interfere with or slow down defibrillation. ▪

Patient Care Cardiac Arrest

(Refer to Skill Summary 9–3 as you read the steps below and on p. 145.)

1. Begin or resume CPR.
2. Determine whether the patient is a candidate for the AED.
   a. If the patient is an adult (defined as at least 12 years old or 90 pounds for the purpose of defibrillation) who has not sustained trauma, proceed with the AED.
   b. If the patient is less than 12 years old and less than 90 pounds OR the patient has sustained trauma, do not attach the AED unless you are ordered to do so by medical direction. Continue CPR and transport.
3. Turn on the defibrillator power.
4. Begin the narrative if the AED has a voice recorder. You should describe who you are, what the situation is, and what you are doing as you do it. However, do not delay your actions in order to describe them.
5. Attach the monitoring-defibrillation pads to the cables.
6. Bare the patient's chest (if not already done) and place the pads so that the one attached to the white cable is in the angle between the sternum and the right clavicle and the one attached to the red cable is over the lower left ribs ("white to right, red to ribs"). Press the pads firmly on the chest to ensure good contact. Once in a while, you may have a male patient whose chest is so hairy that the pads do not make good contact. Use a hospital razor to quickly shave some of the hair away, and use a new pair of pads.
7. Stop CPR and clear the patient (make sure no one is touching the patient).

Note: About half of all patients in cardiac arrest have nonshockable heart rhythms. If this is the case, when you press the analysis button, the AED will give a "No shock" message. In other cases, the AED may give you a "Deliver shock" message and then, after one or more shocks are delivered, will give a "No shock" message on a subsequent try. (When the AED gives a "No shock" message, it may be very bad news: the patient has a non-shockable heart rhythm and cannot be helped by the defibrillator. Or it may be very good news: the electrical rhythm of the patient's heart has responded successfully to earlier shocks. In the latter case, even though the heart's electrical activity has recovered, another stint of CPR may be required to get enough oxygen into the muscle cells of the heart to start it beating again.)

Numbers 8 to 11 of the list below explain how to proceed if you get a "Deliver shock" message every time you press the analysis button.

Number 12 explains how to proceed if you get a "No shock" message when you press the analysis button.

If a "Deliver shock" message is received each time you press the analysis button,

8. When you get a "Deliver shock" message
   - Deliver the first shock.
   - Press the analysis button to reanalyze the rhythm (get a "Deliver shock" message), deliver a second shock.
   - Press the analysis button to reanalyze the rhythm (get a "Deliver shock" message), deliver a third shock.

   The set of shocks you have just delivered is called a set of three stacked shocks— "stacked" because they are delivered with no pause for a pulse check or CPR between the three shocks.

9. After the first set of three stacked shocks, check the carotid pulse. If the patient has a pulse, check breathing.
   a. If the patient is breathing adequately, give high-concentration oxygen by nonrebreather mask and transport.
   b. If the patient is not breathing adequately, provide artificial ventilations with high-concentration oxygen and transport.

10. If the patient does not have a pulse, resume CPR for 1 minute.
   - Press the analysis button to analyze the rhythm (get a "Deliver shock" message), deliver the fourth shock.

Cardiac Arrest Assessment and Management

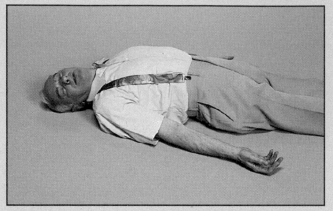

1. On arrival, briefly question those present about arrest events. (If a rescuer already on the scene is performing CPR, direct him to stop CPR.)

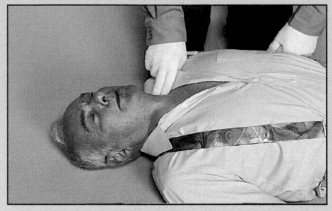

2. Verify absence of spontaneous pulse.

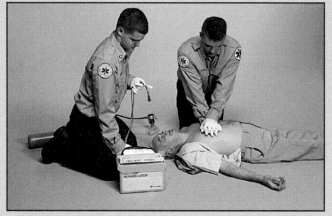

3. One EMT-B provides CPR while other sets up AED (automated external defibrillator).

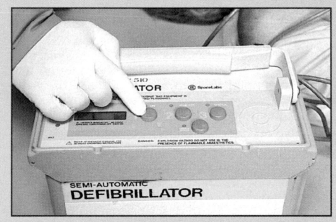

4. Turn on the AED power.

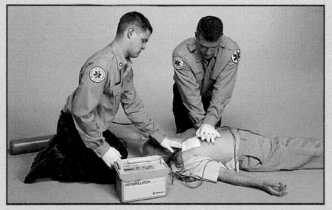

5. Connect two defibrillator pads to cables, following color code. Remove backing. Place one pad on upper right chest, one on lower left ribs.

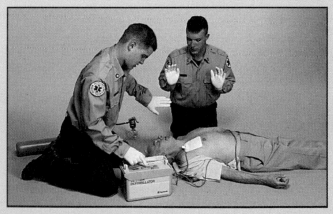

6. Say "Clear!" Ensure that all individuals are clear of patient.

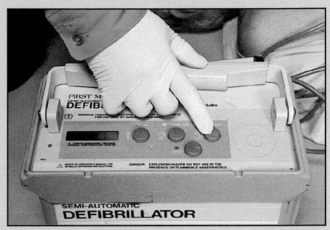

7. After everyone is clear, press the analysis button. Wait for the machine to analyze the rhythm.

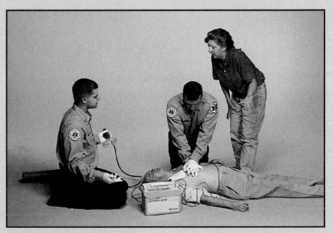

8. If advised by the defibrillator, press button to deliver shock. Repeat analysis and shock delivery until 3 shocks have been delivered.

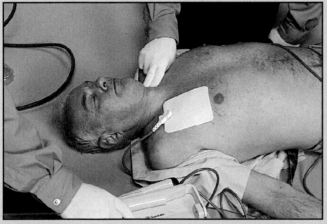

9. Check carotid pulse. Verify presence or absence of spontaneous pulse.

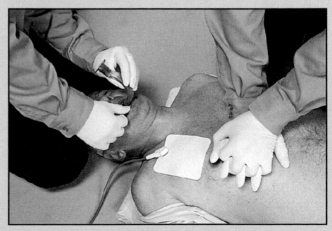

10. If pulse is absent, direct resumption of CPR. Gather additional information on arrest events.

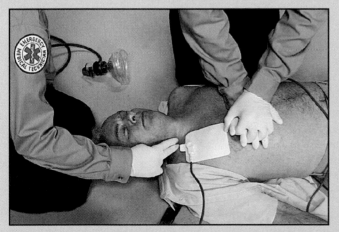

11. Check pulse during CPR to confirm effectiveness of CPR compressions.

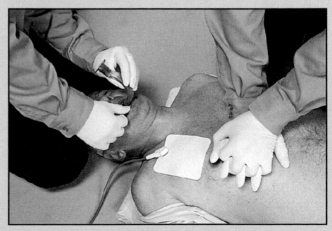

12. Direct insertion of airway adjunct.

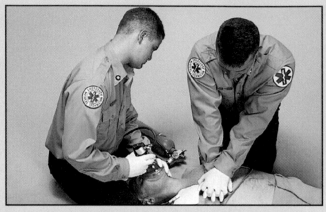

13. Direct ventilation of patient with high-concentration oxygen.

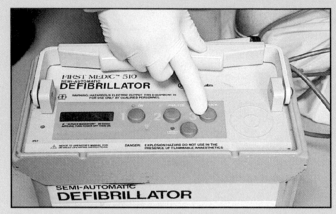

14. After 1 minute of CPR, have all individuals stand clear and repeat sequence of 3 analyses and shocks by AED.

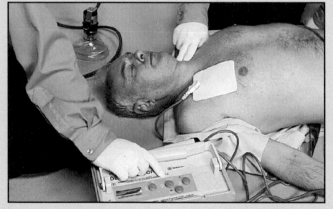

15. Check carotid pulse.

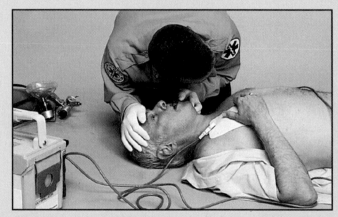

16. If there is a spontaneous pulse, check patient's breathing.

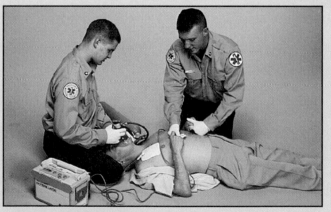

17. If breathing is adequate, provide high-concentration oxygen by nonrebreather mask. If breathing is inadequate, ventilate patient with high-concentration oxygen. Transport without delay.

Note: *At earliest opportunity, call for ALS intercept.*

- Press the analysis button to reanalyze the rhythm (get a "Deliver shock" message), deliver a fifth shock.
- Press the analysis button to reanalyze the rhythm (get a "Deliver shock" message), deliver a sixth shock.

You have now completed the second set of three stacked shocks.

11. Assuming there is no on-scene ALS (such as paramedics), you should transport the patient when *any one* of the following occurs:

   a. The patient regains a pulse (determined during the pulse check before CPR or after the AED gives a "No shock" message), or...

   b. Six shocks have been delivered (two sets of three stacked shocks), or...

   c. The machine gives three consecutive messages (separated by one minute of CPR) that no shock is advised.

If a "No shock" message is received when the analysis button is pressed:

12. After *any* rhythm analysis (whether the first time the analysis button is pushed, or after one or more shocks have already been delivered), if the machine advises "No shock," check the pulse.

   a. If the patient has a pulse, check breathing.

      1. If the patient is breathing adequately, give high-concentration oxygen by nonrebreather mask and transport.

      2. If the patient is not breathing adequately, artificially ventilate with high-concentration oxygen and transport.

   b. If the patient has no pulse, resume CPR for one minute, then...

      1. Analyze the rhythm a second time. If the AED gives a "Deliver shock" message, deliver up to two sets of three stacked shocks (a total of six shocks), with one minute of CPR separating the two sets. (Do not deliver more than a total of six shocks, including those you gave before receiving the "No shock" message. Consider that your first sequence was interrupted by the "No shock" message and now, having received a "Deliver shock" message," you are going to continue the sequence. This will be your second try at completing the sequence of six shocks.)

      2. If you get a "No shock" message at any point during the sequence and there is no pulse, resume CPR for one minute. Analyze the rhythm a third time. If the AED gives a "Deliver shock" message, deliver up to two sets of three stacked shocks separated by one minute of CPR . (Do not deliver more than a total of six shocks, including all those already delivered to this point. This will be your third try at completing the sequence of six shocks.) If you get a "No shock" message again, if there is no pulse, resume CPR and transport. Do not request any further analyses or deliver any further shocks with the AED.

Note: Whenever you do CPR, you should ventilate with 100% oxygen (or as close as you can get). If you are authorized to intubate the trachea also do so at this time. ■

Preceptor Pearl

It is important to remind new EMT-Bs that if at any time they get a "No Shock" message and determine that the patient has a pulse, they should check the patient's breathing. Emphasize the following points:

- If breathing is *adequate,* provide high-concentration oxygen by nonrebreather mask and transport.
- If breathing is *inadequate,* provide artificial ventilations with high-concentration oxygen and transport. ✤

Using an AED

Advantages of Automated External Defibrillation

Use of an AED is an easy skill to learn (in fact, probably easier than CPR), but it still requires an investment of time and energy both initially and later in continuing education. You must know the protocol used in your system so that you can deliver this care quickly and efficiently. The American Heart Association has recommended that anyone who operates an AED should receive continuing education and demonstrate competency in the skill at least every three months.

An AED is very fast. An EMT-B can frequently deliver the first shock within one minute of arrival at the patient's side. This has been shown to be almost a minute faster than EMTs operating manual defibrillators.

Defibrillation with an AED includes the use of adhesive monitoring-defibrillation pads. By making automated defibrillation a "hands-off" skill, the pads improve safety, allow for more consistent electrode placement, and provoke less anxiety among EMT-Bs.

Persistent Ventricular Fibrillation

If you function in a system that does not have ALS or you respond to an arrest patient when ALS is not available, you should prepare the patient for transport after you have:

- delivered six shocks, or
- received three "No shock" messages separated by one minute of CPR, or
- the patient regains a pulse.

Although you can use an AED without ALS and see an increase in survival, having ALS may increase the patient's chance of survival even more. If you work in a system where ALS is available, it is important that you know how and when to call. If you do call for ALS, you should do so as soon as possible. Local protocol will guide you in the decision as to whether it is best to wait for ALS at the scene, arrange an intercept, or transport directly to a hospital. Local protocols will also describe who has the responsibility for coordination of the scene at different stages of the call. Ordinarily, this is the person who is able to give the highest level of care.

Safety

When you operate an AED, it is your responsibility to make sure that the patient is cleared during all rhythm analyses and shocks. This means that no one is touching the patient or anything conductive that the patient is touching. This ensures that during a rhythm analysis the AED is evaluating the patient's rhythm and not someone else's. When a shock is delivered, being clear prevents other rescuers from being injured by a shock.

Clearing a patient means more than just saying "Clear!" It means saying "Clear!" loudly enough for all involved to hear it and looking from the patient's head to his toes to make sure no one is touching him. This is especially important when the patient is in contact with water or something metallic (like the frame of an ambulance stretcher).

Since no one can touch the patient during these times, you must interrupt CPR to allow rhythm analysis and shocks. This can mean no CPR for up to 90 seconds in order to deliver three

shocks. For experienced EMTs who are new to automated defibrillation, this can be a difficult adjustment. But since defibrillation is more effective than just CPR in resuscitating a patient, this interruption of CPR is actually for the patient's benefit. Practicing defibrillation frequently will help experienced EMTs to realize this and to change old habits.

An automated external defibrillator cannot accurately analyze a patient's ECG rhythm when in a moving vehicle. Road bumps cause movement in some of the patient's muscles. This leads to extra electrical signals that can obscure the patient's ECG and even imitate some ECG rhythms.

If a patient goes into cardiac arrest in the ambulance (or arrests again after regaining a pulse previously) you must bring the vehicle to a complete stop in order to analyze the rhythm. It is also unsafe to defibrillate in a moving ambulance, because the driver may have to swerve or stop suddenly in order to avoid a collision. If this happens when you are pressing the shock button, someone can fall on the patient as the shock is being delivered.

Another potential hazard with defibrillation is medication patches. These devices allow for the slow administration of some medications through the skin. The hazard probably lies in the plastic in the patch which can melt and even explode when a shock is delivered. The most common medication delivered by a patch is nitroglycerin, but any medication patch has the potential to become a hazard. The only patches that have caused problems to date have been on patients' chests. For this reason, if you see a patch on a patient's chest, remove it (with gloved hands so you don't absorb the medication through your skin).

Single Rescuer with an Automated External Defibrillator

Since defibrillation is much more likely than CPR to bring a patient back, if you are alone with a patient in cardiac arrest and an AED, you should:

- Perform an initial assessment and assure unresponsiveness, apnea, and pulselessness but do not start chest compressions.
- Turn on the AED.
- Attach the device.
- Press the analysis button.
- Deliver up to three stacked shocks.

After you have delivered three shocks or you have received a "No shock" message,

- Check for a carotid pulse.
- Activate the EMS system.
- Start CPR if there is no pulse.

The shocks are stacked, just as when you were working with a partner, so do not check for a pulse between the stacked shocks.

Post Resuscitation Care

Once you have completed the defibrillation protocol, the patient will be in one of three conditions. The most common situation is he will have no pulse and the AED will give a "No shock" message. Sometimes the patient will have no pulse and the AED will signify that further shocks may be indicated. The third possibility is that he will have a pulse. If this is the case, you must be aggressive in maintaining the airway. If breathing is adequate, administer high-concentration oxygen by nonrebreather mask and transport the patient on his side. If breathing is inadequate, ventilate with 100% oxygen and transport. You should leave the AED on the patient until you arrive at the hospital. As time allows, perform a focused assessment and ongoing assessment en route.

Recurrent Ventricular Fibrillation

A patient who has just recovered a spontaneous pulse is not stable. Despite your attempts to oxygenate and ventilate the patient and transport him promptly, he may go back into cardiac arrest. If the patient is unconscious and you are ventilating him, it may not be immediately obvious that he no longer has a pulse. To avoid this, you should check the patient's pulse frequently (at least every 30 seconds). If a pulse is absent, tell your driver to stop the vehicle, press the analyze button, and deliver shocks as described by your local protocol. Only if the defibrillator is not immediately ready should you start CPR before using it. This should rarely be the case.

Defibrillator Maintenance

A defibrillator can save a life only if it is working properly. You must check the machine frequently and maintain it in accordance with the manufacturer's recommendations. A special task force of the Food and Drug Administration (FDA) has compiled a list of steps to be taken every shift to ensure that a defibrillator is ready when needed (Figure 9–4). The checklist must be completed at least daily if it is to accomplish its purpose.

When the FDA's task force looked at defibrillator failures, they found that the most common cause of problems was improper device maintenance, usually battery failure. As part of completing the checklist, you must make sure that the battery in the AED is charged

The American Heart Association has been very active in promoting early defibrillation and publishes a variety of guidelines and additional information on automated external defibrillation.

Quality Improvement

Quality improvement (QI) is essential to the success of any EMS system, but especially to a defibrillation program. Simply undergoing AED training and buying an AED by no means guarantees success. A good QI program involves both the individuals who use AEDs and the EMS system in which the machines are used.

As someone using an AED, you have the responsibility to use it quickly and efficiently. You must take care to maintain the skills of CPR, airway maintenance, automated defibrillation, and lifting and moving patients. Because skills that are used infrequently deteriorate over time, most systems permit a maximum of 90 days between AED practice sessions.

Medical direction is an essential component of any defibrillation program. Successfully completing AED training in an EMT-Basic course does not necessarily mean you are automatically allowed to use the device. You are subject to the requirements of state laws and rules as well as local medical direction.

One of the roles of the medical director is to review every event in which an AED is used. Depending on the size of your system, the medical director may delegate some or all of this task, but he or she bears responsibility for your actions and should have the authority to match that responsibility.

The medical director may use a number of different sources of information in reviewing AED cases, including your written report, solid-state memory modules, magnetic tape recordings, and voice-ECG tape recordings. The brand of machine you use will determine what information is available.

AUTOMATED DEFIBRILLATORS: OPERATOR'S SHIFT CHECKLIST

Date: _____   Shift: _____   Location: _____

Mfr/Model No.: _____   Serial No. or Facility ID No.: _____

At the beginning of each shift, inspect the unit. Indicate whether all requirements have been met. Note any corrective actions taken. Sign the form.

	Okay as found	Corrective Action/Remarks
1. Defibrillator Unit		
Clean, no spills, clear of objects on top, casing intact		
2. Cables/Connectors		
a. Inspect for cracks, broken wire, or damage b. Connectors engage securely		
3. Supplies		
a. Two sets of pads in sealed packages, within expiration date * g. Spare charged battery b. Hand towel * h. Adequate ECG paper c. Scissors * i. Manual override module, key, or card d. Razor * e. Alcohol wipes * j. Cassette tape, memory module, and/or event card plus spares * f. Monitoring electrodes		
4. Power Supply		

a. Battery-powered units
  (1) Verify fully charged battery in place
  (2) Spare charged battery available
  (3) Follow appropriate battery rotation schedule per manufacturer's recommendations
b. AC/Battery backup units
  (1) Plugged into live outlet to maintain battery charge
  (2) Test on battery power and reconnect to line power		

5. Indicators/*ECG Display		
* a. Remove cassette tape, memory module, and/or event card * e. "Service" message display off b. Power-on display * f. Battery charging; low battery light off c. Self-test ok g. Correct time displayed—set with dispatch center * d. Monitor display functional		
6. ECG Recorder		
a. Adequate ECG paper b. Recorder prints		
7. Charge/Display Cycle		
* a. Disconnect AC plug—battery backup units * e. Manual override functional b. Attach to simulator f. Detach from simulator c. Detects, charges, and delivers shock for "VF" * g. Replace cassette tape, module, and/or memory card d. Responds correctly to non-shockable rhythms		
8. *Pacemaker		
a. Pacer output cable intact c. Inspect per manufacturer's operational guidelines b. Pacer pads present (set of two)		
☐ **Major problem(s) identified (OUT OF SERVICE)**		

* *Applicable only if the unit has this supply or capability*

rev 1.6 auto, 8/8/91

Signature: _____

FIGURE 9–4 An AED checklist from Laerdal.

CHAPTER REVIEW

■ SUMMARY

This chapter described the assessment and management of patients with cardiac problems. Just as important, it described the assessment and care of patients who do not have cardiac problems, but who appear to. Since it is often hard to tell the difference between these two groups, you must treat patients with signs and symptoms of cardiac compromise as though they actually have cardiac problems.

The new interventions described in this chapter demonstrate two of the most important things EMS providers can do: relieve pain and resuscitate someone from cardiac arrest. Under the right circumstances, you may be able to assist a patient in taking his own nitroglycerin and relieve some or all of his pain. You must be familiar with not only how to give the medication, but also when (and when not) to do so.

Using an automated defibrillator may be one of the most important things you can do as an EMT-B. If you understand the use of the device and practice it until you are confident and competent, you may actually be able to save a life. By participating in a quality improvement program, you will increase that likelihood even further.

■ REVIEW QUESTIONS

1. Describe cardiac compromise and the signs and symptoms that would make you suspect it.
2. What is the emergency medical care for a patient with cardiac compromise?
3. What conditions must a patient meet for you to assist him in taking his nitroglycerin?
4. Describe the relationship between the elements in the chain of survival.
5. Describe how to clear a patient before defibrillating.
6. What are "stacked shocks" and how many should you give?
7. Why should someone who is alone with a defibrillator shock a patient in cardiac arrest before starting chest compressions?

Medical Emergencies 10

- *Respiratory*
- *Allergic Reactions*
- *Environmental*

■ *This chapter begins with the significant changes in the way an EMT-B will handle respiratory emergencies. You are no longer required to attempt to differentiate between emphysema, bronchitis, and other pulmonary conditions. The primary emphasis now is on the differentiation between adequate and inadequate breathing. A respiratory complaint is generally called "breathing difficulty." EMT-Bs are now allowed to assist patients with their prescribed inhalers, which*

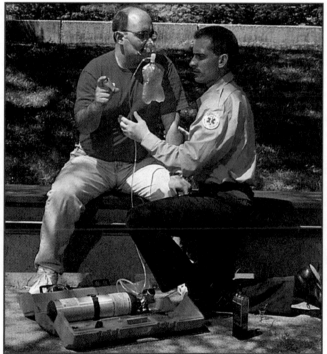

will improve the care you offer to those patients with breathing difficulty.

This chapter also discusses allergies. Allergic reactions are often serious, occasionally fatal. The EMT-B is allowed to assist with another prescribed medication for an allergic reaction—the epinephrine auto-injector.

Finally, this chapter discusses environmental emergencies. These can take the form of exposure to extremes of temperature, immersion in water, or an insect bite or animal sting.

MAKING THE TRANSITION

- The term "breathing difficulty" is used to describe a group of previously diagnosed respiratory conditions.
- How to assist patients with the use of prescribed inhalers and epinephrine auto-injectors is explained.
- Instead of trying to decide whether a patient has heat stroke or heat cramps, the EMT-B should use skin temperature to determine the proper treatment.

OBJECTIVES

The numbered objectives below are from the United States Department of Transportation 1994 EMT-Basic National Standard Curriculum. Objectives with colored bullets that follow in italics are from the EMT-Basic Transitional Program.

■ KNOWLEDGE AND ATTITUDE

At the completion of this chapter, you should be able to:

Respiratory Emergencies

1. List the structure and function of the respiratory system. (pp. 154–155)
2. State the signs and symptoms of a patient with breathing difficulty. (pp. 156–157, 160)
3. Describe the emergency medical care of the patient with breathing difficulty. (pp. 157–160)
4. Recognize the need for medical direction to assist in the emergency medical care of the patient with breathing difficulty. (pp. 157, 158, 159)
5. Describe the emergency medical care of the patient with breathing distress. (pp. 157, 158, 159)
6. Establish the relationship between airway management and the patient with breathing difficulty. (pp. 155–156)
7. List signs of adequate air exchange. (pp. 155, 156)
8. State the generic name, medication forms, dose, administration, action, indications, and contraindications for the prescribed inhaler. (p. 158)
9. Distinguish between the emergency medical care of the infant, child, and adult patient with breathing difficulty. (pp. 157–160)
10. Differentiate between upper airway obstruction and lower airway disease in the infant and child patient. (see Chapter 4)
11. Defend EMT-B treatment regimens for various respiratory emergencies. (p. 155)
12. Explain the rationale for administering an inhaler. (pp. 157–160)
● *Describe the relationship between assessment findings and medical interventions in respiratory emergencies. (pp. 155–157)*

Allergic Reactions

1. Recognize the patient experiencing an allergic reaction. (pp. 160–161)
2. Describe the emergency medical care of the patient with an allergic reaction. (pp. 161–165)
3. Establish the relationship between the patient with an allergic reaction and airway management. (pp. 160–161)
4. Describe the mechanisms of allergic response and the implications for airway management. (pp. 160–161, 163)
5. State the generic and trade names, medication forms, dose, administration, action, and contraindications for the epinephrine auto-injector. (p. 162)
6. Evaluate the need for medical direction in the emergency medical care of the patient with an allergic reaction. (pp. 161, 162, 164)
7. Differentiate between the general category of those patients having an allergic reaction and those patients having an allergic reaction and requiring immediate medical care, including immediate use of the epinephrine auto-injector. (pp. 160–161)
8. Explain the rationale for administering epinephrine using an auto-injector. (pp. 161–165)
● *Describe the relationship between assessment findings and medical interventions in allergic reactions. (pp. 161–165)*

Environmental Emergencies

1. Describe the various ways that the body loses heat. (p. 165)
2. List the signs and symptoms of exposure to cold. (p. 167)
3. Explain the steps in providing emergency medical care to a patient exposed to cold. (pp. 167–170)
4. List the signs and symptoms of exposure to heat. (pp. 171, 172)
5. Explain the steps in providing emergency care to a patient exposed to heat. (pp. 171–172)
6. Recognize the signs and symptoms of water-related emergencies. (pp. 172–173)
7. Describe the complications of near-drowning. (pp. 172–173)
8. Discuss the emergency medical care of bites and stings. (p. 173)

■ SKILLS

Respiratory Emergencies

1. Demonstrate the emergency medical care for breathing difficulty.
2. Perform the steps in facilitating the use of an inhaler.
- *Given medical scenarios, demonstrate the ability to properly assess the patient and demonstrate the ability to properly utilize the intervention of an inhaler.*

Allergic Reactions

1. Demonstrate the emergency medical care of the patient experiencing an allergic reaction.
2. Demonstrate the use of the epinephrine auto-injector.
3. Demonstrate the assessment and documentation of patient response to an epinephrine injection.

4. Demonstrate proper disposal of equipment.
5. Demonstrate completing a prehospital care report for patients with allergic emergencies.
- *Demonstrate the use of an epinephrine auto-injector without missing any critical criteria listed on the skill sheets in the 1994 EMT-Basic Transitional Program.*

Environmental Emergencies

1. Demonstrate the assessment and emergency medical care of a patient with exposure to cold.
2. Demonstrate the assessment and emergency medical care of a patient with exposure to heat.
3. Demonstrate the assessment and emergency medical care of a near-drowning patient.
4. Demonstrate completing a prehospital care report for patients with environmental emergencies.

ON THE SCENE

Your EMS unit is called to the scene of a 38-year-old woman with respiratory distress. The **scene size-up** is uneventful as you arrive and approach the residence. When you enter the residence, you find a woman leaning forward with her hands on her knees. You recognize this as a classic position of a person in respiratory distress. Your **initial assessment** reveals a woman who is oriented. Her breathing is rapid but adequate; her pulse is rapid. She finds it hard to speak full sentences without becoming winded. Your **general impression** is of a patient in considerable respiratory distress. You assign her a high priority.

Your partner has already placed her on oxygen via nonrebreather mask. She feels closed in by the mask

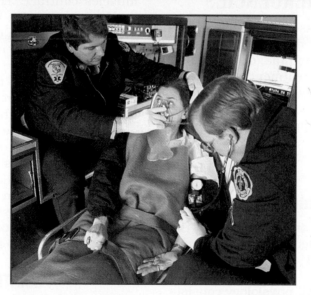

but accepts it. You perform a **focused history** while your partner prepares the stretcher and you place her on it. She advises you that she has asthma and she feels as if she were having an attack. Her distress began while cleaning, and she suspects she has reacted to something in the new cleanser she was using. She describes her breathing difficulty as severe.

The patient's inhaler is on the table next to her. You ascertain whether the inhaler is prescribed to her and ask if she has used it. She explains she has tried it once without relief. Her prescription allows her to try it twice. Your agency's standing orders allow you to facilitate the use of the inhaler up to two times. She would like to try it again and you help. Your role, you realize, is coaching and making sure she breathes the medication in deeply, holding her breath so it will be absorbed. After verifying her vital signs and checking for indications and contraindications, you help her with the medication.

Although the medication helped somewhat, her breathing difficulty is still present. You move the patient to the ambulance. As you reach the ambulance, you prepare to take another set of vitals. En route to the hospital you will contact medical direction for further orders. ■

The patient presented in the scenario is familiar to most experienced EMTs. The tripod position, inability to speak full sentences, and restlessness are all classic signs of respiratory distress. The most common treatment for this patient, the administration of oxygen, is certainly included in the new curriculum. What may be different from your current practice is assisting with, or facilitating, the patient's use of a prescribed inhaler. While the administration of any medication is a serious responsibility, it can provide significant benefit to the patient.

■ RESPIRATORY EMERGENCIES

The new curriculum discusses only one respiratory condition: respiratory distress. The cause, whether it be emphysema, asthma, or bronchitis, is not significant since the treatment is essentially the same. Since this text is condensed, specific respiratory diseases are not covered. However, you are welcome to refer to your prior EMT text for this information if you wish.

Respiratory Anatomy and Physiology

You reviewed the anatomy and physiology of the respiratory system in Chapter 4, Airway. You may wish to refer to Chapter 4 again as you study this section.

Respiratory anatomy and physiology consists of external and internal structures. The nose and mouth are external portions of the respiratory system. The oropharynx and nasopharynx lie posteriorly to the mouth and nose respectively. The trachea, also known as the windpipe, has cartilage rings to support its structure. The structure at the superior portion of the trachea is the larynx, or voice box. It is protected by the epiglottis, which folds over the laryngeal opening to prevent items from being aspirated into the lungs. The cricoid cartilage is a ring-shaped structure that forms the lower portion of the larynx.

The trachea splits or bifurcates into two bronchi. These bronchi continue to divide until they reach the alveoli, the tiny sacs where actual gas exchange with the cells takes place.

The actual act of breathing uses the diaphragm as well as muscles in the chest (Figure 10–1). During inhalation, the diaphragm and intercostal muscles contract. The diaphragm moves downward while the ribs move upward and outward, increasing the size of the thoracic cavity. This increase in the size of the chest cavity draws air into the lungs.

On exhalation, the opposite happens. The diaphragm and intercostal muscles relax, decreasing the size of the chest cavity. The end result is air flowing out of the lungs.

Gases are exchanged at the alveolar level of the lungs. Oxygen is turned over to the red blood cells while carbon dioxide is taken from the cells to be removed from the body. The oxygen-rich blood travels to the capillaries, where oxygen is turned over to the cells of the body and carbon dioxide is picked up for transport to the lungs.

PEDIATRIC HIGHLIGHT

There are differences between the airway anatomy in adult and infant or child patients (Figure 10–2). These differences include:

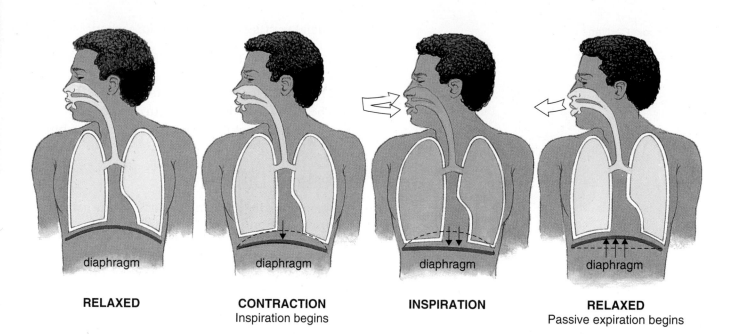

| RELAXED | CONTRACTION
Inspiration begins | INSPIRATION | RELAXED
Passive expiration begins |

FIGURE 10–1 The process of respiration. During inspiration, the diaphragm and rib muscles contract, causing air to flow into the lungs. During expiration, the muscles relax, causing air to flow out of the lungs.

- *All structures are smaller and therefore more easily obstructed.*
- *The tongues of infants and children take up proportionally more space in the mouth than do the tongues of adults.*
- *The tracheas of infants and children are narrower and more flexible than those of adults.*
- *The cricoid cartilage is less developed and therefore less rigid than in adults.*
- *The chest wall of children is softer and they tend to rely more heavily upon the diaphragm for breathing than do adults.* ■

Adequate vs. Inadequate Breathing

Breathing is not an all-or-nothing proposition. In the past, EMS students were taught that the patient would either be breathing or not breathing. Over the years, we have come to realize that this is not always the case. Therefore, the new curriculum uses the terms adequate and inadequate breathing. For example, there are patients who are breathing, but not at a rate or depth adequate to support life. These patients must be treated aggressively with artificial ventilations. The signs of adequate and inadequate ventilations are described in Table 10–1.

Preceptor Pearl

The concept of adequate vs. inadequate breathing is one that must be stressed to new EMT-Bs. The mere thought of providing artificial ventilations to a person who has some respiratory effort is confusing. Ventilating a nonbreathing patient is difficult, let alone one that is breathing. Explain to new EMTs that they should work with the patient's respiratory effort and coach the patient when appropriate. ✛

Recognizing and effectively treating inadequate breathing could be the most important skill you possess as an EMT-B. It is also important to determine if artificial ventilations (pocket face mask or BVM) are being performed adequately.

If these ventilations are being performed *adequately*:

- The chest rises and falls with each ventilation.
- The rate is sufficient (12/minute for adults, 20/min for children and infants).
- The heart rate may return to normal.
- The patient's skin color improves towards normal.

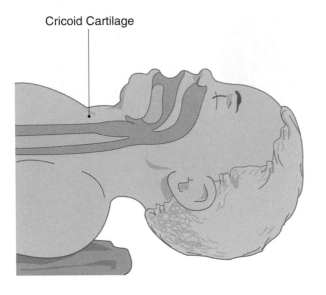

Cricoid Cartilage

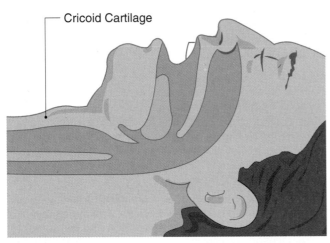

Cricoid Cartilage

FIGURE 10–2 Adult and child respiratory passages.

Artificial ventilation is *inadequate* when:

- The chest does not rise and fall with each ventilation.
- The rate is too slow or too fast.
- The heart rate does not return to normal.
- The patient's skin color becomes gray or blue.

Breathing Difficulty

As noted earlier, the new curriculum combines respiratory conditions into one complaint called "breathing difficulty" (dyspnea). Looking back, whether the patient had congestive heart failure, emphysema, pulmonary embolus, or pneumonia, the care was essentially the same. Continuing with this principle, the process of patient assessment is simplified when compared to that of our initial training.

Patient Assessment **Breathing Difficulty**

The following are signs and symptoms of breathing difficulty:

Signs and Symptoms

- Shortness of breath
- Restlessness
- Increased pulse rate
- Abnormal breathing rate (increased or decreased)
- Skin color changes (cyanotic, pale, flushed)

TABLE 10–1 Adequate and Inadequate Breathing

	Adequate Breathing	Inadequate Breathing
Rate	Adult: 12–20/min Child: 15–30/min Infant: 25–50/min	Above or below normal rates for the patient's age group
Rhythm	Regular	May be irregular
Quality		
Breath sounds	Present and equal	Diminished, unequal, or absent
Chest expansion	Adequate and equal	Inadequate or unequal
Effort of breathing	Unlabored, normal respiratory effort	Labored; increased respiratory effort; use of accessory muscles (may be pronounced in infants and children and involve nasal flaring, seesaw breathing, grunting, and retractions between the ribs and above the clavicles)

- Noisy breathing:
  crowing
  wheezing (whistling sounds)
  gurgling
  snoring
  stridor
- Inability to speak or inability to speak full sentences
- Retractions
- Altered mental status
- Coughing
- Irregular breathing rhythm
- Patient position: tripod, leaning forward
- Unusual anatomy (barrel chest)
- Agonal respirations (slow, gasping breaths) ■

Use the pertinent elements of the OPQRST mnemonic to determine the respiratory history. Since it may be possible to assist the patient with his or her own prescribed medications, be sure to ask which interventions, if any, have been used.

Patient Care Breathing Difficulty

Emergency Care Steps
1. During your patient assessment determine if the patient is breathing adequately.
2. Patients who are breathing adequately can be placed in a position of comfort.
3. Apply high-concentration oxygen and assist ventilations as necessary.
4. Be prepared for changes in respiratory status throughout the call.
5. If the patient has a prescribed inhaler, you may be able to facilitate its use. This is discussed in the next section.
6. Perform an ongoing assessment every five minutes for the unstable patient. ■

Preceptor Pearl

Patients with chronic obstructive pulmonary disease (COPD) may over time lose the normal ability to use the body's blood carbon dioxide levels as a stimulus to breathe. When this occurs, the COPD patient's body may use low blood oxygen as the factor that stimulates him to breathe. Because of this so-called *hypoxic drive*, we have for years been trained to administer only low concentrations of oxygen to these patients for fear of increasing the patient's blood oxygen levels and wiping out their "drive to breathe." However, it is now widely agreed that more harm is done if high-concentration oxygen is withheld. ✤

Prescribed Inhaler

You may be called to a patient complaining of respiratory distress who has a prescribed inhaler. Your EMS system may allow you to assist the patient in the use of the inhaler. Being unable to breathe can be frightening. The use of the inhaler may ease a patient's distress and be a tremendous benefit.

As much of a benefit as medications can be, they may also be a hazard. Administering or facilitating the administration of medications is a major responsibility. It must always be taken seriously and handled responsibly.

Before administering any medication, be sure that it is indicated. The patient must meet certain criteria—in this case signs of respiratory distress must be present (Skill Summary 10–1). The patient must have an inhaler that is actually prescribed to him or her. If your system requires, contact medical direction before you assist with administration of the inhaler.

There are also contraindications to medications—situations in which the medication must not be used. For the prescribed inhaler these include the inability of the patient to use the device, the inhaler not being prescribed to the patient, no consent from medical direction, and the patient already having used the maximum prescribed dose(s). The type of drug contained in prescribed inhalers may cause tremors, nervousness, and increased pulse rate—especially if the maximum dose is exceeded.

Always check the "four rights" as they apply to your situation: right patient, right medication, right route, right dose.

Use of the prescribed inhaler requires the cooperation of the patient (Skill Summary 10–2). This may not be an easy task if the patient is anxious—a condition frequently seen in respiratory distress. It is important to have the patient *exhale* deeply before activating the inhaler. Then, when the inhaler is activated, the patient should *inhale* deeply. Instruct the patient to hold his breath for a reasonable time so the medication may be absorbed. The dose may be repeated if allowed or ordered by medical direction.

You may observe a spacer device attached to the patient's inhaler (Skill Summary 10–2, number 6). The spacer helps the patient inhale more of the medication.

Monitor the patient carefully after administration of any medication. The ongoing assessment should be performed, including vital signs, chief complaint, and effects of the medication.

Prescribed Inhaler

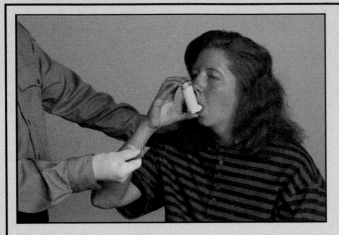

MEDICATION NAME

1. Generic: albuterol, isoetharine, metaproterenol, ipratropium
2. Trade: Proventil, Ventolin, Bronkosol, Bronkometer, Alupent, Metaprel, Atrovent

INDICATIONS

Meets all of the following criteria:
1. Patient exhibits signs and symptoms of respiratory emergency.
2. Patient has physician-prescribed hand-held inhaler.
3. Medical direction gives specific authorization to use.

CONTRAINDICATIONS

1. Patient is unable to use device (e.g., not alert).
2. Inhaler is not prescribed for patient.
3. No permission has been given by medical direction.
4. Patient has already taken maximum prescribed dose prior to EMT-B's arrival.

MEDICATION FORM

Hand-held metered dose inhaler

DOSAGE

Number of inhalations based on medical direction's order or physician's order

ADMINISTRATION

1. Obtain order from medical direction either on-line or off-line.
2. Assure right patient, right medication, right dose, right route, patient alert enough to use inhaler.
3. Check expiration date of inhaler.
4. Check if patient has already taken any doses.
5. Assure inhaler is at room temperature or warmer.
6. Shake inhaler vigorously several times.
7. Have patient exhale deeply.
8. Have patient put her lips around the opening of the inhaler.
9. Have patient depress the hand-held inhaler as she begins to inhale deeply.
10. Instruct patient to hold her breath for as long as she comfortably can so medication can be absorbed.
11. Put oxygen back on patient.
12. Allow patient to breathe a few times and repeat second dose if so ordered by medical direction.
13. If patient has a spacer device for use with her inhaler (device for attachment between inhaler and patient to allow for more effective use of medication), it should be used.

ACTIONS

Beta agonist bronchodilator dilates bronchioles, reducing airway resistance.

SIDE EFFECTS

1. Increased pulse rate
2. Tremors
3. Nervousness

REASSESSMENT STRATEGIES

1. Gather vital signs.
2. Perform focused reassessment of chest and respiratory function.
3. Observe for deterioration of patient; if breathing becomes inadequate, provide artificial respirations.

Prescribed Inhaler— Patient Assessment and Management

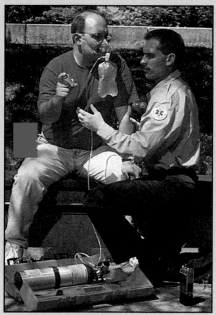

1. The patient has the indication for use of an inhaler: signs and symptoms of breathing difficulty, and an inhaler prescribed by a physician.

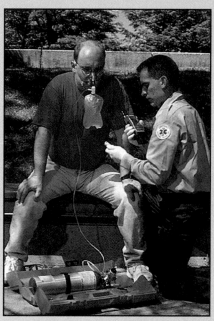

2. The EMT-B contacts medical direction and obtains an order to assist the patient with the prescribed inhaler.

3. The EMT-B assures the four "rights" for administration of a medication:

- Right patient
- Right medication
- Right dose
- Right route

EMT-B checks expiration date, shakes inhaler, makes sure inhaler is room temperature or warmer, makes sure patient is alert.

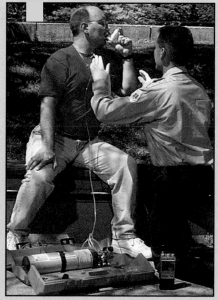

4. The EMT-B coaches the patient in use of the inhaler: Exhale deeply, press inhaler to activate spray, hold breath in so medication can be absorbed.

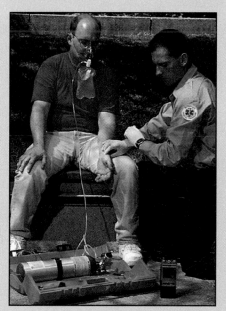

5. After use of inhaler, EMT-B reassesses the patient: takes vital signs, does a focused exam, determines if breathing is adequate.

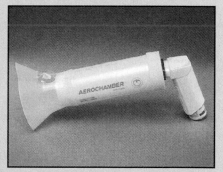

6. A "spacer" device between inhaler (shown inverted) and patient allows more effective use of medication. If the patient has a spacer, it should be attached to the inhaler before use.

Children commonly have prescribed inhalers. The use of the device is the same for children as for adults. The signs and symptoms of respiratory distress in children includes many of those seen in adults, but there are some differences. Intercostal and suprasternal retractions are seen more commonly in children. ■

■ ALLERGIC REACTIONS

An allergic reaction is an exaggerated response of the body's immune system to any substance. Common causes of these reactions include insect bites and stings, foods, plants, and medications, among others (Figure 10–3).

Allergic reactions range from mild to severe, life-threatening **anaphylactic** reactions. In anaphylaxis, exposure to the allergen will cause blood vessels to dilate rapidly, resulting in a drop in blood pressure. The more serious attacks usually begin rapidly after exposure to the allergen, although the reaction can be delayed for up to 30 minutes. There is no way to predict the course of an allergic reaction, so each event must be treated seriously. The greatest danger is compromise of the airway due to swelling and edema (fluid accumulation).

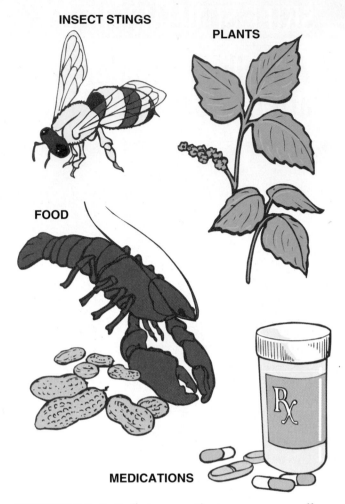

FOOD

INSECT STINGS

PLANTS

MEDICATIONS

FIGURE 10–3 Substances that may cause allergic reaction.

■ Patient Assessment Allergic Reaction

- Perform the focused history and physical exam to determine:
  History of allergies
  What the patient was exposed to
  How the patient was exposed
  What effects the exposure has caused
  The progression of symptoms
  The interventions used by the patient so far
- Assess baseline vital signs and get the remainder of SAMPLE history.

Signs and Symptoms
The signs and symptoms of an allergic reaction vary from person to person. They may range from mild to severe. In mild allergic reactions, the patient may only complain of itchy, watery eyes. Severe allergic reactions include signs and symptoms throughout the body, such as:

Skin
- Itching, hives, flushing, red skin
- Swelling of the face, hands, neck, or tongue
- Cool and clammy to touch if shock (hypoperfusion) present.

Tongue
- Warm or tingling feeling

Respiratory system
- Tightness in the throat, chest
- Rapid, labored, or noisy breathing
- Stridor, hoarseness
- Wheezing, cough

Cardiovascular system
- Increased heart rate
- Decreased blood pressure

Generalized
- Itchy, watery eyes
- Headache
- Runny nose

Level of consciousness
- Altered mental status
- Signs and symptoms of shock ■

Patient Care **Allergic Reaction**

Emergency Care Steps

1. Administer high-concentration oxygen through a nonrebreather mask in the initial assessment if the patient complains of breathing difficulty. Airway assessment and care are very important since respiratory compromise may develop initially or at any time throughout the call.
2. Determine if the patient has an epinephrine auto-injector available. Contact medical direction if necessary to facilitate its use. Be sure to record the administration of the epinephrine auto-injector.
3. Perform an ongoing assessment every five minutes.
4. Transport patient immediately. Consider ALS backup, especially if the patient does not have or does not respond to the epinephrine injection. ■

Some patients exposed to a substance that may cause an allergic reaction will not exhibit signs and symptoms of shock or respiratory distress. These patients should not receive epinephrine. Monitor them carefully in case more serious signs develop.

Epinephrine Auto-Injector

For years, the epinephrine auto-injector has been prescribed to patients who experience severe allergic reactions. The epinephrine works by dilating the bronchioles, which decreases respiratory distress, and constricting blood vessels, thus lessening shock. The auto-injectors come in two sizes: adult and child. The adult syringe contains 0.3 mg of epinephrine while the infant/child injector contains 0.15 mg. The entire syringe is administered. Information about epinephrine auto-injectors is given in Skill Summary 10–3.

The indications for use of an epinephrine auto-injector are:

- Patient exhibits signs and symptoms of a severe/serious allergic reaction (including shock or respiratory distress).
- Medication is prescribed to this patient by a physician.
- Medical direction approves use of the device (on- or off-line).

Since the drug is already prescribed to the patient and is used only in an extreme emergency, there are no contraindications for its use.

There is the possibility of the injector causing side effects such as an increased heart rate, pallor, dizziness, headache, or chest pain. Nausea, vomiting, and excitability have also been reported.

Follow this procedure for administering the auto-injector (Skill Summary 10–4):

1. Determine that the patient shows signs of allergic reaction (including shock or respiratory distress).
2. Obtain permission from medical direction (on-line or off-line).
3. Obtain the patient's auto-injector. Verify that it is prescribed to the patient and the solution is not cloudy.
4. Remove cap from auto-injector.
5. Place auto-injector firmly against the patient's thigh. (The skin should be bared prior to the injection.) Hold in place for 10 seconds to allow the medication to inject.
6. Dispose of injector in a biohazard (sharps) container.
7. Record activity and time.

As with any unstable patient, frequent reassessment is important. The main focus of the reassessment is airway, breathing, and circulation. If the symptoms worsen or don't improve, you may be called upon by medical direction to repeat the use of an auto-injector. The injectors are single-use, so be sure to take any extras the patient has available with you to the hospital in case they are needed. If the patient fails to respond or if the condition continues to worsen, as may happen in serious reactions, call for ALS backup if possible, be prepared to assist ventilations, perform CPR, and use the AED if necessary.

Epinephrine Auto-Injector

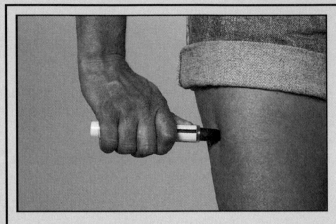

MEDICATION NAME

1. Generic: epinephrine
2. Trade: Adrenalin™, Epi-Pen®

INDICATIONS

Must meet the following three criteria:
1. Patient exhibits signs of a severe allergic reaction, including either respiratory distress or shock (hypoperfusion)
2. Medication is prescribed for this patient by a physician
3. Medical direction authorizes use for this patient

CONTRAINDICATIONS

No contraindications when used in a life-threatening situation

MEDICATION FORM

Liquid administered by an auto-injector—an automatically injectable needle-and-syringe system

DOSAGE

Adult—One adult auto-injector (0.3 mg)
Infant and child—One infant/child auto-injector (0.15 mg)

ADMINISTRATION

1. Obtain patient's prescribed auto-injector. Ensure:
   a. Prescription is written for the patient who is experiencing the severe allergic reaction
   b. Medication is not discolored (if visible)
2. Obtain order from medical direction, either on-line or off-line.
3. Remove cap from auto-injector.
4. Place tip of auto-injector against patient's thigh.
   a. Lateral portion of the thigh
   b. Midway between waist and knee
5. Push the injector firmly against the thigh until the injector activates.
6. Hold the injector in place until the medication is injected (at least 10 seconds).
7. Record activity and time.
8. Dispose of injector in biohazard container.

ACTIONS

1. Dilates the bronchioles
2. Constricts blood vessels

SIDE EFFECTS

1. Increased heart rate
2. Pallor
3. Dizziness
4. Chest pain
5. Headache
6. Nausea
7. Vomiting
8. Excitability, anxiety

REASSESSMENT STRATEGIES

1. Transport
2. Continue focused assessment of airway, breathing, and circulatory status.

   If patient's condition continues to worsen (decreasing mental status, increasing breathing difficulty, decreasing blood pressure):
   a. Obtain medical direction for an additional dose of epinephrine
   b. Treat for shock (hypoperfusion)
   c. Prepare to initiate basic life-support procedures (CPR, AED)

   If patient's condition improves, provide supportive care:
   a. Continue oxygen
   b. Treat for shock (hypoperfusion)

Using the Epinephrine Auto-Injector

FIRST take body substance isolation precautions.

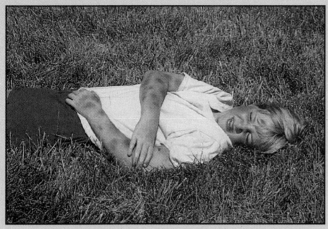

1. Patient suffers severe allergic reaction.

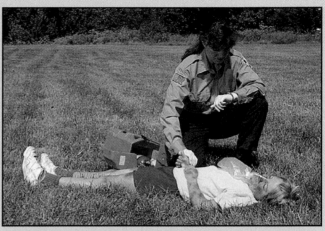

2. Perform an initial assessment. Provide high-concentration oxygen by nonrebreather mask.

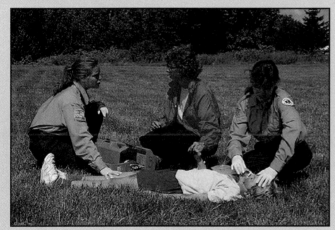

3. Perform a focused history and physical exam and obtain a SAMPLE history.

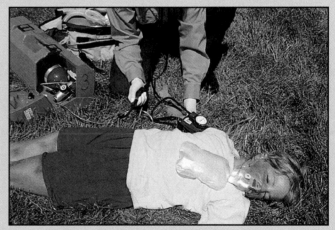

4. Take the patient's vital signs.

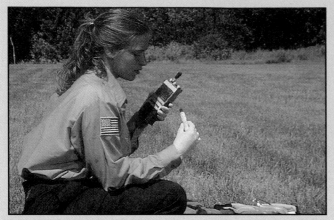

5. Ascertain if the patient has a prescribed epinephrine auto-injector. Check to be sure injector is prescribed for this patient. Check expiration date. Check for cloudiness or discoloration if liquid is visible. Contact medical direction.

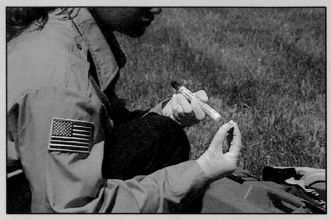

6. If medical direction orders use of the epinephrine auto-injector, prepare it for use. Remove the safety cap.

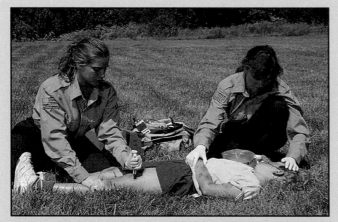

7. Press the injector against the patient's thigh to trigger release of the spring-loaded needle and inject the dose of epinephrine into the patient.

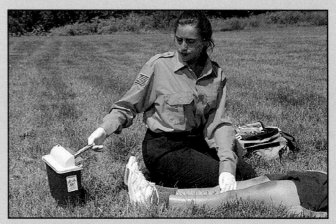

8. After holding the injector against the patient's thigh for at least 10 seconds, dispose of the used injector in a biohazard container.

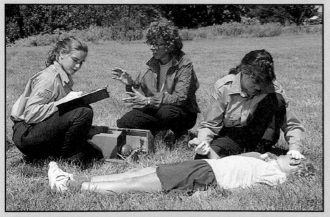

9. Document the patient's response to the medication.

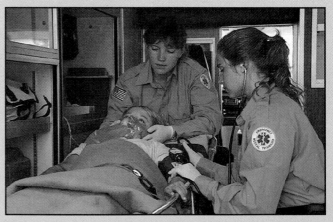

10. Perform ongoing assessment, paying special attention to the patient's ABCs and vital signs, en route to the hospital.

■ ENVIRONMENTAL EMERGENCIES

Environmental emergencies cover a wide range of conditions, including heat exposure, cold exposure, water emergencies, and bites and stings. Some of these problems, like heat exposure, occur more often in some areas of the country than others, but there are certain conditions—like hypothermia—that you may encounter no matter where you are located.

Temperature Regulation

The human body does an amazing job of keeping internal temperature constant despite a bewildering array of environmental conditions. Whether a person lives in the sub-zero Arctic or a tropical jungle, his temperature is kept close to 98.6°F (37°C). The body accomplishes this by balancing the amount of heat generated internally and the amount of heat lost externally.

When someone is exposed to cool or cold temperatures, the body conserves heat by constricting blood vessels, especially the ones in and near the skin surface, thereby limiting the amount of heat given off. At the same time, the person feels cold and puts on clothing to prevent further heat loss. If the temperature dips lower, the person generally puts on more layers of clothing or seeks shelter. If the person's temperature drops below normal despite these measures, the person experiences **hypothermia**.

On the other hand, when someone is exposed to warm or hot temperatures, the body attempts to lose heat through dilation of the blood vessels in and near the skin surface. The person removes clothing to accelerate heat loss. There comes a point, though, when there is no more clothing to remove. Fortunately, there are other means of promoting cooling: conduction, convection, radiation, evaporation, and breathing. If the person's temperature rises above normal despite these efforts, the person experiences **hyperthermia**.

Conduction occurs when two objects of different temperatures touch. The warmer object will transfer heat to the cooler object. An example of this is the summertime hiker who stops and sits on a large rock in the shade. The hiker can become much cooler in a surprisingly short time. For *convection* to work, there must be air currents to carry heat away. This is part of the reason why fans make people feel cooler. *Radiation* of heat occurs when the sun warms the earth or a person stands in the sunshine. There is no need for any medium to carry the heat from the source to the object being warmed. *Evaporative* heat loss occurs through the cooling power of evaporating water or sweat. This is the other reason why fans make people feel cooler in the summer. Finally, *breathing,* or respiration, is the last means of losing heat. This is usually apparent only in colder weather, e.g., the condensation of breath on a cold day.

An understanding of these mechanisms of heat loss can help you not only to protect yourself from extremes of temperature, but also to give your patients better care.

Exposure to Cold

Cold exposure can cause either generalized or localized problems. If the patient's body temperature is lower than normal, he has a generalized condition called **hypothermia**. If only a part of the body is cooled to the point where tissues freeze, this is a localized cold injury commonly called frostbite.

There are many factors that can predispose a patient to cold injury, including the environment, the patient's age and medical condition, and drugs or poisons.

Hypothermia

It is easy to see how a cold environment can induce hypothermia, but what is less obvious is just how easily this can occur. The body temperature of someone who is suddenly immersed in cold water can drop quickly despite all of the body's attempts to prevent it. Less apparent, but more common, is the case of someone old or ill who is exposed to room-temperature air with little clothing for protection. This kind of hypothermia occurs fairly often but can be difficult to recognize because of the subtlety of its presentation.

PEDIATRIC HIGHLIGHT

The extremes of age present another risk factor for hypothermia. Very old and very young patients have a reduced ability to compensate for variations in temperature. Infants and young children, like many elderly people, have thinner skin and less body fat. Shivering may not be as effective because of relatively small muscle mass, especially in infants, who don't shiver at all. Like elderly people who have limited mobility, infants need help putting on additional clothing. Children and infants also have proportionally more body surface area that puts them at additional risk of losing heat. ■

Many medical conditions affect the body's ability to regulate temperature. Shock (hypoperfusion) typically causes sweating, which increases heat loss. So does significant hypoglycemia. A serious head injury sometimes causes a high temperature with significant vasodilation. If the patient is not protected against excessive heat loss, this can eventually cause hypothermia. Burns, because they interfere with the normal function of the skin, prevent the normal mechanisms of heat preservation from working. A generalized infection can cause a fever that leads to so much heat loss that hypothermia develops. An injury to the spinal cord can cause enough vasodilation to produce the same result.

Certain drugs and poisons interfere with the body's ability to respond to changes in temperature. This may be the result of either an overdose or, sometimes, just the proper dose of medication.

The signs and symptoms of hypothermia are progressive. As the patient's core temperature drops, this will usually be reflected in the way he presents. Subtle signs at the beginning of hypothermia become more and more obvious as body temperature continues to go down (Table 10–2).

■ Patient Assessment Hypothermia

For a generalized cold emergency, consider the impact of the following factors: air temperature, wind chill and/or water chill, the patient's age, whether or not the patient's clothing is adequate, health of the patient including underlying illness and existing injuries, how active the patient was during exposure, and whether or not the patient may have used alcohol or drugs.

- Perform an initial assessment.
- Perform a focused history and physical exam of pertinent areas. For all environmental emergencies, in addition to the usual OPQRST information, obtain the following:

  What is the source of the problem (for potentially toxic environmental exposures)?

  If there is alcohol or other drug involvement, what is the exact name of the substance? What route was involved?

  What is the environment like?

  What are the temperature and humidity? Was the patient immersed at any time?

  Was there a loss of consciousness? If so, how long?

  What effects is the patient experiencing?

TABLE 10–2 Stages of Hypothermia

Core Body Temperature		Symptoms
99°F–96°F	37.0°C–35.5°C	Shivering
95°F–91°F	35.5°C–32.7°C	Intense shivering. If conscious, patient has difficulty speaking.
90°F–86°F	32.0°C–30.0°C	Shivering decreases and is replaced by strong muscular rigidity. Muscle coordination is affected and erratic or jerky movements are produced. Thinking is less clear, general comprehension is dulled, possible total amnesia. Patient generally is able to maintain the appearance of psychological contact with surroundings.
85°F–81°F	29.4°C–27.2°C	Patient becomes irrational, loses contact with environment, and drifts into stuporous state. Muscular rigidity continues. Pulse and respirations are slow and cardiac arrhythmias may develop.
80°F–78°F	26.6°C–20.5°C	Patient loses consciousness and does not respond to spoken words. Most reflexes cease to function. Heartbeat becomes erratic.

- Gather a SAMPLE history.
- Obtain a complete set of vital signs.

Signs and Symptoms

The signs and symptoms of hypothermia include the following. Note that decreasing mental status and decreasing motor function both correlate with the degree of hypothermia.

- Shivering in early stages when core body temperature is above 90°F. In severe cases, shivering decreases or is absent.
- Numbness, or reduced-to-lost sensation to touch
- Stiff or rigid posture in prolonged cases
- Drowsiness and/or unwillingness or inability to do even the simplest activities. In prolonged cases, the patient may become irrational, drift into a stuporous state, or actually remove clothing.
- Rapid breathing and rapid pulse in early stages. Slow-to-absent breathing and pulse in prolonged cases. Blood pressure may be low to absent.
- Loss of motor coordination, such as staggering or inability to hold things.
- Joint/muscle stiffness, or muscular rigidity
- Decreased level of consciousness, or unconsciousness. In extreme cases the patient has a "glassy stare."
- Cool abdominal skin temperature. (To assess, place the back of your hand inside the clothing and against the patient's abdomen.)
- Skin may appear red in early stages. In prolonged cases, skin is pale to cyanotic. In most extreme cases, some body parts are stiff and hard (frozen). ▪

During initial assessment, be sure to check an awake patient's orientation to person, place, and time. (Can he tell you his name? where he is? what day it is?) Perform a focused history and physical exam to help you estimate the extent of hypothermia. Assume a case of severe hypothermia if shivering is absent.

Emergency Medical Care Passive rewarming involves simply covering the patient and taking other steps to prevent further heat loss, allowing the body to rewarm itself. **Active rewarming** includes application of an external heat source to the body. All EMS systems permit passive rewarm-

ing. Some EMS systems allow the active rewarming of a hypothermic patient who is alert and responding appropriately. However, many do not.

Active rewarming can prove to be a dangerous process if the patient's condition is more serious than believed. If you are allowed to rewarm a patient with hypothermia who is alert and responding appropriately, do not delay transport. Rewarm the patient while en route. *The emergency care steps listed below assume a protocol that permits active rewarming of a patient who is alert and responding appropriately. Follow your local protocols.*

■ **Patient Care** **Hypothermic Patient Alert and Responding Appropriately**

Emergency Care Steps

For the hypothermic patient who is alert and responding appropriately, proceed with active rewarming.

1. *Remove all of the patient's wet clothing.* Keep him dry, dress him in dry clothing, or wrap him in dry warm blankets. Keep the patient still and handle him very gently. Do not allow the patient to walk or exert himself. Do not massage extremities.

2. *During transport, actively rewarm the patient. Do not warm the patient too quickly.* Gradually and gently apply heat to the patient's body in the form of heat packs, hot water bottles, electric heating pads, warm air, radiated heat, and even your own body heat. Rapid warming will circulate peripherally stagnated cold blood and rapidly cool the vital organs, possibly causing cardiac arrest. If transport is delayed, move the patient to a warm environment if at all possible.

3. *Provide care for shock. Provide oxygen.* The oxygen should be warmed and humidified, if possible.

4. *Give the alert patient warm liquids slowly.* When warm fluids are given too quickly, circulation patterns change, sending blood away from the core to the skin and extremities. Do not allow the patient to eat or drink stimulants.

5. *Except in the mildest of cases (shivering), transport the patient.* Continue to provide high-concentration oxygen and monitor vital signs. *Never allow a patient to remain in, or return to, a cold environment.* ▪

Take the following precautions when actively rewarming a patient.

- *Rewarm the patient slowly.* Handle the patient with great care, the same as you would if there were unstabilized cervical-spine injuries.
- *Use **central rewarming**.* Heat should be applied to the lateral chest, neck, armpits, and groin. You must avoid rewarming the limbs. If they are warmed first, blood will collect in the extremities due to vasodilation (dilation of blood vessels) and may cause a fatal form of shock (see Chapter 12, Bleeding and Shock).
- *If transport must be delayed, a warm bath is very helpful,* but you must keep the patient alert enough so that he does not drown. Again, do not warm the patient too quickly.
- *Keep the patient at rest.* Do not allow the patient to walk, and avoid rough handling of the patient. Such activity may set off severe heart problems, including ventricular fibrillation. Since the patient's blood is coldest in the extremities, exercise or unnecessary movement could also quickly circulate the cold blood and lower the core body temperature.

Patient Care Hypothermic Patient Unresponsive or Not Responding Appropriately

A patient who is unresponsive or not responding appropriately has severe hypothermia. For this patient, provide passive rewarming. Do not try to actively rewarm the patient with severe hypothermia. Remove the patient from the environment and protect him from further heat loss. Active rewarming may cause the patient to develop ventricular fibrillation.

Emergency Care Steps
For the patient with severe hypothermia, you should

1. Assure an open airway.
2. *Provide high-concentration oxygen that has been passed through a warm-water humidifier if possible.* If necessary, the oxygen that has been kept warm in the ambulance passenger compartment can be used. If there is no other choice, oxygen from a cold cylinder may be used.
3. *Wrap the patient in blankets.* If available, use insulating blankets. Handle the patient as gently as possible. Rough handling may cause ventricular fibrillation. Do not allow the patient to eat or drink stimulants. Do not massage extremities.
4. *Transport immediately.* ■

Patient Care Extreme Hypothermia

In extreme cases of hypothermia, you will find the patient unconscious, with no discernible vital signs. In extreme hypothermia, the heart rate can slow to less than 10 beats per minute, and the patient will feel very cold to your touch (core body temperature may be below 80°F). Even so, be aware that it is possible that the patient is still alive or can be resuscitated.

Emergency Care Steps
1. *Assess the carotid pulse* for 30–45 seconds. If there is no pulse, start CPR immediately. (If you detect a pulse, do not start CPR.)
2. *Transport immediately.* ■

Because the hypothermic patient may not reach biological death for over 30 minutes, the staff at the hospital emergency department will not pronounce a patient dead until after he is both rewarmed and resuscitative measures have failed. This means you cannot assume that a severe hypothermia patient is dead on the basis of body temperature and lack of vital signs. As medical personnel point out, "You're not dead until you're warm and dead!"

Local Cold Injury
When the temperature drops low enough, ice crystals form and tissue freezes. This is most likely to occur in cold, windy environments and affect the nose, ears, cheeks, and tips of the fingers and toes. Smoking, like anything that causes constriction of the blood vessels near the skin surface, can increase the risk of local cold injury.

Early or Superficial Local Cold Injury Early or superficial local cold injuries (sometimes called frostnip) are brought about by direct contact with a cold object or exposure of a body part to cold air. Wind chill and water chill also can be major factors. Tissue damage is minor and the response to care is good. The tip of the nose, the tips of the ears, the upper cheeks, and the fingers (all areas that are usually exposed) are most susceptible to

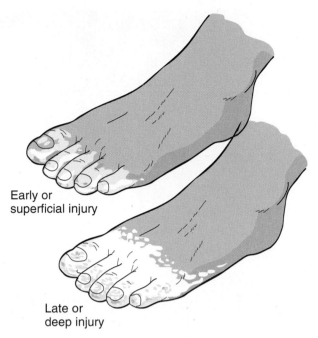

Early or superficial injury

Late or deep injury

FIGURE 10-4 Local cold injuries.

early or superficial local cold injuries. The injury, as its name suggests, is localized, with clear demarcation of its limits.

Patient Assessment Early or Superficial Local Cold Injury

Patients are often unaware of the onset of an early local cold injury until someone indicates that there is something unusual about their skin color.

Signs and Symptoms

● The affected area of patients with light skin at first reddens; dark skin lightens. Both then blanch (whiten). Once blanching begins, the color change can take place very quickly.

● The affected area feels numb to the patient. ∎

Patient Care Early or Superficial Local Cold Injury

Emergency Care Steps

Emergency care for early local cold injury is simple.

1. Get the patient out of the cold environment.
2. Warm the affected area.

3. If the injury is to an extremity, splint and cover it. Do not rub or massage, and do not re-expose to the cold. ∎

Usually, the patient can apply warmth from his own bare hands, blow warm air on the site, or, if the fingers are involved, hold them in the armpits. During recovery from an early local cold injury, the patient may complain about tingling or burning sensations, which is normal. If the condition does not respond to this simple care, begin to treat for a late or deep local cold injury.

Late or Deep Local Cold Injury Late or deep local cold injury (also known as frostbite), develops if an early or superficial local cold injury goes untreated (Figure 10–4). In late or deep local cold injury, the skin and subcutaneous layers of the body part are affected. Muscles, bones, deep blood vessels, and organ membranes can become frozen.

Patient Assessment Late or Deep Local Cold Injury

Signs and Symptoms

● In frostbite, the affected area of the skin appears white and waxy. When the condition progresses to actual freezing, the skin turns mottled or blotchy, the color turns from white to grayish yellow and finally to grayish blue. Swelling and blistering may occur.

● With frostbite, the affected area feels frozen, but only on the surface. The tissue below the surface is still soft and has its normal resilience, or "bounce." With freezing, the tissues are not resilient and feel frozen to the touch. (**Note:** Do not squeeze or poke the tissue. The condition of the deeper tissues can be determined by gently feeling the affected area. Do the assessment as if the affected area had a fractured bone.) ∎

Patient Care Late or Deep Local Cold Injury

Emergency Care Steps

Initial care for late or deep local cold injury—frostbite and freezing—is the same.

1. *Administer high-concentration oxygen.*

2. *Transport to a medical facility without delay,* protecting the frostbitten or frozen area by covering it and handling it as gently as possible.

3. *If transport must be delayed, get the patient indoors and keep him warm.* Do not allow the patient to drink alcohol or smoke, because constriction of blood vessels and decreased circulation to the injured tissues may result. Rewarm the frozen part per local protocol, or request instructions from medical direction. ■

Important: Never listen to myths or folktales about the care of frostbite. Never rub a frostbitten or frozen area. Never rub snow on a frostbitten or frozen area. There are ice crystals at the capillary level; rubbing the injury site may cause them to seriously damage the already injured tissues. Do not break blisters or massage the injured area. Do not allow the patient to walk on an affected extremity. *Do not thaw a frozen limb if there is any chance it will be refrozen.*

Active Rapid Rewarming of Frozen Parts

Active rewarming of frozen parts is seldom recommended. The chance of permanently injuring frozen tissues with active rewarming is too great. Consider it only if local protocols recommend it, if you are instructed to do so by medical direction, or if transport will be severely delayed and you cannot reach medical direction for instructions. If you are in a situation where you must attempt rewarming without instructions from a physician, follow the procedure described here.

You will need warm water and a container in which you can immerse the entire site of injury without the limb touching the sides or bottom of the container. If you cannot find a suitable container, fashion one from a plastic bag supported by a cardboard box or wooden crate (Figure 10–5). Proceed as follows.

1. Heat water to a temperature between 100°F and 105°F. You should be able to put your finger into the water without experiencing discomfort.

2. Fill the container with the heated water and prepare the injured part by removing clothing, jewelry, bands, or straps.

3. Fully immerse the injured part. Do not allow the injured area to touch the sides or bottom of the container. Do not place any pressure on the affected part. Continuously stir the water.

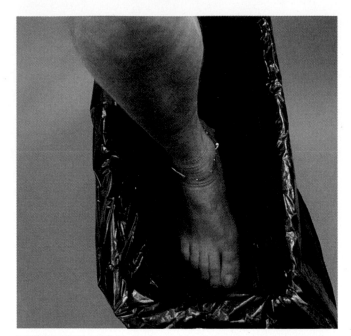

FIGURE 10–5 Rewarming of the frozen part.

When the water cools below 100°F, remove the affected part and add more warm water. The patient may complain of moderate pain as the affected area rewarms or he may experience some period of intense pain. The presence of pain is usually a good indicator of successful rewarming.

4. If you complete rewarming of the part (it no longer feels frozen and is turning red or blue), gently dry the affected area and apply a dry sterile dressing. Place dry sterile dressings between fingers and toes before dressing hands and feet. Next, cover the site with blankets or whatever is available to keep the affected area warm. Do not allow these coverings to come in direct contact with the injured area or to put pressure on the site. It is best if you first build some sort of framework on which the coverings can be placed.

5. Keep the patient at rest. Do not allow the patient to walk if a lower extremity has been frostbitten or frozen.

6. Make certain that you keep the entire patient as warm as possible without overheating. Cover the patient's head with a towel or small blanket to reduce heat loss. Leave the patient's face exposed.

7. Continue to monitor the patient.

8. Assist circulation according to local protocol.

9. Do not allow the limb to refreeze.

10. Transport as soon as possible, with the affected limb slightly elevated.

Exposure to Heat

A patient who is exposed to high temperature is no longer able to lose heat through radiation. This leads to excessive sweating (up to one liter an hour or more) and dehydration. When high temperature is combined with high humidity, the body has even less ability to get rid of excessive heat. In this situation, sweating doesn't work because the air is already saturated with water. This can lead to life-threatening increases in body temperature.

Just as certain conditions increase the risk of cold injury, there are conditions that predispose patients to heat injury. Again, the extremes of age are considerable risk factors—for the reasons mentioned under hypothermia. Pre-existing illnesses such as heart disease, obesity, fatigue, or diabetes also put the patient at increased risk, as do certain medications.

Patient with Moist, Pale, Normal-to-Cool Skin

Prolonged exposure to excessive heat can create an emergency in which the patient presents with moist pale skin that may feel normal or cool to the touch. The individual perspires heavily, often drinking large quantities of water. As the sweating continues, salts are lost by the body, bringing on painful muscle cramps (sometimes called heat cramps). A person who is actively exercising can lose more than a liter of sweat per hour.

Healthy individuals who have been exposed to excessive heat while working or exercising may experience a form of shock brought about by fluid and salt loss. This is seen among firefighters, construction workers, dock workers, and those employed in poorly ventilated warehouses. It is more of a problem during the summer and reaches a peak during prolonged heat waves. This condition is sometimes known as heat exhaustion.

Patient Assessment Heat Emergency Patient with Moist, Pale, Normal-to-Cool Skin

Signs and Symptoms
- Muscular cramps—usually in the legs and abdomen
- Weakness or exhaustion, sometimes dizziness or periods of faintness
- Rapid, shallow breathing
- Weak pulse

- Moist pale skin that may feel normal to cool
- Heavy perspiration
- Loss of consciousness is possible ■

Patient Care Heat Emergency Patient with Moist, Pale, Normal-to-Cool Skin

Emergency Care Steps
1. Remove the patient from the hot environment and place in a cool environment (such as the back of an air-conditioned ambulance).
2. Administer oxygen by nonrebreather mask at 15 liters per minute.
3. Loosen or remove clothing to cool the patient by fanning without chilling him. Watch for shivering.
4. Put patient in supine position with legs elevated. Keep him at rest.
5. If the patient is responsive and not nauseated, have him drink water (Figure 10–6). If he is unresponsive or vomiting, transport to the hospital with patient on his left side.
6. If patient experiences muscular cramps, apply moist towels over cramped muscles.
7. Transport. ■

Patient with Hot Skin (Dry or Moist)

When a person's temperature-regulating mechanisms fail and the body cannot rid itself of excessive heat, you will see a patient with hot, dry or possibly moist skin. When the skin is hot—whether

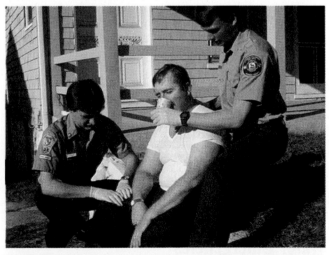

FIGURE 10–6 Give water to the heat emergency patient, if he has moist, pale, normal-to-cool skin and if he is responsive and not nauseated.

dry or moist—this is a true emergency. It is a condition that is sometimes known as heat stroke. The problem is compounded when, in response to loss of fluid and salt, the patient stops sweating, which prevents heat loss through evaporation. Athletes, laborers, and others who exercise or work in hot environments commonly develop this condition. So do the elderly who live in poorly ventilated apartments without air conditioning, and children left in cars with the windows rolled up.

More cases of patients with hot, dry skin are reported on hot, humid days. However, many cases occur from exposure to dry heat.

■ Patient Assessment Heat Emergency Patient with Hot Skin (Dry or Moist)

Signs and Symptoms
- Rapid, shallow breathing
- Full and rapid pulse
- Generalized weakness
- Hot, dry or possibly moist skin
- Little or no perspiration
- Loss of consciousness or altered mental status
- Dilated pupils
- Possible seizures; no muscle cramps ■

■ Patient Care Heat Emergency Patient with Hot Skin (Dry or Moist)

Emergency Care Steps
1. Remove the patient from the hot environment and place in a cool environment (in air-conditioned ambulance with air conditioner running on high).
2. Remove clothing. Apply cool packs to neck, groin, armpits. Keep the skin wet by applying water by sponge or wet towels. Fan aggressively.
3. Administer oxygen by nonrebreather mask at 15 liters per minute.
4. Transport immediately. Should transport be delayed, find a tub or container, immerse the patient up to the neck in cooled water, and monitor vital signs throughout process. ■

Water Emergencies

Drowning occurs when someone dies after being immersed in water. A patient has experienced near-drowning if he has been immersed, but is still alive. In this case, the patient may have no pulse (for the moment), may have a pulse but no breathing, may be unconscious and breathing, or may be alert and in no distress. In all of these cases, you must exercise caution if you decide to rescue the patient. Rescue a patient from the water only if you have the proper training and equipment to do so.

Once you have reached the patient, you must be aggressive in your treatment. This is obvious in the patient who is unconscious, but it is just as important in the patient who is alert and denying any difficulty. A number of patients who look fine shortly after near-drowning episodes deteriorate hours later. Urge all of these patients to accept your offer of treatment and transportation.

■ Patient Assessment Water Emergencies

Learn to look for the following problems in water-related accident victims.

- *Airway obstruction* This may be from water in the lungs, foreign matter in the airway, or swollen airway tissues. Spasms of the larynx may be present in cases of near-drowning.
- *Cardiac arrest* This is often related to respiratory arrest or occurs before the near-drowning.
- *Signs of heart attack* Through overexertion, the patient may have greater problems than the obvious near-drowning. Some untrained rescuers too quickly conclude that chest pains are due to muscle cramps as a result of swimming.
- *Injuries to the head and neck* These are expected to be found in boating, water-skiing, and diving accidents, but they also occur in swimming accidents.
- *Internal injuries* While doing the focused physical exam, stay on the alert for musculoskeletal injuries, soft-tissue injuries, and internal bleeding (which may be missed during the first stages of care).
- *Generalized cooling, or hypothermia* The water does not have to be very cold and the length of stay in the water does not have to be very long for hypothermia to occur. In some cases of near-drowning, the patient may have a better chance for survival in cold water.
- *Substance abuse* Alcohol and drug use are closely associated with adolescent and adult drownings. Elevated blood alcohol levels have been found in over 30 percent of

drowning victims. The screening for drug use has not been as extensive as that done for alcohol, but research indicates that drugs are a contributory factor in many water-related accidents.

- *Drowning or near-drowning* The patient may be discovered under or face down in the water. He may be unconscious and without discernible vital signs or may be conscious, breathing, and coughing up water. ■

Patient Care **Water Emergencies**

Emergency Care Steps
1. Ensure the safety of all rescue personnel.
2. Suspect spine injury if the patient was diving or if diving cannot be ruled out.
3. If the patient has been submerged in cold water, be aggressive in your resuscitation efforts. Any pulseless, nonbreathing patient who has been submerged in cold water should receive resuscitation efforts unless medical direction orders otherwise.
4. If the patient is in the water and you suspect spine injury, apply neutral in-line immobilization of the head and cervical spine. Remove the patient from the water with a backboard (Skill Summary 10–5).
5. If there is no reason to suspect a spine injury, place the patient on his left side to allow water, vomitus, and secretions to drain from the upper airway.
6. Suction as needed.
7. Administer oxygen if you have not already done so during the initial assessment.
8. If you are unable to ventilate the patient because of gastric distention, place the patient on his left side. With suction immediately available, place your hand over the epigastric area of the abdomen and apply firm pressure to relieve the distention. Do this only if the gastric distention interferes with ventilation. ■

Bites and Stings

Animals that bite and sting far outnumber human beings on this planet, and it is only natural to expect some of them to be toxic. Fortunately, most of them cause no more than transient discomfort or mild pain. There are a few, however, that can cause more serious problems—sometimes from an allergic or anaphylactic reaction.

(You reviewed the recognition and treatment of this condition earlier in this chapter.) At other times, the problem results from a poisonous or venomous sting or bite.

The specific signs and symptoms you will see depend not only on the particular animal, but also on the patient and the circumstances surrounding the exposure. A very young or very old patient may react more strongly to a sting, for example, as may someone who has a pre-existing illness. Bites and stings of interest to EMT-Bs commonly result from insects, spiders, snakes, and marine life.

Patient Assessment **Bites and Stings**

- Perform an initial assessment.
- Perform a focused history and physical exam.
- Gather a SAMPLE history.
- Obtain a complete set of vital signs.
- Evaluate the patient for these signs and symptoms:

  History of bite (spider, snake) or sting (insect, scorpion, marine animal)

  Pain, redness, and swelling

  Weakness and dizziness

  Chills and fever

  Nausea and vomiting

  Bite marks

  Stinger ■

Patient Care **Bites and Stings**

Emergency Care Steps
1. If a stinger is present, remove it. Scrape the stinger out, e.g., with the edge of a credit card. Avoid using tweezers or forceps as these can squeeze venom from the venom sac into the wound.
2. Wash the area gently.
3. Remove jewelry from the injured area before swelling begins, if possible.
4. Position the injection site slightly below the level of the patient's heart.
5. Do not apply cold to snakebites.
6. If the wound is a snakebite, consult medical direction about whether to apply a constricting band.
7. Observe the patient for development of signs and symptoms of an allergic reaction. Treat appropriately. ■

Water Rescue—Possible Spinal Injury

1. Splint head and neck with arms.

2. Roll patient over into supine position.

3. Ensure airway and breathing.
- Patient not breathing: Begin rescue breathing (with a mask if possible) and rescue from water as soon as possible.
- Patient breathing: Slide backboard under patient.

4. Apply a rigid extrication collar.

5. Tie down torso, then head and neck with straps or cravats. Float board to edge of water.

6. Remove patient from water (with as much assistance as needed).

Chapter Review

■ SUMMARY

Difficulty breathing (dyspnea) is one of the most common complaints to which EMS agencies respond. On these calls, the EMT-B needs to determine quickly whether the patient is breathing adequately and begin assisting ventilations in those patients who have inadequate breathing. Fortunately, most dyspneic patients are breathing adequately, in spite of their respiratory distress. Oxygen is a treatment the EMT-B can easily and quickly administer and is essential to these patients. If a patient with breathing difficulty has a prescribed inhaler, the EMT-B can now assist the patient in using it.

Truly life-threatening allergic reactions are rare, but EMS is likely to be called when they occur. When this happens, the EMT-B must quickly and carefully assess the patient. Also, if the patient has an epinephrine auto-injector, the EMT-B must determine whether the patient's condition justifies use of the device, in accordance with local protocol.

Environmental emergencies are frequently obvious, but sometimes they are subtle and difficult to detect. The patient who has been in cold water for fifteen minutes should obviously be treated for hypothermia. But so should the confused elderly patient who was found on the floor next to her bed in the morning. Heat exposure is usually apparent from the patient's condition and history. The mainstay of life-saving treatment is to cool the patient who has hot skin. The treatment of bites and stings consists primarily of limiting further injury and transporting the patient.

■ REVIEW QUESTIONS

1. Describe the assessment of an alert patient who is complaining of difficulty breathing.
2. What conditions must a patient meet for you to assist in use of an inhaler?
3. List three body systems and the signs and symptoms of anaphylaxis associated with each.
4. What are the indications for use of an epinephrine auto-injector?
5. When should you rewarm an extremity with a local cold injury?
6. How should you cool a patient who is unconscious and has hot, dry skin?
7. Describe the steps in the management of a patient with a scorpion sting.

11

Medical Emergencies
- *Diabetes*
- *Poisoning and Overdose*
- *Behavioral*

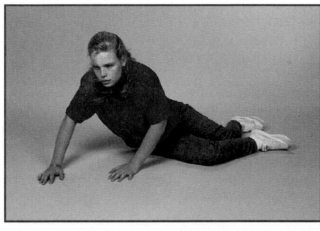

■ *The revised EMT-B curriculum recognizes the need to give EMT-Bs appropriate medical interventions to improve patient outcome in the diabetic or poisoning emergency. With medical direction approval, you will be able to carry and administer oral glucose and activated charcoal. This chapter discusses when you should use these medical interventions.*

As an experienced EMT, you know the importance of a thorough patient assessment. A rapid, well-organized evaluation of your patient's condition helps ensure proper treatment. This chapter

focuses on how to conduct assessments for diabetic, poisoning, and behavioral emergencies. An understanding of how treatment is driven by your assessment findings will also be discussed.

Finally, you will gain a greater understanding of the changing roles, skills, and responsibilities of the EMT-B. Why is this important? Knowing how newly trained EMT-Bs approach

a diabetic, poisoning, or behavioral emergency prepares you to work more effectively as a team member. This cooperative effort leads to improved patient care and improved patient outcomes.

MAKING THE TRANSITION

- Treatment of the medical emergencies involving diabetics, poisoning/overdose, and behavioral problems is driven by assessment findings.
- EMT-Bs are now able to administer oral glucose and activated charcoal.
- Dilution of some ingested poisons is recommended.
- Scene-safety is stressed before an EMT-B treats a behavioral emergency.

177

OBJECTIVES

The numbered objectives below are from the United States Department of Transportation 1994 EMT-Basic National Standard Curriculum. Objectives with color bullets that follow in italics are from the EMT-Basic Transitional Program.

■ KNOWLEDGE AND ATTITUDE

At the completion of this lesson, you should be able to:

Diabetes and Altered Mental Status

1. Identify the patient taking diabetic medication with altered mental status and the implications of a diabetes history. (p. 180)
2. State the steps in the emergency medical care of the patient taking diabetic medicine with an altered mental status and a history of diabetes. (pp. 181, 182, 183)
3. Establish the relationship between airway management and the patient with altered mental status. (pp. 181, 182)
4. State the generic and trade names, medication forms, dose, administration, actions, and contraindications for oral glucose. (p. 183)
5. Evaluate the need for medical direction in the emergency medical care of the diabetic patient. (pp. 181, 182)
6. Explain the rationale for administering oral glucose. (pp. 180, 181)
- *Discuss the general pharmacology of the medications that will be administered by the EMT-Basic. (p. 183)*
- *Describe the relationship between assessment findings and medical interventions for diabetes. (pp. 180–182, 183)*
- *Defend the rationale for the EMT-Basic to carry and assist with medications. (p. 180)*
- *Recognize and respond to the feelings of the patient who may require interventions to be performed. (pp. 180, 181)*

Poisoning and Overdose Emergencies

1. List various ways that poisons enter the body. (p. 182)
2. List signs and symptoms associated with poisoning. (p. 184)
3. Discuss the emergency medical care for the patient with possible overdose. (pp. 184–186)

4. Describe the steps in the emergency medical care for the patient with suspected poisoning. (pp. 184–186, 187–189)
5. Establish the relationship between the patient suffering from poisoning or overdose and airway management. (pp. 184, 187)
6. State the generic and trade names, indications, contraindications, medication forms, dose, administration, actions, side effects, and reassessment strategies for activated charcoal. (p. 185)
7. Recognize the need for medical direction in caring for the patient with poisoning or overdose. (pp. 182, 184, 188, 189)
8. Explain the rationale for administering activated charcoal. (p. 182)
9. Explain the rationale for contacting medical direction early in the prehospital management of the poisoning overdose patient. (pp. 182, 184, 188, 189)
- *Discuss the general pharmacology for the medications that will be administered by the EMT-Basic. (p. 185)*
- *Describe the relationship between assessment findings and medical interventions for poisoning/overdose. (pp. 182–186)*
- *Defend the rationale for the EMT-Basic to carry and assist with medications. (p. 182)*
- *Recognize and respond to the feelings of the patient who may require interventions to be performed. (p. 184)*

Behavioral Emergencies

1. Define behavioral emergencies. (p. 186)
2. Discuss the general factors that may cause an alteration in a patient's behavior. (pp. 186, 190)
3. State the various reasons for psychological crises. (pp. 186, 190)
4. Discuss the characteristics of an individual's behavior that suggests that the patient is at risk for suicide. (pp. 186, 190)
5. Discuss special medical/legal considerations for managing behavioral emergencies. (pp. 186, 190)
6. Discuss the special considerations for assessing a patient with behavioral problems. (pp. 186, 190)

7. Discuss the general principles of an individual's behavior that suggests that he is at risk for violence. (pp. 186, 190)

8. Discuss the methods used to calm behavioral emergency patients. (p. 190)

9. Explain the rationale for learning how to modify your behavior toward the patient with a behavioral emergency. (pp. 186, 190)

■ SKILLS

Diabetes and Altered Mental Status

1. Demonstrate the steps in the emergency medical care for the patient taking diabetic medicine with an altered mental status and a history of diabetes.

2. Demonstrate the steps in the administration of oral glucose.

3. Demonstrate the assessment and documentation of patient response to oral glucose.

4. Demonstrate how to complete a prehospital care report for patients with diabetic emergencies.

● *Given medical scenarios, demonstrate the ability to properly assess the patient and demonstrate the ability to properly utilize the intervention of oral glucose.*

Poisoning and Overdose Emergencies

1. Demonstrate the steps in the emergency medical care for the patient with possible overdose.

2. Demonstrate the steps in the emergency medical care for the patient with suspected poisoning.

3. Perform the necessary steps required to provide a patient with activated charcoal.

4. Demonstrate the assessment and documentation of patient response.

5. Demonstrate the proper disposal of the equipment for the administration of activated charcoal.

6. Demonstrate completing a prehospital care report for patients with a poisoning/overdose emergency.

● *Given medical scenarios, demonstrate the ability to properly assess the patient and demonstrate the ability to properly utilize the intervention of activated charcoal.*

Behavioral Emergencies

1. Demonstrate the assessment and emergency medical care of the patient experiencing a behavioral emergency.

2. Demonstrate various techniques to safely restrain a patient with a behavioral problem.

Your EMS unit is called to a local college dormitory for an unresponsive patient. You arrive, begin your **scene size-up**, and exit the ambulance. College security officers motion you in.

You take the elevator to the third floor. You exit to find a crowd around one of the doors. The crowd is orderly and stands aside to let you access the patient. You don protective gloves and approach the patient.

He is verbally responsive but appears to be speaking incoherently. His roommate tells you that his name is Keith. You perform an **initial assessment** and find Keith breathing adequately and that he has adequate circulation. You find no evidence of trauma. Your general impression is of a 19-year-old male with an altered mental status. He is given a high priority.

Since Keith has an unknown problem, you perform a **rapid trauma assessment** that provides no signs of injury. Your partner interviews the roommate, who cannot provide any medical history. A security guard suggests intoxication, which the roommate denies.

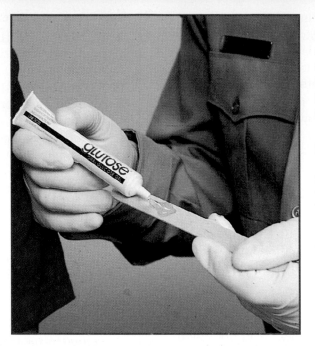

The baseline vitals seem within normal limits with the exception of Keith's skin—it is cool and moist. Although Keith has been placed on oxygen, his level of consciousness has deteriorated slightly.

As you prepare for transport, you ask the college security officers to radio their dispatcher for any information they may have about Keith. You take a last look at the room, but you see no signs of alcohol or drugs. Keith does not have any medical alert devices.

As you work your way back to the ambulance, the security officer has called Keith's parents and reports that Keith is a diabetic. As soon as you reach the ambulance, you verify that Keith is conscious and able to swallow. Your medical director has instituted a standing order for the use of oral glucose. You squeeze oral glucose onto a tongue depressor and insert it into Keith's mouth between his cheek and gum. The oral glucose provides a response in minutes.

It was your diligence that allowed you to provide the necessary care to Keith, who turned out to be a diabetic. This was done while beginning the transportation process. ■

There are many causes of altered mental status—diabetes is only one. This chapter covers diabetes, poisoning and overdose, and behavioral emergencies—all of which may present as "altered mental status."

■ DIABETIC EMERGENCIES

While the old curriculum focused on treatment driven by diagnosis, the On the Scene scenario demonstrates treatment that is driven by your assessment findings. How you manage a diabetic emergency depends on your ability to assess an altered mental status, a history of diabetes, and the patient's ability to swallow. An initial assess-ment and focused history and physical exam are simply a patient plan of action to help you arrive at the most accurate assessment finding.

Your assessment findings also help you determine what type of medical intervention is appropriate. In this situation, the patient received oral glucose, which is the appropriate medical intervention. The revised EMT-B curriculum recognizes what many EMS systems have practiced for years: Early recognition of the diabetic emergency, along with the prompt administration of sugar, is a safe and highly effective medical intervention. Instead of treating oral glucose administration as a special skill learned only after field experience, EMT-Bs are now trained to provide this life-saving medical intervention at the outset of their training/career.

Administering Oral Glucose

As you know, low blood sugar, or **hypoglycemia**, is the most common medical emergency for a diabetic. Hypoglycemia occurs when the diabetic

- takes too much insulin or oral medications used to treat diabetes, or ...
- decreases sugar levels by not eating, or ...
- overexercises and uses sugar faster than normal, or ...
- vomits and empties the stomach of food and sugar.

Oral glucose, which comes as a gel, in toothpaste-type tubes, increases the patient's blood sugar. With the approval of medical direction, oral glucose is given when *all* of the following criteria are met:

- The patient presents with an altered mental status.
- The patient has a history of diabetes.
- The patient is alert enough to swallow.

You administer glucose by squeezing it from the tube onto a tongue depressor. Some patients may be frightened and unsure of your capabilities. If your patient is responsive, explain the procedure you are about to perform. A calm reassuring approach both relaxes the patient and helps instill confidence in your treatment efforts. Next, place the tongue depressor between the patient's cheek and gum. The patient typically responds with an improved level of orientation in several minutes. When oral glucose is given properly, there are no side effects. Aspiration of the glucose into the trachea may occur in patients without a gag reflex. Therefore, make sure that the patient can swallow.

If there is no response to the oral glucose and/or the patient loses consciousness or seizes, remove the tongue depressor. Suction the airway as needed. Contact medical direction about whether to administer additional glucose.

Patient Assessment Diabetic Emergencies

An assessment-based approach to the diabetic emergency means you recognize and treat the condition based on your findings. It is not important that you distinguish the difference between hypoglycemia or hyperglycemia (high blood sugar).

The treatment is the same. To obtain accurate findings for the diabetic emergency

- Perform the initial assessment. Assess for an altered mental status by using AVPU. Assess ABCs. If a life-threatening condition exists, treat it immediately.

Then for the **responsive patient:**

- Perform a focused history and physical exam.
- Assess history of present illness.
- Assess SAMPLE history.

  <u>S</u>igns/<u>S</u>ymptoms   Are there any other symptoms? Has the patient vomited?

  <u>A</u>llergies   Is the patient allergic to anything?

  <u>M</u>edications   Does the patient take any medications? (Insulin might be found in the refrigerator.)

  <u>P</u>ertinent past history   Does the patient have other medical problems? Have similar problems happened before? Who is the patient's doctor?

  <u>L</u>ast oral intake   When did the patient last eat or drink? What did the patient eat or drink?

  <u>E</u>vents leading to the illness   How does the patient feel?

- Assess vital signs: respirations, pulse, skin, pupils, and blood pressure.
- Provide emergency care. (Check with medical direction; in some jurisdictions, oral glucose may be given before the vital signs are taken.)

For the **unresponsive patient:**

- Perform a focused history and physical exam.
- Perform a rapid trauma exam. Assess the head, neck, chest, abdomen, pelvis, extremities, and posterior aspect of the body.
- Assess vital signs: respirations, pulse, skin, pupils, and blood pressure.
- Gather a SAMPLE history from bystanders or family.
- Provide emergency care.

Signs and Symptoms
- Altered mental status; if conscious, may appear intoxicated, anxious, combative
- Slurred speech
- Staggering walk
- Rapid heart rate
- Cold, clammy skin
- Hunger
- Seizures ■

Emergency Care Steps

1. After completing the appropriate assessment steps, obtain order from medical direction either by radio or by protocols to administer oral glucose. Consider request for advanced life support.
2. Assure that the patient

   has altered mental status

   has history of diabetes

   is conscious and can swallow.
3. Administer glucose (Skill Summary 11–1).
4. Perform ongoing assessment.

   If patient loses consciousness or seizures, remove tongue depressor, secure airway, and provide artificial ventilations if necessary. ■

■ SEIZURES

If the normal functions of the brain are upset by injury, infection, or disease, the electrical activity of the brain can become irregular. This irregularity can bring about a sudden change in sensation, behavior, or movement, called a seizure. Some seizures involve the uncontrolled muscular movements called *convulsions.* The most common reason for EMS calls involving seizures in adults is failure to take anti-seizure medication. The most common cause of seizures in infants and children 6 months to 3 years of age is high fever (see Chapter 14.)

The emergency medical care for seizures includes assuring patency of airway, positioning patient on side if no possibility of cervical spine trauma, having suction ready, and transporting. If the patient exhibits signs of inadequate respirations, assure airway and artificially ventilate.

■ POISONING AND OVERDOSE EMERGENCIES

How Poisons Enter the Body

A poison is any substance that can harm the body by altering cell structure or functioning. Poisons may enter the body in four ways:

- Ingestion (swallowing)
- Inhalation (breathing in)
- Absorption (through unbroken skin)
- Injection (through the skin, by a needle, snake fangs, or insect stinger)

Administering Activated Charcoal

Research now suggests that the most effective means for managing many ingested poisons includes the administration of activated charcoal. In some cases, dilution of ingested poisons is also recommended. Poison-control experts no longer consider syrup of ipecac the medication of first choice. Ipecac's disadvantages are slowness and relative ineffectiveness; syrup of ipecac may take longer than 15 or 20 minutes to work. During this delay, a patient can become drowsy or lose consciousness. This increases the chances of aspiration of vomitus in a nonalert patient. Regarding ipecac's effectiveness, studies indicate that, **on the average,** less than a third of the patient's stomach contents are removed following vomiting. Due to these disadvantages, activated charcoal replaces ipecac as the first drug of choice for certain ingested poisons.

How does activated charcoal work? Activated charcoal binds with many ingested poisons and drugs and prevents absorption into the body. Activated charcoal is pre-mixed in water. It typically is available in a plastic bottle. Veteran EMTs may remember the messiness of the powder form of activated charcoal. Powdered charcoal should not be used in the field.

Many poisons are absorbed by activated charcoal, but rather than memorizing all the poisons which activated charcoal effectively absorbs, you should consult medical direction before giving activated charcoal.

Since it may not always be clear which patients should receive activated charcoal, remember these conditions for which activated charcoal is contraindicated:

- A patient who cannot swallow
- Ingestion of acids or alkalis
- Altered mental status
- A patient who swallows gasoline

To provide proper administration of activated charcoal, follow the instructions given to you by medical direction. Occasionally, medical direction may request **dilution** of an ingested poison.

Administering Oral Glucose

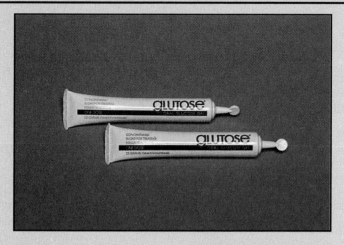

MEDICATION NAME

1. Generic: Glucose, oral
2. Trade: Glutose, Insta-glucose

INDICATIONS

1. Patients with altered mental status with a known history of diabetes mellitus

CONTRAINDICATIONS

1. Unconsciousness
2. Known diabetic who has not taken insulin for days
3. Unable to swallow

MEDICATION FORM

Gel, in toothpaste-type tubes

DOSAGE

One tube

ADMINISTRATION

1. Assure signs and symptoms of altered mental status with a known history of diabetes
2. Assure patient is conscious and able to swallow
3. Administer glucose
   a. Place on tongue depressor between cheek and gum
   b. Self-administered between cheek and gum
4. Perform ongoing assessment

ACTIONS

Increases blood sugar

SIDE EFFECTS

None when given properly. May be aspirated by the patient without a gag reflex.

REASSESSMENT STRATEGIES

If patient loses consciousness or seizes, remove tongue depressor from mouth.

Dilution with water may delay the absorption rates of some poisons; dilution with milk may soothe an upset stomach. As with the administration of activated charcoal, you should consult medical direction before you decide to dilute any ingested poison.

Patient Assessment Poisoning and Overdose Emergencies

A rapid, organized approach to patient assessment is essential in cases of possible ingested poisoning. Before you contact medical direction you should:

- Perform the initial assessment. Look for an altered mental status. Use AVPU to assess mental status. Assess ABCs. If a life-threatening condition exists, treat immediately.

Then for the **responsive patient:**

- Perform a focused history and physical exam.
  Assess history of present illness.
    What substance was ingested?
    When was the substance ingested?
    How much was ingested?
    Over what time period did the ingestion occur?
    What interventions have the patient, family, or bystanders taken?
    How much does the patient weigh?
  Assess SAMPLE history.
    <u>S</u>igns/<u>S</u>ymptoms   Are there any other symptoms? Has patient vomited?
    <u>A</u>llergies   Is patient allergic to anything?
    <u>M</u>edications   Does patient take any medications?
    <u>P</u>ertinent past history   Does patient have other medical problems? Has this problem happened before? Who is the patient's doctor?
    <u>L</u>ast oral intake   When did the patient last eat or drink? What did patient eat or drink?
    <u>E</u>vents leading to the illness   How does the patient feel?
- Assess vital signs: respirations, pulse, skin, pupils, and blood pressure.
- Provide emergency care. (Check with your medical direction. In some jurisdictions, syrup of ipecac may still be the medication of first choice for ingested poisons.)

For the **unresponsive patient:**

- Perform a focused history and physical exam.

Perform a rapid trauma exam. Assess the head, neck, chest, abdomen, pelvis, extremities, and posterior aspect of the body.
Assess vital signs: respirations, pulse, skin, pupils, and blood pressure.
Gather and assess a SAMPLE history from bystanders or family.
- Provide emergency care.

Signs and Symptoms
The following signs and symptoms are associated with the poisoning or overdose emergency.

- Nausea
- Vomiting
- Diarrhea
- Altered mental status
- Abdominal pain
- Chemical burns around or inside the mouth
- Rapid pulse
- Abnormal breath odors ■

Patient Care Poisoning and Overdose Emergencies

Emergency Care Steps
1. Perform the initial assessment. Recognize and treat immediately life-threatening problems discovered during the initial assessment. Request advanced life support when appropriate.
2. Perform a focused history and physical exam. Remove any pills, tablets, or fragments from patient's mouth.
3. Assess baseline vital signs.
4. Consult medical direction. Administer activated charcoal (Skill Summary 11–2) or dilute with water or milk as directed by medical direction.
5. Bring all poison containers, bottles, and labels to receiving facility.
6. Conduct ongoing assessment en route to the emergency department. ■

Preceptor Pearl

Sometimes it can be very difficult to convince a patient to drink a pre-mixed solution of activated charcoal. Providing a covered container and straw to the patient may make it easier to drink a medication that looks like mud. As mentioned previously, it is important to acknowledge any fear and apprehension your patient is experiencing. Your calm, professional demeanor helps gain a patient's trust and respect in your ability to administer medication in the appropriate manner. Remember, too, that activated charcoal can be given to the patient while en route to the receiving facility. ✤

Administering Activated Charcoal

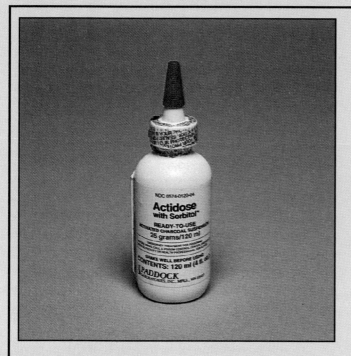

MEDICATION NAME

1. Generic: activated charcoal
2. Trade: SuperChar, InstaChar, Actidose, Liqui-Char, and others

INDICATIONS

1. Poisoning by mouth

CONTRAINDICATIONS

1. Altered mental status
2. Ingestion of acids or alkalis
3. Unable to swallow

MEDICATION FORM

1. Pre-mixed in water, frequently available in plastic bottle containing 12.5 grams of activated charcoal
2. Powder—should be avoided in field

DOSAGE

1. Adults and children: 1 gram activated charcoal/kg of body weight
2. Usual adult dose: 25–50 grams
3. Usual pediatric dose: 12.5–25 grams

ADMINISTRATION

1. Consult medical direction.
2. Shake container *thoroughly*.
3. Since medication looks like mud, patient may need to be persuaded to drink it. Providing a covered container and a straw will prevent patient from seeing the medication and so may improve patient compliance.
4. If patient does not drink the medication right away, the charcoal will settle. Shake or stir it again before administering.
5. Record the name, dose, route, and time of administration of the medication.

ACTIONS

1. Activated charcoal binds to certain poisons and prevents them from being absorbed into the body.
2. Not all brands of activated charcoal are the same; some bind much more than others, so consult medical direction about the brand to use.

SIDE EFFECTS

1. Black stools
2. Some patients, particularly those who have ingested poisons that cause nausea, may vomit. If patient vomits, repeat the dose once.

REASSESSMENT STRATEGIES

1. Be prepared for the patient to vomit or further deteriorate.

For the other types of poison exposures (inhaled, absorbed, or injected poisons) apply the assessment techniques learned in this chapter. Treatment for these poison exposures remains the same (Skill Summaries 3 and 4). Emergency care steps for injected poisons were discussed in Chapter 10.

PEDIATRIC HIGHLIGHT

Accidental ingestion of poison occurs most frequently with children. No matter how horrible something tastes, children will sometimes drink the same poison on more than one occasion. Also, with children it is very difficult to determine how much of a poison has been ingested. Always treat for the worst possible ingestion. Remember, before appropriate care is provided, you will need to give medical direction the child's approximate weight. ■

■ BEHAVIORAL EMERGENCIES

As an experienced EMT, you know that many calls involve situations in which the patient acts in strange, unexpected, and sometimes dangerous ways. However, you are not expected to diagnose these behaviors. The new curriculum does not require you to learn many psychiatric terms used to describe the kind of behavioral emergencies you might encounter. As an EMT-B, it is not critical for you to determine if the patient is schizophrenic, psychotic, or neurotic. You are, however, expected to recognize emotional danger signals which alert you to the possibility of a patient who may be a danger to himself or others. The curriculum lists behavioral emergencies as: **emotional emergencies, psychiatric emergencies, potential or attempted suicide, and aggressive or hostile behavior.**

Occasionally, unusual behavior has a medical cause. Earlier in this chapter, we discussed how a hypoglycemic patient may appear intoxicated. From your experience, you also know that some ingested poisons and overdoses can cause unusual behavior. Once again, appropriate patient care in the behavioral emergency does not depend on a specific diagnosis.

Behavioral emergencies require you to begin your care only when the scene is secure. Once it is safe to approach the patient, you should identify and treat immediately any threats to life.

The revised curriculum also stresses the importance of following local protocols for the safe restraint of the behavioral-emergency patient. Accordingly, your agency's protocols should be consistent with state and local ordinances.

Finally, early recognition of the patient in need of advanced life support care is an important component of the revised curriculum. Of course, not every community has access to advanced life support. If you work in a system that does, remember to contact advanced life support as soon as possible. If your system is without access to ALS, then your primary responsibility is prompt treatment and rapid transport to the nearest appropriate hospital or medical facility.

■ **Patient Assessment** **Behavioral Emergencies**

An assessment-based approach to a behavioral emergency begins with caution. Before you begin your initial assessment, make sure the scene is safe.

● Ask for police assistance if, prior to your emergency response to the scene, you know the patient is displaying destructive behavior.

● Conduct a scene size-up. Ensure personal safety. Ask yourself: Is the patient in an unsafe environment? Are there unsafe objects in the possession of or in reach of the patient?

● Perform the initial assessment only after it is safe to approach the patient. Determine the following:

Is there a life-threatening condition? If so, treat immediately.

How does the patient feel?

Does the patient have suicidal tendencies?

Is the patient a threat to self or others?

Remember to assess mental status using these indicators in behavioral emergencies:

Appearance

Activity level

Speech

Orientation to person, place, and time

For the **responsive patient:**

● Perform a focused history and physical exam.

Assess vital signs: respirations, pulse, skin, pupils, and blood pressure.

● Conduct a SAMPLE history. Consider the following common causes for behavioral changes:

Lack of oxygen

Low blood sugar

Inhaled Poisons

> **SAFETY NOTE:**
>
> In the presence of hazardous fumes or gases, wear protective clothing and self-contained breathing apparatus or wait for those who are properly trained and equipped to enter the scene and bring the patient out.

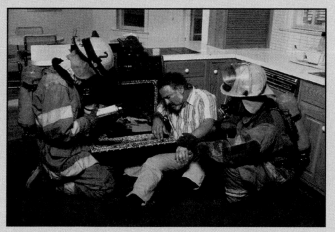

1. Remove patient from source.

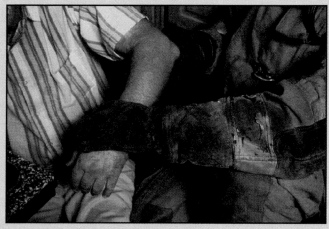

2. Avoid touching contaminated clothing and jewelry.

3. Remember: It is critical to establish and maintain an open airway.

4. Caution: Stay alert for vomiting. Properly position patient and have suction equipment ready.

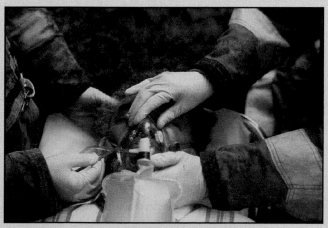

5. Administer a high concentration of oxygen.

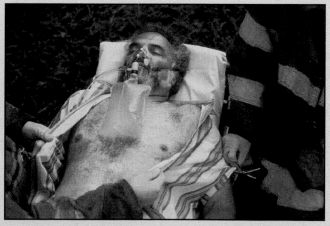

6. Remove contaminated clothing and jewelry.

CHAPTER 11 Medical Emergencies—Diabetes, Poisoning and Overdose, Behavioral

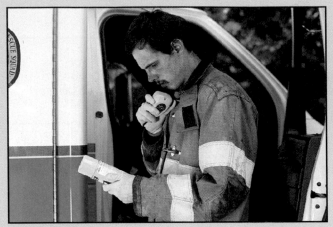

7. Call medical direction. Follow directions.

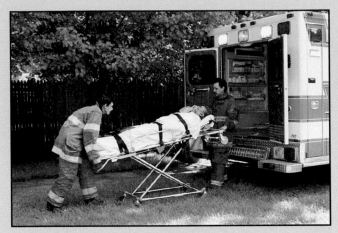

8. Transport as soon as possible.

WARNING:

If called to the scene of a hazardous material incident, do only what you have been trained to do and what your equipment allows. Be careful to protect other rescuers and assure that the patient has been decontaminated by a hazardous materials response team (see Chapter 18). Remember that inhaled poisons can frequently be absorbed through the skin.

Absorbed Poisons

> **SAFETY NOTE:**
>
> Take care to protect your skin from contact with poisonous substances. Wear protective clothing. If necessary, have firefighters or others who are properly protected hose off the patient before you touch him.

FIRST take body substance isolation precautions.

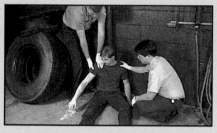

1. Remove patient from source or source from patient. Avoid contaminating yourself with the poison. If a powder, brush it off the patient's skin.

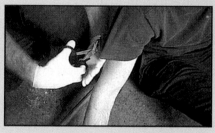

2. Remove contaminated clothing and other articles.

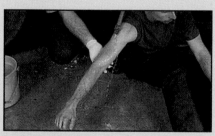

3. Wash with clear water. Call medical direction. Follow directions.

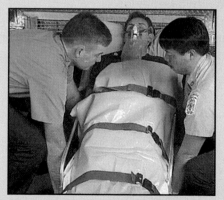

4. Be alert for shock and transport as soon as possible.

> **WARNING:**
>
> If called to the scene of a hazardous material incident, do only what you have been trained to do and what your equipment allows. Be careful to protect other rescuers and assure that the patient has been decontaminated by a hazardous materials response team (see Chapter 18).

Head trauma

Mind-altering drugs

Inadequate blood flow to the brain

Excessive cold or heat

Depression

For the **unresponsive patient:**

● Perform a focused history and physical exam.

  Perform a rapid trauma exam. Assess the head, neck, chest, abdomen, pelvis, extremities, and posterior aspect of the body.

  Assess vital signs: respirations, pulse, skin, pupils, and blood pressure.

  Gather and assess SAMPLE history from bystanders or family.

Signs and Symptoms

Experienced EMTs know that the signs and symptoms of a behavioral emergency are highly variable. Situational stresses, medical illness, psychiatric problems, and alcohol and drugs are all factors that may affect a person's behavior. Look for the following signs and symptoms:

● Panic

● Agitation

● Anxious, combative attitude

● Sadness, crying, depression

● Bizarre thinking and behavior

● Threatening behavior

● Self-destructive behavior ■

Patient Care Behavioral Emergencies

Emergency Care Steps

1. Scene size-up

2. Patient assessment

   Identify yourself, let the person know you are there to help.

   Question the patient in a calm, reassuring, nonjudgmental manner.

   Acknowledge the patient's feelings.

   Listen to what the patient says. Repeat back to patient what you have heard.

3. Calm the patient.

   Tell the patient you wish to help.

   Acknowledge the patient's feelings.

   Encourage the patient to express problems.

   Tell the truth.

   Use good eye contact.

   Do not make quick moves.

   Maintain a comfortable distance.

4. Restrain the patient if necessary. (Follow local protocol for restraint procedures.)

5. Transport. (If overdose patient, bring any drugs or medications found to receiving facility.) ■

Preceptor Pearl

Assessment and care of the behavioral emergency patient require a high level of caution. Experienced EMT-Bs know that anything can happen at any time. Newly certified EMT-Bs should remember to maintain a safe distance when managing all behavioral-emergency patients. Finally, management of the behavioral emergency takes time. As an EMT-B, be prepared to spend time with the behavioral emergency patient. Remember, these types of calls require that you become "patient with the patient." ✤

CHAPTER REVIEW

■ SUMMARY

This chapter stresses the importance of a rapid, organized approach to patient assessment and medical intervention. Your treatment decisions are a direct result of your ability to pull together information from your assessment findings. As demonstrated by the On the Scene scenario, the assessment-based approach quickly identifies any life threats and provides for immediate medical intervention.

For the diabetic emergency, you do not need to spend time gathering diagnostic information to determine if a patient suffers from hypoglycemia or hyperglycemia. The treatment remains the same. Give oral glucose.

Since the practice of emergency medical care constantly changes, care procedures are updated so that medical interventions by EMT-Bs can make a difference in patient outcome. To this end, the revised curriculum includes when and how oral glucose and activated charcoal should be administered. It is possible that after consultation with medical direction, EMT-Bs may be advised to dilute certain ingested poisons with either water or milk. Before giving any medication or assisting with any medication, you must gain the confidence of the patient. Always communicate with the patient in a calm, professional manner.

Finally, scene-safety when managing behavioral emergencies is critical. Assessment of the behavioral-emergency patient occurs only when it is safe to do so. Remember to contact law enforcement if police are not already on the scene.

■ REVIEW QUESTIONS

1. When administered orally, how does glucose affect the blood of a patient who suffers from a diabetic emergency?

2. How does activated charcoal prevent certain poisons from being absorbed into the body?

3. Does your medical intervention change if the patient has hypoglycemia or hyperglycemia?

4. Why should you explain your medical interventions to a responsive patient?

5. Should you give oral glucose to an unconscious diabetic?

6. Decide which assessment findings might guide your decision to administer activated charcoal?

7. List four conditions for which activated charcoal is contraindicated.

8. Before treating the behavioral emergency patient, what should you consider?

9. Police have restrained a hostile 25-year-old male with a history of diabetes. As you conduct your assessment, the patient's friend tells you he has ingested at least 10 aspirin. What medical interventions would you perform?

12

Trauma

- *Bleeding*
- *Shock*
- *Soft Tissue*

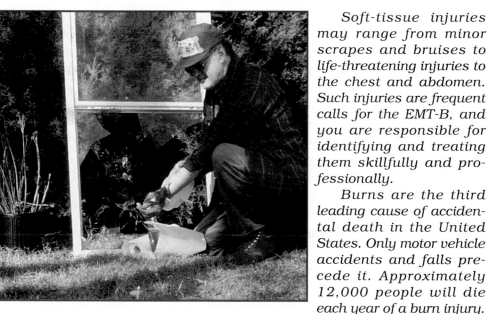

■ As a practicing EMT-B, you have often treated patients who suffered from bleeding, shock, and soft-tissue injuries; therefore, you will be familiar with many of the concepts in this chapter. However, this chapter integrates the 1994 EMT-Basic National Curriculum's revised format for patient assessment and emergency medical care of these trauma emergencies.

In order to treat the trauma patient and prevent or reverse any worsening conditions, you must quickly recognize mechanism of injury (MOI), detect signs and symptoms of bleeding and shock (hypoperfusion), and act swiftly to provide emergency medical care.

Soft-tissue injuries may range from minor scrapes and bruises to life-threatening injuries to the chest and abdomen. Such injuries are frequent calls for the EMT-B, and you are responsible for identifying and treating them skillfully and professionally.

Burns are the third leading cause of accidental death in the United States. Only motor vehicle accidents and falls precede it. Approximately 12,000 people will die each year of a burn injury. Most people think burn injuries only affect the skin; however, they often have an impact on other body systems.

MAKING THE TRANSITION

- Shock is defined as hypoperfusion.
- Pneumatic anti-shock garment (PASG) is recommended for use in the presence of pelvic instability, for controlling bleeding and shock (hypoperfusion), and for stabilizing pelvic, hip, femoral, and multiple-leg fractures.
- Early recognition and transport of patients with life-threatening conditions are emphasized.

The numbered objectives below are from the United States Department of Transportation 1994 EMT-Basic National Standard Curriculum. Objectives with colored bullets that follow in italics are from the EMT-Basic Transitional Program.

■ KNOWLEDGE AND ATTITUDE

At the completion of this chapter, you should be able to:

Bleeding and Shock

1. List the structure and function of the circulatory system. (pp. 197–198)
2. Differentiate between arterial, venous, and capillary bleeding. (p. 198)
3. State methods of emergency medical care of external bleeding. (pp. 199–202)
4. Establish the relationship between body substance isolation and bleeding. (p. 199)
5. Establish the relationship between airway management and the trauma patient. (p. 203)
6. Establish the relationship between mechanism of injury and internal bleeding. (p. 203)
7. List the signs of internal bleeding. (p. 203)
8. List the steps in emergency medical care of the patient with signs and symptoms of internal bleeding. (p. 203)
9. List signs and symptoms of shock (hypoperfusion). (pp. 203–204)
10. List the steps in the emergency medical care of the patient with signs and symptoms of shock (hypoperfusion). (pp. 204, 205)
11. Explain the sense of urgency to transport patients that are bleeding and show signs of shock (hypoperfusion). (p. 204)
● *Describe the use of the PASG as a splint.* (p. 204)

Soft-Tissue Injuries

1. State the major functions of the skin. (p. 211)
2. List the layers of the skin. (p. 211)
3. Establish the relationship between body substance isolation (BSI) and soft-tissue injuries. (pp. 199, 206)
4. List the types of closed soft-tissue injuries. (pp. 204, 206)
5. Describe the emergency medical care of the patient with a closed soft-tissue injury. (p. 206)
6. State the types of open soft-tissue injuries. (pp. 206–211)
7. Describe the emergency medical care of the patient with an open soft-tissue injury. (p. 208)
8. Discuss the emergency medical care considerations for a patient with a penetrating chest injury. (p. 208)
9. State the emergency medical care considerations for a patient with an open wound to the abdomen. (p. 209)
10. Differentiate the care of an open wound to the chest from an open wound to the abdomen. (pp. 208–209)
11. List the classifications of burns. (pp. 211, 213)
12. Define superficial burn. (p. 211)
13. List the characteristics of a superficial burn. (p. 211)
14. Define partial-thickness burn. (p. 211)
15. List the characteristics of a partial-thickness burn. (p. 211)
16. Define full-thickness burn. (p. 211)
17. List the characteristics of a full-thickness burn. (pp. 211, 213)
18. Describe the emergency medical care of a patient with a superficial burn. (pp. 214–218)
19. Describe the emergency medical care of a patient with a partial-thickness burn. (pp. 214–218)
20. Describe the emergency medical care of a patient with a full-thickness burn. (pp. 214–218)
21. List the functions of dressing and bandaging. (pp. 219–220)

22. Describe the purpose of bandaging. (pp. 200, 220)

23. Describe the steps in applying a pressure dressing. (pp. 201–202)

24. Establish the relationship between airway management and the patient with chest injury, burns, and blunt and penetrating injuries. (pp. 208, 209, 211, 215)

25. Describe the effects of improperly applied dressings, splints, and tourniquets. (p. 200)

26. Describe the emergency medical care of a patient with an impaled object. (pp. 209, 210)

27. Describe the emergency medical care of a patient with an amputation. (pp. 210–211)

28. Describe the emergency care for a chemical burn. (p. 217)

29. Describe the emergency care for an electrical burn. (pp. 217, 218)

■ SKILLS

Bleeding and Shock

1. Demonstrate direct pressure as a method of emergency medical care of external bleeding.

2. Demonstrate the use of diffuse pressure as a method of emergency medical care of external bleeding.

3. Demonstrate the use of pressure points and tourniquets as a method of emergency medical care for external bleeding.

4. Demonstrate the care of the patient exhibiting signs and symptoms of internal bleeding.

5. Demonstrate the care of the patient exhibiting signs and symptoms of shock (hypoperfusion).

6. Demonstrate completing a prehospital care report for the patient with bleeding and/or shock (hypoperfusion).

Soft-Tissue Injuries

1. Demonstrate the steps in the emergency medical care of closed soft-tissue injuries.

2. Demonstrate the steps in the emergency medical care of open soft-tissue injuries.

3. Demonstrate the steps in the emergency medical care of a patient with an open chest wound.

4. Demonstrate the steps in the emergency medical care of a patient with open abdominal wounds.

5. Demonstrate the steps in the emergency medical care of a patient with an impaled object.

6. Demonstrate the steps in the emergency medical care of a patient with an amputation.

7. Demonstrate the steps in the emergency medical care of an amputated part.

8. Demonstrate the steps in the emergency medical care of a patient with superficial burns.

9. Demonstrate the steps in the emergency medical care of a patient with partial-thickness burns.

10. Demonstrate the steps in the emergency medical care of a patient with full-thickness burns.

11. Demonstrate the steps in emergency medical care of a patient with chemical burns.

12. Demonstrate completing a prehospital care report for patients with soft-tissue injuries.

You and your partner have just finished cleaning and restocking the ambulance after a cardiac arrest call. You're looking forward to going home for some rest and a hot dinner. But moments later, you are dispatched to a scene described as a "reported eight-year-old patient with a gunshot injury to the chest. Patient is breathing and does have a pulse." The dispatcher advises you that police are en route and should arrive ahead of your unit. While en route, you and your partner discuss the possible types of chest wound the patient may have, as well as the need for rapid transport, especially since the victim is a child.

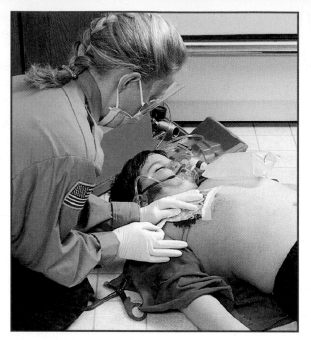

Since the scene is ten minutes away from the trauma center, you call the hospital on the cellular phone. You relay that you are en route to a reported young patient with a gunshot wound to the chest and most likely will transport to their facility. The emergency department acknowledges, advises that they will prepare, and asks you to provide more details as they become available.

The dispatcher relays that the police have secured the scene. However, as you respond, you approach the scene cautiously, as well as take BSI precautions. Your partner grabs a backboard for quick evacuation of the patient, as you get the oxygen, portable suction, and jump kit. You ask the police officer on the scene if the gun has been secured. She advises you that they have recovered a .38 caliber pistol. As you enter the kitchen door, you note only one patient appears to have suffered a gunshot wound. You think about ALS backup, but you know they are fifteen minutes away; the hospital is only ten minutes away.

You begin your **initial assessment** by looking at the patient. The child is unconscious, "looks bad," and has a wound to his upper right chest near the collarbone; he also has a laceration on the right cheek. His airway is open, and he is breathing rapidly. You ask your partner to get a pediatric nonrebreather mask and

put oxygen on high flow. You check for a radial pulse on the right side but cannot feel one. You check the carotid pulse and palpate a very rapid rate. There is not much blood on the floor, so you suspect there is air and/or blood in the victim's chest. You quickly apply an occlusive dressing over the chest wound. It appears he is in shock (a state of hypoperfusion). You consider the patient high priority and use the backboard to move him quickly to the ambulance.

Once the patient is on the ambulance stretcher, you have your partner begin transport to the hospital. Because the patient is still unconscious, you begin a limited **focused history and physical exam.** You cut off the child's clothing and look for other wounds but do not find any. You again attempt to take a radial pulse on the right side but cannot feel one. However, you do get a carotid pulse. You try the radial pulse on the left side and feel a faint, thready, rapid pulse around 140. You palpate a blood pressure of 80 mmHg. You radio the hospital to inform them of the patient's condition and your ETA.

En route, you perform the **ongoing assessment** every five minutes by rechecking ABCs and vital signs and making sure the oxygen is flowing. As you arrive at the hospital, you give the triage staff a quick report of what has taken place and the emergency medical care you have provided. The patient is wheeled away to the trauma room. As you start your prehospital care report, you question if you performed the correct interventions and if you should have called ALS.

Later, you learn that the bullet had severed the child's right axillary artery and he had lost about three units of blood. Perhaps this explains why you could not get a pulse on his right side. Shock (hypoperfusion), as well as the severed artery, caused his absent pulse. The ED physician explains that, without your prompt care and transport, the patient would probably have died. ■

■ CIRCULATORY SYSTEM REVIEW

The circulatory system is responsible for circulating blood throughout the body in order to supply it with nutrients and rid it of wastes. It has three major components: the heart (pump), the blood vessels (pipes), and the blood (fluid).

The Heart

The heart is a four-chambered, muscular pump about the size of a fist, lying beneath and slightly to the left of the sternum. The right side of the heart receives oxygen-depleted blood from the body and pumps it to the lungs. The left side receives oxygen-rich blood from the lungs and pumps it throughout the body. The two upper chambers of the heart are called the **atria**; the lower chambers are called the **ventricles**.

The Blood Vessels

There are three major types of blood vessels—arteries, veins, and capillaries (Figure 12–1). **Arteries** are blood vessels that carry oxygen rich blood *away* from the heart and supply it to the body. The exception is the pulmonary artery, which carries oxygen-depleted blood to the lungs. Arteries are composed of three different layers containing muscle and elasticized tissue that allow for dilation or constriction depending on the system's needs.

Veins are the blood vessels that carry oxygen-depleted blood *back* to the heart. The exception is the pulmonary vein, which carries oxygen-rich blood from the lungs to the left atrium. Since blood in the veins is under less pressure than the blood in the arteries, the veins contain valves at various points to prevent back flow of blood.

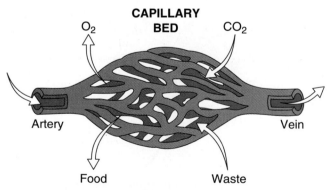

FIGURE 12–1 The blood vessels.

The larger arteries gradually branch to smaller and smaller vessels called **arterioles**, which *lead to* the **capillaries**—a functional network of tiny, one-celled blood vessels that are found in all parts of the body. The **venules**, the smaller branches of larger veins, *lead away* from the capillaries. This thin-walled capillary network that connects arterioles and venules allows for the exchange of oxygen and nutrients for carbon dioxide and other wastes, thus ensuring that all body cells are nourished and wastes are removed.

Blood Composition

Approximately $\frac{1}{12}$ to $\frac{1}{15}$ of a person's body weight is blood. A person weighing 150 pounds has about 10 to 12 pints of total blood volume. Blood is composed of red blood cells, white blood cells, plasma, and platelets. **Red blood cells** give the blood its color, carry oxygen *to* the body's cells, and pick up carbon dioxide and carry it *away* from the body's cells and back to the lungs. **White blood cells** are part of the body's immune system, which defends against infections. **Plasma** is the serum, or fluid, that carries the blood cells and nutrients to the body's cells. Plasma also carries away the waste products that are the result of cell metabolism. **Platelets** are essential to blood clotting and aid in the prevention of blood loss. Normal clotting of the blood takes six to seven minutes.

The Pulse

As the heart's left ventricle contracts, it sends a wave, or pulsation, of blood through the arteries. A **pulse** can be felt, or palpated, at any location where an artery passes over a bone near the skin surface. The most common "pulse points" are found in the wrist over the radial artery (Figure 12–2) and in the neck over the carotid artery. Other pulse points include the brachial artery in the upper arm, the femoral artery in the groin, the popliteal artery behind the knee, the dorsalis pedis on the top of the foot, and the posterior tibial found behind the medial ankle.

Blood Pressure

Blood pressure is defined as the pressure exerted against the arterial walls during circulation. The **systolic pressure** is the pressure exerted against

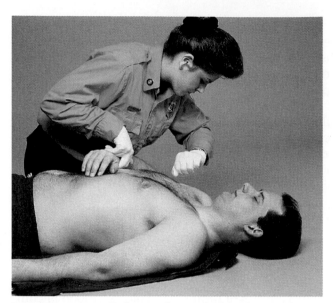

FIGURE 12–2 Palpate the radial pulse at the wrist.

the arterial wall during *contraction* of the left ventricle. The **diastolic pressure** is the pressure exerted against the arterial wall during *relaxation* of the left ventricle.

Perfusion

Perfusion is the supply of oxygen to and removal of wastes from the cells and tissues of the body as a result of the flow of blood through the capillaries. **Hypoperfusion**, or shock, is the inadequate perfusion of the cells and tissues of the body caused by insufficient flow of blood through the capillaries. The two major causes of hypoperfusion are low blood volume (hypovolemia) or insufficient pumping action by the heart (pump damage).

■ BLEEDING

Since all parts of the body require some level of perfusion, a loss of blood volume as a result of bleeding has a devastating effect on perfusion. No body part can exist for indefinite periods without receiving its normal level of nutrients and ridding its wastes. The heart requires a constant flow of blood, or it will not function properly. The brain and spinal cord cannot withstand a lack of perfusion for more than 4 to 6 minutes before irreversible damage begins. Lack of perfusion in the kidney for more than 45 minutes leads to kidney damage. Skeletal muscle can withstand lack of

perfusion for about 2 hours before permanent damage begins to occur.

External Bleeding

There are three types of external bleeding: arterial, venous, and capillary (Figure 12–3). **Arterial bleeding** is characterized by bright-red, spurting blood, which indicates that an artery has been damaged or severed. In some cases, arterial bleeding is difficult to control because of the higher pressure in the arteries. **Venous bleeding** is characterized by dark-red, steady-flowing blood and indicates that a vein is severed or damaged. Venous bleeding can be profuse and life threatening; however, it is usually easier to control due to the lower pressure in the veins. Dark-red blood oozing slowly from a wound is a sign of **capillary bleeding**. Damage to the capillaries usually is not life threatening; however, if there is an extensive amount of capillary damage due to injury to a large body surface area, blood loss may be severe.

PEDIATRIC HIGHLIGHT

Because of the differences in total circulating blood volume in adults and children, pediatric patients are at greater risk for serious bleeding. The sudden blood loss of ½ liter (500 cc) in children and 100 to 200 cc in infants is

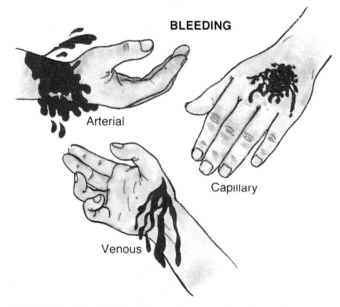

FIGURE 12–3 The three types of external bleeding.

considered serious. For example, a one-year-old child has a total of only 800 cc blood volume. A loss of 150 cc is considered significant, since this represents approximately 20% of the child's total blood volume. ■

Importance of BSI

Before caring for bleeding patients, body substance isolation must be taken to avoid contact with the victim's blood or other body fluids. By using gloves, eye protection, mask, gown, and proper hand washing techniques, you can dramatically reduce your chances for contracting an infectious disease from exposure to blood or body fluids. The amount of personal protective equipment (PPE) needed correlates directly to the degree of exposure to blood and other body fluids. If there is a slight chance of exposure, then only gloves are needed. If there is a greater potential for exposure, such as occurs in emergency childbirth, endotracheal intubation, or major trauma, all PPE must be worn. Always wash your hands after every call.

Severity of Bleeding

To get a general impression of the severity of a patient's bleeding, assess:

- *Severity of blood loss*   The loss of one liter or 1000 cc of blood is considered serious (Figure 12–4).
- *Signs or symptoms*   If the patient is presenting with signs or symptoms of shock (hypoperfusion), the bleeding is considered serious.

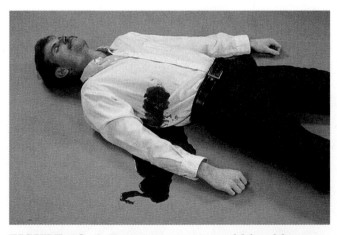

FIGURE 12–4 Estimating external blood loss: ½ liter (approximately 1 pint).

- *Rate of blood flow*   The larger the blood vessel, the more bleeding.
- *Type of bleeding*   Arterial bleeding is more rapid and profuse; venous is slower.

■ **Patient Assessment** **External Bleeding**

In general, assessment of external bleeding has not changed. However, the "assessment format" has been realigned to reflect more realistic out-of-hospital practices.

● Begin the assessment with scene size-up, considering the need for body substance isolation, making sure the scene is safe, determining the mechanism of injury and number of patients, and calling for additional resources if needed. Upon arrival at the scene, the EMT-B should quickly consider the mechanism of injury and if there are multiple victims. Consider questions such as:

What caused the patient's injury?

Did the patient fall and is there a possibility for spine injury?

Is there a weapon or other item that caused the patient's injury?

● The next step, the initial assessment, includes rapidly identifying and treating-as-you-go any life-threatening problems, assessing the ABCs, mental status, and the need for spine stabilization. Form a general impression of the patient to assist you in setting priorities and making early transport decisions for critical patients. Severe or profuse arterial or venous bleeding is usually detected and controlled immediately in the initial assessment.

● Treatment of shock (hypoperfusion) and bleeding is performed following the initial assessment and a rapid transport decision is made. Any non-life-threatening bleeding will, generally, be detected and treated during the rapid trauma exam, which is part of the focused history and physical exam—trauma patient. ■

■ **Patient Care** **External Bleeding**

The steps in the emergency medical care of external bleeding have not changed from past practices. Always use appropriate body substance isolation techniques and wear personal protective equipment when controlling bleeding. Remember to always expose the wound area to completely assess the injury.

The major steps for bleeding control are direct pressure, elevation of an extremity, and use of pressure points (Skill Summary 12–1). Other methods include the use of splints or pneumatic pressure devices and, as a last resort, tourniquets.

Remember that since blood loss reduces perfusion and the supply of oxygen to the tissues, the use of supplemental oxygen is vital. Oxygen should be administered after the bleeding has been controlled. Never delay the manual methods of bleeding control to set up or deliver oxygen to the patient.

Direct pressure involves applying pressure directly over a wound with a sterile gauze pad, or **dressing**. If a dressing is not readily available, use your gloved hand. Use a **bandage** to snugly hold the dressing in place and to provide pressure over the wound. A large gaping wound may require extra dressing material to pack it in order to control bleeding.

Combine **elevation** of an injured extremity with direct pressure to control bleeding. Raise the injured extremity above the level of the heart to slow the flow of blood. However, if the extremity is painful, swollen, or deformed, avoid this technique.

Use **pressure points** if direct pressure and elevation fail to control bleeding. A pressure point is a site where a main artery lies near the surface of the body and directly over a bone (Figure 12–5). Compressing the artery over the bone slows or reduces the blood flow to the injured area. The two most commonly used pressure points are on the brachial and femoral arteries.

Use **splints and pneumatic pressure devices** to control bleeding from painful, swollen, or deformed extremities (suspected fractures). Bleeding occurs when the jagged bone ends or fragments damage the tissue and blood vessels that surround the bone. Splinting the body part stabilizes the bone ends or fragments and thus aids in controlling bleeding. Pneumatic pressure devices, such as an air splint or pneumatic anti-shock garment (PASG), apply pressure over a wound area. Use a PASG in the presence of massive soft-tissue injury to the lower extremities by inflating the leg compartments.

Use **tourniquets** to control bleeding only when all other bleeding control methods fail. Tourniquets have the potential to cause nerve damage and injure soft tissue and may result in the loss of the limb to which the tourniquet is applied. Remember, once a tourniquet is applied, it should never be loosened or removed without approval from medical direction. ■

Special Considerations

When a trauma patient is bleeding from the ears or nose, suspect a possible skull fracture. Do not try to stop the flow of blood, because the skull is incapable of expanding; therefore, attempting to control bleeding would increase pressure inside the skull. Instead, place a loose dressing over the area to collect any drainage and to reduce the risk of further contamination.

FIGURE 12–5
The use of pressure points can stop profuse bleeding from an arm or leg.

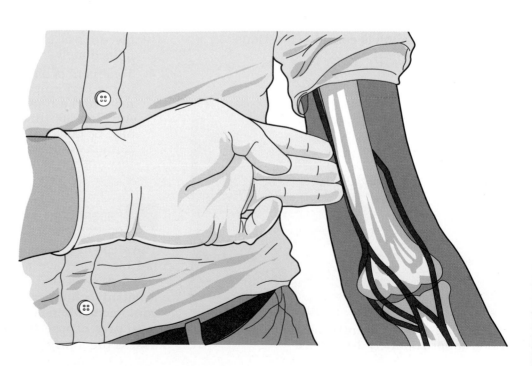

Bleeding Control

FIRST take body substance isolation precautions.

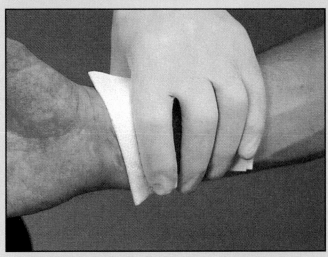

1. Apply direct pressure to the wound. You may cover the wound with a gauze pad. In cases of profuse bleeding, *do not* waste time looking for a pad. Provide pressure directly to the wound with your gloved hand.

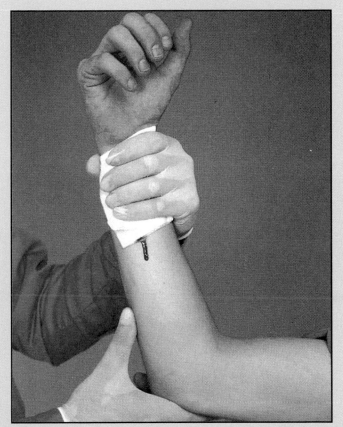

2. Elevate the extremity above the level of the heart.

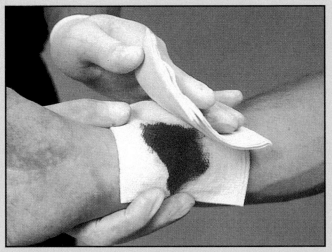

3. Apply a dressing to the wound. If the wound continues to bleed, apply additional dressings.

Skill Summary 12–1 *(continued)*

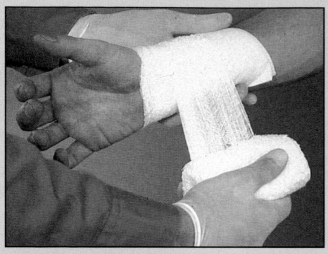

4. Bandage the dressing in place.

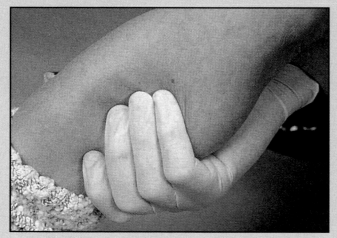

5. If the wound still continues to bleed, apply pressure to appropriate arterial pressure point. Press the brachial artery pressure point to control bleeding from the arm.

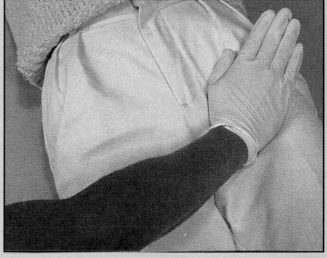

Press the femoral artery to control bleeding from the leg.

Internal Bleeding

Internal bleeding, while not always evident, results from blunt and penetrating trauma, abnormal clotting mechanisms within the body, rupture of a blood vessel, or long bone or pelvic fractures. It may progress into life-threatening shock. The severity of the internal bleeding depends on its source as well as the patient's overall medical condition and age. The blood loss from internal bleeding can ultimately lead to death. During the scene size-up, you should have a high index of suspicion for internal bleeding based upon the patient's mechanism of injury (MOI).

◼ Patient Assessment Internal Bleeding

- During the scene size-up, evaluate the scene, looking for mechanism of injury such as impact marks, fallen ladders, or other sights and smells.

- Your general impression and ABC assessment during the initial assessment will also lend support to a suspicion for internal bleeding.

- When you perform the rapid trauma exam during the focused history and physical exam—trauma patient, look for: pain, tenderness, swelling, or discoloration at the suspected injury site (Figure 12–6); bleeding from the mouth, rectum, vagina or other orifice; bright-red blood or dark, coffee-ground colored blood in vomitus; dark, tarry stools or stools with bright-red blood; tender, rigid, and/or distended abdomen; and other signs of hypovolemic (low-volume) shock. ◼

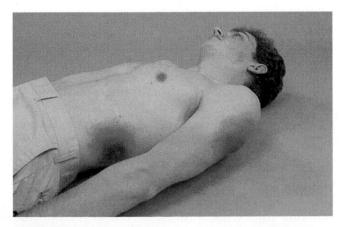

FIGURE 12–6 Bruising is one sign of internal bleeding.

◼ Patient Care Internal Bleeding

While the steps for the emergency medical care for internal bleeding have not changed, there is renewed emphasis on early recognition and early transport decisions.

Emergency Care Steps

1. Take body substance isolation precautions.
2. Maintain airway and breathing; provide artificial ventilations when necessary.
3. Administer high-flow oxygen.
4. Splint any painful, swollen, or deformed extremities and control any external bleeding with direct pressure.
5. Provide immediate transport for critical patients with signs and symptoms of shock. During transport, continually re-evaluate the critical patient with ongoing assessments every five minutes. ◼

◼ SHOCK

As you know, the term shock is now used interchangeably with the term hypoperfusion, which more accurately describes the condition. Shock is essentially a result of inadequate or low perfusion (hypoperfusion) of the body's cells and tissues caused by insufficient blood flow through the capillaries. This condition ultimately leads to death of the tissue. In cases of shock, peripheral perfusion is reduced due to inadequate circulating volume or heart (pump) failure. Victims with blood loss from internal or external bleeding may be at risk for shock.

The urgency in transporting shock patients is due to the fact that most injuries require surgical interventions to correct. The term "golden hour" has been used to describe the maximum time period between the time of injury and surgery. EMT-Bs should keep scene times to less than 10 minutes (unless extrication is required). This is referred to as the "platinum ten minutes."

◼ Patient Assessment Shock

Follow these steps to assess for shock:

- During the initial assessment evaluate the patient's mental status. A patient who is restless, anxious, has a "feeling of impending doom," or exhibits any altered mental status

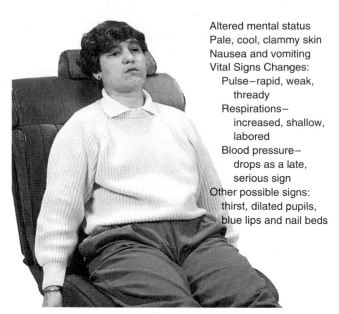

Altered mental status
Pale, cool, clammy skin
Nausea and vomiting
Vital Signs Changes:
   Pulse—rapid, weak,
      thready
   Respirations—
      increased, shallow,
      labored
   Blood pressure—
      drops as a late,
      serious sign
Other possible signs:
   thirst, dilated pupils,
   blue lips and nail beds

FIGURE 12–7 Signs and symptoms of shock.

may be experiencing the early stages of shock. As you assess circulation, look for a weak, thready, or absent pulse in the distal extremities, which can be an indicator of decreased peripheral perfusion. Also, the skin may be pale, cool, and clammy.

- During the focused history and physical exam—trauma patient, complete a rapid trauma exam, looking for any signs of further injury. Abnormal vital signs, such as increased pulse rate, with or without signs of external bleeding, may also indicate a patient at risk for shock. Also, a patient's breathing rate may increase and become labored, shallow, and irregular. The blood pressure may remain normal for some time; however, a late sign of shock is a decreasing pulse. Other signs to look for are dilated pupils, marked thirst, nausea or vomiting, and pallor with cyanosis (Figure 12–7). ■

PEDIATRIC HIGHLIGHT

When infants and children under six are experiencing shock, capillary refill (blanching of the skin and recording the time it takes for color to return) will be greater than 2 seconds in normal ambient air temperature. Unfortunately, however, infants and children can maintain (compensate) their blood pressure until half of their blood volume is depleted. Therefore, if an infant or child's blood pressure is dropping, it is an ominous sign that the child may be close to death. ■

Patient Care **Shock**

The steps for the emergency care of shock are essentially unchanged and are similar to those for internal bleeding. Study Skill Summary 12–2 and the steps below.

1. Take body substance isolation and use appropriate personal protective equipment.
2. Maintain airway and ventilation with high-concentration oxygen through either a nonrebreather or bag-valve mask assist.
3. Control any external bleeding.
4. Elevate the lower extremities 8 to 12 inches if no suspected spinal injury.
5. Splint all painful, swollen, or deformed extremities. (Do not delay transport of high-priority patients.)
6. Maintain body temperature and keep the patient warm.
7. Make an early transport decision and transport rapidly to an appropriate facility. ■

Use of the PASG

While the use of PASG (pneumatic antishock garment) for the treatment of shock has been controversial, its use is indicated in the presence of pelvic fractures or instability accompanied by shock (blood pressure < 90 mmHg) and to control bleeding in massive soft-tissue injuries to the lower extremities. Medical experts agree that PASG should *not* be used with thoracic trauma. Also, the garment is not recommended for shock caused by medical emergencies. Apply the PASG in accordance with local medical direction and protocols. Remember to remove the patient's clothing before applying the garment.

■ SOFT-TISSUE INJURIES

A wound is caused by trauma, which disrupts the normal structure of the tissues, an organ, or a bone. Wounds are categorized as open or closed.

Closed Wounds

Closed wounds are beneath the skin, but the skin remains intact, or unbroken. The three specific types of closed injuries are contusions, hematomas, and crushing injuries. A **contusion**, or bruise,

Shock Management

FIRST take body substance isolation precautions.

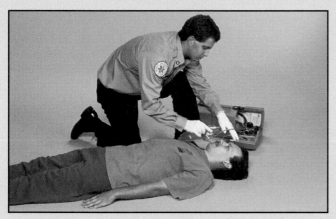

1. Maintain an open airway. Give high-concentration oxygen by nonrebreather mask. Control external bleeding. Assist ventilations and perform CPR as necessary.

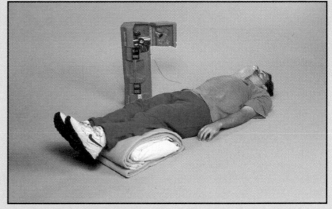

2. Properly position the patient. If there is no serious injury, usually position the patient supine with legs elevated 8 to 12 inches.

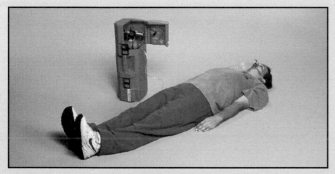

3. If there is any possibility of serious injuries to head, neck, spine, chest, abdomen, pelvis, hip, or extremities, position patient supine with NO elevation of extremities.

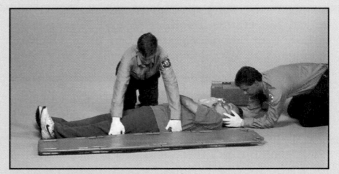

4. Splinting of bone and joint injuries can help control shock but should be done en route. Meanwhile, placing the patient on a spine board will have the effect of splinting the whole body.

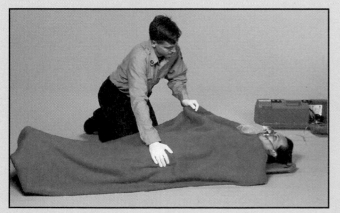

5. Protect the patient from heat loss.

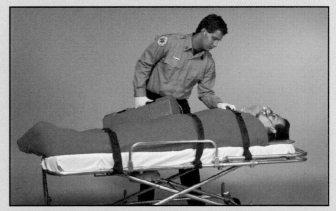

6. Transport immediately.

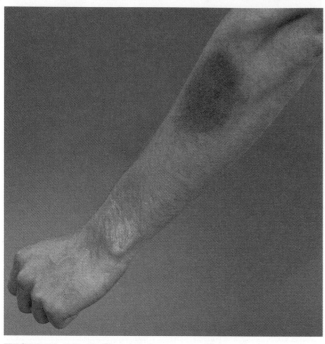

FIGURE 12–8 Contusions are the most common form of closed wounds.

results when the epidermis remains unbroken; however, the cells and blood vessels contained within the dermis are injured, causing an accumulation of blood in surrounding tissues that is evidenced by discoloration (Figure 12–8). A contusion causes localized swelling and pain at the injury site.

A **hematoma** is also a collection of blood beneath the epidermis, but in larger amounts, due to damage of a larger blood vessel.

A **crush injury** results from a severe crushing force and may be serious, depending on its location and the underlying tissue or organ damage. Crush injuries are associated with internal injuries and shock (hypoperfusion).

Patient Assessment Closed Wounds

Contusions are the most frequently encountered closed wounds. Most simple bruises will not require emergency care in the field. However, bruising may also be a sign of internal injury and bleeding. ■

Patient Care Closed Wounds

Emergency Care Steps
1. Take appropriate body substance isolation precautions.

2. Manage the patient's airway, breathing, and circulation. Apply high-concentration oxygen by nonrebreather mask.
3. MANAGE AS IF THERE IS INTERNAL BLEEDING, AND CARE FOR SHOCK if you believe that there is a possibility of internal injuries.
4. Splint extremities that are painful, swollen, or deformed.
5. Stay alert for the patient to vomit.
6. Continue to monitor the patient for the development of shock and transport as soon as possible. ■

Open Wounds

An **open wound** is any injury that damages the integrity of the skin. This break in the skin increases the chances for blood loss and the risk for infection.

An **abrasion** is a scrape (caused by friction), rubbing, or shearing of the outermost layer of the skin (Figure 12–9). Although an abrasion is con-

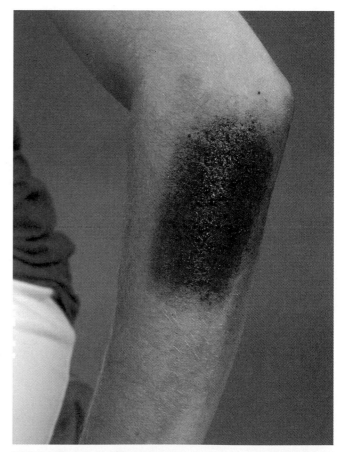

FIGURE 12–9 Abrasions are the least serious form of open wound.

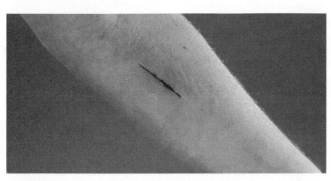

FIGURE 12–10 Some lacerations have smooth edges.

sidered a superficial injury, it can be extremely painful because it involves the nerve endings. In most cases bleeding will be minimal and easily controlled. However, when a larger body surface area is injured, such as the "road rash" that results when a motorcyclist falls off of a cycle, blood loss may be severe.

A **laceration** is a linear (regular) or stellate (irregular) tearing of the skin caused by sharp objects (Figures 12–10 and 12–11). A laceration's depth may vary. Lacerations tend to bleed profusely, due to the severing of larger blood vessels.

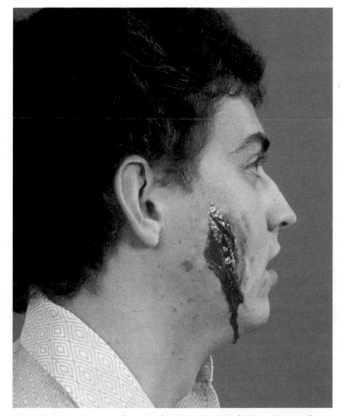

FIGURE 12–11 Some lacerations have jagged edges.

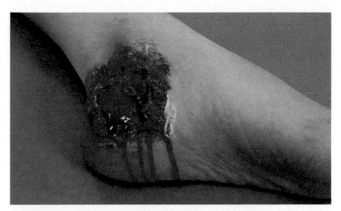

FIGURE 12–12 Avulsed skin.

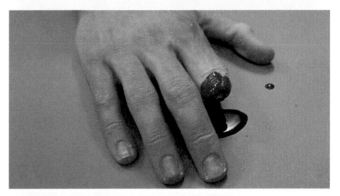

FIGURE 12–13 An amputation.

An **avulsion** and an **amputation** are the ripping or tearing of skin and soft tissue that cause complete or incomplete detachment of a body part (Figures 12–12 and 12–13). Avulsions generally involve soft tissue only; amputations involve bones as well. The amount of bleeding from these types of injuries can range from profuse (due to damage to large blood vessels) to negligible (due to retraction of the blood vessels).

A **penetration** or **puncture** is caused by a sharp object, such as a pencil or ice pick, being pushed into the soft tissue (Figures 12–14 and 12–15). External bleeding is usually minimal, but internal injury can be severe if the wound is located over a major blood vessel or organ. Apply a sterile dressing and be prepared to treat for shock of the puncture to the torso or neck.

▮ Patient Assessment **Open Wounds**

Airway, breathing, circulation, and severe bleeding are identified and treated in the initial assessment. Once the initial assessment and the appropriate physical examination have been completed, care for the individual wounds begins. ▪

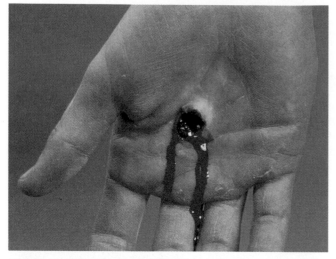

FIGURE 12–14 A penetrating puncture wound.

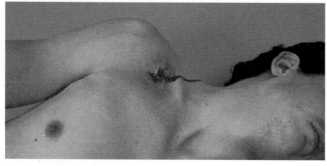

A.

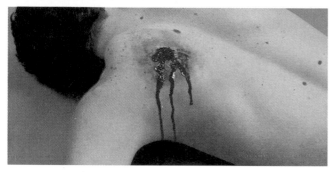

B.

FIGURE 12–15 A perforating puncture wound has an entrance and an exit.

Patient Care **Open Wounds**

Care for open wounds as follows.

1. *Expose the wound.* Clothing that covers a soft-tissue injury must be lifted, cut, or split away. For some articles of clothing, this is best done with scissors or a seam cutter. Do not attempt to remove clothing in the usual manner. To do

so may aggravate existing injuries and cause additional damage and pain.

2. *Clean the wound surface.* Do not try to pick out embedded particles and debris from the wound. Simply remove large pieces of foreign matter from its surface. When possible, use a piece of sterile dressing to brush away large debris from the surface while protecting from contact with your soiled gloves. Do not spend much time cleaning the wound. Control of bleeding is the priority.

3. *Control bleeding.* Start with direct pressure or direct pressure and elevation. When necessary, employ pressure point procedures. Remember, a tourniquet is used only as a last resort.

4. *Care for shock.* For all serious wounds, care for shock, including the administration of a high-concentration of oxygen.

5. *Prevent further contamination.* Use a sterile dressing, if possible. When none is available, use the cleanest cloth material at the scene.

6. *Bandage the dressing in place after bleeding has been controlled.* If an extremity is involved, check for a distal pulse to make certain that circulation has not been interrupted by the application of a tight bandage. With the exception of a pressure dressing, bleeding must be controlled before bandaging is started. Periodically recheck the bandage to make certain that bleeding has not restarted.

7. *Keep the patient lying still.* Any patient movement will increase circulation and could restart bleeding.

8. *Reassure the patient.* This will help ease the patient's emotional response and perhaps lower his pulse rate and blood pressure. In some cases this may help to reduce the bleeding rate. Also, a patient who feels reassured will usually be more willing to lie still, reducing the chances of restarting controlled bleeding. ■

Patient Care **Penetrating Chest Injuries**

The chest provides a closed, airtight system for respiration. When chest injuries occur, air may leak from the wound and disrupt respiration (Figure 12–16). When treating penetrating chest injuries, use an occlusive dressing to prevent air from entering the chest, which could cause a **pneumothorax.** Leave one side or corner of the dressing unsecured to allow air to escape as the patient exhales in order to prevent a **tension pneumothorax** (Figure 12–17). ■

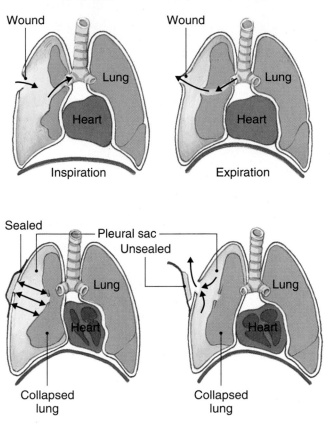

Open chest wound with punctured lung

Wound

Wound

Lung

Lung

Heart

Heart

Inspiration

Expiration

Sealed

Pleural sac

Unsealed

Lung

Lung

Heart

Heart

Collapsed lung

Collapsed lung

Sealing wound can cause increase in pressure within thoracic (chest) cavity.

If patient's condition declines after sealing puncture wound, open the seal immediately.

FIGURE 12–16 Open chest wound with punctured lung.

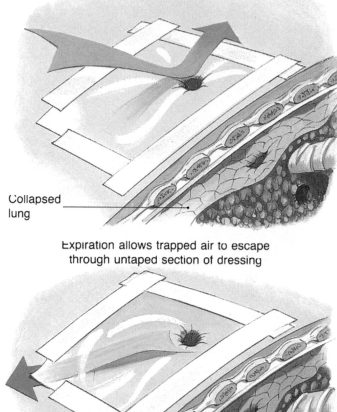

On inspiration, dressing seals wound, preventing air entry

Collapsed lung

Expiration allows trapped air to escape through untaped section of dressing

FIGURE 12–17 Creating a flutter valve to allow air to escape from the chest cavity.

Patient Care Evisceration

When abdominal injuries result in an **evisceration** (an organ or part of an organ protruding through a wound opening), do not touch or attempt to push the organ back into the abdominal cavity. Cover the exposed organ(s) with a sterile, moist dressing or an occlusive dressing large enough to cover all of the protruding organs. Avoid using an absorbent material, since it may adhere to the organs. Keep the dressing in place with a large bandage or clean sheet to protect the site and prevent heat loss. If there is no suspected spinal injury, transport the patient with the hips and knees flexed to decrease tension on the abdominal muscles (Figure 12–18). ■

Preceptor Pearl

Plastic wrap is preferred over aluminum foil as an occlusive dressing because the sharp edges of the aluminum foil may cause further damage to abdominal organs. ✦

Patient Care Impaled Objects

Manually secure **impaled objects** in place to prevent movement that could cause further damage. Expose the area and control any bleeding with direct pressure around the wound edges. Stabilize the object with bulky dressings and secure in place (Figure 12–19). ■

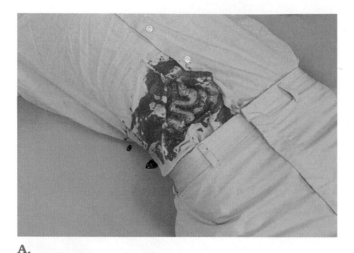

A.

B.

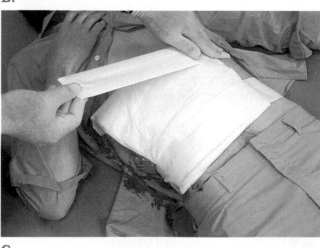

C.

FIGURE 12–18 A. Open abdominal wound with evisceration. **B.** Cut away clothing from wound. Apply a sterile saline-soaked dressing. Apply an occlusive dressing over the moist dressing if local protocols recommend. **C.** Cover the dressed wound to maintain warmth. Secure covering with tape or cravats tied above and below position of exposed organ.

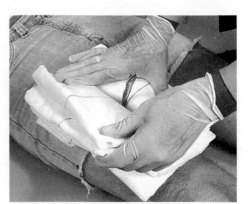

A.

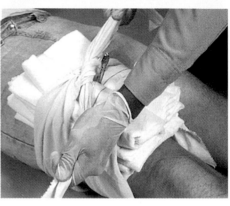

B.

FIGURE 12–19 Impaled objects. **A.** Expose the wound and control bleeding. **B.** Stabilize the impaled object.

Patient Care Amputations

Amputations create situations in which the EMT–B must care for not only the patient but the detached body part as well. However, always focus emergency medical care on the patient rather than expending valuable time looking for the amputated part. If, however, the amputated part is located, wrap it in dry, sterile dressings. Some EMS systems recommend moistening the dressing material with saline solution; check with medical direction to determine your local protocols. Place the wrapped body part in a plastic bag or wrap and label the bag with the date, the time the part was bagged or wrapped, and the patient's name. Place the bagged part into a cooler or other suitable container on top of an ice pack or ice. Never place an unwrapped body part directly on the ice pack or ice since this will freeze the body part. Never place the tissue in water as this will lead to tissue damage. If possible, transport the body part with the patient. If you are unable to locate the body part in time, transport the patient immediately and make arrangements to have the body part, if it is found, transported to the same hospital. ■

Patient Care Open Wounds to the Neck

Because major blood vessels are located in the neck, a large open wound to the neck is susceptible not only to life-threatening bleeding but also to an air embolism. An **air embolism**, or bubble, can travel by veins to the heart and cause abnormal functioning of the heart, including cardiac arrest. Arterial bleeding from the neck is a grave sign; venous bleeding may be profuse. Focus your care on establishing an adequate airway and breathing. Apply direct pressure with an occlusive dressing. Avoid pressing over the carotid pulse. (Skill Summary 12–3). ■

Burn Injuries

As you know, the skin is made up of three layers: the epidermis (outermost), the dermis (middle), and subcutaneous (deepest). Its thickness may range from one cell to several layers, and it serves multiple functions. The skin provides a barrier against infection and protection from pathogens, such as bacteria or other harmful agents found in the environment; insulates and protects underlying structures and body organs from injury; aids in the regulation of body temperature; provides for sensation transmission (hot, cold, pain, and touch); aids in elimination of some of the body's wastes; and contains fluids necessary to the proper functioning of other organs and systems. Any or all of these functions can be impaired or destroyed by a burn injury.

Patient Assessment Burns

Classifying Burn Injuries
During the scene size-up and in your more detailed evaluation during the focused history and physical exam—trauma patient, the first step in assessing a burn injury is to classify it according to the depth of injury to the skin. Burns are classified as superficial, partial-thickness, or full-thickness burns (Figure 12–20).

A **superficial burn**, or first-degree burn, is a painful injury that involves the epidermis and is caused by a flame, scald, or the sun. The skin will be dry and will appear pink to red. In some

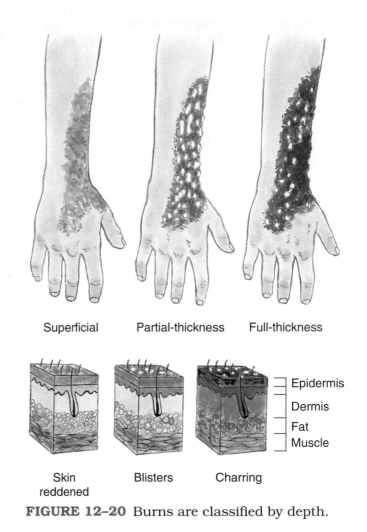

FIGURE 12–20 Burns are classified by depth.

cases, there may be a slight swelling, but an absence of blisters. A superficial burn may take several days to heal.

A **partial-thickness burn**, or second-degree burn, involves not only the epidermis, but portions of the dermis. Partial-thickness burns are caused by contact with a fire flame or flash, hot liquids or hot solid objects, chemical substances, or the sun. The skin may appear white to cherry red, moist, and mottled. Partial-thickness burns are characterized by blisters, a result of damage to the blood vessels, which causes plasma and tissue fluid to rise to the top layer of the skin. Because the nerve endings are damaged, partial-thickness burns will cause intense pain. They will usually heal on their own in 2 to 4 weeks. However, if a large skin surface area or depth is involved, specialized interventions may be required.

Full-thickness burns, or third-degree burns, damage the entire dermis and can extend beyond it to the subcutaneous layer and into the muscle, bone, or organs below. Full-thickness burns are a

Open Neck Wound—Occlusive Dressing

FIRST take body substance isolation precautions.

Dressing must be heavy plastic, sized to be 2 inches larger in diameter than wound site.

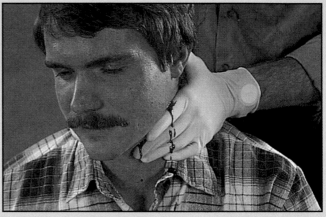

1. Do not delay! Place your gloved palm over the wound.

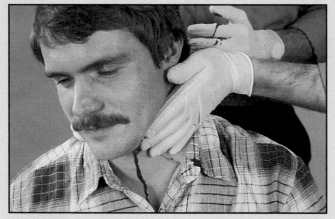

2. Occlusive dressing is placed over wound site.

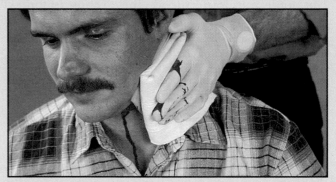

3. A dressing is placed over the occlusive dressing. (A roll of gauze can be placed between the trachea and the dressing to help keep pressure off the airway.)

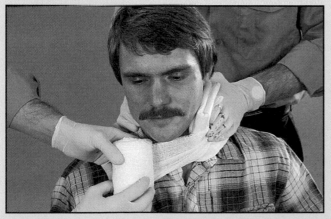

4. Start a figure-eight, bringing bandage over dressing.

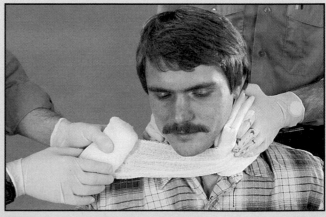

5. Cross over the shoulder.

Note: For demonstration purposes, the patient is upright.

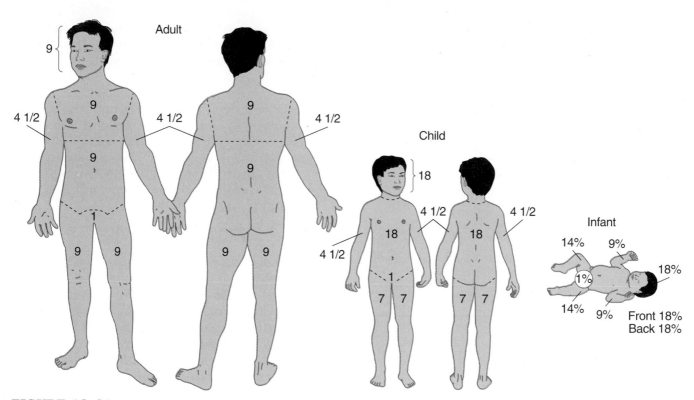

FIGURE 12–21 The Rule of Nines.

result of contact with extreme heat sources. The skin will become dry, hard, tough, and leathery and may appear white-waxy to dark brown or black charred. Most full-thickness burns are not very painful since nerve ending destruction is complete. However, most full-thickness burns are accompanied by partial-thickness burns, which can cause intense pain. Full-thickness burns usually require specialized surgical intervention and skin grafting. The length of the healing process depends on the size of the injured area and can take anywhere from two months to years. Scarring may be extensive, depending on the extent of the burn.

Determining Severity of Burn Injuries

In addition to classifying a burn during the focused history and physical exam—trauma patient, you also need to determine the burn's severity. The severity of a burn is dependent upon the percentage of **body surface area (BSA)** involved, the burn's location, the depth of the burn, and the patient's age and other preexisting medical conditions. Determining the source agent, or cause, of the burn is also helpful.

To quickly identify the amount of burned skin surface, you can use the **Rule of Nines.** In this system, specific body surface areas are assigned certain percentages to determine the amount of

BSA involved in the burn (Figure 12–21). The Rule of Nines is not only helpful in estimating a burn's severity, but also enables you to appropriately triage, or categorize, the patient and alert the receiving facility about the severity of the patient's condition.

PEDIATRIC HIGHLIGHT

Since the body proportions of infants and children differ from those of adults, the BSA percentages assigned to a child's body regions also differ (Figure 12–21). Since a child's head is much larger in relationship to the rest of the body, the child's head is counted as 18% of the entire body surface. The chest and abdomen are counted as 18%, the entire back as 18%, each upper extremity as 9%, each lower extremity as 14%, and the genital region as 1%. ■

Preceptor Pearl

An alternate way to determine the BSA estimate is the "Rule of Palm," which uses the patient's palm surface area as a unit of measurement. The patient's palm is considered equal to approximately 1% of the BSA. You can mentally estimate a burn area on any age patient. For example, if the burn area is equal to "7 palm surface areas," then the burn would be estimated at 7% BSA. ✛

TABLE 12-1 Agents and Sources of Burns

Agents	Sources
Thermal	Including flame; radiation; excessive heat from fire, steam, hot liquids, hot objects
Chemicals	Including various acids, bases, caustics
Electricity	Including AC current, DC current, lightning
Light (typically involving the eyes)	Including intense light sources, ultraviolet light (includes sunlight)
Radiation	Usually from nuclear sources; ultraviolet light can also be considered to be a source of radiation burns

The **location** of a burn injury is a major factor in determining burn severity. Burns to the face are considered critical because of their potential to cause respiratory compromise and eye injuries. Burns to the hands and feet are critical because they can lead to loss of function. Genital or groin region burn injuries can compromise genitourinary function and increase the chances for infection.

Circumferential burns are those that encircle a particular body area, such as an arm, a leg, or the chest. The constriction or swelling of tissue over the joints of the extremities caused by circumferential burns can lead to circulatory compromise and nerve damage. Burns that encircle the chest may impede respiratory function by limiting chest expansion.

As an EMT-B, you know that a minor burn in a healthy adult can turn out to be a severe burn for a patient with preexisting medical conditions, such as diabetes. A patient with an existing respiratory illness or condition may be adversely affected if there is further respiratory compromise from a burn injury. A patient with an existing cardiovascular problem may have increased complications from a burn injury and the resulting fluid loss.

The **source**, or **agent**, that causes a burn is also important in determining burn severity. See Table 12–1 for a summary.

PEDIATRIC HIGHLIGHT

In addition to BSA percentage differences, infants and children face other challenges from burns; children have the potential for greater fluid loss and the scarring from burns can impede the growth process. ■

In order for you to provide optimal emergency medical care, to make early transport decisions, and to give an accurate receiving facility report, it is imperative for you to be able to classify the severity of a burn injury. Table 12–2 summarizes **critical**, **moderate**, and **minor burn injuries**.

PEDIATRIC HIGHLIGHT

The classification of burn injury severity differs for children under five years old. Any full- or partial-thickness burn injury greater than 20%, or any burn involving hands, feet, face, or genitalia is considered a critical burn. Any partial-thickness burn of 10% to 20% is considered a moderate burn. Any partial-thickness burn less than 10% is considered a minor burn. ■

Patient Care Burn Injuries

Essentially, the emergency medical care for burn injuries has not changed. However, specific treatment may depend on your local medical direction, protocols, and practices. Always check your local area's specific treatment guidelines.

The two major goals in the treatment of burn injuries are to stop the burning process and to prevent further injury or contamination.

Emergency Care Steps

1. During the scene size-up, in addition to beginning patient assessment by determining the mechanism of injury, you must consider your own well-being. If you are not trained to enter a scene or cannot make it safe, then wait for additional specially trained and equipped resources to arrive.

2. In the initial assessment, focus on stopping the burning process. Because burns may continue to injure the skin even after the burn source is removed, "cool" the burn with water or saline for the first ten minutes after the injury. If the burn injury is thermal, wetting down the burned area will aid in stopping the burning process. If the burn source is a semi-solid or liquid (tar, grease, or oil), cool the burn to stop the burning process. Do not attempt to

TABLE 12–2 Classifying Burn Severity

Critical Burn Injuries

- Any burn injury complicated by respiratory tract injuries or other accompanying major traumatic injury (soft tissue or bone).
- Full- or partial-thickness burns involving the face, hands, feet, genitalia, or respiratory tract.
- Any full-thickness burn injury covering 10% or more BSA.
- Any partial-thickness burn injury covering 30% or more BSA.
- Burn injuries complicated by painful, swollen, or deformed extremities.
- Any moderately classified burn in children less than five or adults older than fifty-five.
- Any burn that encircles a body part, such as an arm, leg, or chest.

Moderate Burn Injuries

- Full-thickness burns covering 2% to 10% BSA, excluding the face, hands, feet, genitalia, or respiratory tract.
- Partial-thickness burns with 15% to 30% BSA involvement.
- Superficial burns greater than 50% BSA.

Minor Burn Injuries

- Full-thickness burns involving less than 2% BSA.
- Partial-thickness burns involving less than 15% BSA.

remove the substance, since this could cause further tissue damage. Attempt to remove any smoldering clothing, which still will be emitting heat, and any jewelry, whose metal retains heat. If any clothing remains adhered to the patient, cut around the area. DO NOT attempt to remove the adhered portion, since this may cause further damage to soft tissues.

3. Assess for any indications that the airway may be injured or compromised, such as sooty deposits in the mouth or nose, singed facial or nose hairs, signs of smoke inhalation, or any facial burns. Assessing the airway is of prime importance since the first reaction when one is frightened or startled and in a confined space in which there is an explosion or fire is to deeply inhale. In such a situation, the air is superheated and has an adverse effect on the airway and respiratory function. Provide high-concentration oxygen via a nonrebreather mask or BVM assist. Since most burns do not bleed, if profuse bleeding is evident, look for other causes or injuries and treat the patient for any signs or symptoms of shock.

4. After treating all life-threatening injuries during the focused history and physical exam—trauma patient, reassess the mechanism of injury. During the rapid trauma exam, evaluate the burn injury by assessing its depth, BSA

percentage, and severity. Once you have stopped the burning process, cover the wounds with dry, sterile dressings or a burn sheet to prevent further injury or contamination.

5. During the ongoing assessment, repeat the initial assessment and vital signs, and check interventions. En route to the hospital, complete the ongoing assessment every five minutes for unstable patients and every fifteen for stable patients. Continually evaluate the airway especially when there are burns to the face. ■

Preceptor Pearl

Continual use of a wet or moist dressing may cause hypothermia in the burn patient because the burned area is no longer capable of heat regulation. However, for partial- or full-thickness burns of 10% or less BSA, some EMS systems recommend use of moist, saline-soaked dressings to decrease the patient's pain. Always check with medical direction regarding the use of wet or moist dressings.

When using dry, sterile dressings, avoid using any material that shreds or leaves particles, since these can cause further contamination of the burn area. Never apply any type of ointments, lotions, or antiseptics to burn injuries since they can lead to heat retention. Never attempt to break or drain blisters, since this action may cause further contamination and fluid loss. ✢

Care for Thermal Burns

FIRST take body substance isolation precautions.

STOP THE BURNING PROCESS!

1. Flame—Wet down, smother, then remove clothing.
   Semi-solid (grease, tar, wax)—Cool with water ... do **not** remove substance.
2. Ensure an open airway. Assess breathing.
3. Look for airway injury: soot deposits, burnt nasal hair, and facial burns.
4. Complete the initial assessment.
5. Treat for shock. Provide a high concentration of oxygen. Treat serious injuries.
6. Evaluate burns ⟨ Depth / Rule of Nines or Rule of Palm / Severity

   Decide if special transport is needed.
   Remove clothing if necessary.

	Tissue Burned					
Type of Burn	Outer Layer of Skin	2nd Layer of Skin	Tissue below Skin	Color Changes	Pain	Blisters
Superficial	Yes	No	No	Red	Yes	No
Partial-Thickness	Yes	Yes	No	Deep red	Yes	Yes
Full-Thickness	Yes	Yes	Yes	Charred black or white	Yes/No	Yes/No

7. **Do not** clear debris. Remove clothing and jewelry.
8. Wrap with dry sterile dressing.
9A. Burns to hands or toes—Remove rings or jewelry that may constrict with swelling. Separate digits with sterile gauze pads.
9B. Burns to the eyes—Do not open eyelids if burned. Be certain burn is thermal, not chemical. Apply sterile gauze pads to **both** eyes to prevent sympathetic movement of injured eye if only one eye is burned. If burn is chemical, flush eyes for 20 minutes en route to hospital.

FOLLOW LOCAL BURN CENTER PROTOCOL, AND TRANSPORT ALL BURN PATIENTS AS SOON AS POSSIBLE.

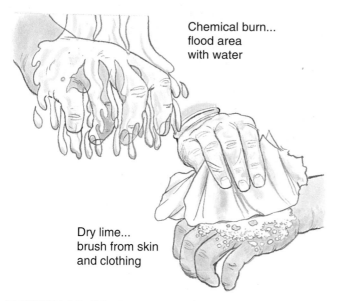

Chemical burn...
flood area
with water

Dry lime...
brush from skin
and clothing

FIGURE 12–22 Emergency care of chemical burns.

Patient Care Thermal Burns

Skill Summary 12–4 summarizes the care for thermal burns. ■

Patient Care Chemical Burns

Chemical burns require immediate care because the longer a chemical is in contact with the skin the more severe a burn becomes. Use the following steps to treat chemical burn injuries.

Emergency Care Steps

1. Protect yourself first. Chemical burns are often the result of a hazardous material incident that you may not be trained to handle.

2. Always wear gloves and eye protection. In cases where there is a danger of greater exposure to a chemical, you may need to wear an impervious (fluid-proof) gown to prevent further contamination.

3. Most chemical burns can be flushed with copious amounts of water. Always ensure that the chemical may be diluted with water; some chemicals when mixed with water may produce combustion. Minimize further wound contamination by ensuring that the fluid used to flush the burn flows away from rather than towards any uninjured areas. Remove all clothing and jewelry.

4. Brush off dry chemicals such as lime before flushing with water (Figure 12–22).

5. Continue to flush for at least twenty minutes while en route to the hospital.

6. Cover the injured area with a sterile dressing, treat for shock, keep the patient warm, and transport. ■

Patient Care Electrical Burns

Electrical burns including those caused by electrical current and lightning can cause severe damage not only to soft tissue, but to the entire body as well (Figure 12–23). Because electricity always seeks the path of least resistance to "ground," any tissues or organs in the energy flow tract from entrance to exit is suspect for injury. Since the body, especially the heart, produces its own electrical energy from chemical reactions, an outside electrical current can disturb or destroy these functions and can cause heart "rhythm" disturbances or cardiac arrest. Because of the extremely hazardous nature of electricity, scene safety is an important consideration.

Emergency Care Steps

Use these guidelines for electrical burn injuries:

1. Never attempt to remove a victim from an electrical source unless trained and equipped to do so.

2. Never touch a victim still in contact with the electrical source.

3. Always assess for the burn's entrance and exit wounds. All tissue between these wounds, even if not readily visible, may be injured. Treat entrance and exit injuries the same as for thermal burns.

4. Monitor the patient for respiratory and cardiac arrest. Use the automated external defibrillator, if necessary.

5. Assess the patient for muscle tenderness, which may or may not be accompanied by muscle twitching or seizure activity.

6. Transport the patient as soon as possible. Most electrical burn injuries will have a slow onset, and underlying tissue or organ damage may not be readily apparent. ■

Special Areas of Concern

Because the eyes, hands, and feet represent special areas of concern, use the following guidelines when treating burns to these areas.

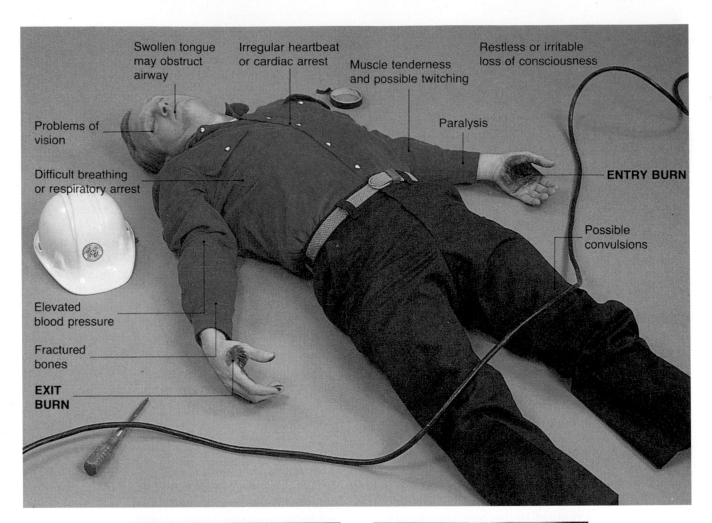

Swollen tongue may obstruct airway

Irregular heartbeat or cardiac arrest

Muscle tenderness and possible twitching

Restless or irritable loss of consciousness

Problems of vision

Paralysis

Difficult breathing or respiratory arrest

ENTRY BURN

Elevated blood pressure

Possible convulsions

Fractured bones

EXIT BURN

Electrical burn—contact with source

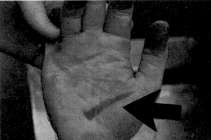

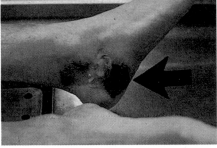

Electrical burn—exit

FIGURE 12–23 Injuries due to electrical shock.

- *Burns to the Eyes* Don't attempt to open burned eyelids. Assure that the burn is thermal, not chemical. Apply dry sterile dressing to BOTH eyes to prevent simultaneous movement of both eyes. Flush chemical burns with water for at least 20 minutes while en route to the hospital. Flush from the medial to the lateral side of the eye to avoid injury to the opposite eye.

- *Burns of the Hands and Toes* Remove all rings and jewelry since they retain heat and the swelling from the burn may cause them to be constrictive. Separate all digits with dry, sterile dressings to prevent the digits from adhering to each other.

Examples of General Dressing and Bandaging

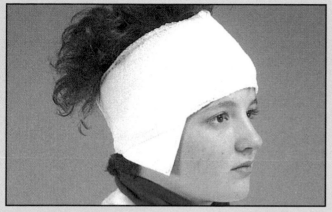

FOREHEAD (NO SKULL INJURY) OR EAR
Place dressing and secure with self-adherent roller bandage.

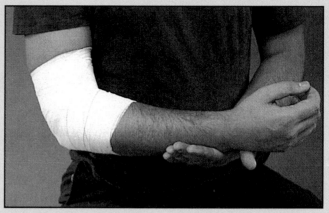

ELBOW OR KNEE Place dressing and secure with cravat or roller bandage. Apply roller bandage in figure 8 pattern.

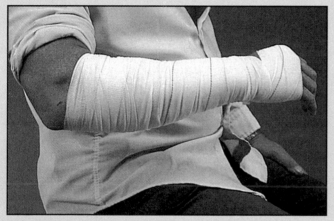

FOREARM OR LEG Place dressing and secure with roller bandage, distal to proximal. Better protection is offered if palm or sole is wrapped.

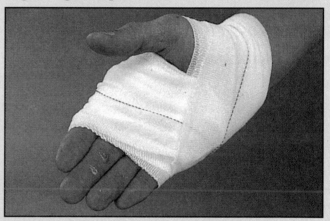

HAND Place dressing, wrap with roller bandage, and secure at wrist. When possible, bandage in position of function.

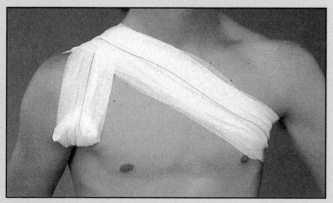

SHOULDER Place dressing and secure with figure 8 of cravat or roller dressing. Pad under knot if cravat is used.

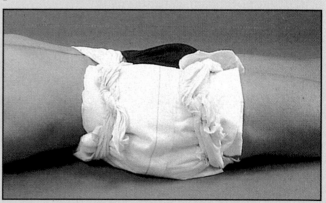

HIP Place bandage and large dressing to cover hip. Secure with first cravat around waist and second cravat around thigh on injured side.

Note: Always leave fingertips or toes showing to assess circulation.

Dressing and Bandaging

Dressing and bandaging procedures are essentially unchanged. The purpose of dressings is to cover open wounds and prevent further contamination. Dressings must be sterile or clean in order to prevent infection. Most dressings will come in various sizes in commercially wrapped or prepared packages. Use will vary depending on specific injured body area. Bandages hold or secure dressings in place and also are available in various sizes. While a bandage should be secure enough to hold the dressing in place, it should not restrict circulation distal to the wound. Use will depend on the type and location of the injured body area. Skill Summary 12–5 summarizes various types of dressing and bandaging.

CHAPTER REVIEW

■ SUMMARY

In order to effectively treat trauma injuries, an understanding of the anatomy and physiology of the circulatory system is necessary.

Trauma injuries can result in significant external or internal blood loss. The methods for controlling external bleeding include direct pressure, elevation, and the use of pressure points. Tourniquets are a last resort and rarely necessary. Emergency care for internal bleeding should focus on the prevention and treatment of shock. Shock, or hypoperfusion, is the inability of the body to supply, or perfuse, the cells and tissues of the body with oxygen and nutrients due to insufficient blood flow through the capillaries. This lack of perfusion also leads to the inadequate removal of waste products from the cells. The emergency care for shock includes maintaining the airway, administering oxygen, attempting to stop what is causing the shock, and attempting to maintain perfusion.

Soft-tissue injuries range from minor scrapes and bruises to life-threatening injuries to the chest and abdomen. Soft-tissue injuries are classified as closed or open. Closed wounds are internal injuries for which there is no open pathway from outside the body to the injury site. Open injuries are those in which the skin is broken, exposing the tissues underneath. Treatment for both open and closed injuries includes taking appropriate BSI precautions, determining the mechanism of injury, protecting the patient's airway and breathing, administering high-concentration oxygen, stopping bleeding, treating for shock, and transporting.

To determine the severity of a burn injury, you must consider the burn's source (thermal, chemical, electrical), depth (superficial, partial-thickness, full-thickness), and extent (determined by location on the body and percent of body surface involved), as well as the patient's age and other preexisting illnesses. Treatment varies depending on the burn's severity.

■ REVIEW QUESTIONS

1. List and describe the three types of bleeding.
2. Define *hypoperfusion*.
3. List and explain the emergency care steps for the treatment of external bleeding.
4. Differentiate between the early and late signs of shock.
5. List the types of closed and open soft-tissue injuries.
6. Describe how you would determine the severity of a burn injury.
7. Differentiate between a dressing and a bandage.

Trauma
- *Musculoskeletal*
- *Head and Spine*

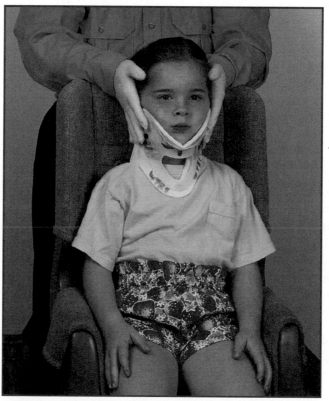

■ As an experienced EMS provider, you are aware that injuries to the musculoskeletal system are very common in our high-paced, action-oriented society. Injuries to muscles and bones can range from a low-priority injury in which the patient returns home from the hospital wearing a cast to an injury that can cause permanent disability or death. This chapter covers the entire spectrum of musculoskeletal injuries, with an emphasis on those injuries that can threaten a patient's life or limbs.

Throughout this text, you have constantly read, "Assess the airway" with the added caveat, "keeping in mind the possibility of an injury to the spine." Although fortunately not as common as less harmful bone injuries, a spinal injury, if not handled appropriately, may result in permanent disability or death. Second only to proper assessment and care for the ABCs, proper assessment and care for head and spinal injuries is your most important responsibility as an EMT-B.

MAKING THE TRANSITION

- ■ The assessment and emergency care of a painful, swollen, or deformed extremity are explained.
- ■ The use of the PASG as a splint is described.
- ■ The procedure of rapid extrication and when it is used is described.

OBJECTIVES

The numbered objectives below are from the United States Department of Transportation 1994 EMT-Basic National Standard Curriculum. Objectives with colored bullets that follow in italics are from the EMT-Basic Transitional Program.

■ KNOWLEDGE AND ATTITUDE

At the end of this chapter, you should be able to meet the following objectives:

Musculoskeletal Injuries

1. Describe the function of the muscular system. (p. 225)
2. Describe the function of the skeletal system. (p. 225)
3. List the major bones or bone groupings of the spinal column, the thorax, the upper extremities, and the lower extremities. (pp. 226–227)
4. Differentiate between an open and a closed painful, swollen, deformed extremity. (p. 228)
5. State the reasons for splinting. (p. 229)
6. List the general rules of splinting. (pp. 229–230)
7. List the complications of splinting. (p. 230)
8. List the emergency medical care for a patient with a painful, swollen, deformed extremity. (pp. 229–252)
9. Explain the rationale for splinting at the scene versus load and go. (pp. 229–230)
10. Explain the rationale for immobilization of the painful, swollen, deformed extremity. (p. 229)

Injuries to the Head and Spine

1. State the components of the nervous system. (pp. 253–255)
2. List the functions of the central nervous system. (pp. 253–255)
3. Define the structure of the skeletal system as it relates to the nervous system. (pp. 253–254)
4. Relate mechanism of injury to potential injuries of the head and spine. (pp. 255–256, 260–261)
5. Describe the implications of not properly caring for potential spinal injuries. (p. 260)
6. State the signs and symptoms of a potential spinal injury. (pp. 261–262)
7. Describe the method of determining if a responsive patient may have a spinal injury. (p. 262)
8. Relate the airway emergency medical care techniques to the patient with a suspected spinal injury. (p. 262)
9. Describe how to stabilize the cervical spine. (p. 263) *(See also Chapter 6.)*
10. Discuss indications for sizing and using a cervical spine immobilization device. (p. 263) *(See also Chapter 6.)*
11. Establish the relationship between airway management and the patient with head and spinal injuries. (pp. 258, 262)
12. Describe a method for sizing a cervical spine immobilization device. (p. 263) *(See also Chapter 6.)*
13. Describe how to log roll a patient with a suspected spinal injury. (pp. 265, 269)
14. Describe how to secure a patient to a long spine board. (pp. 270–271)
15. List instances when a short spine board should be used. (pp. 272–273)
16. Describe how to immobilize a patient using a short spine board. (pp. 272–273, 276–278)
17. Describe the indications for the use of rapid extrication. (p. 272)

18. List steps in performing rapid extrication. (pp. 274–275)

19. State the circumstances when a helmet should be left on the patient. (pp. 262–263)

20. Discuss the circumstances when a helmet should be removed. (p. 263)

21. Identify different types of helmets. (p. 262)

22. Describe the unique characteristics of sport helmets. (p. 262)

23. Explain the preferred methods to remove a helmet. (pp. 262–263, 264)

24. Discuss alternative methods for removal of a helmet. (pp. 262–263, 264)

25. Describe how the patient's head is stabilized to remove the helmet. (pp. 263, 264)

26. Differentiate how the head is stabilized with a helmet compared to without a helmet. (pp. 262–263, 264)

27. Explain the rationale for immobilization of the entire spine when a cervical spine injury is suspected. (p. 262)

28. Explain the rationale for utilizing immobilization methods apart from the straps on the cot. (pp. 262–273)

29. Explain the rationale for utilizing a short spine immobilization device when moving a patient from the sitting to the supine position. (p. 272)

30. Explain the rationale for utilizing rapid extrication approaches only when they indeed will make the difference between life and death. (p. 272)

31. Defend the reasons for leaving a helmet in place for transport of a patient. (pp. 262–263)

32. Defend the reasons for removal of a helmet prior to transport of a patient. (pp. 262–263)

• *Describe the use of the PASG as a splint.* (pp. 240, 242–243)

■ SKILLS

Musculoskeletal Injuries

1. Demonstrate the emergency medical care of a patient with a painful, swollen, deformed extremity.

2. Demonstrate completing a prehospital care report for patients with musculoskeletal injuries.

Injuries to the Head and Spine

1. Demonstrate opening the airway in a patient with suspected spinal cord injury.

2. Demonstrate evaluating a responsive patient with a suspected spinal cord injury.

3. Demonstrate stabilization of the cervical spine.

4. Demonstrate the four-person log roll for a patient with a suspected spinal cord injury.

5. Demonstrate how to log roll a patient with a suspected spinal cord injury using two people.

6. Demonstrate securing a patient to a long spine board.

7. Demonstrate using the short spine board immobilization technique.

8. Demonstrate procedure for rapid extrication.

9. Demonstrate preferred methods for stabilization of a helmet.

10. Demonstrate helmet removal techniques.

11. Demonstrate alternative methods for stabilization of a helmet.

12. Demonstrate completing a prehospital care report for patients with head and spinal injuries.

Eighteen-year-old Lisa Sparks works the midnight shift at a 24-hour gas station min-market. For some time, her boyfriend has been concerned about her late-night hours, since the neighborhood around the station has started to deteriorate. About 5:30 A.M. you respond to a call for a woman who has been assaulted. Upon your **scene size-up**, you find that the police are on the scene, it is secure, and apparently a robber struck Lisa on the back of the head with a pistol and made off with the money from the cash register.

As you begin your **initial assessment**, you get a general impression of a young woman who is conscious but still lying supine on the floor where a police-officer first responder has advised her to remain. Pending your arrival, he has manually stabilized Lisa's head. Your partner takes over manual stabilization as you introduce yourself.

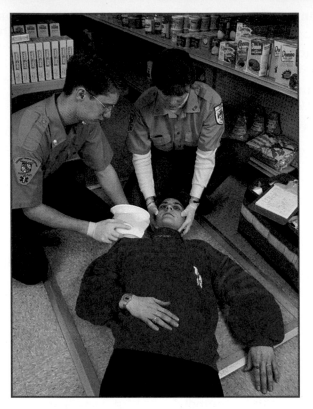

You: Hi. We're emergency medical technicians from the town ambulance service. We're here to help you. I'm Jim Freeman. What's your name?
Lisa: Lisa Sparks.
You: What happened, Lisa?
Lisa: I must have gotten hit on the head when I turned around to get the guy some cigarettes.
You: Did you pass out?
Lisa: I'm not sure. The police officer said I was out of it when he got here. But I don't remember getting hit.
You: Do you know where you are and the day of the week?
Lisa: I am in the gas station where I work. I'm not sure which day it is...is it Tuesday?
You: No, it's Sunday morning.

From her responses, it is obvious that Lisa has an open and clear airway, is breathing OK, is verbally responsive, and knows her name and where she is, but she is not oriented to day. As your partner continues to stabilize Lisa's head and neck, you check her pulse, which is strong and slightly rapid, and her skin, which remains warm, pink, and dry. There is no evidence of blood loss.

You begin your **rapid trauma exam**, since Lisa does have an altered mental status. While examining Lisa's head, you discover a painful swelling on the left side but no bleeding. As soon as you finish examining her neck, you measure and apply a rigid cervical collar and then continue with your physical exam. Your partner knows that the collar doesn't replace manual stabilization, so she continues to hold Lisa's head still. Examination of the rest of Lisa's torso and extremities reveals no additional injury other than an obvious right-side arm and leg weakness. With the assistance of a police officer, you carefully log roll her, place a spine board under her, and then roll her onto the board. You ask the SAMPLE history and get a quick set of vital signs.

Finding nothing else out of the ordinary, you and your partner load Lisa and the board onto the stretcher and then into the ambulance. En route to the hospital, you have time for a **detailed physical exam, ongoing assessment,** and a quick radio call to the hospital alerting them of Lisa's condition. Upon arrival, your reassessment of her mental status reveals that she is getting better, not worse, and you carefully document this outcome on the PCR before leaving the hospital. ■

THE MUSCULOSKELETAL SYSTEM

Some textbooks separate the musculoskeletal system into two body systems—the muscular system and the skeletal system. However, since both systems function to give the body its shape, provide for movement of the body, and protect the body, they are often described as one complex system.

The Muscles

Muscles are classified into three types: skeletal, cardiac, and smooth muscles (Figure 13–1). The skeletal, or voluntary, muscles are under conscious control, which means you can direct them to move the body. Voluntary muscles, which are attached to the long bones, account for the bulk of the body mass. Cardiac muscle is comprised of specialized involuntary muscle cells that provide contraction and electrical stimulation of the heart. Smooth, or involuntary, muscles control movement of materials through the gastrointestinal tract, lungs, blood vessels, and urinary system. For example, when constriction of the blood vessels is needed to compensate for blood loss, such as occurs in compensated shock, the smooth muscles see to it that the job gets done.

As an experienced EMT-B, you are familiar with the names of a number of the major muscles in the body. Muscles are usually named in reference to the bones they support and their insertion points on the bone. For example, one of the accessory muscles that moves the chest when a patient in respiratory distress attempts to breathe is the sternocleidomastoid muscle. This muscle is positioned from the <u>stern</u>um, over the <u>c</u>lavicle, and inserts into the <u>mastoid</u> area of the skull, the slight depression on the lateral sides of the back of your skull.

The Bones

Bones are classified with words that describe their appearance—long, short, flat, or irregular. The bones in the arms and legs are long bones. The majority of the short bones are in the hands and feet. The sternum, shoulder blades, and ribs are flat bones. The vertebrae are considered irregular-shaped bones. A bone is covered with a strong, white, fibrous membrane called **periosteum**, which contains the bone's blood supply and nerves. It is the periosteum that bleeds and causes swelling of the soft tissue when a bone is injured.

PEDIATRIC HIGHLIGHT

When fractures occur near the ends of long bones in children, they must be managed carefully. A bone's growth plates are located at the ends of the bone. A serious fracture in these locations can result in the permanent shortening of a limb. ■

There are two major divisions of the skeleton—axial and appendicular (Figure 13–2). The **axial** division includes the skull, spine, and ribs. The **appendicular** division includes the bones of the arms and legs as well as the bones that comprise the joints that hold the limbs in place, such as the pelvis and the shoulder.

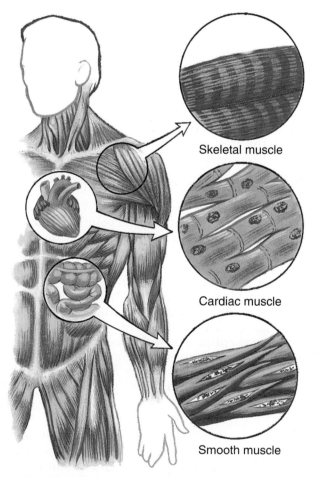

Skeletal muscle

Cardiac muscle

Smooth muscle

FIGURE 13–1 There are three types of muscles in the human body.

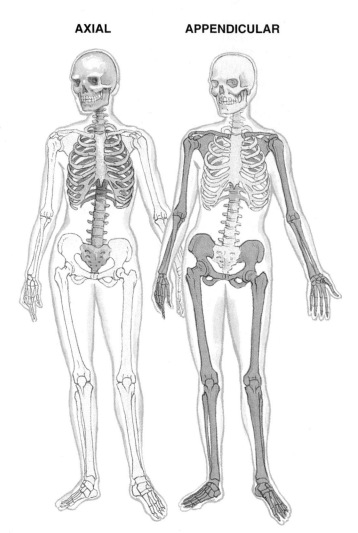

AXIAL   **APPENDICULAR**

FIGURE 13–2 The two major divisions of the human skeleton.

As an experienced EMT-B, you frequently refer to the bones by their medical names. The following is a quick review of the body's major bone groupings (Figure 13–3).

- The **skull** consists of the facial bones anteriorly and the **cranium** on the lateral, posterior, and superior sides. The upper jaw is the **maxilla**; the lower moveable jaw is the **mandible**. When we refer to the regions of the cranium, we refer to top as the **parietal**, the sides as the **temporal**, the forehead as **frontal**, and the back as **occipital**.

- The **spinal column** consists of 33 vertebrae stacked one on top of another. The vertebrae are broken down into five divisions: the seven **cervical** vertebrae found in the neck, the twelve **thoracic** vertebrae corresponding with the ribs and upper back, the five **lumbar** vertebrae in the

lower back, the five fused **sacral** vertebrae that make up the posterior wall of the pelvis, and the four fused **coccyx** vertebrae, or tailbone.

- The **thorax**, or chest, is made up of the twelve pairs of ribs, the **sternum** (breast bone), and the thoracic spine that surround and protect the heart, lungs, and great vessels. All twelve pairs of **ribs** attach to the spine in the back, yet only ten pair attach to the sternum in the front. The two remaining bottom pairs are called "floating ribs." The sternum is a flat bone with three sections: the **manubrium** or superior portion, the **body**, or center, and the **xiphoid** process, which is the inferior tip.

- The **pelvis** is a bowl-shaped structure composed of three major pairs of fused bones: the **ilium**, or major bone that your belt rests on laterally, the **ischium** in the inferior posterior section, used as the attachment point for the traction splint, and the **pubis** in the anterior, which protects the urinary bladder. The ilium joins with the sacral spine posteriorly to support the spinal column. The hip joints are formed laterally by the pelvic bones which create the socket called the acetabulum to which the ball-shaped head of the femur connects.

- The **upper extremities** include your shoulder, which is made up of the **clavicle**, or collarbone on the anterior surface, the **scapula**, or shoulder blade, in the posterior, and the **acromion**, the highest portion of the shoulder which with the clavicle forms the **acromioclavicular joint**. The arm consists of three bones which meet at the elbow: the **humerus**, or upper arm, the **radius** on the thumb side of the forearm, and the **ulna** on the pinky side of the forearm. The wrist bones are the **carpals**; the hand is made up of the **metacarpals**, and the fingers are the **phalanges**.

- The **lower extremities** include your leg which is made up of the **femur**, or thigh bone, the **tibia**, or long bone that forms the anterior surface of your lower leg, and the **fibula**, the thin bone on the lateral surface of your lower leg. The knee cap is called the **patella**; the bony prominence on the outside of the ankle is the **lateral malleolus**; the one on the inside of your ankle is the **medial malleolus**. The ankle joint itself is made up of the **tarsal** bones and the distal tibia and fibula; the foot includes the tarsal and **metatarsal** bones; and the toes, like the fingers, are called **phalanges**.

The connective tissue that helps to support the bones and muscles, especially where they join together, consists of cartilage, tendons, and ligaments. **Cartilage** is tough tissue that covers the

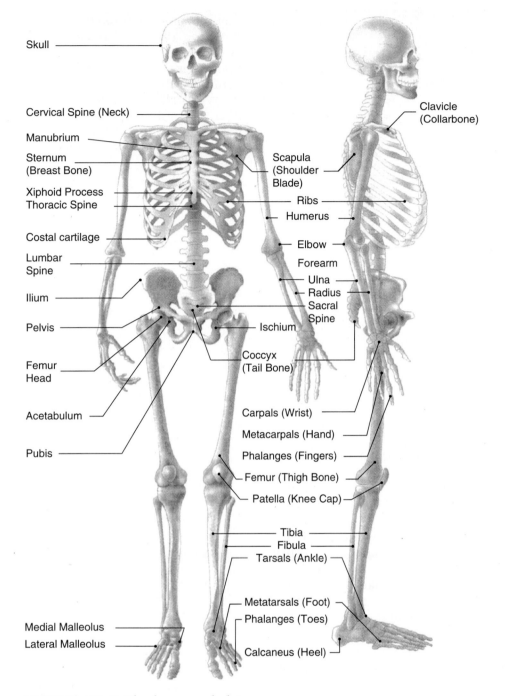

FIGURE 13–3 The human skeleton.

joint ends of bones as well as helps to form certain body parts such as the ear. **Tendons** are designed to connect the muscles to the bones. **Ligaments** act as fibrous elastic bands binding bones to bones.

For our purposes in the field we treat all painful, swollen, deformed extremities (PSDE) as if they were fractures by immobilizing them.

■ MUSCULOSKELETAL INJURIES

As you know, the new EMT-B curriculum focuses on the assessment-based, or complaint-based, approach rather than the diagnosis-based approach used in the past. For example, in the past, if a patient complained of a painful, swollen, deformed extremity, we called the injury either a

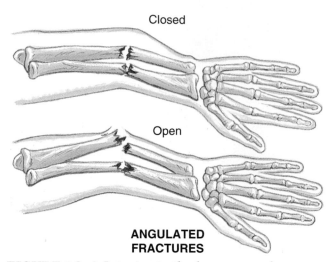

Closed

Open

ANGULATED FRACTURES

FIGURE 13–4 Injuries to the bones may be open or closed. A broken bone may be angulated (bent).

"possible fracture" or an actual fracture if the extremity was severely angulated (bent) or if a bone was actually protruding. We also attempted to diagnose the injury. In fact, EMT texts of the past often showed X-ray pictures of various fractures that were named greenstick, oblique, comminuted, or transverse. Today's assessment-based approach uses the complaint to name a musculoskeletal injury as a painful, swollen, deformed extremity (PSDE). Since in the field the treatment for a fracture, dislocation, sprain, or strain is basically the same, there is no longer a need to distinguish among these injuries.

However, to ensure that you will understand the Emergency Department physician and other health professionals when they use medical terminology that refers to musculoskeletal injuries, let's review some common terms. A **fracture** is any break in a bone. It can be **angulated** (broken bone is bent at an angle) and either open or closed (Figure 13–4). A **dislocation** is the disruption of the joint due to the tearing of the joint capsule and the soft tissue that surrounds it, such as occurs in a dislocated shoulder. A **sprain** is the stretching or tearing of muscles or ligaments.

It is important that you be able to differentiate between an open and a closed PSDE. The **open** PSDE has a laceration at the site of the injury, which is usually due to the bone breaking through the skin. In some instances, the bone may be protruding, but in others, the bone may pop back into place on its own. With a **closed** PSDE, there is no evidence that the bone ends have broken through the skin. To set a fracture, a physician

first realigns the broken bone ends. This is called **reducing** the fracture. At times, when you are attempting to move the bones of an angulated fracture into a splintable position, you may accidentally reduce it.

When treating a closed PSDE, it is important that you splint the injury where you find the patient by immobilizing the bone ends and two adjacent joints. This will prevent the fracture from breaking through the skin and becoming an open fracture. Through gentle handling and splinting of closed fractures, EMT-Bs can help reduce the patient's pain, prevent lengthy hospital stays, and lower health care costs.

■ **Patient Assessment** **Musculoskeletal Injuries**

When assessing a musculoskeletal injury, you often need to expose the injury by removing at least part of the patient's clothing. The decision to expose an injury depends on weather conditions, the patient's degree of modesty, the severity of the injury, and patient refusal.

Signs and Symptoms
The signs and symptoms of a musculoskeletal injury include:

- Pain and tenderness
- Deformity or angulation
- Grating, or **crepitus**, which is the sound or feeling caused by broken bone ends rubbing together
- Swelling (Don't forget to remove the patient's jewelry before it needs to be cut off.)
- Bruising (**ecchymosis**, or large black-and-blue discoloration of the skin, which indicates an injury that is hours to days old)
- Exposed bone ends
- Joints locked into position
- Nerve or blood vessel compromise
- Inability to move the extremity ■

Preceptor Pearl

Do not allow a grotesque PSDE to distract you from performing the initial assessment and rapid trauma exam and making a priority decision. Also, always expose the injury. If you fail to expose the injury prior to splinting, what you thought was a closed injury might actually be an open injury and the protruding bone ends may "grab a woman's stockings" and pull them into the wound! ✤

Patient Care Musculoskeletal Injuries

Most fractures, though painful and disabling, are rarely fatal. Make sure you manually stabilize the trauma patient's cervical spine, assess the airway and breathing, provide oxygen, and assure that breathing is adequate. Assess pulses and skin color. Control bleeding and manage shock.

Emergency Care Steps

Assure that the scene is safe and that you will not become a victim of the same mechanism of injury as the patient.

1. Take body substance isolation precautions.

2. Perform the initial assessment and rapid trauma exam and attend to any life-threatening priorities. Determine patient priority. High-priority patients may need to be splinted with a total body splint on a long backboard rather than taking time to splint individual fractures. Control bleeding, apply sterile dressings if needed, and attempt to maintain body temperature. If the patient is low priority, apply individual splints, apply a cold pack to the injury site to minimize swelling, and elevate the splinted extremity.

3. Always be sure to assess the distal MSC (movement, sensation, circulation) *before* and *after* application of a splint and document your findings on your PCR. ■

Preceptor Pearl

Keep in mind that when a bone breaks, it bleeds. Therefore, a patient with multiple breaks can easily be in shock from significant blood loss. In the first two hours of an uncomplicated simple fracture of the tibia and fibula, a patient can lose a pint of blood. A fractured femur can cause a two-pint blood loss; a pelvic fracture can cause a three- to four-pint loss. ✤

Splinting

The purpose of splinting is simple—your goal is to immobilize the bone ends and the adjacent joints. Doing so minimizes the movement of the disrupted joints or broken bone ends, decreases the patient's pain, and helps to prevent any additional damage to nerves, arteries, veins, and muscles. A properly applied splint can prevent a closed fracture from becoming an open one, as well as minimize blood loss. In addition, splinting on a

backboard prevents injury to the spinal cord and helps to prevent permanent paralysis.

Although the thought of realigning an extremity can be a frightening one, the experienced EMT-B knows that if the extremity is not realigned, the splint is often ineffective and can cause increased pain and possible further injury to the patient.

When the distal circulation is compromised, as in an angulated fracture or a cyanotic or pulseless extremity, the lack of circulation causes oxygen-starved tissues to begin to die.

To realign a PSDE, the first EMT-B grasps the distal extremity while a partner places one hand above and one hand below the injury site. The partner supports the site while the first EMT-B pulls gentle traction in the direction of the long bone axis of the extremity. If resistance is felt or it appears as if the bone ends will come through the skin, stop realignment and splint in the position found. If no resistance is felt, maintain gentle traction until the extremity is splinted.

Preceptor Pearl

Always immobilize a stable patient in the spot where he or she is found. However, the actual extremity will need to be moved into a "splintable" position, which is straight enough to fit on a padded board. As the saying goes "immobilize them where they lie *not* as they lie." ✤

Splinting Rules

Keep in mind these general rules of splinting:

- If the patient is unstable, do not waste time splinting. Care for life-threatening problems first. Align the injuries in anatomical position and immobilize the patient's entire body on a long spine board.

- The method of splinting is dictated by the patient's status and priority for transport. If the patient is a high priority for "load and go," choose a rapid method of splinting such as a long backboard (fastest method but only slightly better than no splinting) or the PASG, or MAST, for multiple-fractured legs. If the patient is a lower priority, use a slower but more effective splinting method.

- If a patient must be rapidly removed from a car prior to splinting, try to immobilize the injured leg to the uninjured leg until you have the time to do the splinting en route.

- Before moving the injured extremity, expose it and control bleeding.

- Examine for and record MSCs before and after splinting.
- To be effective a splint must immobilize the bone ends and two adjacent joints.
- If severe deformity exists or distal circulation is compromised, align long bone injuries to anatomical position under gentle traction.
- Do not attempt to push protruding bones back into place. If they accidentally slip back into place during realignment, inform the ED staff and document this occurrence on your prehospital care report.
- Pad the voids between the body part and the splint to increase patient comfort and ensure proper immobilization. Many rigid splints do not conform to body curves and allow too much movement of the limb.
- The exception to the rules of splinting long bones is the femur, which is splinted using a traction splint. (See Splinting Application: Lower Extremities on p. 240.)

Splinting Complications

Occasionally there are complications from splinting. Carefully observe for the following:

- The EMT-B who forgets that the patient is high priority. If the patient has a life-threatening problem, remember to expedite the splinting and concentrate on airway, breathing, and circulation problems.
- A splint that is applied too tightly. This can compress soft tissue and injure nerves, blood vessels, and muscles.
- A splint that is applied too loosely. This may allow too much movement and has the potential to convert a closed fracture to an open fracture or cause further soft-tissue damage.
- A splinted extremity that is not realigned. This can create further damage.

There are many types of splints for long bones such as rigid, formable, and traction splints. No matter what type of splint is used, the general procedures and rules remain the same. The procedure for immobilizing a long bone is shown in Skill Summary 13–1. The procedure for immobilizing a joint is shown in Skill Summary 13–2.

Splint Application: Upper Extremities

Patients with a clavicle injury complain of pain in the shoulder, and you may observe a dropped shoulder (Figure 13–5). The patient is often found

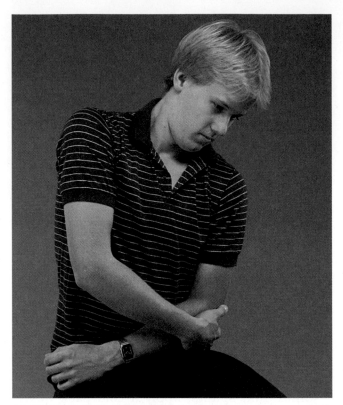

FIGURE 13–5 A fractured clavicle may be noted by a "dropped" shoulder.

holding the injured arm against the chest. Sometimes a sharp blow to the shoulder blade injures the scapula. If, upon palpation of the entire shoulder, the head of the humerus is felt in front of the shoulder, this may indicate an anterior shoulder dislocation or fracture.

If a dislocation occurs, tie a blanket roll under the arm and around the body to give the patient something on which to rest the injured arm. Then apply a sling and swathe. Do not attempt to straighten or reduce any dislocations. Occasionally, some patients may pop their shoulder back into place. If this occurs, be sure to assess MSCs, note the self-reduction on your PCR, and report it to the ED.

The sling and swathe is very useful for splinting a number of upper extremity PSDEs. The procedure for applying a sling and swathe is reviewed in Skill Summary 13–3 and is shown as a means of splinting an injury to the humerus in Skill Summary 13–4. The sling and swathe can also be combined with the use of board splints, as shown in the care of the arm and elbow injuries (Skill Summary 13–5) and in the care of injuries to the forearm, wrist, and hand (Skill Summary 13–6).

Immobilizing a Long Bone

FIRST take body substance isolation precautions.

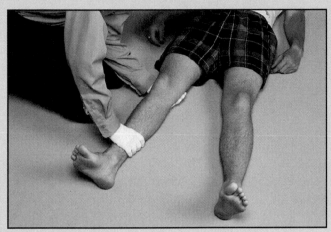

1. Direct application of manual stabilization.

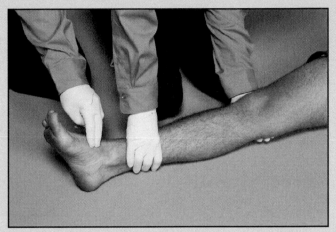

2. Assess distal motor ability, sensory response, and circulation (MSC).

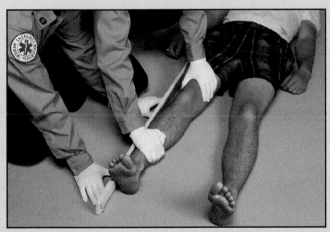

3. Measure splint. It should extend several inches beyond joints above and below injury.

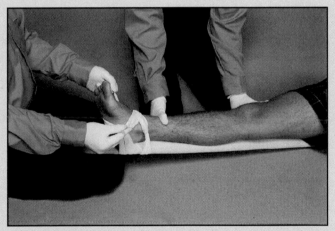

4. Apply splint and immobilize joints above and below injury.

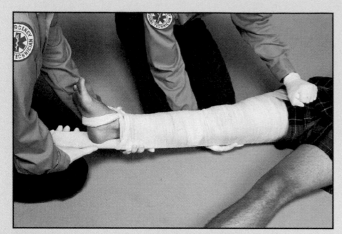

5. Secure the entire injured extremity.

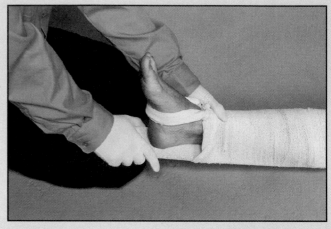

6.a. Secure foot in position of function as shown ...

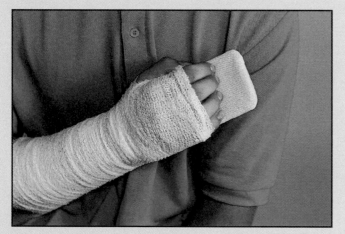

6.b. ... or if splinting an arm, secure hand in position of function. This is the position the hand would be in if the patient were holding a palm-sized ball. A roll of bandage can be placed in the patient's hand to help maintain the position of function.

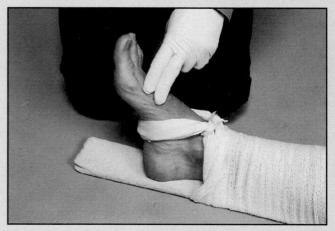

7. Reassess distal MSC function.

Immobilizing a Joint

FIRST take body substance isolation precautions.

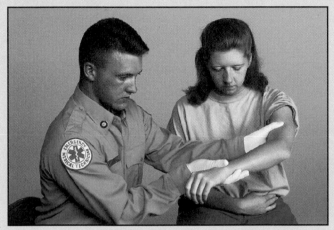

1. Direct application of manual stabilization.

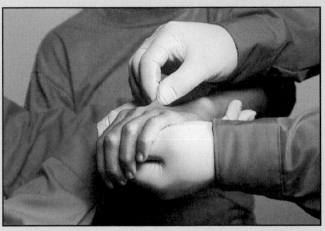

2. Assess distal motor ability, sensory response, and circulation (MSC).

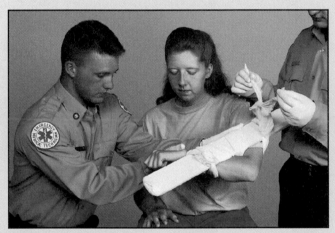

3. Select proper splint material. Immobilize site of injury and bones above and below.

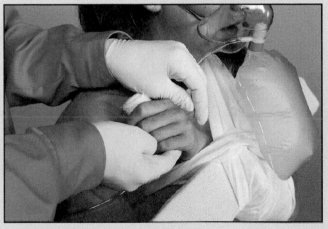

4. Reassess distal MSC function.

Sling and Swathe

A sling is a triangular bandage used to support the shoulder and arm. Once the patient's arm is placed in a sling, a swathe can be used to hold the arm against the side of the chest. Commercial slings are available. Velcro straps can be used to form a swathe. Use whatever materials you have on hand, provided they will not cut into the patient.

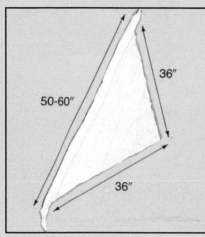

1. The sling should be in the shape of a triangle.

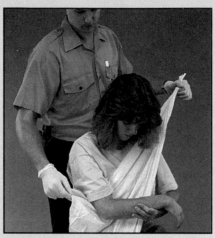

2. Position the sling over the top of the patient's chest as shown. Fold the patient's injured arm across the chest.

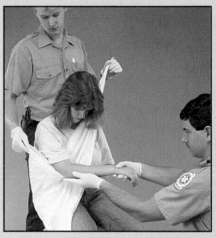

3. If the patient cannot hold her arm, have someone assist until you tie the sling.

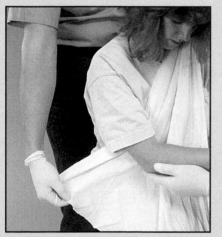

4. One point of the triangle should extend behind the elbow on the injured side.

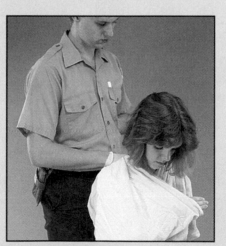

5. Take the bottom point of the triangle and bring this end up over the patient's arm. When you are finished, this point should be taken over the top of the patient's injured shoulder.

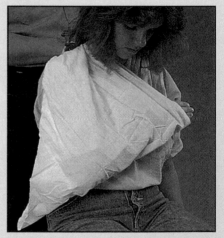

6. Draw up on the ends of the sling so that the patient's hand is about four inches above the elbow (exceptions are discussed later).

Note: Assess distal motor ability, sensory response, and circulation (pulse) both before and after immobilizing or splinting an extremity.

Skill Summary 13–3 *(continued)*

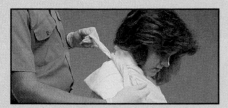

7. Tie the two ends of the sling together, making sure that the knot does not press against the back of the patient's neck. The area can be padded with bulky dressings or sanitary napkins.

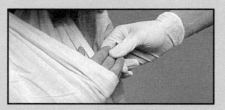

8. Leave the patient's fingertips exposed to permit check of motor and sensory function and circulation.

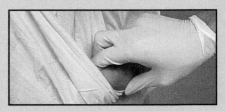

9. Check motor and sensory function. Check for radial pulse. If the pulse has been lost, take off the sling and repeat the procedure. Repeat sling procedure if necessary.

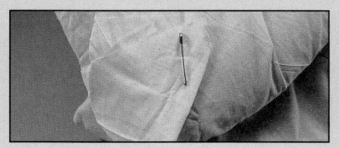

10A. Take hold of the point of material at the patient's elbow and fold it forward, pinning it to the front of the sling. This forms a pocket for the patient's elbow.

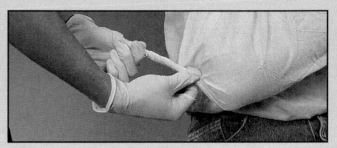

10B. If you do not have a pin, twist the excess material and tie a knot in the point.

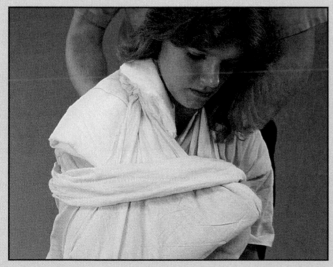

11. A swathe can be formed from a second piece of triangular material. This swathe is tied around the chest and the injured arm, over the sling. Do not place this swathe over the patient's arm on the uninjured side.

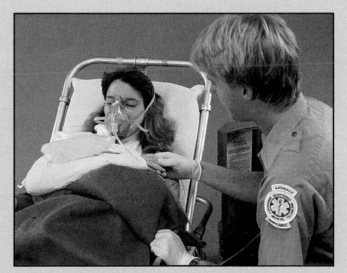

12. Assess distal motor and sensory function and circulation. Treat for shock. Provide a high concentration of oxygen. Take vital signs. Perform detailed and ongoing assessments as appropriate.

Note: If the patient has cervical spine injury, do not tie sling around neck.

Injuries to Humerus—Soft Splinting

SIGNS:

Injury to the humerus can take place at the proximal end (shoulder), along the shaft of the bone, or at the distal end (elbow). Deformity is the key sign used to detect fractures to this bone in any of these locations; however, assess for all signs of skeletal injury. Follow the rules and procedures for care of an injured extremity.

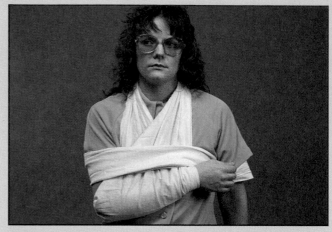

1. Fracture at proximal end. Gently apply a sling and swathe. If you have only enough material for a swathe, bind the patient's upper arm to her body, taking great care not to cut off circulation to the forearm.

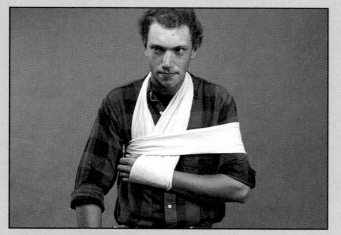

2. Fracture of the shaft. Use rigid splints whenever possible; otherwise, gently apply a sling and swathe. The sling should be modified so that it supports the wrist only.

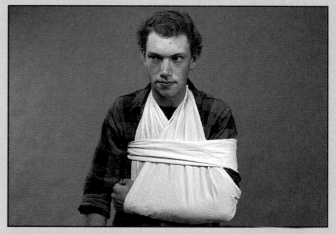

3. Fracture at distal end. Gently apply full sling and swathe. Do not draw the hand upward to a position above the elbow. Instead, keep elbow flexion as close to a 90° angle as possible.

Warning: Before applying a sling and swathe to care for injuries to the humerus, check for distal motor and sensory function and circulation. If you do not feel a pulse, attempt to straighten any slight angulation if the patient has a closed fracture (follow local protocol). Otherwise, prepare for immediate immobilization and transport. Should straightening of the angulation fail to restore the pulse or function, splint with a medium board splint, keeping the forearm extended. If there is no sign of circulation or sensory or motor function, you will have to attempt a second splinting. If this fails to restore distal function, transport immediately. Do not try to straighten angulation of the humerus if there are any signs of fracture or dislocation of the shoulder or elbow.

Note: Assess distal motor ability, sensory response, and circulation (pulse) both before and after immobilizing or splinting an extremity.

Arm and Elbow Injuries

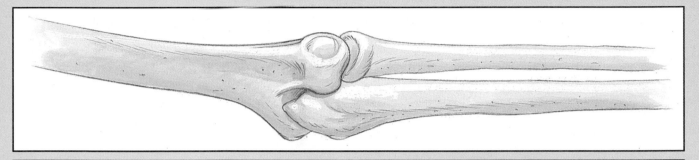

The elbow is a joint and not a bone. It is composed of the distal humerus and the proximal ulna and radius, forming a hinge joint. You will have to decide if the injury is truly to the elbow. Deformity and sensitivity will direct you to the injury site.

CARE: If there is a distal pulse, the dislocated elbow should be immobilized in the position in which it is found. The joint has too many nerves and blood vessels to risk movement. When a distal pulse is absent, make one attempt to slightly reposition the limb after contacting medical direction. Do not force the limb into anatomical position.

Elbow in or Returned to Bent Position

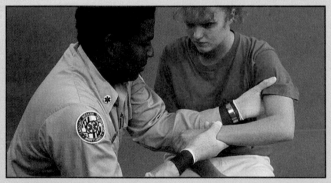

1. Move limb only if necessary for splinting or if pulse is absent. **Do not** continue if you meet resistance or significantly increase the pain.

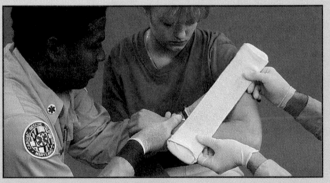

2. Use a padded board splint that will extend 2 to 6 inches beyond the arm and wrist when placed diagonally.

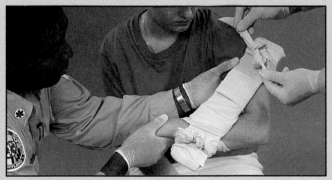

3. Place the splint so it is just proximal to the elbow and to the wrist. Use cravats to secure to the forearm, then the arm.

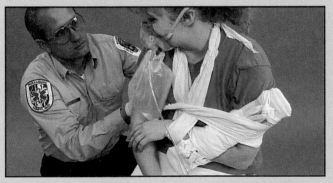

4. A wrist sling can be applied to support the limb; keep the elbow exposed. Apply a swathe if possible.

237

Elbow in Straight Position

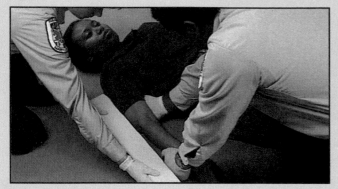

1. Assess distal motor and sensory function and circulation (pulse).

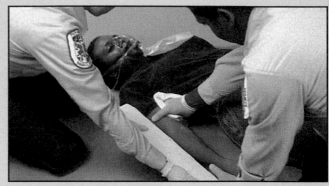

2. Use a padded board splint that extends from under the armpit to a point past the fingertips. Pad the armpit.

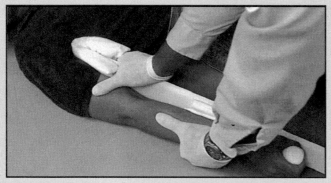

3. Place a roll of bandages in the patient's hand to help maintain position of function. Place padded side of board against medial side of limb. Pad all voids.

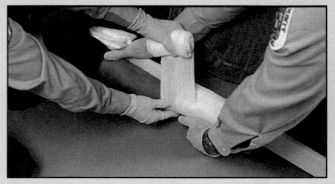

4. Secure the splint. Leave fingertips exposed.

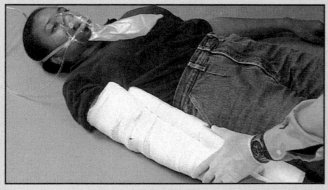

5. Place pads between patient's side and splint.

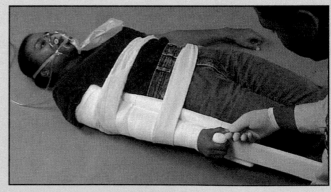

6. Secure splinted limb to body with two cravats. Avoid placing over suspected injury site. Reassess distal motor, sensory, and circulatory function.

Note: Assess distal motor ability, sensory response, and circulation (pulse) both before and after immobilizing or splinting an extremity.

Injuries to the Forearm, Wrist, and Hand

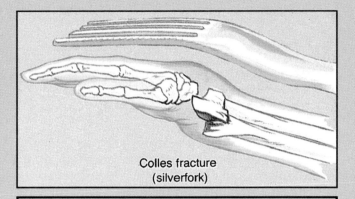

Colles fracture
(silverfork)

SIGNS:

- Forearm—deformity and tenderness. If only one bone is broken, deformity may be minor or absent.
- Wrist—deformity and tenderness, with the possibility of a Colles (KOL-ez) fracture that gives a "silverfork" appearance to the wrist.
- Hand—deformity and pain. Dislocated fingers are obvious.

Note: Assess distal motor ability, sensory response, and circulation (pulse) both before and after immobilizing or splinting an extremity.

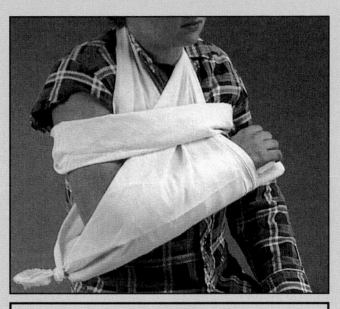

CARE: Injuries occurring to the forearm, wrist, or hand can be splinted using a padded rigid splint that extends from the elbow past the fingertips. The patient's elbow, forearm, wrist, and hand all need the support of the splint. Tension must be provided throughout the splinting. A roll of bandage should be placed in the hand to ensure the position of function. After rigid splinting, apply a sling and swathe.

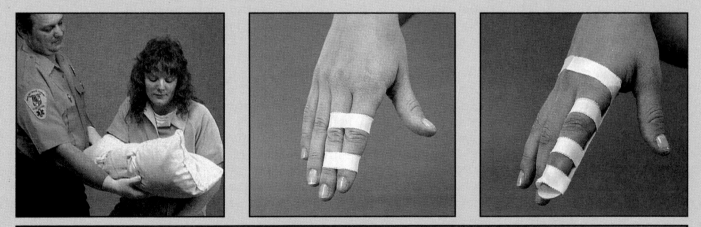

ALTERNATIVE CARE: Injuries to the hand and wrist can be cared for with soft splinting by placing a roll of bandage in the hand to maintain position of function, then tying the forearm, wrist, and hand into the fold of one pillow or between two pillows. An injured finger can be taped to an adjacent uninjured finger or splinted with a tongue depressor. Some emergency department physicians prefer that care be limited to a wrap of soft bandages. **DO NOT** try to "pop" dislocated fingers back into place.

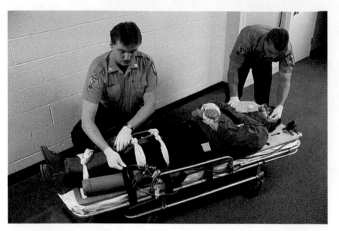

FIGURE 13–6 Immobilizing a patient with hip or pelvis injury on a long spine board.

Preceptor Pearl

If a patient has a possible neck injury, never wrap a sling around the patient's neck. ✤

Splinting Application: Lower Extremities

Injuries to the pelvis can be very serious because of the potential for extreme blood loss and internal organ injury. The patient with a pelvic injury may complain of pain in the pelvis, hips, groin, or lower back. Often there is no deformity, but the mechanism of injury leads you to suspect a pelvic injury. The patient may have pain upon palpation of the iliac wings or the pubic bone or an unexplained pressure on the urinary bladder accompanied by a feeling of the need to urinate. The patient may be unable to lift the leg when supine; the foot on the injured side may turn outward (lateral rotation). This rotation may also indicate a hip fracture.

It is difficult to distinguish between a fractured pelvis and a fracture of the upper femur; if in doubt, treat the patient for a pelvic fracture. Move the patient as little as possible and never log roll to place him on a long spine board. Straighten both of the patient's legs and place a folded blanket between them extending from the groin to the feet. Bind the legs and the blanket together with a series of cravats (Figure 13–6).

Some EMS systems use the PASG for pelvic injuries as well as to control shock and splint hip, femoral, and multiple-leg fractures. A PASG is strongly indicated for use with a pelvic fracture accompanied by hypotension (blood pressure below 90). If this is your system's procedure,

follow the application of the device shown in Skill Summary 13–7. A physician must order the removal of a PASG.

Preceptor Pearl

When splinting multiple fractures, consider the "whole patient" before deciding on the immobilization device. If a patient is stable and has a fractured tibia and femur, a long board splint is appropriate. However, if the patient has signs and symptoms of shock or has sustained other multiple injuries, the use of the PASG is more appropriate, since both the shock and the fracture can be treated at the same time. ✤

A hip dislocation (Figure 13–7) occurs when the head of the femur moves out of its socket. (It is difficult to tell the difference between a hip injury and a proximal femur injury.) Patients who have had a surgical hip replacement are at greater risk for a dislocation. In an anterior dislocation, the hip is flexed and the leg is externally rotated. In a posterior dislocation, the leg is dislocated inward, the hip is flexed, and the knee is bent. Often there is a lack of sensation in the limb due to injury to the sciatic nerve. This type of injury often occurs in a motor vehicle collision when the occupant's knees strike the dash. A patient with a hip dislocation can be splinted on a long spine board (as described above for a pelvis injury), or a padded board that extends from the armpit to the foot can be placed between the patient's legs and secured with cravats.

Splint the patient with a PSDE that obviously involves the femur with a traction splint. The injured leg will often appear shortened due to the overriding of the bone ends, and the patient may have intense pain. The traction splint is needed because the large muscles surrounding the femur—the quadriceps and the hamstrings—go into spasm and literally grind down the ends of the broken bone. This causes severe pain, additional soft tissue injury, and bleeding. The traction counteracts the muscle spasms and reduces the pain. There are two types of devices frequently used— the bipolar, with two poles, such as the Hare or Fernotrac traction splint, and the unipolar, with one pole, such as the Sager traction splint. The unipolar units are less likely to lose traction when the patient is lifted. The application of the bipolar (Fernotrac) traction splint is shown in Skill Summary 13–8. A variation of the traction splint is

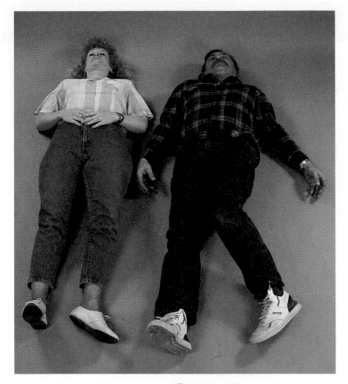

Posterior view

Posterior dislocation

FIGURE 13–7 Signs of anterior and posterior hip dislocation.

shown in Skill Summary 13–9, and the unipolar (Sager) device is shown in Skill Summary 13–10.

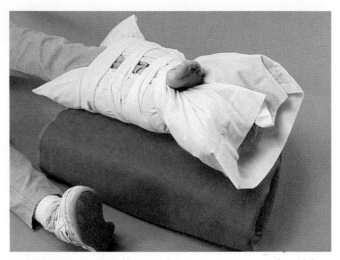

FIGURE 13–8 Pillow splinting an injured ankle.

If you suspect a fracture to the knee or tibia/fibula, do not use the traction splint. Apply the ankle hitch as shown in Skill Summary 13–11.

Knee injuries can be very complex. The patella can become displaced when the lower leg is twisted and can cause ligament damage. A knee dislocation occurs when the tibia itself is forced either anteriorly or posteriorly in relation to the distal femur. Always check for a distal pulse, since the dislocated knee joint can compress the popliteal artery and stop the major blood supply to the lower leg. If there is no pulse, contact medical control for permission to gently move the leg anteriorly to allow for a pulse and transport the patient immediately. The splinting of a bent knee using a technique called triangulation with two long board splints is shown in Skill Summary 13–12, and the splinting of the straight knee is shown in Skill Summary 13–13.

Injuries to the tibia or fibula are very common. They are usually splinted with two boards as shown in Skill Summary 13–14. An air splint can also be used on a straight arm or lower leg as shown in Summary 13–15.

Injuries to the ankle or foot can be splinted using a pillow splint (Figure 13–8). However, remember that a pillow does not immobilize the knee; therefore, the patient must be placed on a stretcher with the knee strapped down in place. Keep the toes exposed so the patient's circulation can be monitored. For an ankle injury, use a commercial Velcro-closure type splint with both a foot section and a leg section that extends above the knee.

Application of an Anti-Shock Garment

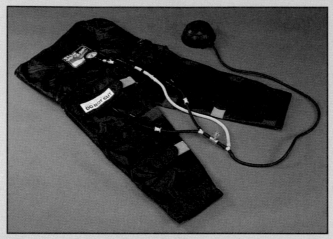

Adult garment and inflation pump.

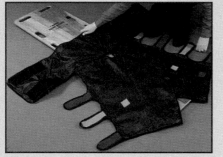

1. Unfold the garment and lay it flat on a backboard. It should be smoothed of wrinkles.

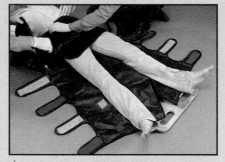

2. Slip garment under patient. The upper edge of the garment must be just below the rib cage.

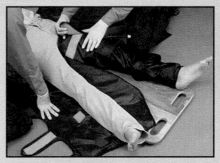

3. Enclose the left leg, securing the Velcro straps.

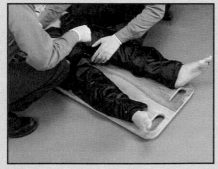

4. Enclose the right leg, securing the Velcro straps.

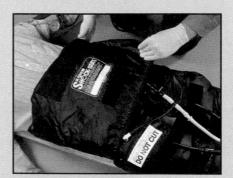

5. Enclose the abdomen and pelvis, securing the Velcro straps.

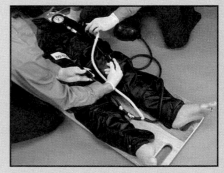

6. Check the tubes leading to the compartments and the pump.

Note: Patient's clothing remains on for demonstration purposes. In actual use, clothing should be removed. Anti-shock garment can be placed over traction splint.

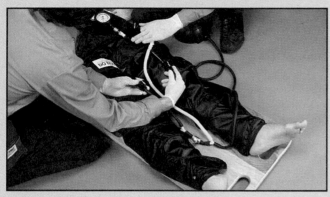

7. Open the stopcocks to the legs and close the abdominal compartment stopcock.

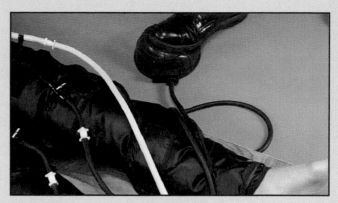

8. Use the pump to inflate the lower compartments simultaneously, or the required lower extremity compartment. Inflate until air exhausts through the relief valves, the Velcro makes a crackling noise, or the patient's systolic blood pressure is stable at 90 mm Hg or higher.

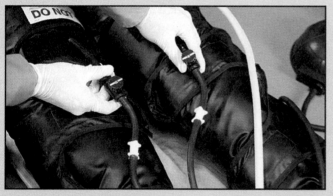

9. Close the stopcocks.

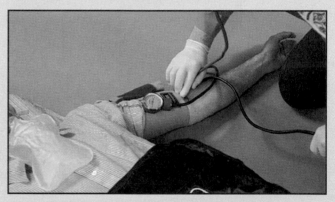

10. Check the patient's blood pressure.

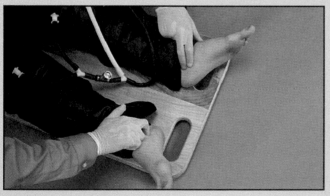

11. Check both lower extremities for a distal pulse.

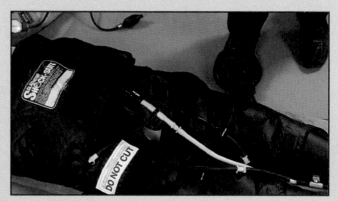

12. If BP is below 90, open the abdominal stopcock and inflate abdominal compartment. Close stopcock.

Note: Monitor and record vital signs every 5 minutes. If the garment loses pressure, add air as needed. Some protocols call for the inflation of all three compartments of the garment simultaneously.

The Fernotrac Traction Splint— Preparing the Splint

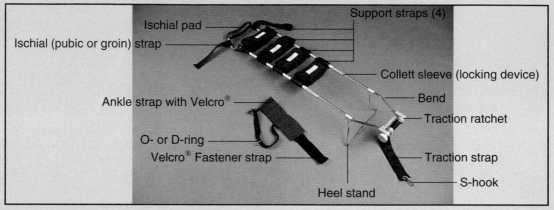

Support straps (4)
Ischial pad
Ischial (pubic or groin) strap
Collett sleeve (locking device)
Bend
Ankle strap with Velcro®
Traction ratchet
O- or D-ring
Velcro® Fastener strap
Traction strap
S-hook
Heel stand

1. The Fernotrac Traction Splint

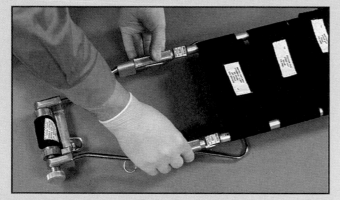

2. Loosen sleeve locking device.

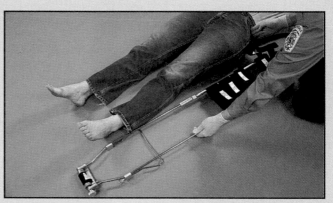

3. Place next to uninjured leg—ischial pad next to iliac crest.

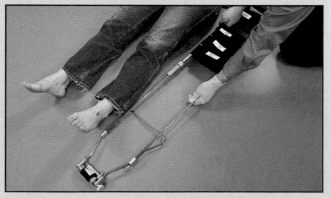

4. Hold top and move bottom until bend is at heel.

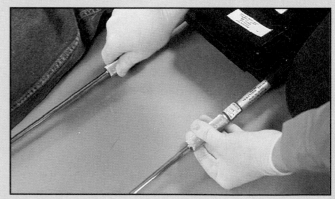

5. Lock sleeve.

Notes: Some splints in use are measured by placing the ring at the level of the bony prominence that can be felt in the middle of each buttock (ischial tuberosity) and the distal end of the splint placed 8 to 10 inches beyond the foot. Assess distal motor ability, sensory response, and circulation (pulse) both before and after immobilizing or splinting an extremity.

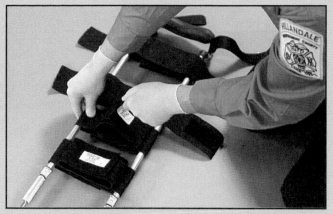

6. Open support straps.

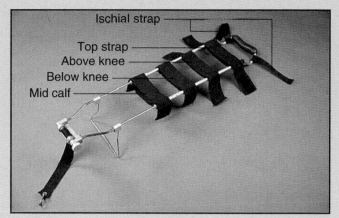

Ischial strap
Top strap
Above knee
Below knee
Mid calf

7. Place straps under splint.

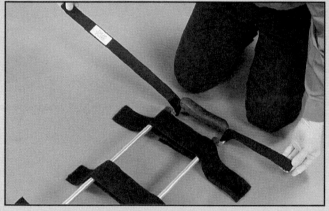

8. Release ischial strap. Attached ends should be next to ischial pad.

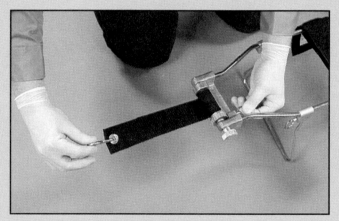

9. Pull release ring on ratchet and ...

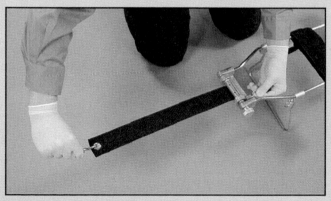

10. ... release the traction strap.

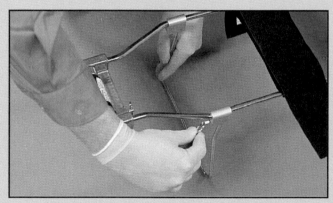

11. Extend and position heel stand after splint is in position under patient.

Note: Traction splints vary depending on the manufacturer. Learn to use the equipment supplied in your area and keep up to date with new equipment as it is approved for use.

CHAPTER 13 Trauma—Musculoskeletal, Head and Spine

Traction Splinting—Variation

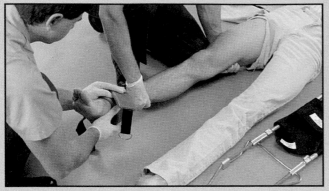

1. Some systems attach the ankle hitch prior to applying manual traction (tension). EMT-B 1 should apply the hitch while EMT-B 2 stabilizes the limb.

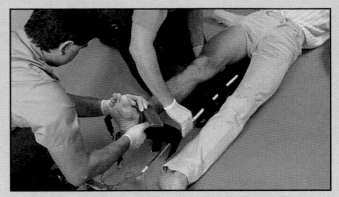

2a. While EMT-B 1 applies manual traction (tension), EMT-B 2 can position the splint.

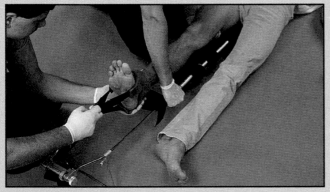

2b. Some systems allow manual traction to be applied by grasping the D-ring and ankle.

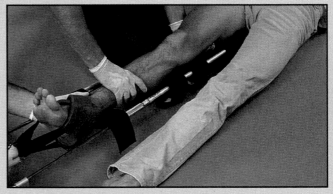

3. EMT-B 1 maintains manual traction (tension) and lowers the limb onto the cradles of the splint.

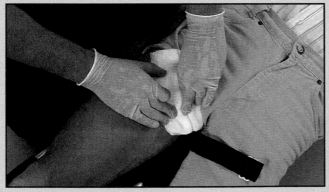

4. While EMT-B 1 maintains manual traction, EMT-B 2 applies padding to the groin area before securing the ischial strap. **Note:** Some EMS systems do not apply padding in order to reduce slippage.

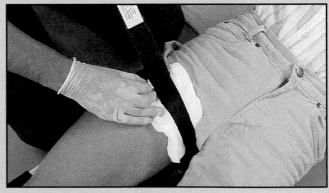

5. EMT-B 2 secures the ischial strap, connects the ankle hitch to the windlass, tightens the ratchet to equal manual traction (tension), and secures the cradle straps.

Note: Assess distal motor ability, sensory response, and circulation (pulse) both before and after immobilizing or splinting an extremity.

The Sager Traction Splint

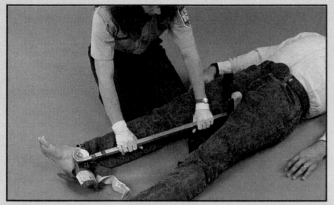

1. Splint will be placed medially.

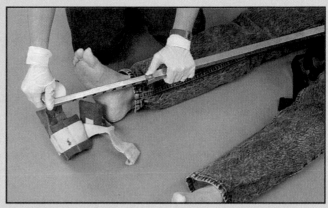

2. Length should be from groin to 4 inches past heel. Unlock to slide.

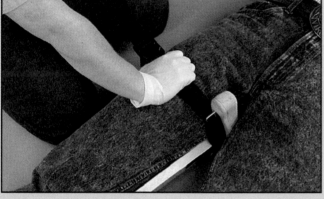

3. Secure thigh strap.

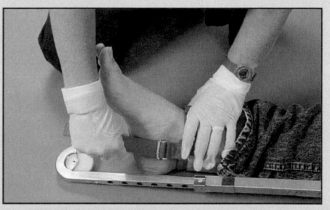

4. Wrap ankle harness above ankle (malleoli) and secure under heel.

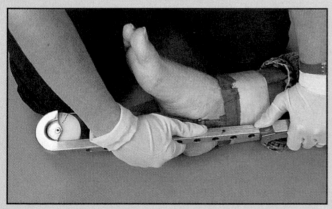

5. Release lock and extend splint to achieve desired traction (in pounds on pulley wheel).

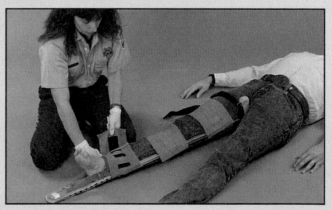

6. Secure straps at thigh, lower thigh and knee, and lower leg. Strap ankles and feet together. Secure to spine board.

Note: Assess distal motor ability, sensory response, and circulation (pulse) both before and after immobilizing or splinting an extremity.

The Ankle Hitch

The ankle hitch can be used with a single padded board splint to immobilize injured knees and legs. It is made with a 3-inch wide cravat.

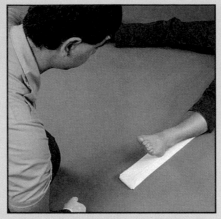

1. Kneel at distal end of limb.

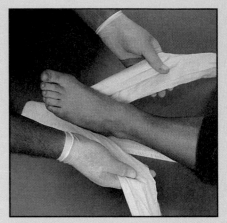

2. Center cravat in arch.

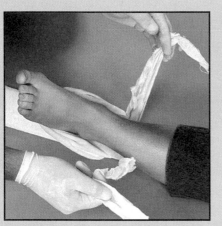

3. Place cravat along sides of foot and cross cravat behind ankle.

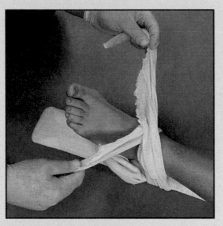

4. Cross cravat ends over top of ankle.

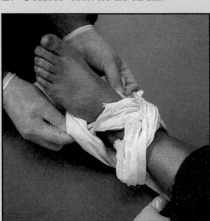

5. A stirrup has been formed.

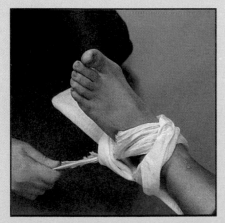

6. Thread ends through stirrup.

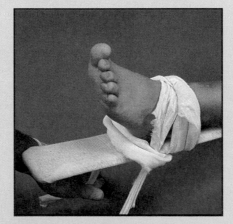

7. Pull ends downward to tighten.

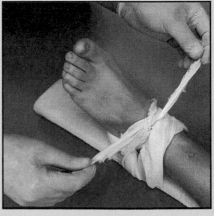

8. Pull upward and tie over ankle wrap.

Note: *Assess distal motor ability, sensory response, and circulation (pulse) both before and after immobilizing or splinting an extremity.*

Knee Injuries—Knee Bent—Two-Splint Method

If there is a distal pulse and nerve function, or the limb cannot be straightened without meeting resistance or causing severe pain, knee injuries should be splinted with the knee in the position in which it is found.

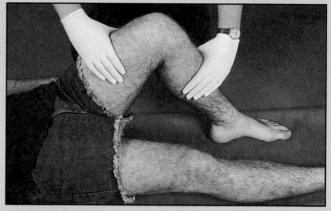

1. One EMT-B stabilizes the knee above and below the injury site as shown.

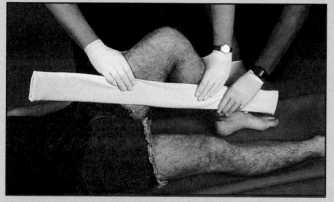

2. The splints should be equal and extend 6-12 inches beyond the mid thigh and mid calf.

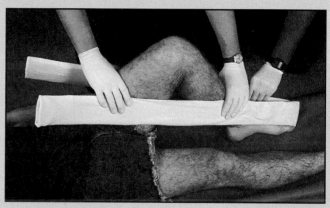

3. Place padded side of splints next to extremity.

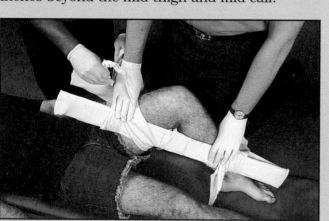

4. Place a cravat through the knee void and tie the boards together.

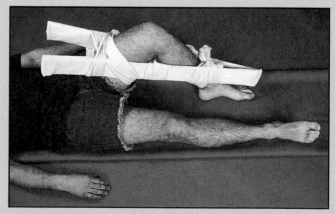

5. Using a figure eight, secure one cravat to the ankle and the boards; secure the second cravat to the thigh and the boards.

Note: *Assess distal motor ability, sensory response, and circulation (pulse) both before and after immobilizing or splinting an extremity.*

Knee Injuries—Knee Straight or Returned to Anatomical Position—Two-Splint Method

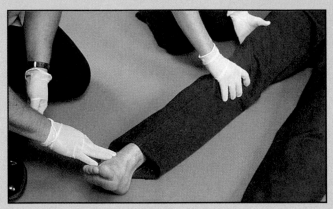

1. Assess distal motor and sensory function and circulation (pulse).

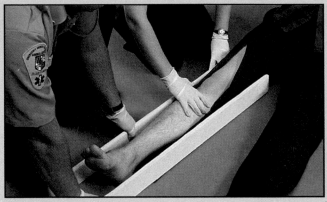

2. Padded board splints, medial from groin, lateral from iliac crest, both to 4 inches beyond foot.

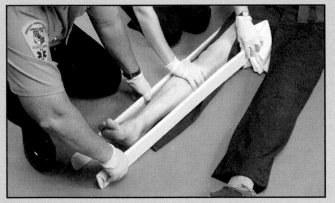

3. Stabilize the limb and pad groin.

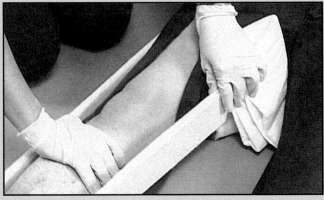

4. Position splints.

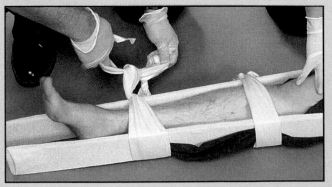

5. Secure splints at thigh, above and below knee, and at mid calf. Pad voids.

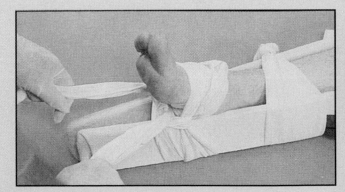

6. Cross and tie two cravats at the ankle or hitch the ankle.

Reassess distal function, care for shock, and provide high-concentration oxygen.

Note: *Assess distal motor ability, sensory response, and circulation (pulse) both before and after immobilizing or splinting an extremity.*

Leg Injuries—Two-Splint Method

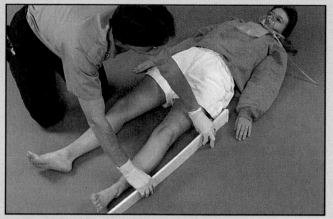

1. Measure splint. It should extend above the knee and below the ankle.

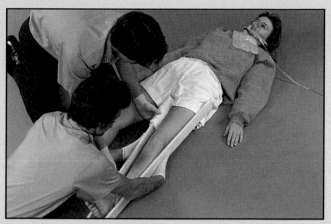

2. Apply manual traction (tension) and place one splint medially and one laterally. Padding is toward the leg.

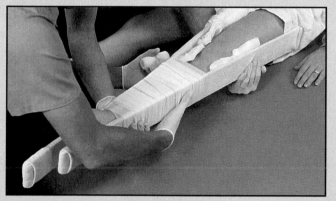

3. Secure splints, padding voids.

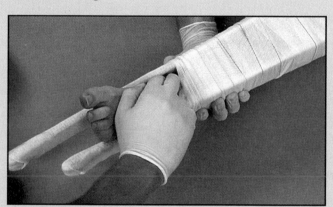

4. Reassess distal motor and sensory function and circulation (pulse).

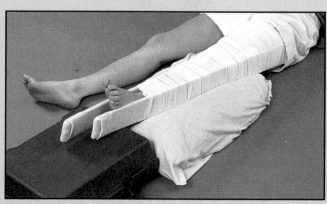

5. Elevate, once immobilized.

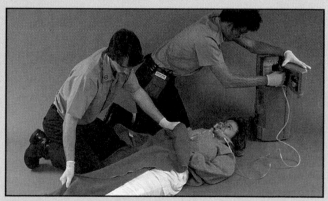

6. Treat for shock and administer high-concentration oxygen. Transport on a long spine board.

Note: Assess distal motor ability, sensory response, and circulation (pulse) both before and after immobilizing or splinting an extremity.

Air-Inflated Splints

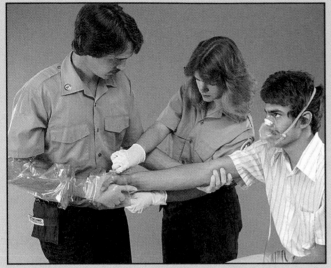

1. Slide the inflated splint up your forearm, well above the wrist. Use the same hand to grasp the hand of the patient's injured limb as though you were going to shake hands and apply steady tension.

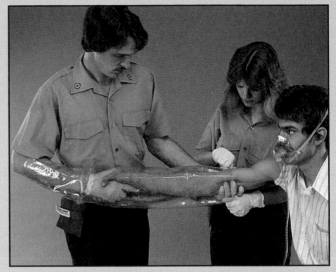

2. While you support patient's arm, your partner gently slides the splint over your hand and onto the patient's injured limb. The lower edge of the splint should be just above his knuckles. Make sure the splint is free of wrinkles.

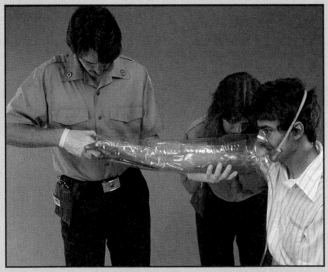

3. Continue to support the arm while your partner inflates the splint by mouth to a point where you can make a slight dent in the plastic when you press it with your thumb.

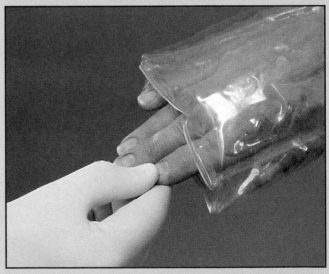

4. Continue to assess distal motor and sensory function and circulation.

Warning: Air-inflated splints may leak. When applied in cold weather, an inflatable splint will expand when the patient is moved to a warmer place. Variations in pressure also occur if the patient is moved to a different altitude. Frequently monitor the pressure in the splint with your fingertip. Air-inflated splints may stick to the patient's skin in hot weather.

> **Note:** Assess distal motor ability, sensory response, and circulation (pulse) both before and after immobilizing or splinting an extremity.

■ HEAD AND SPINAL INJURIES

In order to understand injuries to the head and the spine, knowledge of the anatomy and physiology of the nervous system and skeleton is necessary.

The Nervous System

Anatomically and physiologically, the nervous system (Figure 13–9) is divided into three sub-systems: 1) the central nervous system (CNS), 2) the peripheral nervous system, and 3) the auto-nomic nervous system. The **central nervous system** consists of the brain and the spinal cord. The **peripheral nervous system** includes the pairs of nerves that enter and exit the spinal cord between each vertebrae, all the branches of these nerves that are responsible for sensation and motion throughout the body, and the twelve pairs of cranial nerves that travel between the brain and structures of the head and neck without passing through the spinal cord.

The **autonomic nervous system** connects the brain and spinal cord to many organs including the heart, lungs, glands, muscles in the walls of hollow organs, and blood vessels in the skin. The autonomic system controls involuntary functions, or those we cannot consciously control, such as increasing or decreasing the rate and strength of heart contractions, constricting or dilating blood vessels in skeletal muscles, skin, and abdominal organs, changing bronchial diameter, contracting and relaxing the urinary bladder, and increasing or decreasing the secretion of saliva and digestive juices. The autonomic nervous system is also referred to as the "fight or flight" system, which, when the body is stressed, will allow you to run away or stay and fight something or someone who threatens you!

Messages of sensation—such as those of light, sound, touch, heat, and cold—are carried from the sense organs to the brain over a network of **sensory nerves**. The brain then interprets the messages and sends back orders for action to the muscles over another network of nerves called **motor nerves**. Motor nerves control voluntary movements such as walking or grasping.

As the motor nerves exit the brain and extend into the spinal cord, they cross over to the oppo-site side of the body. This is why an injury to the right side of the brain is exhibited by weakness or lack of sensation on the left side of the body. Since the cranial nerves exit the brain above this

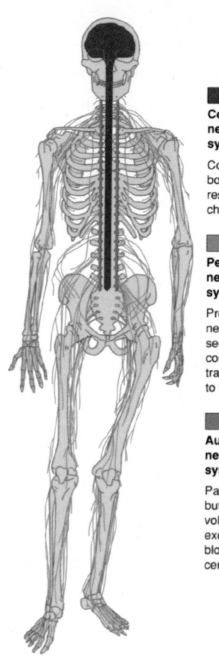

Central nervous system

Controls all basic bodily functions, and responds to external changes

Peripheral nervous system

Provides a complete network of motor and sensory nerve fibers connecting the cen-tral nervous system to the rest of the body

Autonomic nervous system

Parallels spinal cord but is separately in-volved in control of exocrine glands, blood vessels, vis-cera and genitalia

FIGURE 13–9 Anatomy of the nervous system.

crossover, they control the same side of the body on which they are located.

The Brain

The brain is the master organ of the body, the center of consciousness, self-awareness, and thought. It controls basic functions, including breathing and, to some degree, heart activity. Messages from all over the body are received by the brain, which decides how to respond to chang-ing conditions both inside and outside the body.

The brain sends messages to the muscles so that we can move or to a particular organ so that it will carry out a desired function.

The brain is divided into three major sections: the cerebrum, the cerebellum, and the brain stem. The **cerebrum** is the largest part of the brain and contains the centers for hearing, seeing, touching, tasting, and smelling, which receive messages from the body's main sense organs and sends messages to the muscles so that we can move. The **cerebellum** coordinates the body's muscle movements, and if it is injured, control over the muscles is greatly disturbed. The **brain stem** connects the cerebrum with the spinal cord. Nerves on their way to and from the higher centers of the brain pass through the brain stem. The lowest part of the brain stem, the **medulla oblongata**, helps regulate vegetative functions such as breathing, digestion, and circulation.

The soft, spongy mass of tissue that makes up the brain is covered by three **meninges**, or membranes, which also cover the spinal cord. The outermost membrane is called the **dura matter**, the middle layer, the **arachnoid**, and the inner layer, the **pia**. Collections of blood (hematomas) around or within the brain are named in relationship to these membranes. You will read more about hematomas under brain injuries later in this section.

The brain and spinal cord are bathed in cerebrospinal fluid (CSF). When the continuity of the skull is broken due to a basilar (base of the skull) fracture, CSF may exit through the nose, ears, or throat. When a patient in an automobile collision tells you that he has hit his head on the dash and has a salty taste in his mouth, this is most likely due to CSF, which is high in salt content. In order for the fluid to exit the ears, it must exit the brain through a tear in the meninges, travel through the eustachian tube (the tube which equalizes pressure in your head when you are in an airplane), rupture the eardrum, and then flow from the external ear. This clear fluid mixes with blood. Therefore you will be unable to distinguish if the mixture contains cerebrospinal fluid unless you gently absorb some of the mixture onto a gauze dressing and watch as the clear fluid separates from the blood. This is called the halo test, although it is not always reliable nor practical to conduct in the field.

The Spinal Cord

The spinal cord is a relay between most of the body and the brain. A large number of the mes-

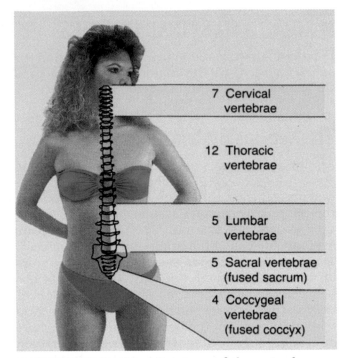

FIGURE 13–10 The divisions of the spinal column.

sages to and from the brain are sent through the spinal cord. Damage to the cord can isolate a part of the body from the brain, and function of this part can be lost, possibly forever.

The spinal cord is also the center of reflex activity. Reflexes allow us to react quickly to such things as pain and excessive heat without orders sent by the brain. In a reflex action, sensory nerves flash a message to the spinal cord. In turn the spinal cord, acting as a relay center, flashes back a message to motor nerves in the muscle telling it to move at once—and it also sends another message to the brain about the original message.

The spinal cord is protected by the spine, 33 separate irregular-shaped bones called vertebrae which sit on top of one another (Figure 13–10). Each vertebra has a spinous process which is one of the lumps you can palpate on a patient's back. Two transverse processes are located on the sides of each vertebra. The body of the vertebra forms a channel approximately 15 mm in diameter. The spinal cord is about 10 mm in diameter. Between each vertebrae is a fluid-filled cartilage disk which provides some cushioning of the bones and allows for flexibility of the spine.

The areas of the spine that are most often injured are those areas where the natural curvature of the spine changes its direction as well as those areas that are not supported by a bone structure such as the ribs and pelvis. This is why cervical and lumbar injuries are very common.

The healing power of the brain and nerve tissue is limited. Once this tissue is damaged, to a certain extent, function is lost and cannot be restored. As an EMT-B your initial care can often prevent additional damage to the brain, spinal cord, and major nerves of the body.

Injuries to the Head

Skull Injuries

Skull injuries include fractures to the cranium and facial bones. Severe injuries to the skull can also injure the brain. Cuts to the scalp and other soft-tissue injuries to the skull are covered in Chapter 12.

Skull injuries can be either open or closed. The words *open* and *closed* refer to the skull bones. When the bones of the cranium are fractured, and the scalp overlying the fracture is lacerated, the patient has an *open head injury.* In other cases, there may be a laceration of the scalp; however, if the cranium is intact, or free of fractures, the term *closed head injury* is used. In practice, it may not be possible for the EMT-B to determine if a head injury is open or closed. It is safest for you to assume that there may be an open head injury beneath any laceration of the scalp.

Brain Injuries

Brain injuries are classified as direct or indirect. *Direct injuries* occur when the brain is lacerated, punctured, or bruised by the broken bones of the skull, by bone fragments, or by foreign objects.

An *indirect injury* to the brain can be the result of closed injuries to the skull and certain types of open skull injuries. In other words, the impact of the injury to the skull is transferred to the brain.

Like any other mass of tissue, the brain swells when it is injured. This swelling is serious since there is little room for the brain to expand within the rigid skull. Swelling makes it more difficult for blood to get to the brain. This leads to lowered oxygen levels and increased carbon dioxide levels in the brain tissue. The presence of high carbon dioxide levels further increases the swelling.

Indirect injuries to the brain include concussions and/or contusions. When a person strikes his head in a fall, or is struck by a blunt object, a certain amount of the force is transferred through the skull to the brain, which causes a **concussion**. A concussion may be so mild that the patient is unaware of the injury. Usually there is no detectable damage to the brain and the patient may or may not lose consciousness. Most patients who sustain a concussion will feel a little "groggy" after receiving a blow to the head and usually suffer from headaches. The patient with a concussion may experience a period of altered level of consciousness, but if there is a loss of consciousness, it usually lasts only a brief period and it does not tend to reoccur. Witnesses of auto collisions often describe the victim who sustains a concussion as a person who "just sat there staring off into space for a few minutes." Some short-term memory loss concerning the events that surrounded the accident is fairly common. Long-term memory loss associated with concussion is rare. Memory loss, whether short- or long-term, is called amnesia.

A **contusion**, or a bruise of the brain, can occur when the force of a blow to the head is great enough to rupture small blood vessels found on the surface of, or deep within, the brain. Since there is little space in which the brain can move before it strikes the walls of the cranial cavity, a contusion often appears on the side of the brain opposite the point of impact to the skull. A contusion is usually caused by an acceleration/deceleration injury in which the brain hits the one side of the cranial cavity on acceleration, bounces off the opposite side on deceleration, and then rebounds to strike the first side of the cranial cavity again. Bruising of the brain on the same side of the skull injury, is called a *coup;* bruising that occurs on the side opposite the injury is called a *contrecoup.*

The inside of the skull has many sharp, bony ridges that can lacerate a moving brain. The brain can also be lacerated by a penetrating or perforating wound to the cranium. Not only is there the problem of direct injury, but there may also be severe indirect injury due to hematoma formation. For example, a subdural hematoma would be a collection of blood below the dura, yet outside the brain tissue itself.

The brain is supplied with a rich supply of blood through four major arteries, two vertebral arteries, which travel through the spine, and two carotid arteries. An acute blockage to any one of these four arteries can have a catastrophic effect on the brain. One very important artery is the middle meningeal artery. Since this artery is located in a very thin area of the skull above the ear, it is easily damaged. When severed, it causes a hematoma in the epidural space (outside the dura and inside the skull). A patient with an epidural hematoma is usually knocked unconscious, then proceeds to regain consciousness (this period is referred to as a lucid interval); and then consciousness begins to decrease in the next few minutes to hour.

Preceptor Pearl

An epidural hematoma is often associated with severe blows to the head. If you recognize an epidural hematoma in its early stages and promptly transport the patient to a trauma center, it can make the difference between life and death. Be aggressive if you suspect an epidural hematoma. ❖

The brain's venous flow is very close to the brain's surface. When the brain is bruised, lacerated, or punctured, blood from ruptured vessels can flow between the brain and its meninges. When a hematoma develops in the subdural space, this is often due to venous bleeding and it has very serious ramifications. Often, this bleeding is a slow venous flow. Even when the bleeding stops, the hematoma will continue to grow in size as it absorbs tissue fluids. Since there is no room for expansion in the skull, severe pressure can be placed on the brain. Death can occur if vital brain centers are damaged. This type of hematoma may occur rapidly or over a prolonged period of time.

An intracerebral hematoma occurs when blood pools within the brain itself, pushing tissues against the bones of the cranium. This can develop into a fatal injury in minutes to hours depending on the area of the brain that is damaged and the extent of bleeding. When the brain is injured and begins to bleed or swell, intracerebral pressure (ICP) rises.

When assessing for signs and symptoms of injury to the skull or brain, also be alert for the strong possibility of cervical spine injury as well.

Patient Assessment Head Injury

Signs and Symptoms

Unless accompanied by an open head injury, a penetrating injury, a CSF leak, or a hematoma, a skull fracture is generally not considered critical. Brain injuries that result in increased ICP and a hematoma are very serious.

Consider the possibility of a brain injury or a skull fracture whenever you note any of these signs or symptoms:

- *Visible bone fragments* and perhaps bits of brain tissue. These are the most obvious signs of skull fracture, but the majority of skull fractures do not produce these signs.
- *Decreased level of consciousness*, confusion, or unconsciousness.
- *Short term memory loss*, in which the patient keeps asking the same questions over and over again.
- *Deep laceration or severe bruise* to the scalp or forehead. Do not probe into the wound or separate the wound opening to determine wound depth.
- *Severe pain or swelling* at the site of a head injury. Pain may range from a headache to severe discomfort. Do not palpate the injury site since this could push bone fragments into the brain.
- *Depressions* or *deformity of the skull*, large swellings ("goose eggs"), or anything that looks unusual about the shape of the cranium.
- *"Battle's Sign,"* a bruise or swelling behind the ear. This is a late sign of a basilar (base of skull) fracture.
- *Unequal pupils* that may not react to light. This is a late sign caused by compression of the cranial nerve that controls pupil constriction.
- *"Raccoon's Eyes,"* black eyes, or discoloration of the soft tissues under both eyes. This is usually a delayed finding indicating a basilar skull fracture.
- *One eye that appears to be sunken.*
- *Bleeding from the ears and/or the nose.*
- *CSF flowing* from the ears and/or the nose.
- *Personality changes* ranging from irritable to irrational behavior.
- *Cushing's syndrome*, the combination of an increased blood pressure and a decreased pulse rate.
- *Irregular breathing patterns* such as Cheyenne Stokes (increasing rate of respirations followed by periods of apnea).
- *Increased or decreased temperature*, a late sign that indicates damage to temperature-regulating centers in the brain.
- *Blurred or multiple-image vision* in one or both eyes.
- *Impaired hearing*, ringing in the ears.
- *Equilibrium problems* in which the patient is unable to stand still with the eyes closed or stumbles when attempting to walk. (Do not test for this.)
- Forceful or projectile *vomiting*.

FIGURE 13–11
The Glasgow Coma Scale.

The Glasgow Coma Scale			
Eye Opening Response	Spontaneous	4	
	To voice	3	
	To pain	2	
	None	1	
Best Verbal Response	Oriented	5	(Knows name, date, place)
	Confused	4	
	Inappropriate words	3	(Often patient curses)
	Incomprehensible sounds	2	(Mumbling, moans, groans)
	None	1	
Best Motor Response	Obeys command	6	
	Localizes pain	5	
	Withdraws (pain)	4	
	Flexion (pain)	3	
	Extension (pain)	2	
	None	1	
	Total	3 – 15	

- *Neurological posturing* when painful stimulus is applied, such as flexing the arms and wrists and extending the legs and feet (called decorticate posture), or extending the arms with the shoulders rotated inward and the wrists flexed, legs extended (called decerebrate posture). These postures may also be assumed spontaneously, without painful stimulus.
- *Paralysis on one side of the body* (hemiplegia).
- *Deteriorating vital signs.* ▨

PEDIATRIC HIGHLIGHT

Shock is rarely a sign of head injury, except in infants. This is due to their proportionately larger heads and the still unfused soft spots. There simply is not enough room in the adult skull to permit enough bleeding (over 25% to 30% of the blood volume) into the head to cause shock. In an adult, if a head injury is accompanied by shock, look for indications of blood loss at some other place on the body. ■

Neurological Assessment/The Glasgow Coma Scale

All patients who sustain head injury or suspected brain damage must be continually and carefully monitored and reassessed during transport. Always be prepared for the patient to vomit or have a seizure. The early signs of deterioration are subtle changes in mental status that can be easily overlooked if you fail to look for them. What you observe and report to the ED staff can have a great bearing on the initial actions they take.

Many EMT-Bs use the Glasgow Coma Scale (GCS) in addition to AVPU for ongoing neurological assessment as well as triage (Figure 13–11). For a patient with a GCS of 8 or less, some systems would immediately triage directly to the trauma center if they are within 30 minutes' transport time. You should become familiar with the GCS if it is used in your EMS system. When using this score, remember to consider the following:

- Note if there are eye injuries or injuries to the face that prevent the patient from opening the eyes. If the injuries are more than minor ones, do not ask the patient to open his eyes.
- Spontaneous eye opening means that the patient has the eyes open without your having to do anything. If his eyes are closed, then you should say, "Open your eyes" to see if the patient will obey this command. Try a normal level of voice. If this fails, shout the command. Should the patient's eyes remain closed, apply an accepted painful stimulus (e.g., pinch a toe, scratch the palm or sole, rub the sternum).
- When evaluating the patient's verbal responses, use the following criteria.
  1. Oriented—The patient, once aroused, can tell you who he is, where he is, and the day of the week. A person who can answer all three of these questions appropriately is said to be alert on the AVPU scale.
  2. Confused—The patient cannot answer the above questions, but he can speak in phrases and sentences.
  3. Inappropriate words—The patient says or shouts a word or several words at a time. Usually this requires physical stimulation.

The words do not fit the situation or a particular question. Often, the patient curses.

4. Incomprehensible sounds—The patient responds with mumbling, moans, or groans.

5. No verbal response—Repeated stimulation, verbal and physical, does not cause the patient to speak or make any sounds.

- The following are the criteria used to evaluate motor response.

1. Obeys command—The patient must be able to understand your instruction and carry out the request. For example, you can ask (when appropriate) for the patient to hold up two fingers.

2. Localizes pain—Should the patient fail to respond to your commands, apply pressure to one of the nail beds for 5 seconds or firm pressure to the sternum. Note if the patient attempts to remove your hand. Do not apply pressure over an injury site. Do not apply pressure to the sternum if the patient is experiencing difficulty breathing.

3. Withdraws—after painful stimulation. Note if the elbow flexes, he moves slowly, there is the appearance of stiffness, he holds his forearm and hand against the body, or the limbs on one side of the body appear to be paralyzed (hemiplegic position).

4. Posturing—after painful stimulation. Note if the legs and arms extend, there is apparent stiffness with these moves, and if there is an internal rotation of the shoulder and forearm.

▌Patient Care Head Injuries

Emergency Care Steps

1. Take body substance isolation precautions.

2. Assume a cervical spine injury and use the jaw-thrust maneuver to open the airway.

3. Maintain an open airway. Monitor the conscious patient for changes in breathing. For the unconscious patient, insert an oropharyngeal airway without hyperextending the neck.

4. Provide resuscitative measures if needed.

5. Apply a rigid collar and immobilize the neck and spine and evaluate the method of extrication, either normal or rapid (see algorithm in Figure 13–12).

6. Be prepared for vomiting. Have your suction unit ready. It may be necessary to flip the long backboard on its side, which allows the patient's airway to drain if vomiting occurs.

Make sure the patient is securely immobilized and a suction unit is available.

7. Administer oxygen via nonrebreather mask and evaluate the need for positive pressure ventilations. This is critical should there be any brain damage. If the patient shows signs of a brain injury (i.e., increased blood pressure and decreased pulse, altered level of consciousness), hyperventilate with oxygen-assisted ventilations (bag-valve mask or positive pressure) at the rate of 25+ per minute rather than the usual 12 ventilations per minute. This will help reduce brain-tissue swelling by lowering carbon dioxide levels and raising oxygen levels. It should be noted that in some EMS systems, the use of hyperventilation is no longer recommended for head injuries.

8. Control bleeding. Do not apply pressure if the injury site shows bone fragments, depression of the bone, or if the brain is exposed. Do not attempt to stop the flow of blood or cerebrospinal fluid from the ears or the nose. If the skull is fractured, you may increase intracranial pressure and may also increase the risk of infection. Use a loose gauze dressing.

9. Keep the patient at rest. (This can be a critical factor.)

10. Monitor vital signs every five minutes en route to the hospital.

11. Talk to the conscious patient, providing emotional support. Ask questions so that the patient will have to concentrate. This will also help you detect changes in the patient's level of consciousness.

12. Dress and bandage open wounds. Stabilize any penetrating objects. (Do not remove any objects or bone fragments.)

13. Elevate the head of the spine board slightly if there is no evidence of shock. ▪

If you are unsure of the severity of the patient's injuries and there is evidence of cervical spine injury, or the head-injured patient is unconscious, apply a rigid cervical or extrication collar and position the patient on a long spine board. This full-body immobilization will allow you to rotate the patient on the board into a lateral position so that blood and mucus can drain freely; it also prevents vomitus from causing an airway obstruction. Some patients will vomit without warning. Many vomit without first experiencing nausea. If other injuries prevent such positioning, constant monitoring and frequent suctioning are necessary.

FIGURE 13–12
Choose appropriate
extrication and immobi-
lization procedures.

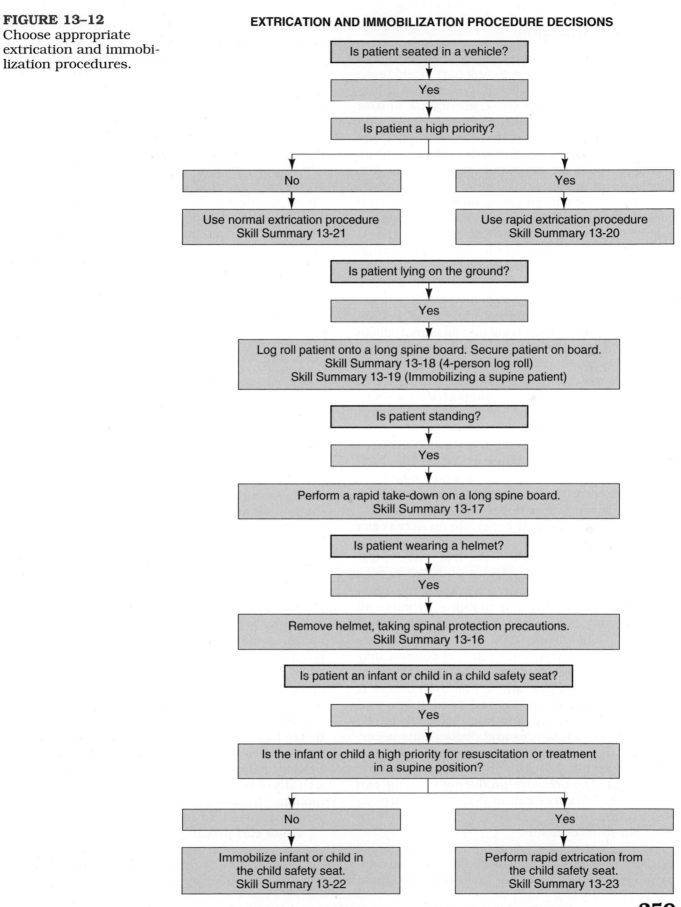

EXTRICATION AND IMMOBILIZATION PROCEDURE DECISIONS

Is patient seated in a vehicle?

Yes

Is patient a high priority?

No

Use normal extrication procedure
Skill Summary 13-21

Yes

Use rapid extrication procedure
Skill Summary 13-20

Is patient lying on the ground?

Yes

Log roll patient onto a long spine board. Secure patient on board.
Skill Summary 13-18 (4-person log roll)
Skill Summary 13-19 (Immobilizing a supine patient)

Is patient standing?

Yes

Perform a rapid take-down on a long spine board.
Skill Summary 13-17

Is patient wearing a helmet?

Yes

Remove helmet, taking spinal protection precautions.
Skill Summary 13-16

Is patient an infant or child in a child safety seat?

Yes

Is the infant or child a high priority for resuscitation or treatment
in a supine position?

No

Immobilize infant or child in
the child safety seat.
Skill Summary 13-22

Yes

Perform rapid extrication from
the child safety seat.
Skill Summary 13-23

CHAPTER 13 Trauma—Musculoskeletal, Head and Spine

Injuries to the Spine

Injuries to the spine must always be considered whenever there is trauma to any part of the body. Do not overlook the possibility of spinal injury when dealing with head, chest, abdominal, and/or pelvic injuries. Even injuries to the upper and lower extremities caused by intense impact can produce spinal injury. You must *always* do an initial assessment and rapid trauma exam and then determine the priority of the patient. Failure to complete the patient assessment and to determine the most appropriate immobilization method could lead to further injuries. In the field, always "uptriage" or overtreat patients with potential spinal injuries because the costs in terms of pain, suffering, disability, and dollars soar when a spine-injured patient is not immobilized.

Injuries to the spinal column include: fractures, with and without bone displacement; dislocations; ligament sprains; and disk injury, including compression. When the disk fluid leaks out, this is referred to as a herniated, or ruptured, disk. Since the vertebrae are supported by a series of muscles and ligaments, if the spine is hyperflexed or hyperextended, it is possible to injure a muscle or ligament allowing the vertebrae to dislocate or move out of alignment. When this happens, it is possible to stretch, tear, or compress the spinal cord. Most voluntary motor messages from the brain travel down the spinal cord to peripheral nerves. A pair of peripheral nerves exit between each vertebrae. These control sensory and motor functions of the body. When the cord is damaged, it can render the peripheral nerves below the injury inoperable. A cervical spine injury can cause quadriplegia or inability to move all four extremities whereas a lumbar or thoracic injury can cause paraplegia or inability to move the lower extremities. The vertebral column may be injured without damage to the spinal cord or spinal nerves. For example, a fractured coccyx is below the level of the spinal cord. Ligament sprains are relatively simple injuries. However, when displaced fractures and dislocations occur, the cord, disk, and spinal nerves may be severely injured. Serious contusions and lacerations, accompanied by pressure-producing swelling, can take place. The entire column can become unstable, leading to cord compression that may produce paralysis or death.

Some parts of the spine are more susceptible to injury than others. Because it is somewhat supported by the attached ribs, the thoracic segment of the spine is not usually damaged except by the most violent accidents or by gunshot wounds. The pelvic-sacral spine attachment helps to protect the sacrum in the same way. On the other hand, the cervical and lumbar vertebrae are susceptible to injury because they are not supported by other bony structures.

The experienced EMT-B knows to maintain a high degree of suspicion for spinal injury when finding any of the following: 1) an MVA, 2) a struck pedestrian, 3) a fall, 4) a blunt injury to the spine or above the clavicles, 5) penetrating trauma to the head, neck, or torso, 6) a diving accident, 7) a hanging, 8) loss of consciousness due to trauma.

Preceptor Pearl

There is a simple rule you can follow. If the mechanism of injury exerts great force on the upper body or if there is any soft-tissue damage to the head, face, or neck due to trauma (e.g., from being thrown against a dashboard), then assume that there is a possible cervical spine injury. Any blunt trauma above the clavicles may damage the cervical spine. ❖

The spine is most often injured by compression or excessive flexion, extension, or rotation. EMS workers often injure the spine by using incorrect lifting techniques. An excessive pull on the spine, such as occurs in a hanging, is called a **distraction** injury. Years ago rescuers were taught to pull traction on the neck of an injured patient sitting in an automobile, which actually had the potential to cause further injury. Now, EMT-Bs are taught to manually stabilize the head and neck or, basically, to hold them still.

The adult skull weighs more than 17 pounds, and it rests on a very small area of the cervical spine, somewhat like a pumpkin on a broom handle. Because of this weight and positioning, when a vehicle strikes another vehicle or a fixed object head on, the occupant's head can whip quickly back and forth. Although the vehicle decelerates abruptly, the occupant's head continues to travel forward at the same rate of speed at which the vehicle was traveling, even if the body is held by safety restraints. This head movement usually exceeds the neck's normal range of motion. Virtually the same thing occurs when the vehicle is struck from behind.

A fall can produce spinal injury if the victim strikes an object, the ground, or the floor. The force generated during a fall may be enough to fracture, crush, or dislocate vertebrae.

Preceptor Pearl

| As a rule of thumb, assume any fall three times the patient's height or with enough force to cause open PSDEs to the ankles will also be accompanied by a spinal injury. ✤

Today more and more people are participating in sports of all kinds: in-line skating, bicycling, surfing, rock climbing, and others too numerous to mention. Many sports accidents can cause spinal injury. A sledding or skiing accident may hurl a person into a tree or other fixed object, twisting or compressing the spinal column. There may be no PSDE, or signs of injury may be hidden by bulky clothing. As a result, improper care may be rendered as the victim with a possible spinal injury is placed on a stretcher without adequate examination and immobilization.

Diving accidents often produce injury to the cervical spine. When the diver strikes the diving board, the side or bottom of the pool, or an underwater object, the head can be severely forced beyond its normal limits of motion. Cervical vertebrae may be fractured or dislocated, ligaments may be severely sprained, and the spinal cord may be compressed or otherwise traumatized in the cervical region and at other spots along its length.

Football and other contact sports can cause accidents severe enough to produce spinal injury. Spear tackling, using the head, has been outlawed in grade schools and high schools for a number of years due to the incidence of cervical compression fractures. Whenever the injury involves player contact or falling to the ground, be on the alert for spinal injury.

Patient Assessment Spinal Injury

You must do a complete initial assessment and physical exam of the patient. You should assume that all unconscious trauma patients have spinal injury. Whenever you are in doubt, assume that there are spinal injuries and immobilize the torso and the head and neck.

Signs and Symptoms
- *Paralysis, pain without movement, pain with movement, and tenderness anywhere along the spine* These are reliable indicators of possible spinal injury in the conscious patient. If these are present, you have sufficient reason to immobilize the patient before proceeding with the assessment. If immediate immobilization is

not possible, use extreme care in handling the patient. In the field, it is not possible to rule out spinal injury, even in cases in which the patient has no pain and is able to move his limbs. The mechanism of injury alone may be the deciding factor to immobilize.
- *Pain without Movement* The pain is not always constant and may occur anywhere from the top of the head to the buttocks. Pain in the leg is common for certain types of injury to the lower spinal cord and vertebral column. Other painful injuries can mask this symptom of spinal injury.
- *Pain with Movement* The patient normally tries to lie perfectly still to prevent pain on movement. You should not request the patient to move just to determine if pain is present. However, if the patient complains of pain in the neck or back experienced with voluntary movements, you must consider this to be a symptom of possible spinal injury. Pain with movement in apparently uninjured shoulders and legs is another good indicator of possible spinal injury.
- *Tenderness* Gentle palpation of the injury site, when accessible, may reveal point tenderness.
- *Impaired Breathing* Neck injury can impair nerve function to the chest muscles. Watch the patient breathe. If there is only a slight movement of the abdomen, with little or no movement of the chest, it is safe to assume that the patient is breathing with the diaphragm alone (diaphragmatic breathing). The nerve that controls the diaphragm is located high in the cervical area and is often unharmed, but the intercostal nerves that control the chest muscles are often damaged in cervical and thoracic injuries.
- *Deformity* The removal of clothing to check the back for deformity of the spine is not recommended. Obvious spinal deformities are rare. However, if you note a gap between the spinous processes (bony extensions) of the vertebrae or if you can feel a broken spinous process, you must consider the patient to have serious spinal injuries. It is also possible to feel tight muscles in spasm.
- *Priapism* A nonemotionally justified, persistent erection of the penis is a reliable sign of spinal cord injury affecting nerves to the external genitalia.
- *Posturing* In some cases of spinal injury, motor nerve pathways to the muscles that extend the arm can be interrupted, but those that lead to the muscles that bend the elbow and lift the arm remain functional. The patient may be found on his back, with the arms extended above the head, which may indicate a cervical

spine injury. Arms flexed across the chest or extended along the sides with wrists flexed also signal spinal injury.

- *Loss of Bowel or Bladder Control*
- *Nerve Impairment to the Extremities* The patient may have loss of use, weakness, numbness, or tingling in the upper and/or lower extremities.
- *Paralysis of the Extremities* This is probably the most reliable sign of a spinal injury in a conscious patient.
- *Severe Spinal Shock* This may occur even when there are no indications of external or internal bleeding. It can be caused by the failure of the nervous system to control the diameter of blood vessels (neurogenic shock). Remember that the pulse rate may be normal because the message to "speed up" the heart may never have reached the heart due to the spinal injury. ■

When assessing the responsive spine-injured patient, be sure to ask questions about the mechanism of injury. Question the patient to determine if there is any pain in the back or neck and determine if he is able to move and feel a light touch on all four extremities. If the patient describes a feeling of "pins and needles" in the legs, this is a positive sign of a potential spinal injury. Observe for contusions, lacerations, and deformities to the neck and back. Check by palpating for tenderness or muscle spasm in the neck and back. Also compare the strength of the arms by a simple hand grip and the legs by asking the patient to push against your hands. If the patient is unresponsive, do not spend time attempting to exclude a spinal injury—immobilize the patient if a mechanism for spinal injury exists.

Preceptor Pearl

If there is a potential mechanism for a spinal injury, treat for one by immobilizing the patient. Also, always assess and document the neurological function in all four extremities before and after immobilizing the spine. ✤

■ Patient Care **Spinal Injury**

Regardless of where in the neck or back the apparent spinal injury is located, care is the same. First take body substance isolation and do the initial assessment and rapid trauma exam. Determine the patient's priority since this affects how he will be immobilized.

Emergency Care Steps

For all patients with possible spinal injury and for all accident victims when there is doubt as to the extent of injury, you should:

1. Provide manual stabilization for the head and neck. Apply an extrication or rigid collar and continue to maintain manual stabilization.

2. Quickly assess the MSCs in all four extremities if the patient is responsive.

3. Based on the patient's priority, apply the appropriate spinal immobilization device at the appropriate speed (Figure 13–12).

4. Administer oxygen via nonrebreather mask and evaluate the need for positive pressure ventilations. This is critical should there be any cord damage. If the patient shows signs of spinal shock, edema to the cord may impair oxygen delivery to the cord. When this occurs, cellular death can take place.

5. Reassess MSCs in four extremities if the patient is responsive. ■

Immobilization Issues

Patients Found with a Helmet On

Helmets are worn in many sporting events and by many motorcycle riders. A sporting helmet is typically open on the front and provides easier access to the patient's airway than does a motorcycle helmet, which has a shield and often a full-face section that is not removable. Facial, neck, and spinal injury care and airway management may call for the removal of the helmet. The helmet should not prevent you from reaching the patient's mouth or nose if resuscitation efforts are needed. Protection shields can be lifted and face guards can be cut away. If the face guard is to be cut, one EMT must steady the patient's head and neck with manual stabilization. The other EMT should snap off the guard or unscrew it.

Do not attempt to remove a helmet if doing so causes increased pain or if the helmet proves difficult to remove, unless there is a possible airway obstruction or ventilatory assistance must be provided (i.e., hyperventilation of the head-injured patient). The indications for leaving the helmet in place include the following:

1. The helmet has a snug fit that provides little or no movement of the patient's head within the helmet.

2. There are absolutely no impending airway or breathing problems nor any reason to hyperventilate the patient.

3. Removal would cause further injury to the patient.

4. Proper spinal immobilization can be done with the helmet in place.

5. There is no interference with the EMT-B's ability to assess and reassess airway or breathing.

It is important to note that if an injured football player is wearing shoulder pads, you should either remove the pads or pad behind the head to make up for the fact that his shoulders are off the ground. This will prevent the head from falling into a hyperextended position when the helmet is removed and the head is slowly lowered to the ground. When a helmet must be removed, it is a two-rescuer procedure (Skill Summary 13–16).

Preceptor Pearl

Many EMS providers put the controversy of helmet removal vs. nonremoval into the following perspective. If your child's neck was injured in a football accident, would you want the trainer and the EMT-B to work together to remove the helmet at the scene or would you prefer that this be left to the emergency department staff, who probably will not have assistance of the trainer or the benefit of frequent practice in the helmet-removal technique? ✣

Tips for Applying a Cervical Collar

Cervical spine immobilization devices, or extrication collars, have come a long way since the early days of EMS. Originally, ambulance personnel would borrow soft collars from the hospital's emergency department. Unfortunately most early ambulance personnel did not realize that soft collars were put on patients who had been X rayed in the emergency department and whose X-ray films determined that they had no fracture or dislocation. These soft collars were applied merely to remind patients not to move their necks so muscle strain could heal. The patients who had fractures were admitted and placed in traction.

Preceptor Pearl

Soft collars, or "neck warmers," have no place in the field! ✣

The collars of today are rigid and are designed to limit flexion, extension, and lateral movement when combined with an immobilization device such as a long backboard or a vest-style device. Even though there have been marked improvements in collars, there is still no collar that completely eliminates movement of the spine. For this reason, when applying a collar, always maintain the neck and head in a neutral position in alignment with the rest of the body. (See Chapter 6.)

Do not stop short in immobilizing the patient after applying the collar! Always continue to hold the neck and head until a short or long backboard is applied to the patient.

Since the sizing of a collar depends upon the brand, make sure you are familiar with the collar application procedure for collars used by your service. Make certain that you assess the patient's neck prior to placing the collar. Take special care to look at the neck for tracheal deviation, distended jugular veins, and injuries prior to covering it. Ensure that the collar neck is not so tight that it obstructs the patient's breathing or the opening of the airway.

Make sure the collar is the right size for the patient. A large patient may not require a large collar; whereas, a small patient with a long neck may need the largest collar. The front width of the collar should fit between the point of the chin to the chest at the suprasternal (jugular) notch. Once in place, the collar should rest on the clavicles and support the lower jaw.

When applying a collar be sure to remove the patient's necklaces and large earrings. Also keep the head in the anatomical position when applying manual stabilization and the collar. Be certain to keep the patient's hair out of the way, maintain manual stabilization while the collar is secured, and continue to manually immobilize the head and neck until the patient is secured to a long spine board.

If a collar does not fit, try using a rolled towel and tape to secure the head to the board after the torso is immobilized. An improperly fitting collar can cause more harm than good; have a full set of various sizes.

Preceptor Pearl

Remember, airway maintenance always takes the highest priority. Therefore, if you cannot do a jaw thrust and are unable to adequately ventilate your patient because the collar is obstructing your ability to open the airway, then remove the collar. In this case, you will need to manually stabilize the patient while doing a two-handed jaw thrust to open the airway. A second EMT-B will need to ventilate the patient with a bag-valve mask unless the patient has an endotracheal tube in place. ✣

Helmet Removal from Injured Patient

1

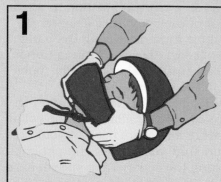

EMT-Basic A is positioned at the top of the patient's head and maintains manual stabilization with two hands holding the helmet stable while the finger tips hold the lower jaw.

2

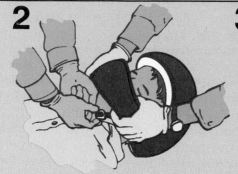

EMT-Basic B opens, cuts, or removes the chin strap.

3

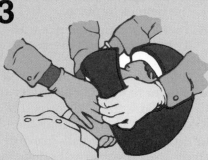

EMT-Basic B then places one hand on the patient's mandible and, using the other hand, reaches in behind the neck and applies stabilization at the occipital region. Using the combination of the hand in front of the chin and the hand behind the neck, this EMT-Basic should be able to hold the head very secure. *If the patient has glasses on, they should be removed now, prior to removal of the helmet.*

4

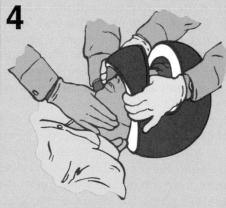

EMT-Basic A can now release manual stabilization and slowly remove the helmet. The lower sides, or ear cups, of the helmet will have to be gently pulled out to clear the ears.

5

The helmet should come off straight without tilting it backwards, which could cause unnecessary flexion of the neck. If it is a full-face helmet, it may be necessary to tilt the helmet backwards just a bit to clear the nose with the chin guard. EMT-Basic B should be prepared to take the full weight of the head without allowing the head to move as the helmet is removed.

6

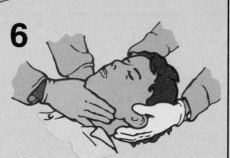

EMT-Basic A, after removing the helmet, re-establishes manual stabilization and maintains an open airway by using the jaw thrust.

7

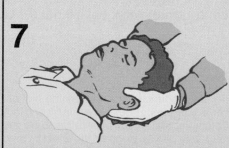

EMT-Basic B can now release manual stabilization and apply an extrication collar. The patient should then be fully assessed, and torso, then head, secured to a long spine board.

Note: If the patient has shoulder pads and you are removing a football helmet, remember to pad behind the head to keep it aligned with the padded shoulders.

From John E. Campbell, M.D., and Alabama Chapter, American College of Emergency Physicians, *BTLS Basic Prehospital Trauma Care,* The Brady Company, 1988.

Tips for Dealing with the Standing Patient

When you approach a vehicle and see the tell-tale sign of a spider-cracked windshield, this is evidence that whoever sat behind that windshield will need full spinal immobilization. Sometimes, such a patient will be up and walking around at the collision scene. It can be very dangerous to have such a patient sit or lie down on the long backboard. Therefore, use a backboard to carefully, but rapidly, take him down to the supine position without compromising his spine. Some EMS providers advocate using the long board application while the patient is standing; however, this procedure is often not practical in the field. It works in the classroom because the simulated patients are not in shock, intoxicated, head injured, combative, or dizzy!

The easiest technique to utilize is the rapid takedown, which like all skills in this text should be demonstrated by a qualified instructor and practiced in the classroom setting prior to use in the field. The procedure takes three EMT-Bs, a set of collars, and a long backboard (Skill Summary 13–17).

Tips for Applying a Long Backboard

The following tips will help you round out your knowledge of the application of the devices used for immobilization of the supine patient:

- Log roll the patient to apply the long backboard (Skill Summaries 13–18 and 13–19). This procedure must be done carefully, keeping the patient's spine aligned. Whenever a move is done involving neck stabilization, the EMT-B holding the neck calls for the move (i.e., we will turn on three...one...two...three).

- When a patient is secured to a long spine board, the order of straps goes from chest to foot. A backboard with Velcro straps or quick-hook clip straps (Figure 13–13) makes the job easier. Secure the head last, using 3-inch hypoallergenic adhesive tape. The tape offers support, especially if the patient and board are to be tilted to allow for drainage. However, blood on the patient's skin and hair may make using tape impractical. You should learn to use cravats or Kling as a backup method. Do not tape or tie the cravats across the patient's eyes.

- When immobilizing a child six years old or younger, it is necessary to provide padding beneath the shoulder blades to compensate for the child's proportionally large head.

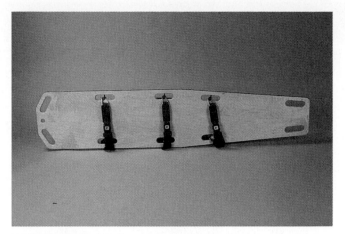

FIGURE 13–13 Long spine board with quick-hook straps.

- Additional immobilization for the head and neck can be provided with light foam-filled sandbags, a commercial head-immobilization device (Ferno Washington head immobilizer, Bashaw CID, or the Laerdal Head Bed), or a blanket roll. If used, apply these after securing the patient's body to the long backboard but before securing the head with tape.

- If you are treating a full-term pregnant patient, after immobilizing her on the back board, prop the board on its side (right side up, left side down) to minimize the uterus compressing the vena cava, which can cause hypotension and dizziness.

- Unless the spine board has specific directions for straps intended to criss-cross the shoulder/chest area, it is best to strap across the upper chest including the arms, the pelvis excluding the hands, and the thighs. If the patient needs to be stood up in order to carry him through a narrow hallway, up a basement stairwell, or into a small elevator, make sure the chest strap is secure under the axilla (arm pits) and tight on the thighs to prevent shifting on the board.

- If your service transports to a helicopter, make sure that your selected backboard will fit inside it. Depending on the helicopter loading configuration, there are some restrictions on the size or taper of the long backboard. Be sure you are aware of this configuration in advance.

- For a water-rescue or diving injury, various specialty back boards, such as the Miller board, are designed to float up beneath the patient and utilize Velcro closures for ease of application.

Rapid Takedown of a Standing Patient

FIRST take body substance isolation precautions.

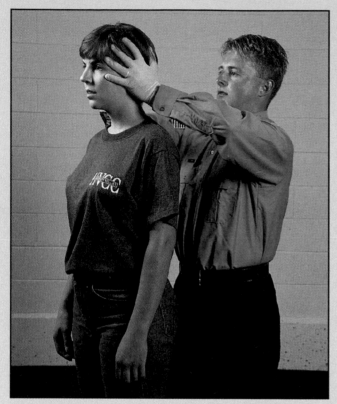

1. Position your tallest crew member (EMT-Basic A) behind patient and hold manual in-line stabilization of the head and neck. This person's hands will not leave the patient's head until entire procedure is complete and head is secured to the long spine board.

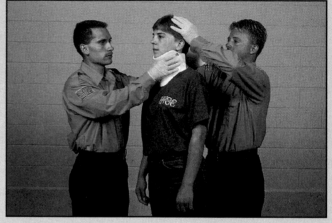

2. EMT-Basic B applies a properly sized cervical collar to patient. EMT-Basic A continues manual stabilization (collar aids, but does not replace manual stabilization).

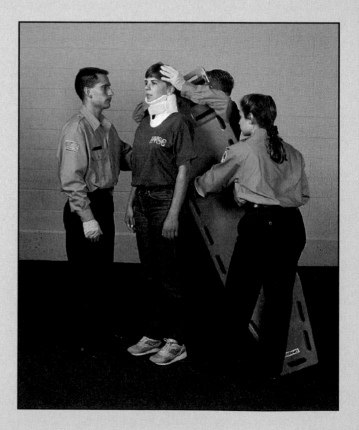

3. EMT-Basic A continues manual stabilization as EMT-Basic B positions a long spine board behind the patient, being careful not to disturb EMT-Basic A's manual stabilization of patient's head. It will help if EMT-Basic A spreads elbows to give EMT-Basic B more room to maneuver the spine board.

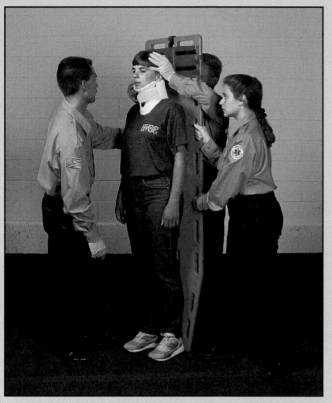

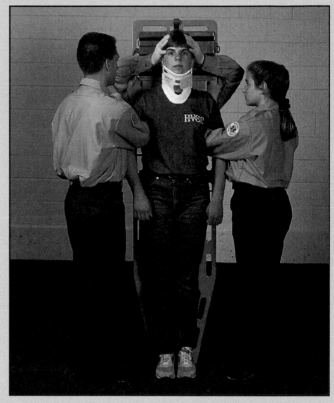

4. EMT-Basic A continues manual stabilization. EMT-Basic B looks at the spine board from the front of the patient and does any necessary repositioning to be sure it is centered behind the patient.

5. EMT-Basic A continues manual stabilization. EMT-Basic B and a third rescuer or helper reach with arm that is nearest patient under patient's armpits and grasp the spine board. (Once the board is tilted down, patient will actually be temporarily suspended by armpits.) To keep patient's arms secure, they use other hand to grasp patient's arm just above elbow and hold it against patient's body.

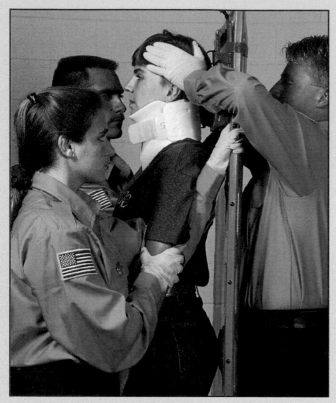

6. EMT-Basic B and third rescuer, when reaching under patient's armpits, must grasp a handhold on the spine board at patient's armpit level or higher.

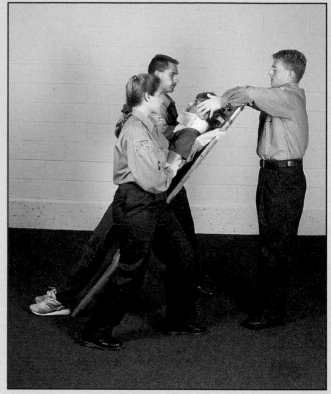

7. EMT-Basic A continues manual stabilization. EMT-Basic B and third rescuer maintain their grasp on the spine board and patient. EMT-Basic A explains to patient what is going to happen, then gives signal to begin slowly tilting board and patient backward to lower to the ground. As board is lowered, EMT-Basic A walks backward and crouches, keeping up with the board as it is lowered. As patient is lowered, EMT-Basic A must allow patient's head to slowly move back to the neutral position against the board. EMT-Basic A must accomplish all this without holding back or slowing the lowering of the board. EMT-Basic A may need to rotate somewhat so that once the board is almost flat he or she is holding the head down on the board. *Once patient's head comes in contact with the board, it must not be allowed to leave the board, to avoid flexing the neck.* The job of the two persons doing the lowering is to control it so that it is slow and even on both sides. They should also move into a squatting position as they lower the board to avoid injuring their backs.

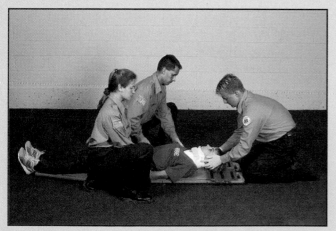

EMT-Basic A continues manual in-line stabilization throughout the procedure.

The Four-Rescuer Log Roll

FIRST take body substance isolation precautions.

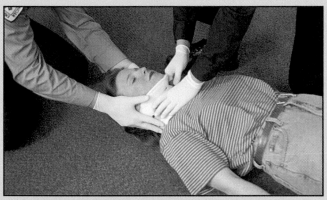

1. Stabilize the head and apply a rigid collar.

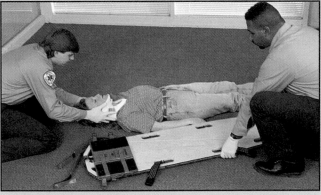

2. Place the board parallel to the patient.

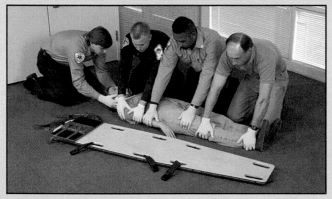

3. Three rescuers will kneel at the patient's side opposite the board, leaving room to roll the patient toward them. Place one rescuer at the shoulder, one at the waist, and one at the knee. One EMT-B will continue to stabilize the head. The rescuers will reach across the patient and take proper hand placement before the roll.

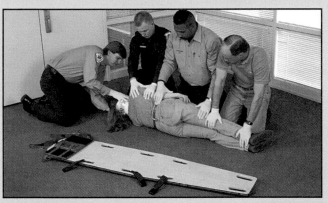

4. The EMT-B at the head and neck will direct the others to roll the patient as a unit.

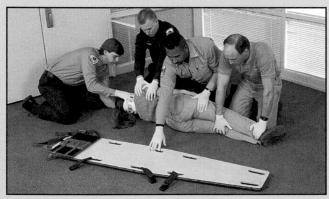

5. The EMT-B at the patient's waist will grip the spine board and pull it into position against the patient. (This can be done by a fifth rescuer.)

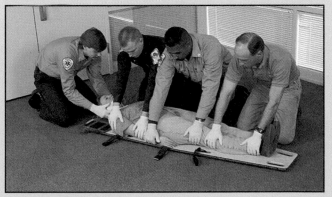

6. Roll the patient onto the board.

269

Spinal Immobilization of a Supine Patient

FIRST take body substance isolation precautions.

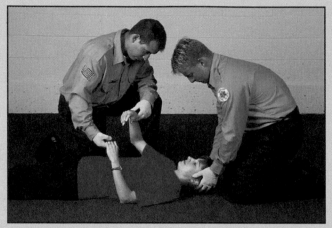

1. Place head in neutral, in-line position and maintain manual immobilization of head. Assess distal motor and sensory function and circulation.

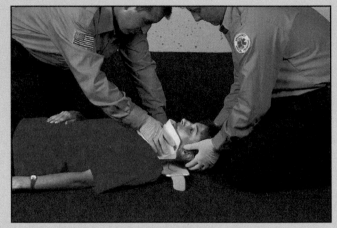

2. Apply appropriate size cervical collar.

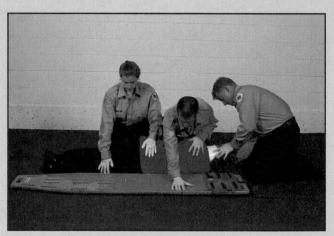

3. Position immobilization device.

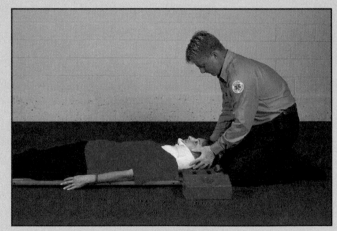

4. Move patient onto device without compromising integrity of spine. (Apply padding to voids between torso and board as necessary.)

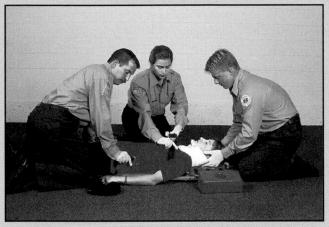

5. Immobilize patient's torso to the board.

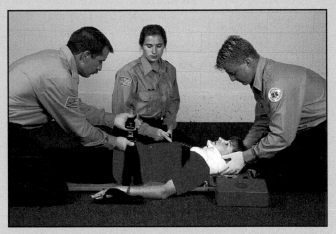

6. Secure torso straps.

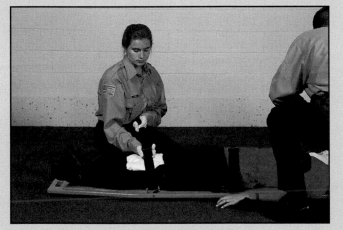

7. Secure patient's legs to board.

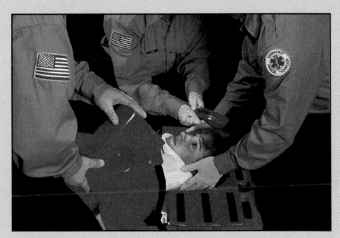

8. Pad and immobilize patient's head.

Reassess distal motor and sensory function and circulation.

PEDIATRIC HIGHLIGHT

If you do not carry a pediatric long spine immobilization device, then practice immobilizing a child using adult equipment and plenty of towels or blankets to pad around the child. EMT-Bs are usually very good at improvising; however, in this case, your first improvisation should be in the classroom so you respond quickly in the field! ■

Tips for Immobilizing the Seated Patient

When a patient is found in the sitting position, decide if he or she is high or low priority. In high priority use the **rapid extrication technique** (Skill Summary 13–20).

Preceptor Pearl

| Only use the rapid extrication technique on high-priority patients. This is not a technique for use on stable patients! ✤

If the patient is stable and low priority, use the normal procedure for spinal immobilization (Skill Summary 13–21). In such situations, when time is not of the essence, secure the patient to a short spine board or extrication device that will immobilize the head, neck, and torso until the patient can be transferred to a long spine board or other full-body immobilization device.

First, manually stabilize the patient's head and neck and quickly assess sensory and motor function to all four extremities. Next apply a rigid collar. Then secure the patient to the short spine board or extrication device.

The short spine board is just a shortened version of a long spine board. This original extrication device has been used for many years and although still often used, it is used less frequently now, not because of loss of popularity among users, but due to narrow bucket seats.

Today's automobiles have fewer bench-type seats and more bucket-type seats whose contoured backs do not accommodate a flat board. Also, the conventional short spine board is often too wide and too high to be used effectively in a small car. In these cases, a vest-style extrication device, a flexible piece of equipment, is useful for immobilizing patients with possible cervical spine injury. It can be used when the patient is found in a bucket seat, in a short compact car seat, in a seat with a contoured back, or in a confined space. It is also useful when the short spine board cannot be inserted into a car because of obstructions. A number of commercial vest-style extrication devices such as the Kendrick Extrication Device (KED), Kansas backboard, XP-1, and the LSP Vest are available. Use the devices approved by your EMS system.

Preceptor Pearl

| Don't be afraid to call for rescue to remove the vehicle's roof if there simply is not enough room to work inside the car. Remember, vehicle damage is much less expensive than the cost of caring for or being sued by a patient whose spinal cord was severed due to excessive movement during his removal from the car. ✤

Whether you are applying a short spine board or a flexible extrication device, a particular sequence must be followed. You must secure the torso first and the head last. This approach offers greater stability throughout the strapping process and may help prevent compression of the cervical spine. If the patient has suffered abdominal injuries or displays diaphragmatic breathing that prevents adequate securing of the torso, the torso straps must still be used, but care must be taken to prevent interfering with the patient's breathing.

There are a number of special considerations when applying a short board to the patient.

- Any assessment or reassessment of the back, scapulae, arms, or clavicles must be done before the device is placed against the patient.

- The EMT-B applying the board must angle it to fit between, without striking or jarring, the arms of the rescuer who is stabilizing the head from behind the patient.

- You must push a spine board as far down into the seat as possible. If you do not, the board may shift and the patient's cervical spine may compress during application of the board. To provide full cervical support, the top of the board should be level with the top of the patient's head. The uppermost holes must be level with the patient's shoulders. The base of the board should not extend past the coccyx.

- Never place a chin cup or chin strap on the patient. Such devices may prevent the patient from opening his mouth if he has to vomit.

- When applying the first strap to secure the torso, do not apply the strap too tightly. This could aggravate existing abdominal injury or limit respirations for the diaphragmatic breathing patient.

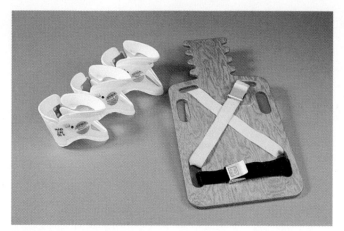

FIGURE 13–14 Short spine board.

- Some short spine boards have buckles with release mechanisms that can be accidentally loosened during patient transfer. This is true of "quick-release" buckles. These should be taped closed after the final adjustment of the straps.

- Do not pad between collar and board unless it is needed. To do so will create a pivot point that may cause the hyperextension of the cervical spine when the head is secured. Instead, padding should be placed at the occipital region, but only pad enough to fill any void. This will help keep the head in a neutral position. Often if the shoulders are rolled back to the board, the head will also come back to the board, which eliminates the need for padding.

- The placement of straps for the short spine board is somewhat complex (Figure 13–14). Most services carry these devices as a last-call backup for a collision involving numerous patients. Make sure you occasionally review the application of this device so you will be comfortable using it.

Preceptor Pearl

Never use excessive padding behind the head because, once the patient is removed from the vehicle, he or she will be placed in a supine position. At that point, the shoulders will fall back, but the head, if it is excessively padded, will not. This will place the patient's head in a position of flexion rather than the desired neutral position. ❖

Tips for Immobilizing Pediatric Patients

Spinal immobilization of pediatric patients can be another challenge for EMT-Bs. Try to utilize the skills you learned for immobilizing an adult patient with a child. Practice adapting adult equipment to the child patient in the classroom to gain the needed experience prior to treating a child in the field.

When a child is found in an intact child restraint seat, he or she can be immobilized right in the seat (Skill Summary 13–22) or rapidly extricated from the seat as shown in Skill Summary 13–23. The key decision point is that if a child would have to be in a supine position in order to be treated, then the patient must be rapidly extricated from the seat. This makes it easier to resuscitate the patient. When attempting to lay the seat back in a supine position, the patient's legs would be raised, which creates abdominal pressure on the diaphragm and restricts ventilation.

Rapid Extrication Procedure—
For High-Priority Patients Only

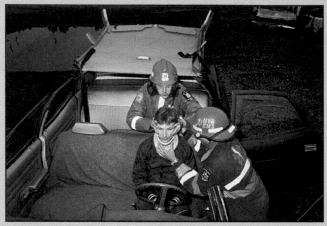

1. Manually stabilize the patient's head and neck and have a second EMT-B apply a cervical collar.

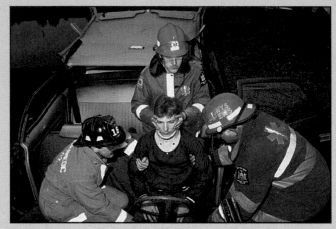

2. At the direction of the EMT-B stabilizing the head and neck, two EMT-Bs each lift the patient by his armpits and buttocks/thighs just enough for a bystander or additional rescuer to slide a long spine board between the patient and the vehicle seat.

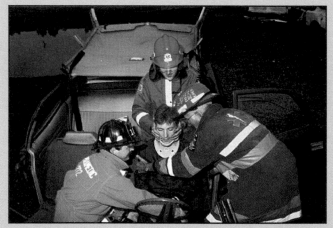

3. The EMT-Bs reposition their hands so the EMT-B on the front seat inside the vehicle holds the patient's legs and pelvis while the EMT-B outside the vehicle holds the upper chest and arms.

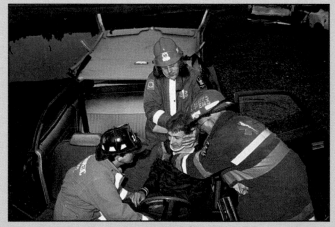

4. At the direction of the EMT-B holding the head and neck, carefully turn the patient a quarter turn so his back is facing the side door of the vehicle.

Note: In the photos, the roof of the vehicle has been removed to allow for easier illustration of the positions of the EMT-Bs. In most cases, this procedure will be done and should be practiced with the roof intact.

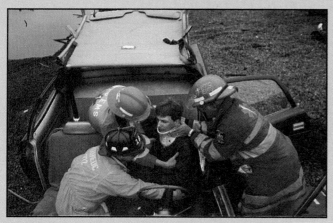

5. The EMT-B who was holding the pelvis temporarily holds the chest so the EMT-B who was holding the chest can take over head and neck stabilization. The EMT-B in the back seat can then reach over the seat and assist with the chest, and the EMT-B inside on the front seat can move his hands back to the pelvis.

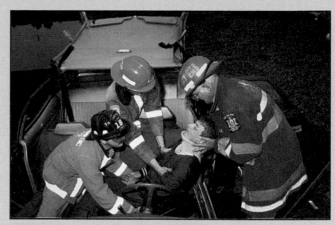

6. At the direction of the EMT-B at the head and neck, gently lower the patient to the spine board. **Note:** Sometimes it may be necessary to move the patient inside the vehicle a few inches so there is ample room to lay him down without touching the upper door opening.

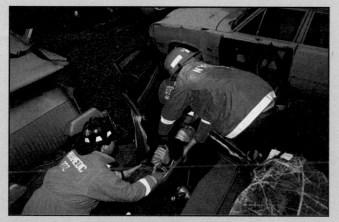

7. As a bystander or additional rescuer holds the end of the spine board, the EMT-Bs slide the patient to the head end of the board.

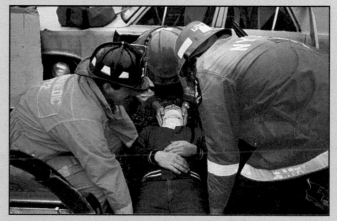

8. Quickly apply straps to the patient's chest, pelvis, and legs and remove the patient to a stretcher or the ground, under the direction of the EMT-B stabilizing the head and neck. **Note:** Since the patient's head is not yet fully immobilized (it is only being manually held stable by the EMT-B and collar), DO NOT walk more than a few steps with the patient. Once on stable ground or the stretcher, apply a head immobilizer or blanket roll and wide tape.

Note: The rapid extrication procedure is only for critical or unstable high-priority patients who must be moved in less time than would be required to apply a short board or extrication vest inside the vehicle before moving the patient to the long spine board. The normal extrication procedure is shown in Skill Summary 13–21.

Spinal Immobilization of a Seated Patient Using a KED

FIRST take body substance isolation precautions.

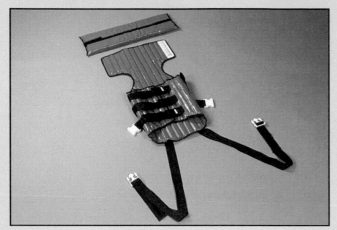

1. Select immobilization device.

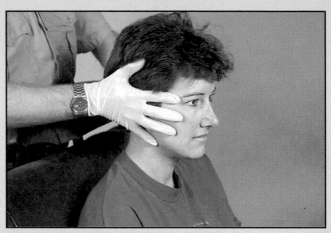

2. Manually immobilize patient's head in neutral, in-line position.

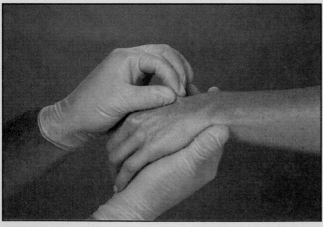

3. Assess distal motor and sensory function and circulation.

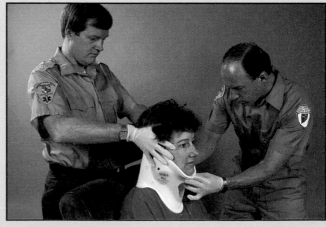

4. Apply appropriate size extrication collar.

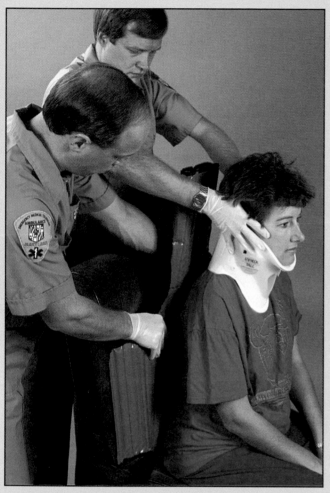

5. Position immobilization device behind patient.

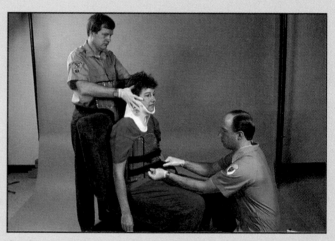

6. Secure device to patient's torso.

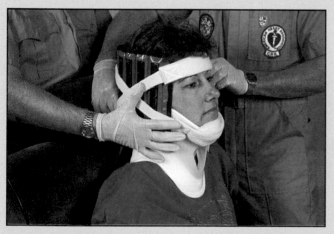

7. Evaluate and pad behind patient's head as necessary. Secure patient's head to device.

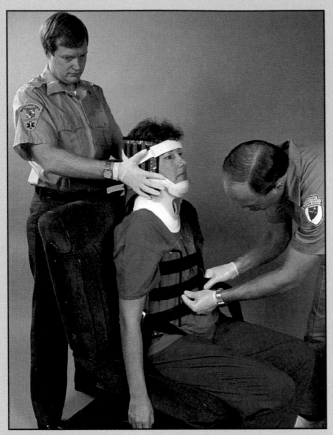

8. Evaluate and adjust straps. They must be tight enough so device does not move excessively up, down, left, or right—not so tight as to restrict patient's breathing.

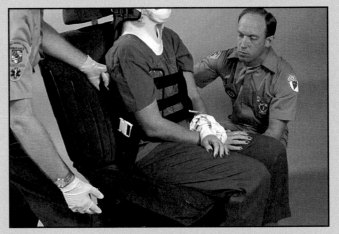

9. As needed, secure patient's wrists and legs and transfer the patient to the long board.

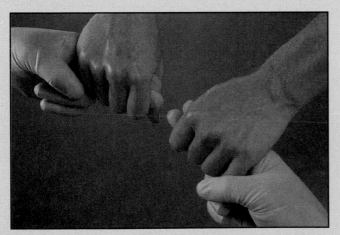

10. Reassess distal motor and sensory function and circulation.

Immobilizing in a Child Safety Seat

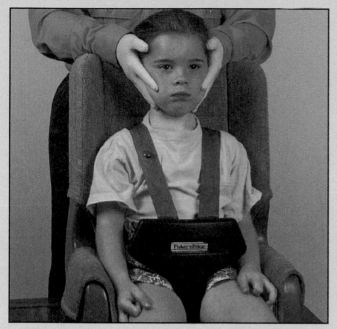

1. EMT-Basic A stabilizes car seat in upright position, applies manual head/neck stabilization ...

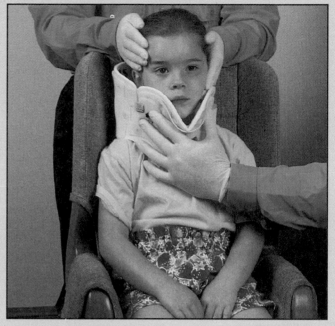

... as EMT-Basic B prepares equipment, then applies cervical collar, or improvises with rolled hand towel for the newborn or infant.

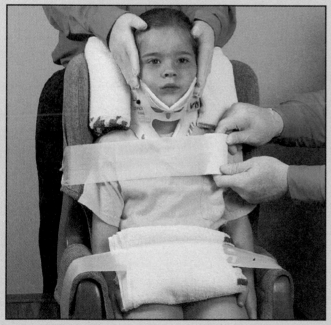

2. As EMT-Basic A maintains manual head/neck stabilization, EMT-Basic B places small blanket or towel on child's lap, then straps or uses wide tape to secure pelvis and chest area to seat.

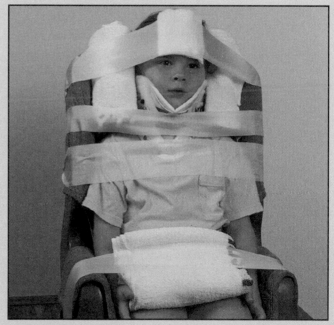

3. EMT-Basic A maintains manual head/neck stabilization as patient and seat are carried to ambulance and strapped onto stretcher with stretcher head raised. EMT-Basic B places a towel roll on both sides of head to fill voids, tapes forehead in place, then tapes across collar or maxilla. (Avoid taping chin, which would place pressure on child's neck.)

Rapid Extrication from a Child Safety Seat

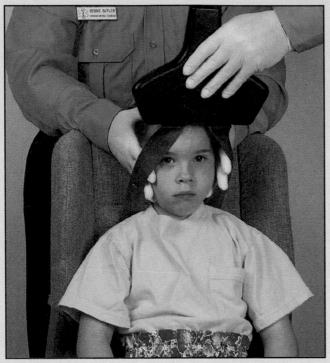

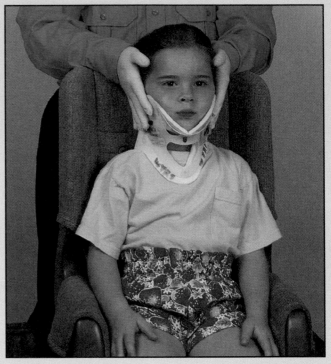

1. EMT-Basic A stabilizes car seat in upright position, applies manual head/neck stabilization as EMT-Basic B prepares equipment, then loosens or cuts the seat straps and raises the front guard.

2. Cervical collar is applied to patient as EMT Basic A maintains manual stabilization of the head and neck.

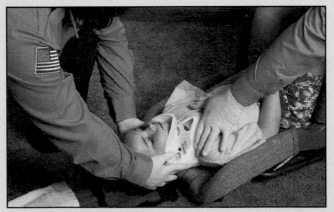

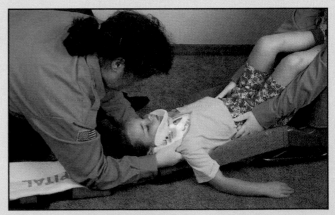

3. As EMT-Basic A maintains manual head/neck stabilization, EMT-Basic B places child safety seat on center of backboard and slowly tilts it into supine position. EMT-Bs are careful not to let child slide out of chair. For child with large head, place a towel under area where shoulders will eventually be placed on the board to prevent head from tilting forward.

4. EMT-Basic A maintains manual head/neck stabilization and calls for a coordinated long axis move onto backboard.

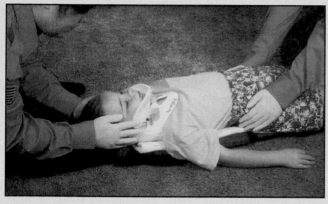

EMT-Basic A maintains manual head/neck stabilization as move onto board is completed, child's shoulders over the folded towel.

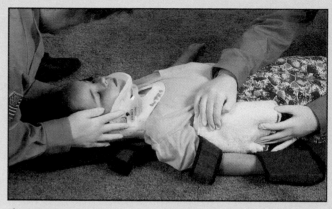

5. EMT-Basic A maintains manual head/neck stabilization as EMT-Basic B places rolled towels or blankets on both sides of patient.

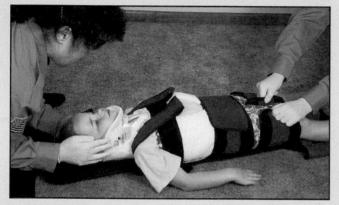

6. EMT-Basic A maintains manual stabilization as EMT-Basic B straps or tapes patient to board at level of upper chest, pelvis, and lower legs. DO NOT STRAP ACROSS ABDOMEN.

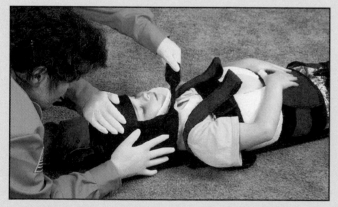

7. EMT-Basic A maintains manual head/neck stabilization as EMT-Basic B places rolled towels on both sides of head, then tapes head securely in place across forehead and maxilla or cervical collar. DO NOT TAPE ACROSS CHIN TO AVOID PRESSURE ON NECK.

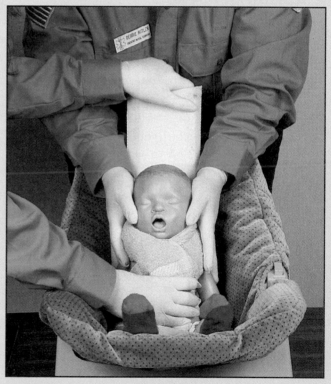

The newborn and infant procedure is exactly the same as for a child, except that an armboard is inserted behind the child in Step Two. If the infant is very small, the armboard may actually be used as the spine board.

CHAPTER REVIEW

■ SUMMARY

Although musculoskeletal injuries are usually not life-threatening, if treated improperly, many of these injuries can result in permanent disability. In the field, patients with a painful, swollen, or deformed extremity (PSDE) should be treated as though they have a fracture. Proper splinting of a PSDE can prevent further damage to soft tissues, organs, nerves, and muscles, and also keep a closed injury from becoming an open one. When caring for a PSDE, always check and record distal, motor, sensory, and circulation function both before and after splinting.

After proper assessment and care for the ABCs, proper assessment and care for head and spinal injuries are your most important responsi-bilities as an EMT-B. Always assume a head or spinal injury whenever there is a mechanism of injury of sufficient force or an injury to the head, neck, or upper body. If there is a head injury, suspect a brain injury as well as a spinal injury. Provide high-concentration oxygen, immobilize, and transport.

When caring for a spine-injured patient, manually stabilize the head and neck and apply a cervical collar. Continue the manual stabilization until the patient is fully immobilized on a long spine board.

Always monitor and document any changes in the mental status of a head- or spine-injured patient.

■ REVIEW QUESTIONS

1. Name the major bones of the spine, thorax, and upper and lower extremities.

2. What are the functions of the skeletal system?

3. Why is it important that you gently handle and properly immobilize PSDEs?

4. What are the goals of splinting?

5. Explain how you would splint an ankle, femur, humerus, and tibia (use a different patient for each explanation).

6. Explain why a head-injured patient can have a hematoma and bruise on the right side of the head but exhibit left-sided arm and leg weakness.

7. List ten signs and symptoms of brain injury and explain which is the most important sign.

8. Explain the four conditions that make a head injury worse and why hyperventilation is a helpful treatment for the head-injured patient.

9. List six examples of mechanism of injury that could cause a spinal injury.

10. List ten signs and symptoms of a spinal injury and explain the significance of a patient feeling "pins & needles" in the extremities.

CHAPTER 14

Pediatric Patients

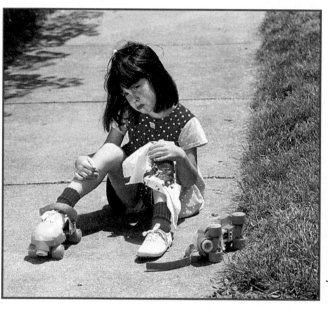

■ In the past, the quality of out-of-hospital care of children was less than desirable. Two principal factors led to this outcome —inadequate coverage of the topic in the old curriculum and EMS providers' lack of understanding of the growth and development patterns of healthy children. Both factors hindered the EMT-B's ability to deal with the emotional and physical needs of injured or ill children. Add to these the fact that most EMS personnel, like most people, consider children to be "special" and they tend to become emotionally involved in their care. Being extra attentive to children's needs just because they are children is understandable; but this extra attention should not overshadow your major goals—proper assessment and emergency medical care. To accomplish these goals, the new curriculum takes the position that EMT-Bs need to be properly trained to manage not only the assessment and care of young children, but the tumultuous feelings that accompany providing this care. To this end, the curriculum calls for increased course time for the study of pediatric emergency care. This chapter contains the information from the new curriculum, which describes the differences in assessment and management of pediatric patients as compared to adults. In addition, it offers support and provides tips for dealing with the overwhelming emotions that often accompany the treatment of these "special" patients.

MAKING THE TRANSITION

- ■ Developmental differences between the five pediatric age groups are described.
- ■ Differences between pediatric anatomy and physiology and that of an adult are explained.
- ■ Recognizing and managing pediatric respiratory emergencies are emphasized.
- ■ Treatment of special needs of pediatric patients at home is explained.

OBJECTIVES

The numbered objectives below are from the United States Department of Transportation 1994 EMT-Basic National Standards Curriculum. (Asterisked objectives are also included in the transitional curriculum.) The objective with a colored bullet that follows in italics is also from the EMT-Basic Transitional Program.

■ KNOWLEDGE AND ATTITUDE

At the completion of this chapter, you should be able to:

*1. Identify the developmental considerations for the following age groups: infant, toddler, preschool, school age, and adolescent. (pp. 285–287)

2. Describe differences in anatomy and physiology of the infant, child, and adult patient. (pp. 287–289)

3. Differentiate the response of the ill or injured infant or child (age specific) from that of an adult. (pp. 286–287)

4. Indicate various causes of respiratory emergencies. (pp. 290–291)

5. Differentiate between respiratory distress and respiratory failure. (pp. 291–293)

6. List the steps in the management of foreign body airway obstruction. (pp. 290–291)

7. Summarize emergency medical care strategies for respiratory distress and failure. (pp. 292–293)

8. Identify the signs and symptoms of shock (hypoperfusion) in the infant and child patient. (pp. 294–295)

9. Describe the methods of determining end organ perfusion in the infant and child patient. (p. 295)

10. State the usual cause of cardiac arrest in infants and children versus adults. (p. 292)

11. List the common causes of seizures in the infant and child patient. (p. 296)

12. Describe the management of seizures in the infant and child patient. (pp. 296–297)

13. Differentiate among the injury patterns in adults, infants, and children. (p. 294)

14. Discuss the field management of the infant and child trauma patient. (pp. 295–296)

15. Summarize the indicators of possible child abuse and neglect. (pp. 295–296)

16. Describe the medical-legal responsibilities in suspected child abuse. (p. 296)

17. Recognize the need for EMT-B debriefing following a difficult infant or child transport. (pp. 299–300)

*18. Explain the rationale for having knowledge and skills appropriate for dealing with the infant and child patient. (pp. 299–300)

*19. Attend to the feelings of the family when dealing with an ill or injured infant or child. (p. 299)

*20. Understand the provider's own response (emotional) to caring for infants or children. (pp. 299–300)

● *Describe the assessment and intervention strategies that are unique to infants and children in medical and trauma situations.* (pp. 285–300)

■ SKILLS

1. Demonstrate the techniques of foreign body airway obstruction removal in the infant.

2. Demonstrate the techniques of foreign body airway obstruction removal in the child.

*3. Demonstrate the assessment of the infant and child.

4. Demonstrate bag-valve mask artificial ventilations for the infant.

5. Demonstrate bag-valve mask artificial ventilations for the child.

6. Demonstrate oxygen delivery for the infant and child.

Three-year-old Billy Johnson has had a fever for the last few hours. His father has given him liquid Tylenol® and has been monitoring Billy's temperature. When Mr. Johnson checked on his son just before bedtime, he found him sitting on the edge of the bed with his chest heaving and he realized Billy was having difficulty breathing. Billy's latest temperature was 103°F and he appeared exhausted. Mr. Johnson called 911.

Upon your arrival to the quiet suburban home, you **size-up** the scene and then don body substance isolation as you are led to the child. Your **initial assessment** begins at the doorway of Billy's room. As you approach, you notice that the child is in respiratory distress; he is leaning forward and working hard to breathe. You try to involve Mr. Johnson in the care of his child in order to calm both of them.

You: Hi, Billy. My name is Jonathan. I'm here to help you because your dad says you feel very hot. It looks like you are having trouble breathing. I'll bet that's scary. You're a pretty brave young man!

Billy: (Nods his head yes but does not look at you. He is concentrating on his breathing and not your presence in the room.)

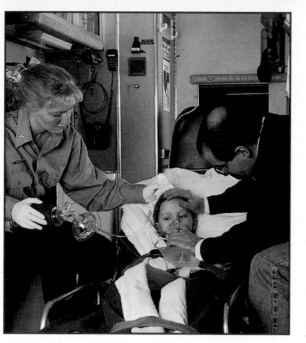

You: Your dad is going to wrap you up and carry you out to the ambulance. We are going to go for a short ride to see the doctor at the hospital so he can help you feel better.

Once in the ambulance, you place Billy on the stretcher with his father nearby to calm him. You pull out a pediatric nonrebreather mask, the BVM, and a suction unit just in case they are needed. As you begin to apply the nonrebreather mask, Billy becomes frightened. So you switch to "blow-by" oxygen, using oxygen tubing poked through the bottom of a plastic comic character cup. This seems to calm him.

By radio, you alert the ED of Billy's condition and your ETA. During the ride to the hospital, you offer Billy a stuffed animal, which he cradles with one arm, and you perform a toe-to-head **physical exam**. Meanwhile, your partner obtains a SAMPLE history from Billy's father. You perform **ongoing assessment** every five minutes, focusing on Billy's airway and breathing, while attempting a rendezvouz with ALS while en route to the ED.

At the hospital, you transfer Billy to the ED staff. When you check back later in your shift, you learn he has a serious upper respiratory infection, but is doing much better now. His father's prompt call to 911 saved the day for Billy. ■

■ APPROACHING THE PEDIATRIC PATIENT

Determining a Pediatric Patient's Age

Physicians usually consider children up to the age of 15 as pediatric patients. Yet it is not unusual for pediatricians to treat young adults through-out their college years and beyond. The American Heart Association defines an *infant* as any child up to a year old, and the term *child* is used for children from 1 to 8 years old. This age grouping is based on the patient's physical development and the procedures recommended for rescue breathing and CPR. In emergency care, the following age groups are used to classify children and are based upon anatomical and emotional development:

TABLE 14–1 Developmental Characteristics of Infants and Children

Age Group	Characteristics	Assessment and Care Strategies
Newborns and infants—birth to 1 year	• Infants do not like to be separated from their parents. • There is minimal stranger anxiety. • Infants are used to being undressed but like to feel warm, physically and emotionally. • The younger infant follows movement with his eyes. • The older infant is more active, developing a personality. • They do not want to be "suffocated" by an oxygen mask.	• Have the parent hold the infant while you examine him. • Be sure to keep them warm—warm your hands and stethoscope before touching the infant. • It may be best to observe their breathing from a distance, noting the rise and fall of the chest, the level of activity, and their color. • Examine the heart and lungs first and the head last. This is perceived as less threatening to the infant and therefore less likely to start them crying. • A pediatric nonrebreather mask may be held near the face to provide "blow-by" oxygen.
Toddlers—1 to 3 years	• Toddlers do not like to be touched or separated from their parents. • Toddlers may believe that their illness is a punishment for being bad. • Unlike infants, they do not like having their clothing removed. • They frighten easily, overreact, have a fear of needles, pain. • Toddlers may understand more than they communicate. • They begin to assert their independence. • They do not want to be "suffocated" by an oxygen mask.	• Have a parent hold the child while you examine him. • Assure the child that he was not bad. • Remove an article of clothing, examine, and then replace the clothing. • Examine in a trunk-to-head approach to build confidence. (Touching the head first may be frightening.) • Explain what you are going to do in terms the toddler can understand (taking the blood pressure becomes a squeeze or a hug on the arm). • Offer the comfort of a favorite toy. • Consider giving the toddler a choice: "Do you want me to look at your belly or your chest first?" • A pediatric nonrebreather mask may be held near the face to provide "blow-by" oxygen.

- Newborn and infant—newborn (birth to 6 months) and infant (6 months to a year)
- Toddler—1 to 3 years
- Preschool—3 to 6 years
- School age—6 to 12 years
- Adolescent—12 to 18 years

Tips For Assessing Each Age Group

Since a child's age is not always accessible or evident, you should practice determining children's ages based upon their physical and developmental characteristics. Table 14–1 should be helpful in the assessment and management of children in each age group. Keep a card handy with the childrens' normal vital signs, weights, and other information you may need in treating pediatric patients (Table 14–2).

Remember, putting the child at ease is an important part of the care you must provide. Always kneel or sit at the child's eye level (Figure 14–1). Let the child see your face and make eye contact without staring at the child.

Age Group	Characteristics	Assessment and Care Strategies
Preschool—3 to 6 years	• Preschoolers do not like to be touched or separated from their parents. • They are modest and do not like their clothing removed. • Preschoolers may believe that their illness is a punishment for being bad. • Preschoolers have a fear of blood, pain, and permanent injury. • They are curious, communicative, and can be cooperative. • They do not want to be "suffocated" by an oxygen mask.	• Have a parent hold the child while you examine him. • Respect their modesty. Remove an article of clothing, examine, and then replace the clothing. • Have a calm, confident, reassuring, respectful manner. • Be sure to offer explanations about what you are doing. • Allow the child the responsibility of giving the history. • Explain as you examine. • A pediatric nonrebreather mask may be held near the face to provide "blow-by" oxygen.
School age—6 to 12 years	• This age group cooperates but likes their opinions heard. • They fear blood, pain, disfigurement, and permanent injury. • School age children are modest and do not like their bodies exposed.	• Allow the child the responsibility of giving the history. • Explain as you examine. • Present a confident, calm, respectful manner. • Respect their modesty.
Adolescent—12 to 18 years	• Adolescents want to be treated as adults. • Adolescents generally feel that they are indestructible but may have fears of permanent injury and disfigurement. • Adolescents vary in their emotional and physical development and may not be comfortable with their changing bodies.	• Although they wish to be treated as adults, they may need as much support as children. • Present a confident, calm, respectful manner. • Be sure to explain what you are doing. • Respect their modesty. You may consider assessing them away from their parents. Have the physical exam done by an EMT-B of the same sex as the patient if possible.

■ ANATOMY AND PHYSIOLOGY DIFFERENCES

The Head

Up until about 6 years of age, children's heads are proportionately larger than those of adults. This disproportional size increases children's potential for head trauma. Unfortunately, when children are struck by an automobile or accidentally fall from a window, they fly, like a javelin, with the heavier end (the child's head) first. Also, when spinal immobilization of a child in this age group is required, it is necessary to pad behind the child's shoulders to avoid flexing the neck.

A baby is born with a skull that has not yet fully fused, which allows for override of the cranial bones so the baby's head can pass through the birth canal. The membranous spaces at the anterior and posterior junctions of these unfused cranial bones are called *fontanelles,* or "soft spots." Cranial bones fuse over the posterior fontanelle

TABLE 14–2 Normal Vital Sign and Weight Ranges, Infants and Children

Normal Pulse Rate (beats per minute, at rest)	
Newborn	120 to 160
Infant 0–5 months	90 to 140
Infant 6–12 months	80 to 140
Toddler 1–3 years	80 to 130
Preschooler 3–5 years	80 to 120
School age 6–10 years	70 to 110
Adolescent 11–14 years	60 to 105

Normal Respiration Rate (breaths per minute, at rest)	
Newborn	30 to 50
Infant 0–5 months	25 to 40
Infant 6–12 months	20 to 30
Toddler 1–3 years	20 to 30
Preschooler 3–5 years	20 to 30
School age 6–10 years	15 to 30
Adolescent 11–14 years	12 to 20

Blood Pressure Normal Ranges		
	Systolic Approx. 80 plus 2 × age	Diastolic Approx. ⅔ Systolic
Preschooler 3–5 years	average 99 (78 to 116)	average 65
School age 6–10 years	average 105 (80 to 122)	average 57
Adolescent 11–14 years	average 115 (94 to 140)	average 59

Normal Weight Ranges	
Newborn/Young Infant	Approx. 3.5 to 7 Kg
Older Infant	Approx. 8 to 11 Kg
Toddler 1–3 years	Approx. 10 to 15 Kg
Preschooler 3–5 years	Approx. 15 to 20 Kg
School age 6–10 years	Approx. 22 to 37 Kg
Adolescent 11–14 years	Approx. 50 to 65 Kg

Notes: A high pulse in an infant or child is not as great a concern as a low pulse. A low pulse (heart rate) may indicate imminent cardiac arrest (stoppage of heart function). Blood pressure is usually not taken on a child under 3 years. In cases of blood loss or shock, a child's blood pressure will remain within normal limits until near the end, then fall swiftly.

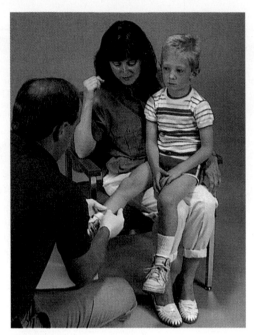

FIGURE 14–1 Kneel or sit at the child's eye level.

between the ages of 4 and 6 months, but it takes 18 months for bones to fuse and close the anterior fontanelle. These "soft spots" are usually flat and soft while the child is quiet. However, a sunken fontanelle may indicate dehydration; a bulging fontanelle may indicate that the infant is crying or has increased intracranial pressure.

Preceptor Pearl

Always *gently* palpate the fontanelle with the tips of your fingers to avoid trauma to the fontanelle. ✤

The Respiratory System

Like adults, airway is the highest priority. This importance is highlighted in children because of certain anatomic factors. Remember these key differences:

- The mouth and nose of a child are smaller and more easily obstructed.
- The child's tongue is proportionately larger and takes up more space in the mouth.
- Newborns and infants are obligate nose breathers; therefore nasal congestion makes it difficult from them to breathe.
- The smallest diameter of the child's airway is located at the cricoid ring in the trachea. The

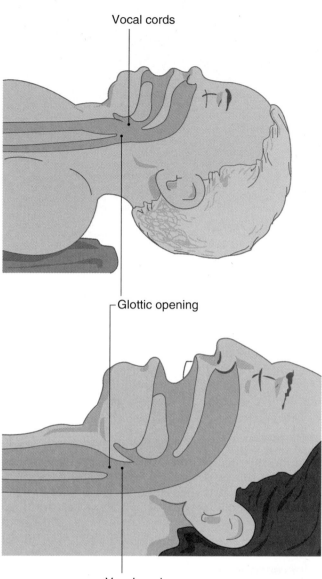

Vocal cords

Glottic opening

Vocal cords

FIGURE 14–2 Adult and child airways compared.

adult's is smallest at the vocal cords (Figure 14–2). The child's cricoid ring forms a physiologic cuff. Due to the diameter of the opening of the cricoid ring, when an endotracheal tube is inserted in a small child an uncuffed tube is used. Since the trachea is relatively narrower than in adults, it is more easily obstructed. This is why "blind" finger sweeps are never used on an infant or child. You could easily push an obstruction further down the narrow trachea.

- Children have a softer, more flexible trachea than do adults. Hyperextension or flexion of the

neck can actually cause airway obstruction. Therefore, as mentioned earlier, place a folded towel under the shoulders of an infant or toddler to keep the airway in a neutral position (Figure 14–3).

- Since the chest wall is softer, children depend more on the diaphragm for breathing. Therefore, respiratory muscle fatigue occurs more rapidly.

Chest and Abdomen

The muscles and bones in the child's chest and the muscles of the abdomen are not well developed and therefore provide only minimal protection for the underlying organs. Since the chest wall is more elastic, when a child in respiratory distress breathes, the movement of the ribs, sternum, and intercostal muscles makes a dramatic and easily observable general impression. Since young children are abdominal breathers, who rely heavily on the movement of the diaphragm, injuries to the chest or abdomen can decrease tidal volume (the amount of inspired air). This is one reason why the abdominal section of the PASG is no longer recommended for use with children.

Preceptor Pearl

When a child is struck by a vehicle you may observe tire marks on his chest. Since the child's chest is so flexible, there may be no evidence of broken ribs. However, there is a strong likelihood that there will be contusions and other injuries to the underlying lung and heart that could be devastating. ❖

The Skin

Since a child's body surface is larger in proportion to body mass, children are more prone to heat loss through the skin. Whenever small children are taken out in the cold, they should be wrapped in a blanket; their heads should be covered since they lose so much heat from their proportionately larger heads. The "Rule of Nines" for calculating the total body surface covered by a burn is different for children too (see Chapter 12). The head accounts for a larger percentage of body surface area, the legs for a lower one. Most EMT-Bs carry a pocket guide with the pediatric Rule of Nines or use the Rule of Palm, which indicates that the size of the child's palm is equal to one percent of the body surface area.

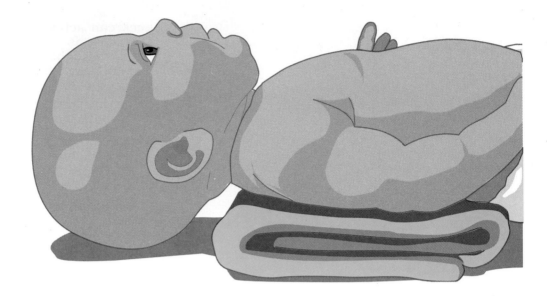

FIGURE 14–3
Use a folded towel to keep the infant's or young child's airway aligned.

■ PEDIATRIC RESPIRATORY EMERGENCIES

Maintaining an Open Airway

As noted earlier, it is important to place the child's head and neck in a neutral position to properly open the airway and to align the spine. Use the folded-towel technique and perform a head-tilt, chin-lift if there is no trauma, or a jaw thrust with spinal immobilization if trauma is suspected.

Be prepared to suction the child's airway with a properly sized catheter, but avoid stimulating the gag reflex in the back of the throat. Stimulating the back of the child's throat can cause the patient to vomit or slow the heart rate.

Children often have considerable amounts of secretions that block their narrow airways and require suctioning. Never suction for more than 15 seconds (which is roughly equal to the amount of time you can hold your own breath), and hyperventilate the child after suctioning.

Foreign Body Airway Obstruction

If you suspect a child's airway is blocked by a foreign body, follow these current American Heart Association guidelines:

- *Conscious child with good air exchange who is choking* Encourage the patient to continue to cough, and monitor closely.

- *Conscious infant patient with poor to no air exchange* Perform a series of 5 back blows and 5 chest thrusts until effective or the patient loses consciousness (Figure 14–4).

- *Conscious child (from age 1 to 8) with poor to no air exchange* Perform abdominal thrusts until effective or the patient loses consciousness.

- *Unconscious infant with poor to no air exchange* Establish unresponsiveness, open the airway, and attempt ventilation; if unsuccessful, reposition the airway and reattempt ventilation, give 5 back blows then 5 chest thrusts, perform a tongue-jaw lift, and remove an object only if you can see it. Repeat these steps continuously, starting with opening the airway, until help arrives or as you begin transport to and en route to the hospital.

- *Unconscious child with poor to no air exchange* Establish unresponsiveness, open the airway, and attempt ventilation; reposition the airway and reattempt ventilation, give 5 abdominal thrusts, perform a tongue-jaw lift, and remove an object only if you can see it. Repeat these steps continuously, starting with opening the airway, until help arrives or as you begin transport to and en route to the hospital.

Never do "blind" finger sweeps in the mouth of an infant or child. Look in the mouth for an obstruction and use your fingers only to remove an obstruction you can actually see.

Oral Airway Insertion

Remember, due to its larger size, the tongue of an infant or child is likely to fall back into and block the airway. If this occurs when the patient is unconscious and does not have a gag reflex, you may insert an oropharyngeal airway to prevent the tongue from blocking the airway. To insert the airway, use a tongue depressor or gloved finger to push the tongue down against the floor of the mouth while placing the properly sized airway straight into the pharynx. Unlike the procedure for adults, do not "flip the airway" over the tongue, since this may damage the uvula or soft palate or cause bleeding in a young child (Figure 14–5).

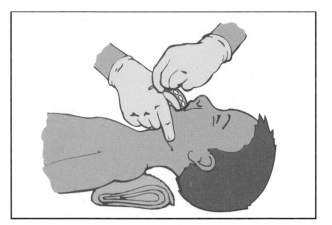

FIGURE 14–5 In an infant or child, the airway is inserted with the tip pointing toward the tongue and throat, in the same position it will be in after insertion.

Respiratory Problems

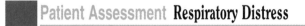

Patient Assessment **Respiratory Distress**

As you begin to assess a child in respiratory distress, ask yourself "Is the child alert and calm?" Children in respiratory distress (Figure 14–6) usually are not alert and calm. Then ask yourself, "Is the child agitated or sleepy?" **Hypoxemia**, too little oxygen in the blood, can make a child agitated. **Hypercarbia**, too much carbon dioxide in the blood, can make a child sleepy. Hypoxemia is more common in children.

Next evaluate the child's skin color by asking the parent to remove the child's shirt so you can examine the skin and look for chest wall movement. Severe hypoxemia can cause cyanosis; poor perfusion can cause mottling of the skin. Pallor or a grayish hue can indicate severe hypoxemia, which signals impending respiratory collapse.

Next assess the respiratory rate by comparing it to the normal rates listed on page 82. Is the rate elevated for the child's age? Increased respiratory effort is always an indicator of some level of airway compromise. The signs of increased respiratory effort include:

● *Nasal flaring*—the dilation of the child's nares in an attempt to decrease airway resistance and increase air flow

● *Stridor*—a high-pitched sound usually heard upon inspiration

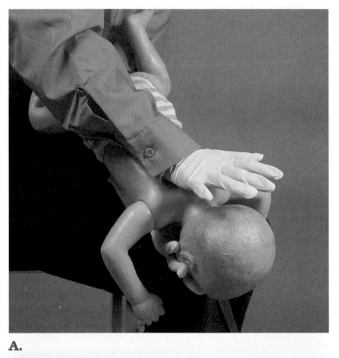

A.

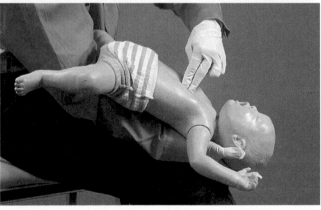

B.

FIGURE 14–4 For a complete airway obstruction in an infant, alternate **A.** back blows and **B.** chest thrusts.

FIGURE 14–6
Signs of respiratory distress.

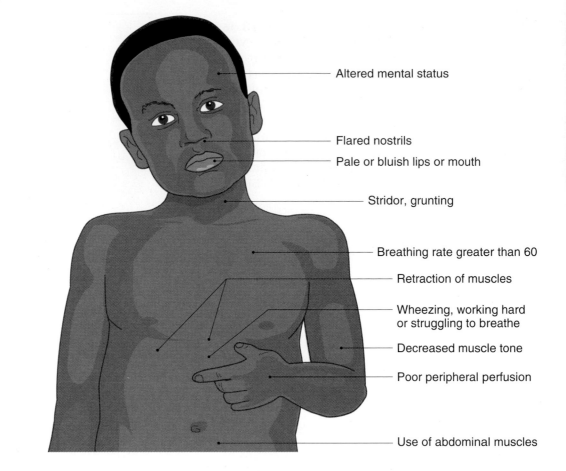

- Altered mental status
- Flared nostrils
- Pale or bluish lips or mouth
- Stridor, grunting
- Breathing rate greater than 60
- Retraction of muscles
- Wheezing, working hard or struggling to breathe
- Decreased muscle tone
- Poor peripheral perfusion
- Use of abdominal muscles

- *Retractions*—visible movements of the muscles that assist the movement of the rib cage in breathing
- *Wheezing*—an audible sound heard over the chest during the expiratory phase of breathing
- *Grunting*—heard in infants on exhalation when air is pushed against a closed glottis to keep the airway open

Next ask yourself, "Is the child flaccid or agitated by your approach?" A flaccid child is seriously ill and may be close to respiratory arrest. An agitated child may be hypoxemic.

Finally, to complete your assessment, feel for air movement at the nose. If there is minimal air movement, this indicates depression of respiratory efforts. Check the child's peripheral perfusion for delayed capillary refill, an indicator of severe hypoxemia and hypoventilation.

A child in respiratory distress quickly slides down a slippery slope that degenerates from respiratory distress to respiratory failure, then from ventilatory failure to respiratory arrest, and finally to cardiopulmonary arrest. *Respiratory failure* is oxygenation difficulty severe enough to cause obvious physical tiring, with increased ventilatory effort and rate. When a child can no longer compensate and becomes physically exhausted, the child deteriorates into severe hypoxia.

Pre-respiratory arrest signs include cyanosis, which degenerates to a grayish hue to the skin. Bradycardia, slowness of the heart manifested in a pulse rate usually under 60 per minute (or 80 in a younger child), is a poor sign that signals severe hypoxemia and acidosis. Generally when children in respiratory distress wear out from breathing efforts, they have shallow breathing and apnea (cessation of breathing) followed by cardiac arrest.

Children do not generally die from primary cardiac causes; the few exceptions are due to congenital heart defects. However, children can suffer primary respiratory arrests that result in cardiac arrests. ■

Patient Care **Respiratory Distress**

Emergency care for the child in respiratory distress must begin immediately with proper airway management, suctioning, and administering 100% oxygen (humidified if available) by mask, and evaluating the need for ventilatory assistance with a BVM. Never increase the child's agitation, as this will quickly make matters worse. ■

Preceptor Pearl

Pediatric care experts emphasize that the priority of children in respiratory distress is "AAA," not just "ABC." In other words, if you manage the patient's airway and oxygenate, circulation improvement will follow! ❖

Providing Supplemental Oxygen and Ventilations

High-concentration oxygen should be administered to children in respiratory distress or with inadequate respirations or possible hypoperfusion. Hypoxia is the underlying reason for many of the most serious pediatric medical problems. Inadequate oxygen immediately affects the heart and the brain, as evidenced by a slowed heart rate and an altered mental status.

Since infants through preschoolers are often afraid of an oxygen mask, try a "blow-by" technique. Have a parent hold the mask 2 inches from the child's face so the oxygen will pass over it and be inhaled. Some children respond well when the tubing is pushed through the bottom of a paper cup or plastic comic character cup. Hand the cup to the child, who will instinctively explore it and hold it near the face, which accomplishes the desired result.

Preceptor Pearl

Do not use styrofoam cups since they are made of particles that can easily flake apart and cause choking if they get into the airway. ❖

It may become necessary to hyperventilate a child, to assist a child's ventilations, or to actually resuscitate the nonbreathing child. The AHA guidelines for ventilating the infant and the child are shown in Table 14–3. It is essential that you be well practiced in the use of the pediatric-sized pocket mask and a BVM using the correct size device (either infant/newborn or child size). Follow these guidelines when ventilating the infant or child patient:

- Avoid breathing too hard through the pocket face mask or using excessive bag pressure and volume. Use only enough to make the patient's chest rise.

- Use properly sized face masks to assure a good mask seal.

- Do not use flow-restricted, oxygen-powered ventilation devices since they are contraindicated in infants and children.

- If ventilation is not successful in raising the patient's chest, perform the procedures for clearing an obstructed airway; then try to ventilate again.

- The AHA standards do not allow the use of a "pediatric pop-off valve" on any size BVM. If your service has one of these valves, replace the BVM with a new one.

TABLE 14–3 Artificial Ventilation and Clearing the Airway

	Child over 8	Child 1 to 8	Infant
Age	8 years and older	1–8 years	birth–1 year
Initial ventilation	1½ to 2 sec.	1 to 1½ sec.	1 to 1½ sec.
Ventilation rate	10–12 breaths/min	20 breaths/min.	20 breaths/min.
Obstructed Airway—Conscious	abdominal thrusts	abdominal thrusts	alternate 5 back blows with 5 chest thrusts
Obstructed Airway—Unconscious	5 abdominal thrusts, finger sweep, ventilate	5 abdominal thrusts, remove visible objects, ventilate	5 back blows, 5 chest thrusts, remove visible objects, ventilate
Working alone: when to call for help	After establishing unresponsiveness—before beginning resuscitation	After establishing unresponsiveness and 1 minute of resuscitation	After establishing unresponsiveness and 1 minute of resuscitation

PEDIATRIC TRAUMA

Childhood injury is the principal childhood public health problem in the United States today, causing more deaths than all childhood disease combined and contributing greatly to childhood disability. Nearly half of all pediatric trauma deaths result from motor vehicles, followed by drowning, burns, firearms, and falls. Blunt trauma far exceeds penetrating trauma in children—by 85% to 15%. Because of their curiosity, children are often injured investigating their environment. Their constant explorations lead to a range of injuries from accidental falls, things falling on them, burns, entrapment, and crushing, to sporting and recreational activities, and other mechanisms of injury.

Injury Patterns

Because of their anatomical and physiological differences, children's injury patterns differ from those of adults. During motor vehicle collisions, unrestrained child passengers tend to sustain head and neck injuries, while restrained passengers tend to sustain abdominal and lower spine injuries. Head, spine, and abdominal injuries are common when children are struck by an automobile while riding a bicycle. The child who has been struck by a vehicle may present with the combination of head, chest/abdominal, and lower extremity injuries. Other common injuries include diving injuries with associated head and spinal injuries. Sports activities also account for a considerable number of musculoskeletal injuries to children.

Patient Assessment Hypoperfusion (Shock)

Trauma is a major cause of hypoperfusion, or shock, in children. Hypoperfusion is the inadequate circulation of blood and oxygen throughout the body.

The circulating blood volume in a healthy child is approximately 8% of the total body weight; an adult's is 6% to 7%. Despite the higher proportion of blood volume in the child, the total volume is much less because of the child's size. An infant has 340 cc of blood, a toddler 1,300 cc, and a school-age child 1,900 cc.

Preceptor Pearl

One way to remember how little blood children have is to envision that an infant's total blood volume would fill only a soda can and a school-age child's a six-pack. ✜

Dehydration from diarrhea is the leading cause of childhood death in the world. Both diarrhea and vomiting can cause dehydration and may lead to life-threatening hypoperfusion. The younger the child, the more quickly dehydration can occur. Therefore, if an infant or toddler has a history of diarrhea and vomiting for more than a day, this is cause for concern.

The most important thing to understand about hypoperfusion in infants and children is that their bodies are able to compensate for it for a long time. Then the compensating mechanisms fail and decompensated hypoperfusion develops very rapidly. Children do not turn the corner from compensated to decompensated hypoperfusion, with an accompanying drop in systolic blood pressure until they have lost about 30% of their blood volume. This is because they have excellent vasoconstriction, which helps maintain their blood pressure.

Preceptor Pearl

Use the mnemonic "60 – 70 – 80 – 90" to help you remember the lower limits of the normal systolic BP in an infant, preschooler, grade schooler, and adolescent. The formula 70 + (2 × the child's age) can be used to estimate the lower limit of a normal systolic BP. The mnemonic "160 – 140 – 120 – 100" can help you remember the upper limits of the normal heart rates in the infant, preschooler, grade schooler, and adolescent. The formula 150 – (5 × the child's age) can be used to estimate this value in a child. ✜

Because of the broader range and greater variability in children's vital signs, and the fact that these signs do not change significantly until moments before circulation fails, they are not the best indicators of whether a child is in hypoperfusion. Assessment should be based on clinical signs of inadequate tissue perfusion. These signs develop as the body attempts to compensate for the decreased circulating blood volume by shunting blood from the peripheral tissues to core organs.

The early signs of hypoperfusion are

- Tachycardia
- Tachypnea
- Delayed capillary refill time
- Mottling

The late signs are

- Marked tachycardia
- Markedly delayed tachypnea
- Marked capillary refill time
- Peripheral cyanosis ■

Preceptor Pearl

The key indicators of inadequate perfusion and severe shock in a child are weak or absent peripheral pulses as compared to central pulses and/or delayed capillary refill. ✣

Patient Care Hypoperfusion

The goal of the treatment for hypoperfusion is to maintain perfusion to the core organs (i.e., brain, heart, lungs, kidneys) for as long as possible. The definitive treatment, regardless of the cause, is restoration of the circulating blood volume. For most pediatric patients this means replacing the blood or fluid that has been lost, and in some instances, surgical control of bleeding.

Emergency Care Steps

The keys to improving the survival rate of pediatric trauma patients include the following:

1. Rapid airway management with a jaw thrust, if you suspect trauma
2. Oxygenation with a nonrebreather mask
3. Evaluation of the need to ventilate with a BVM
4. Hyperventilation of head trauma
5. Immobilization of the spine
6. Maintaining body heat
7. Elevation of the legs
8. Immediate transport to the hospital
9. ALS backup, if available ■

In some EMS systems, the PASG may be used for the treatment of shock. If used, it must fit the patient. Never place the infant in one leg of an adult garment. Do not inflate the abdominal section since it may compromise breathing. A PASG is indicated for the pediatric trauma patient with signs of severe hypoperfusion and pelvic instability.

Nonaccidental Pediatric Trauma: Child Abuse

Authorities agree that the incidence of trauma caused by child abuse is unknown. There is no question that many cases go unrecognized and unreported. Sixty to sixty-five percent of reported abuse is categorized as physical. Current estimates are that there may be as many as 2,000 abuse-related deaths per year in the United States alone.

Since infants often develop the chronic abdominal pain of infancy called colic, they often undergo periods of irritability and incessant crying. These children are often at risk for child abuse from shaking baby syndrome, pinching, or forced bottle feeding. Other children at risk of physical or psychological injury include those with learning disorders, seizures, feeding difficulties, chronic respiratory complaints, and developmental delays. Since these children often require constant special care and attention, their parents or other caretakers often run out of patience and turn to abuse as a way of dealing with their frustration.

After completing your initial assessment and focused physical exam on a child you suspect may have been physically abused, compare your findings to information the parent or caretaker supplied. In some cases, a parent or caretaker will actually describe a history of injuries he or she has inflicted on the child; such a parent or caretaker is begging for help. In other situations, there is a remarkable absence of any history that would pinpoint the cause of the injury. Such unexplained events should trigger a heightened degree of suspicion on your part. At times, parents' explanations of the cause of their child's injury differ. These conflicting histories should be documented in "quotes" on the prehospital care report (PCR).

The location of an injury may also heighten your degree of suspicion. Anatomical sites for accidental injuries include the shins, hips, knees, lower arms, back, forehead, and under the chin. Inflicted wound sites are most often on the upper arms, torso, upper legs, side of the face, ears, neck, genitalia, and buttocks.

When a child exhibits bruises in various stages of healing, especially in the inflicted wound areas listed above, consider the possibility of abuse. Bruises undergo recognizable stages of healing. In the first 24 hours after a bruise is sustained, the color will be red or reddish blue. Over the next 1 to 4 days the wound will turn dark blue or purple color. Over the next 5 to 10 days, color turns green to yellow green to brown. By 1 to 3 weeks the bruise should disappear.

Specific patterns are created on the skin from rope burns, scalds, cigarette burns, dipping injuries, a belt or paddle, pinching, and slaps. Learn to recognize these patterns.

Serious central nervous system damage without any evidence of external trauma is often the result of forcible shaking of a child. The shaking shears veins in the skull causing internal bleeding and altered mental status.

In addition to physical abuse, children are also subjected to emotional abuse, neglect, and sexual abuse. Remember that child abuse is a crime and your goal in the treatment of children who have been abused is to ensure their safety. Never accuse anyone of hurting a child, since you cannot be absolutely sure who the perpetrator was and the person in charge may react to accusations by refusing to allow you to treat the child. Treat the child and recognize that gaining the parent's permission to do so will enable you to transport the child to the Emergency Department where the facts can be sorted out by the proper authorities.

In many states, EMT-Bs are not legally required to report suspicions of child abuse.

Preceptor Pearl

The Emergency Department physician is required to report cases of child abuse. Therefore, complete your PCR with factual information that you observed about the child's home environment, the condition of the home, the reaction of the parents or other caretakers, the child's hygiene, and general interaction of all family members involved, and call it to the attention of the physician. ❖

Many EMT-Bs who are employed by hospitals are required by law to report incidents of child abuse. Learn the laws of your state concerning the reporting of child abuse.

Injury Prevention

EMT-Bs can do their part in reducing injuries to children by becoming role models in their community and advocates for injury prevention. Many injuries are predictable and/or preventable. Examples of causes to promote in your community include:

- Use of protective equipment—Encourage the use of helmets for bicycling and helmets, knee and elbow pads for skate boarding and in-line skating.
- Playground safety—Clean up the glass in the community playground.
- Use of child safety restraints—Do you always use an infant seat or seat belts?

- Water safety—Encourage diving into swimming pools feet first to test the water's depth, which can significantly reduce the number of spinal injuries. Install fences around swimming pools and always provide adult supervision of children around water. Ensure that children wear personal floatation devices when near the water or boating. Teach children to swim.
- Avoid bus mishaps—A knapsack worn on a child's back for books and papers will help decrease the possibility that he or she will drop them under the school bus and try to retrieve them.
- Burn prevention—Use smoke and carbon monoxide detectors and encourage fire prevention education. Keep children away from wires and stoves. Adjust hot water heater (120 degrees or <).
- Poisons—Properly label and safely store poisons.
- Guns—Lock guns in the home in a safe place out of children's reach.
- Prevent falls—Encourage use of window gates on high-rise buildings.

■ PEDIATRIC MEDICAL EMERGENCIES

Seizures

High fever, epilepsy, infections, poisoning, hypoglycemia, trauma (including head trauma,) or decreased levels of oxygen can bring on seizures. Some seizures in children are of unknown cause. They may be brief or prolonged and are rarely life-threatening in children who have them frequently. However, EMT-Bs should consider childhood seizures, including those caused by fever, life-threatening.

Interview the patient or family member to determine if the child has a history of seizures and takes any anti-seizure medication. You should be able to describe the seizure for the ED physician, as this may help determine the cause.

Emergency care of a seizure includes airway management, suctioning, administering 100% oxygen and ventilations as needed, maintaining body heat, monitoring vital signs, and transport. If local protocols allow, consider cooling a child who had a febrile seizure (caused by a rapid rise in body temperature) by removing the child's clothing and covering the child with a towel soaked with tepid water. Carefully monitor the child for shivering, since overcooling the child can result in hypothermia. The significance of fever varies with age. Even the slightest fever in a newborn may be indicative of a life-threatening infection. A fever in an older child may not be as significant.

Poisoning

Children are often poisoned accidentally by ingestion of household products or medications. Poisons can quickly depress the respiratory system and cause respiratory arrest or life-threatening conditions of the circulatory and nervous system. The airway and gastrointestinal track can be burned by corrosive substances ingested or vomited. Some types of poisonings not often associated with adults but common to children are:

- Aspirin—Watch for hyperventilation, vomiting, and sweating. The skin may feel hot. Severe cases cause seizures, coma, and shock.
- Acetaminophen—Many non-prescription medications contain this compound, which causes nausea, vomiting, and heavy perspiration.
- Lead—This poisoning is caused by ingestion of lead-based paint chips or chronic buildup of lead in the body. Watch for nausea with abdominal pain and vomiting. The child may have muscle cramps, headache, muscle weakness, and irritability.
- Cyanide—Apple seeds contain cyanide.
- Petroleum products—The child's vomit or cough will have a distinctive distillate odor (e.g., gasoline, kerosene, heating fuel).

The management of a poisoning involves airway management and oxygen administration; medical control may be contacted for additional advice. Activated charcoal, as discussed in Chapter 11, should be given only with the permission of the ED physician or poison-control center.

Croup and Epiglottitis

Croup is a range of viral illnesses that cause inflammation of the larynx, trachea, and bronchi. Tissues of the upper airway become swollen and restrict the passage of air. It is typically an illness of children 6 months to 4 years of age. It often gets worse at night following an upper respiratory infection. The child will have a mild fever, some hoarseness that develops into a loud "seal bark" cough, and signs of respiratory distress. Patients may also have nasal flaring, retraction of the muscles between the ribs, tugging at the throat, difficulty breathing, restlessness, and cyanosis.

Treatment includes administering humidified oxygen and placing the patient in a position of comfort. Cool night air is helpful to the patient because it reduces the edema in the airway tissues.

Epiglottitis is most commonly caused by a bacterial infection that produces swelling of the epiglottis and partial airway obstruction. The typical patient is between 3 and 7 years old. Because of vaccinations, epiglottitis is occurring much less frequently in children than it did several years ago.

Children with epiglottitis present with a sudden onset of high fever and painful swallowing that causes drooling as the patient attempts to avoid swallowing. The patient often assumes the "tripod" position, sitting upright and leaning forward with the chin thrust outward in a sniffing position, and opens the mouth widely to maintain an open airway.

Epiglottitis can be life-threatening, and all effort should be taken to prevent further aggravation of the patient. Prepare for immediate transport, on the parent's lap if necessary, and provide "blow-by" humidified oxygen. Monitor closely to ensure that the respiratory distress does not degenerate to respiratory failure or arrest. Advise the hospital that you suspect epiglottitis.

Of utmost concern in this instance is that you do not place anything in the child's mouth, including a thermometer, tongue blade, or oral airway. To do so may set off spasms of the larynx and swelling of tissues in the upper airway, causing total obstruction.

Sudden Infant Death Syndrome

Every year in the United States, from 6,500 to 7,500 babies die from **sudden infant death syndrome** (SIDS), which is the unexplained death during sleep of an apparently healthy baby in its first year of life. The peak incidence of SIDS is between 2 and 3 months of age. It is rarely seen in infants older than 6 months and there is often a family history. The greatest incidence occurs during the winter months; there is often a history of a viral illness that was noted 1 to 2 weeks prior to the SIDS. Infants who were premature and who are small for gestational age are at a greater risk for SIDS, as are infants who underwent a stressful delivery that resulted in birth asphyxia, birth trauma, and CNS impairment. Recent studies show that positioning an infant on its side or back rather than face down in the crib reduces the likelihood of SIDS.

When asleep, the typical SIDS patient will show periods of cardiac slowdown and temporary cessation of breathing known as sleep apnea. Eventually, the infant will stop breathing and will not start again on its own. The condition is most commonly discovered in the early morning when the parents attempt to wake the baby.

It is not up to you to diagnose SIDS. Your signal will be that the child is in respiratory or cardiac arrest, and you should treat the child as you would any other patient. Unless there is rigor mortis, severe dependent lividity, decomposition, an obvious mortal injury, decapitation, or an advanced directive, provide resuscitation and let the pronouncement of death come from the hospital.

Ensure that the parents receive emotional support and that they believe that everything possible is being done for the child at the scene and during transport. Parents who lose a child to SIDS often suffer intense guilt feelings from the moment they find the child. Remind them that SIDS occurs to apparently healthy babies who are receiving the best parental care. Never speak with a suspicious or accusative tone, as this may add to their guilt feelings.

Meningitis

Meningitis, which is caused by either a bacterial or a viral infection, is an inflammation of the meninges, the three layers of membranes that cover the brain and spinal cord. It is more common in children than adults, and the majority of the cases are between the ages of 1 month and 5 years. The patient presents with a high fever, lethargy, irritability, headache, stiff neck, and a sensitivity to light. The child may have an accompanying rash. In infants, the fontanelles may be bulging, unless the child is dehydrated. Any movement may be painful, and seizures may occur.

Emergency care of these patients involves managing the ABCs and the symptoms to make the patient more comfortable. Since meningitis is a TRUE emergency, transport the patient to the hospital as soon as possible. Make sure you take body substance isolation precautions; avoid oral secretions by using a mask and eye shield. If you are exposed to meningitis, check with your service's infection-control liaison to find out if the hospital ED recommends that you receive follow-up care.

■ DEALING WITH "SPECIAL NEEDS"

Over the years, medical care has improved significantly, allowing many children who would formerly have died to live. Oftentimes, however, these children have special needs that must be met. Children with special needs are those premature infants with lung disease and children with heart disease, neurological disease, chronic diseases, or altered function from birth.

Often these children are able to live at home with their parents and with the aid of various medical devices. When things go wrong, EMT-Bs are called to respond and often they must deal with complicated medical technologies such as tracheostomy tubes, artificial ventilators, central IV lines, gastrostomy tubes and gastric feeding, and shunts. The children's parents will be familiar with the devices and will be a useful resource to you.

Tracheostomy Tubes

Children who have been placed on a ventilator for a prolonged period often have a tracheostomy tube in place. The tube is placed in the trachea and is designed to create an open airway. The typical complications include obstruction, bleeding from or around the tube, an air leak around the tube, an infection, or a dislodged tube. Emergency care consists of assuring an open airway, suctioning the tube, allowing the child to remain in a position of comfort, and transport to the hospital.

Home Artificial Ventilators

More and more ventilators are being placed in the home for use by special-needs patients. Often, parents face mechanical problems accompanying the use of these devices that lead to a call for EMS. Emergency care includes maintaining an open airway, artificially ventilating with a BVM and oxygen, and then transport to the hospital. Some communities are also prepared for power outages and arrange for emergency power for patients on home ventilators.

Central Intravenous Lines

Unlike peripheral IV lines (IVs in the arms, legs, or external jugular vein), central IV lines may be left in place for long-term use. Used for medication administration, a central IV line is placed close to the heart. Possible complications of central lines include an infection, bleeding, clotting, or a cracked line. Emergency care includes applying pressure, if there is bleeding, and transporting the patient.

Gastrostomy Tubes and Gastric Feeding

A gastrostomy tube is placed through the abdominal wall directly into the stomach. The tube is used to feed a patient who cannot eat anything by mouth. Emergency care includes being alert for altered mental status in a diabetic patient. When unable to eat, diabetic children can quickly become hypoglycemic. Emergency care includes assuring an open airway, suctioning as needed, providing oxygen, and transporting the patient in either a sitting position or lying on the right side with the head elevated to reduce the risk of aspiration.

Shunts

Patients who have excess cerebrospinal (CSF) in the brain often have a drainage device called a shunt inserted. Most all shunts drain from the brain to the abdominal cavity. Should there be a malfunction of the shunt or an infection, pressure inside the skull will rise, causing headache, vomiting, and/or an altered mental status. These patients are prone to respiratory arrest. Emergency care includes maintaining an open airway, ventilating with a BVM and high-concentration oxygen, and transporting.

■ EMOTIONAL RESPONSE OF THE FAMILY AND EMT-B

Parents may react in one of many ways when confronted with a sudden illness or injury of a child. Their first reaction may be one of denial or shock. Some parents will react by crying, screaming, or becoming angry. Another reaction is self-blame and guilt. In all instances, be calm, reassuring, and supportive. Use simple language to explain what has happened and what is being done to and for the child.

If the parents are able to do so, use them to help you provide care and talk to their child

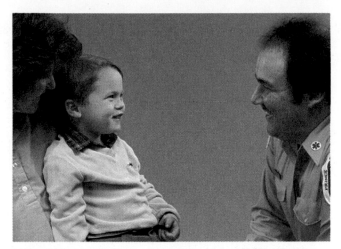

FIGURE 14–7 Have the parent hold the child in a position of comfort to involve the parent and soothe the child.

(Figure 14–7). The most effective method may be to have the parent hold the child in a position of comfort in the lap, if appropriate, during assessment and treatment. Offer as much emotional support as possible to the parent. However, don't forget that your patient is the child, not the parent. Avoid allowing communications with the parent to distract you from the child's care.

It is well known that pediatric calls can be among the most stressful for EMT-Bs, even when they are uneventful. EMT-Bs who have children often identify their patients with their own children. Other EMT-Bs have no experience with children and feel anxiety about talking to and treating them. However, the skills of communicating and treating children can be learned and applied. Often the EMT-B who starts out knowing nothing about children turns out to have a real knack for dealing with them. Most of the care of children consists of applying what you have learned about the care of adult patients and combining it with knowledge of key differences in the developmental characteristics and the anatomy and physiology of children.

Often the most serious stresses an EMT-B faces result from pediatric calls that involve a critically ill, critically injured, or abused child. Calls involving an accidental death of a child or an MCI with numerous children are very stressful. Such calls are, fortunately, rare and can be prepared for with additional training.

When you have had an experience like this, talk with other EMT-Bs. You may first think that you can handle the stress or sorrow by yourself, but as an experienced EMT-B you know better. Unless you resolve the impact of stressful events, the problems created will compound and could lead to "burn out." Contact your local Critical Incident Stress Debriefing (CISD) team for assistance after these incidents.

CHAPTER REVIEW

■ SUMMARY

The preparers of the new curriculum realized that pediatric emergencies pose special problems for the EMT-B and have increased course time for the study of pediatric emergencies. Although children often have the same medical problems as adults, the difference in treating pediatric patients often lies in understanding the differences in their anatomy, physiology, mental development, and psychology. In addition, learning to deal with the strong emotions that accompany the treatment of children can help you treat them more effectively.

■ REVIEW QUESTIONS

1. Explain how the anatomy and physiology of infants and children differ from that of adults.
2. Discuss the different strategies used for dealing with children of each age group.
3. Describe the treatment of a foreign body airway obstruction in an infant versus a child.
4. Explain why suspicion of child abuse should not affect the care you provide for an infant or child.
5. Discuss the cause of shaken baby syndrome.
6. Describe the care of the pediatric patient who is in shock.
7. Define SIDS and describe how it is caused.
8. What is the difference between croup and epiglottitis?
9. Explain why meningitis can be a hazard to the EMT-B.
10. Describe what a shunt is and why it would be used.

CHAPTER 15

Obstetrics and Gynecology

■ *Time has changed many of the things we have practiced as EMTs. The theories behind the use of PASG and capillary refill have changed, as have our patient assessment practices. One thing that has not*

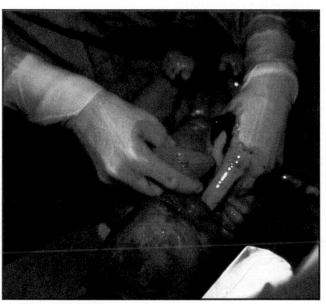

changed significantly (over thousands of years) is the process of childbirth. This chapter will review the anatomy relating to childbirth, childbirth procedures, complications, and other special considerations.

MAKING THE TRANSITION

- ■ There are no significant changes in the procedures involving childbirth.
- ■ The EMT-B may call on medical direction for assistance in normal and abnormal delivery situations.
- ■ The curriculum includes identification of and treatment for meconium (fecal matter) in amniotic fluid.

OBJECTIVES

The numbered objectives below are from the United States Department of Transportation 1994 EMT-Basic National Standard Curriculum.

■ KNOWLEDGE AND ATTITUDE

At the completion of this lesson, you should be able to:

1. Identify the following structures: uterus, vagina, fetus, placenta, umbilical cord, amniotic sac, perineum. (pp. 303, 304)
2. Identify and explain the use of the contents of an obstetrics kit. (p. 306)
3. Identify predelivery emergencies. (pp. 303–305)
4. State indications of an imminent delivery. (p. 306)
5. Differentiate the emergency medical care provided to a patient with predelivery emergencies from a normal delivery. (pp. 303–309)
6. State the steps in the predelivery preparation of the mother. (pp. 306, 307, 309)
7. Establish the relationship between body substance isolation and childbirth. (pp. 306, 307)
8. State the steps to assist in the delivery. (pp. 307–309)
9. Describe care of the baby as the head appears. (p. 307)
10. Describe how and when to cut the umbilical cord. (p. 307, 309)
11. Discuss the steps in the delivery of the placenta. (p. 309)
12. List the steps in the emergency medical care of the mother post-delivery. (p. 309)
13. Summarize neonatal resuscitation procedures. (p. 310)
14. Describe the procedures for the following abnormal deliveries: breech birth, prolapsed cord, limb presentation. (pp. 310–311)
15. Differentiate the special considerations for multiple births. (p. 312)
16. Describe special considerations of meconium. (pp. 312–313)
17. Describe special considerations of a premature baby. (p. 312)
18. Discuss the emergency medical care of a patient with a gynecological emergency. (pp. 312–313)
19. Explain the rationale for understanding the implications of treating two patients (mother and baby). (pp. 305–306, 309–310, 311)

■ SKILLS

1. Demonstrate the steps to assist in the normal cephalic delivery.
2. Demonstrate necessary care procedures of the fetus as the head appears.
3. Demonstrate infant neonatal procedures.
4. Demonstrate post-delivery care of infant.
5. Demonstrate how and when to cut the umbilical cord.
6. Attend to the steps in the delivery of the placenta.
7. Demonstrate the post-delivery care of the mother.
8. Demonstrate the procedures for the following abnormal deliveries: vaginal bleeding, breech birth, prolapsed cord, limb presentation.
9. Demonstrate the steps in the emergency medical care of the mother with excessive bleeding.
10. Demonstrate completing a prehospital care report for patients with obstetrical/gynecological emergencies.

Your EMS unit is dispatched to a call for a woman who is full-term and experiencing labor pains. Although you have delivered babies before, your heart races as you suspect it always will on maternity calls. Your partner shares your excitement.

Your **scene size-up** is uneventful. No signs of danger are noted as you approach with BSI equipment, the first-in bag, and an OB kit. Your excitement is dashed when the first words from the mother are "Help me, please, something is wrong!"

You and your partner move the patient to a supine position. Your partner begins a history of the pregnancy. It is her third child; two others were delivered without problems. The mother's physician was concerned about the baby's position and was considering a Cesarean section if there was no change by next week.

She is approximately 40 weeks pregnant, feels the urge to move her bowels, and has strong contractions about 4 minutes apart.

Your heart sinks even further when you observe the umbilical cord, which is prolapsed from the woman's vagina.

Your experience kicks in as you don sterile gloves and move your hand into the patient's vagina. You must get the head off the cord in order for the baby to have a chance. You are able to move the head back slightly and feel pulsation in the cord. Your partner prepares the stretcher so the patient will be in a head-lower-than-pelvis position. He applies oxygen, and transport is begun immediately. Your partner radios medical control at the receiving hospital. A team is waiting for your arrival. A short time later a baby girl is born. ■

■ ANATOMY OF CHILDBIRTH

The **uterus** is the organ which contains the **fetus**, or developing child. Contractions of the uterus expel the infant during labor. Within the uterus is the **amniotic sac**, which contains fluid (amniotic fluid) in which the fetus "floats" for protection during development. The **placenta** is attached to the wall of the uterus. The placenta is responsible for distribution of oxygen, nutrients, and other substances between the mother and fetus. It also serves to remove waste products from the fetus. The fetus and placenta are connected by the **umbilical cord**. The **cervix** is the inferior opening of the uterus. The birth canal includes the cervix and the **vagina**, from which the baby is born. The **perineum** is the area of skin between the vagina and anus which may be torn during delivery. The anatomy of childbirth is shown in Figure 15–1.

The part of the infant that appears at the vaginal opening first is called the **presenting part**. In most cases this is the head. In abnormal delivery, an arm, leg, the buttocks, or umbilical cord may present first. **Crowning** is when the presenting part presses against the vaginal opening. This causes the vagina to appear as if it were bulging and is the first appearance of the infant. At some time around the beginning of labor a "bloody show" may be seen. This mixture of blood and mucus comes from the cervix and is considered normal.

Labor is a process in which uterine muscles begin a series of contractions resulting in the delivery of the infant and eventually the placenta. The stages of labor are shown in Figure 15–2.

■ PREDELIVERY EMERGENCIES

There are several emergencies that may occur during the nine months of pregnancy before the actual delivery. These include miscarriage, seizures during pregnancy, and trauma.

Miscarriage (Spontaneous Abortion)

A **miscarriage** is a delivery of the fetus (or products of conception) before the baby could live outside the mother's body. If this happens on its own, it is called a **spontaneous abortion**. Induced abortions are those in which intentional actions are taken to terminate the pregnancy.

■ Patient Assessment **Miscarriage**

Signs and Symptoms
- Abdominal pain which may resemble labor pains
- Vaginal bleeding
- Discharge of tissue and blood from the vagina ■

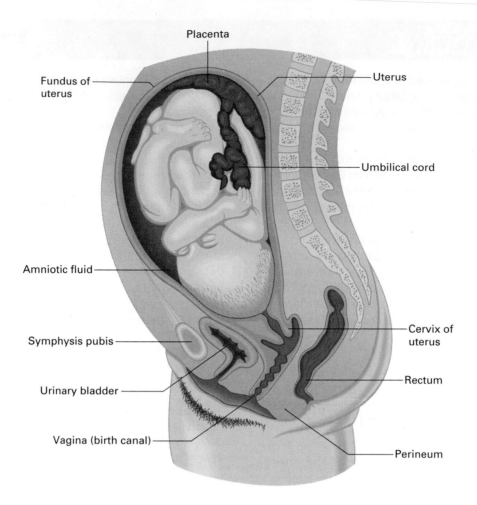

FIGURE 15–1 Anatomy of childbirth.

Patient Care **Miscarriage**

Emergency Care Steps
1. Complete a patient assessment including vital signs.
2. Apply high-concentration oxygen. Be alert for shock.
3. Use vaginal pads to absorb blood. Do not pack vagina.
4. Transport as soon as possible.
5. Save all tissue that has been expelled from the vagina and bring it to the hospital.
6. Provide emotional support. ■

Seizures During Pregnancy
Seizures may occur during pregnancy. They usually occur late in the course of the pregnancy and are associated with elevated blood pressure and fluid accumulation, which may be seen in the extremities. Although it is not included as part of the new EMT-B curriculum, you will recognize these signs and symptoms as part of a condition called **eclampsia**.

Patient Assessment **Seizures During Pregnancy**

Signs and Symptoms
- Watch for elevated blood pressure. The risk of **abruptio placentae** (the placenta prematurely separating from the uterine wall) increases with elevated blood pressure.
- Excess weight gain
- Extreme swelling of the face, hands, ankles, and feet
- Headache ■

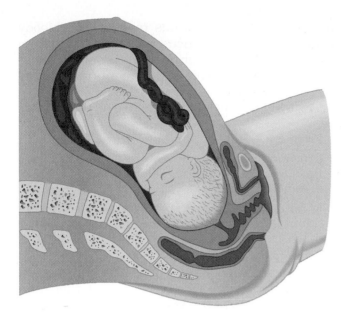

FIRST STAGE:
First uterine contraction to dilation of cervix

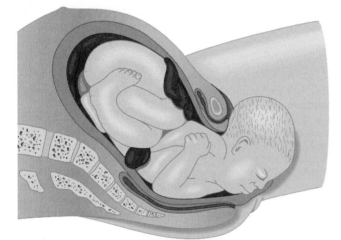

SECOND STAGE:
Birth of baby or expulsion

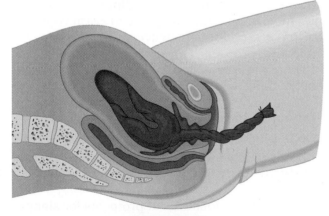

THIRD STAGE
Delivery of placenta

FIGURE 15–2 Three stages of labor.

■ **Patient Care** Seizures During Pregnancy

Emergency Care Steps
1. Maintain an open airway. Administer oxygen.
2. Complete a full patient assessment.
3. Transport patient positioned on her left side.
4. Handle gently. Rough handling may increase the chance of seizure.
5. Have suction and a delivery kit ready. ■

Trauma During Pregnancy

Trauma may occur to anyone, including those who are pregnant. There are few differences in patient assessment or emergency care simply because the patient is pregnant.

■ **Patient Assessment** Trauma During Pregnancy

● Perform the full patient assessment sequence.
● You may be able to observe a patient and determine if she is pregnant. The fact that a woman is pregnant will usually be volunteered out of concern for the baby.
● Shock (hypoperfusion) may be more difficult to assess in the pregnant patient. The pulse may be naturally 10–15 beats per minutes faster than in the non-pregnant female. Additionally, due to an increase in blood volume of up to 48%, signs of shock may not appear until a considerable blood volume has been lost. ■

■ **Patient Care** Trauma During Pregnancy

Emergency Care Steps
1. Perform emergency care based on the signs and symptoms exhibited by the patient. A general rule is "What's good for the mother is good for the baby."
2. Since the patient's oxygen demand is higher (due to pregnancy), administer high-concentration oxygen by nonrebreather mask.
3. Transport as soon as possible. The patient should be transported on her left side. This is because a near-term fetus will press against the mother's inferior vena cava which runs along the right side of the spine. Compression of this major vein will reduce blood flow to the heart with a resulting decrease in blood pressure. Placing the mother on the left eliminates this potential complication. If the mother must be immobilized, as is often the case, secure the

mother firmly to the spine board and place padding under the right side of the board, which causes a shift to the left but still maintains immobilization.

4. Provide emotional support. The mother will naturally worry about her unborn child. ■

■ CHILDBIRTH

Normal Delivery

Childbirth is a natural process. Unlike many other situations encountered by an EMT-B, childbirth is not a result of a disease state or injury. At the scene of a call for impending childbirth, your main functions will be determining whether there is time for transport to the hospital before delivery and/or supporting and assisting the mother during delivery.

Predelivery Considerations

In general, it is best to transport the mother and have the delivery occur at a hospital. This will be done in many cases. However, delivery will be performed at the scene for two reasons: The delivery is imminent or there are situations such as severe storms that prevent you from transporting the patient to the hospital in a reasonable time. Asking the questions below and performing a brief physical examination will help you make a transportation decision.

- What is your name?
- Are you pregnant? How long have you been pregnant? Is this your first pregnancy?
- Have there been any complications with this pregnancy?
- Are there any contractions or pain?
- Have you observed any bleeding or discharge?
- Do you feel the need to push?
- Do you feel as if you are having a bowel movement?

During first pregnancies, women may be in labor for 16 hours or longer. However, not all first pregnancies will take that long. Subsequent pregnancies generally have shorter periods of labor. When labor pains are two or three minutes apart and last 30 seconds to one minute, delivery of the baby may be imminent.

It will not be unusual to find clear or slightly bloody fluid coming from the vagina during the process of labor. The fluids may be the "bloody show," which is the mucus plug separating from the cervix, or the rupturing of the amniotic sac or "bag of waters." These are both normal events during pregnancy.

You will also need to examine the patient for:

- Frequency and duration of contractions.
- Crowning or bulging of the presenting part from the vagina during contractions. *This is a sign of imminent delivery.*
- Rigidity of the uterus that may be felt through the skin. This area will feel more rigid as the delivery of the baby nears.

Remember that your actions may cause alarm or be embarrassing for the mother, father, and anyone else present. Do your best to explain everything you do and to protect the patient's modesty.

With few exceptions, it will not be necessary to place your hand or fingers in the vagina. It is never necessary to check for cervical dilation.

Preceptor Pearl

It is not uncommon to find patients and family members who are very nervous. This is to be expected. This emotion will make examination of the patient and subsequent decision making very difficult. The patient or her family may want to rush to the hospital; or they may have the opposite feeling that there just isn't time. Encourage new EMT-Bs to carefully and objectively examine the patient and obtain a history. This is the proper basis for a transportation decision. Assure the patient and family that you are equipped and trained both to evaluate the situation and to handle the delivery at home or in the ambulance. ❖

When preparing for delivery, use body substance isolation precautions. Gloves, eye protection, face mask, and a gown are appropriate. Also have a childbirth delivery kit at your side (Table 15–1).

There are a few "don'ts" involved in the delivery of a child:

- Do not let the mother go to the bathroom.
- Do not hold the mother's legs together.
- Do not touch the patient's vaginal area except during delivery and with a partner present.

Remember to follow local protocols for signs of impending delivery. Medical direction should be consulted if required by protocol or for advice when needed.

TABLE 15–1 Contents of a Sterile, Disposable Obstetric Kit

Surgical scissors

Hemostats or cord clamps

Umbilical tape or sterilized cord

Bulb syringe

Towels

2 × 10 gauze sponges

Sterile gloves

One baby blanket

Sanitary napkins

Plastic bag

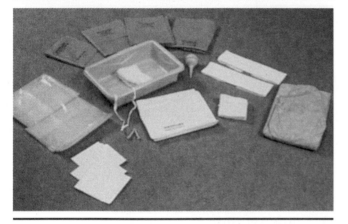

Delivery

The following steps outline the procedure for assisting with childbirth (Figure 15–3).

1. Take body substance isolation precautions (gloves, mask, eye protection, and gown).
2. Have the mother lie with knees drawn up and spread apart. Elevate the buttocks with a blanket or pillow.
3. Create a sterile field around the vaginal opening. This may be done with drapes or towels found in the OB kit (Figure 15–4).
4. When the infant's head appears (crowning), place your fingers on the bony part of the infant's skull. This will prevent an explosive delivery. Do not place your fingers on the soft fontanelles or face.
5. As the infant's head appears, make sure the amniotic sac is broken. If it is intact, break the membrane and pull it away from the infant's face. As the head continues to emerge, make sure the umbilical cord is not wrapped around the infant's neck. If this is the case, slip the cord over the infant's shoulder. If this is not

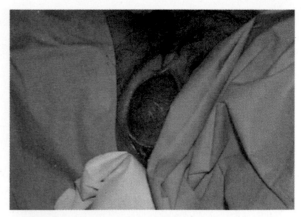

A. Crowning.

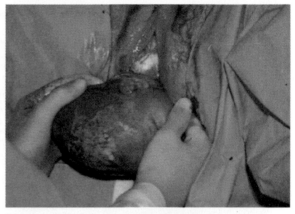

B. Head delivers and turns.

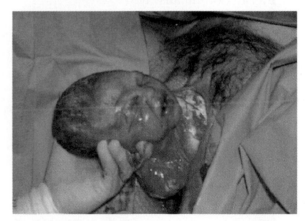

C. Shoulders deliver.

FIGURE 15–3 Process of normal childbirth. *(continued on next page)*

possible, clamp the cord in two places and cut between, and unwrap the cord immediately.

6. After the infant's head delivers, support the head and suction the mouth two or three times, then the nostrils. It is important to suction the mouth before the nose. Suctioning the nose first may cause the infant to gasp and suck fluid from the mouth into the lungs.

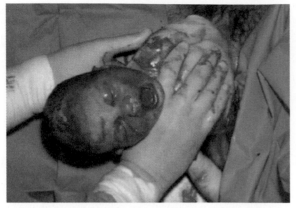

D. Chest delivers.

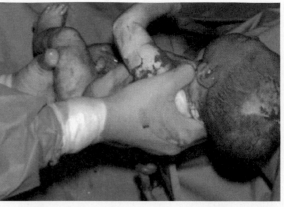

E. Infant delivered.

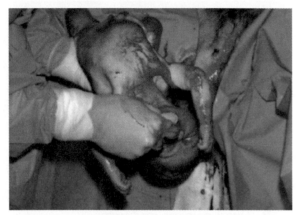

F. Suctioning airway.

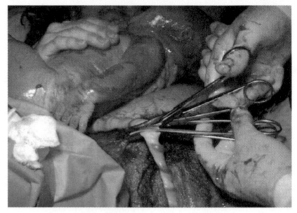

G. Cutting of cord.

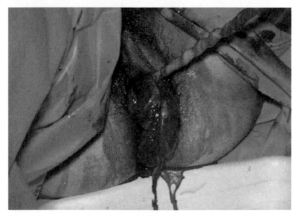

H. Placenta begins delivery.

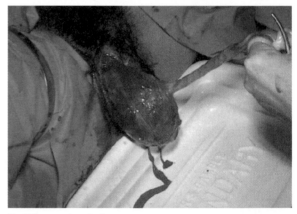

I. Placenta delivers.

FIGURE 15–3 *(continued)*

Use the bulb syringe found in the OB kit. Expel air from the bulb syringe before introducing it into the infant's nose or mouth.

7. Support the torso, body, and legs of the infant as each appears. Use both hands. Securely hold the baby and wipe the blood and mucus from the mouth and nose of the infant. Use the bulb syringe again on the mouth and nose (Figure 15–5).

8. Warmth is very important. Wrap the infant in a warm blanket and place it on its side, at the level of the vagina until the cord is cut. The infant's head should be slightly lower than its trunk.

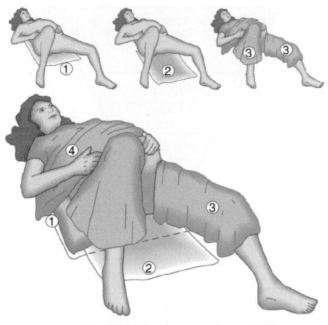

PLACEMENT OF SHEETS OR TOWELS
① One under the buttocks
② One under the vaginal opening
③ One over each thigh
④ One over the abdomen

FIGURE 15–4 Preparing the mother for delivery.

9. When the pulsations cease in the umbilical cord, place two clamps (or thick ties) on the cord, the first being approximately four finger widths from the infant. Cut between the clamps. Your partner should continue to monitor and care for the infant.

10. While preparing for transportation, watch for delivery of the placenta. If it delivers, wrap it in a towel, then place it in a plastic bag. Bring

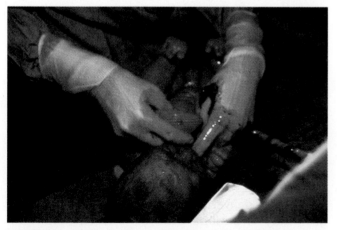

FIGURE 15–5 Suction the mouth, then the nose, of the newborn.

Control Bleeding

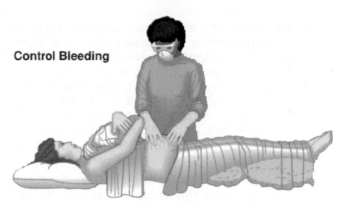

FIGURE 15–6 After delivery of the placenta, massaging the uterus helps control vaginal bleeding.

the placenta to the hospital with the mother and infant.

11. There may be vaginal bleeding after delivery. Some experts state that up to 500 cc is not unusual. Do not let normal amounts of bleeding place undue stress on you and the new family. Place a sterile pad over the vagina and have the mother lower and hold her legs together.

12. Record time of delivery and begin transport.

13. If bleeding is profuse, massaging the uterus may help control the bleeding (Figure 15–6). Place your open hand on the mother's abdomen above the pubis. Massage in a kneading motion over the area. Treat for shock (hypoperfusion) and transport, performing the massage en route.

Care of the Newborn

Care of the newborn after delivery is very important. Although a seemingly small task, drying and keeping the infant warm is crucial. Wrap the infant in blankets and cover the top of the head. Place the infant in a position on its side with the head slightly lower than the trunk. Repeat suctioning as necessary.

Assessment of the Newborn

There are five areas in which the newborn should be assessed. Ideally, this should be done one minute after birth and again five minutes after birth. *This assessment should not take the place of resuscitation or care of the newborn.* This may be performed by yourself or by a partner while care is ongoing.

- Appearance—The infant may be pink, blue, or some combination of the two colors. A baby that is all blue should be evaluated carefully for the need for resuscitation. Some infants are born with a pink torso and blue extremities. This will usually correct itself in a few minutes. Most important is the change over time: A baby who was bluish and becomes pink is doing better, while a baby who shows no change or becomes bluer requires urgent care.

- Pulse—The pulse may be determined with a stethoscope over the heart. An infant should have a pulse of at least 100/minute, but this may be as high as 180/min. It is considered a problem when the pulse gets below 100/min. The section below on resuscitation of the newborn explains this further.

- Grimace—When the infant is flicked on the foot, there should be some response. The ideal response is vigorous motion and crying. You may see some motion or crying or no response at all.

- Activity—There should be some movement of the extremities. This may range from no movement to some slight flexion to active motion.

- Respiratory effort—This is an observation of the ease of breathing. The infant's crying helps make this determination. Strong crying requires air movement and indicates adequate breathing. Notice chest expansion and the effort required by the baby to breathe.

Resuscitation of the Newborn

True resuscitation of the newborn is rarely required. In most cases, some very simple measures will cause the newborn to respond and thrive.

An inverted pyramid is used to describe the actions taken, in order, during resuscitation (Figure 15–7). The pyramid shape is broader on the top indicating that the most commonly successful interventions are the least invasive. As you work down through the levels of the pyramid, the procedures become more invasive. The following steps outline the procedure for resuscitation of the newborn.

1. The infant should begin breathing within about 30 seconds. If breathing does not begin spontaneously, stimulate the infant to breathe by gently, but vigorously, rubbing the infant's back. If this fails, flick the soles of the infant's feet with your finger.

2. If the infant's breathing is absent, shallow, or slow, begin artificial respiration. Use gentle

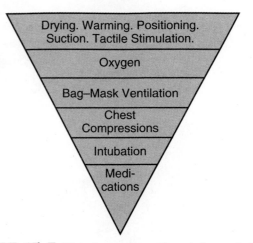

FIGURE 15–7 The American Heart Association's inverted pyramid of neonatal resuscitation showing approximate relative frequencies of neonatal resuscitative efforts. Note that a majority of infants respond to simple measures. (Source: American Heart Association).

puffs if using a mouth-to-mask technique, or a gentle squeeze on an infant BVM. Ventilate at a rate of 40 to 60 per minute. Reassess the infant's respiratory effort frequently.

3. Assess the infant's heart rate. If the infant's heart rate is below 100/min., assist ventilations. If the heart rate is below 80/min. and hasn't increased after ventilations, begin chest compressions. Begin compressions immediately at a rate of 120/min. on any infant with a pulse below 60 (Figure 15–8).

    It may seem unusual providing compressions in the presence of a pulse. The low pulse rates are dangerous for an infant, and compressions will help maintain circulation. The infant may regain adequate pulse and respirations after ventilations and compressions.

4. In cases where there are adequate pulse and respirations but the infant has cyanosis (especially of the torso), use oxygen tubing to deliver 10 to 15 lpm by the "blow-by" method. Place the tubing near, but not directly into, the infant's face. This provides supplemental oxygen to the infant.

■ ABNORMAL DELIVERIES

While most deliveries are considered normal, there are many situations that are termed abnormal. These include prolapsed umbilical cord, breech birth, and limb presentation.

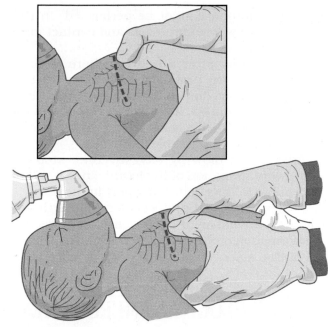

FIGURE 15-8 Chest compressions in the newborn should be delivered at a rate of 120 compressions per minute, midsternum, with two thumbs, fingers supporting the back, at a depth of ½ to ¾ inch.

Prolapsed Umbilical Cord

Patient Assessment Prolapsed Umbilical Cord

When the umbilical cord presents through the birth canal before delivery of the head this is known as a **prolapsed umbilical cord**. This is a serious emergency which endangers the life of the unborn fetus. ■

Patient Care Prolapsed Umbilical Cord

Emergency Care Steps
1. Position the mother in a head-down position. Administer high-concentration oxygen to the mother.
2. Insert a sterile, gloved hand into the vagina. This is one of the few situations where it is appropriate to do this. The purpose is to push the presenting part of the fetus off the cord. When this is successful you should be able to feel pulsations in the cord. This action is critical to the survival of the baby.
3. Immediately transport the patient. Do not release pressure until relieved at a medical facility. ■

Breech Presentation

Patient Assessment Breech Presentation

A breech birth occurs when the buttocks or lower extremities are the presenting part. While it is not impossible for a breech baby to deliver, the complication rate is high. The risk of prolapsed cord is greater in a breech delivery. ■

Patient Care Breech Presentation

Emergency Care Steps
1. Place the mother in a head-down position. If a prolapsed cord exists, begin care for that emergency.
2. Place the mother on high-concentration oxygen and begin immediate transportation. ■

Limb Presentation

Patient Assessment Limb Presentation

This condition is identified by a single limb (arm or leg) protruding from the vagina. Limb presentation requires immediate intervention by an obstetrician. Delivery should not be attempted in the field. ■

Patient Care Limb Presentation

Emergency Care Steps
1. Place the mother in a head-down position. Administer high-concentration oxygen.
2. Initiate immediate transportation. ■

■ CHILDBIRTH COMPLICATIONS

Meconium

Normal amniotic fluid is clear in color. You may observe a green or brownish-yellow thick substance in the amniotic fluid. This is **meconium**. Meconium is the result of fetal defecation and is usually a sign of fetal distress.

Meconium must be suctioned immediately. If this substance is observed, suction the baby's mouth, then nose, thoroughly before any more of the infant delivers. Never stimulate breathing until the infant has been suctioned thoroughly. Infants born with meconium in the amniotic fluid are at greater risk for respiratory complications after birth.

Multiple Births

Multiple births are not a complication of pregnancy, provided the deliveries are normal. It is a normal condition when more than one fetus is to be delivered. When a woman has been under a doctor's care, she will very likely be aware that she is carrying more than one baby. Other indicators of impending multiple births are an abnormally large abdomen or an abdomen that remains abnormally large after the delivery of the first infant.

Twins are the most frequent multiple birth. The procedure for delivery of each infant is identical to that of a single birth. The mother may remain in labor to deliver the second child. With twins, you may find that there are one or two placentas. After each delivery, clamp and cut the umbilical cord.

An infant who is one of multiple births may have a smaller birth weight than a single birth. Make sure that the infants are kept warm. In the event that they require resuscitation, remember that you may have to resuscitate two (or more) infants and care for the mother. Additional help may be required: Call for assistance early if necessary.

Premature Births

Premature births are those that occur before the 37th week of gestation or when infants are born weighing less than 5½ pounds. You may determine the birth is premature from information the mother tells you and your observation of the infant. Premature infants have heads that are larger in proportion to the rest of their bodies than are those of full-term infants. Their bodies are also smaller, thinner, and redder.

Premature infants are at increased risk for hypothermia, even more so than a full-term infant. Many systems use foil or insulating plastic wrap in addition to blankets for warmth. However, never let sharp surfaces of the foil come in contact with the infant's skin.

Provide resuscitation as needed, based in the inverted pyramid described earlier. There may be some cases where an infant is so premature

that resuscitation cannot be performed. In this situation, follow local protocols and contact medical direction.

Occasionally after a delivery there is some blood loss from the umbilical cord. Since the premature infant has limited blood supply, this blood loss must be stopped. If blood is leaking from the end of the cord, tie the cord again, this time closer to the infant to stop the bleeding.

Administer blow-by oxygen. Take steps to reduce contamination of the infant since it will be susceptible to infection. Transport immediately.

Follow your local protocols for childbirth and delivery. Remember to contact medical direction for information on delivery of normal births, abnormal births, and complications you may encounter.

■ GYNECOLOGICAL EMERGENCIES

Vaginal Bleeding

■ Patient Assessment Vaginal Bleeding

Bleeding from the vagina may range from very minor to severe. Vaginal bleeding may occur in non-pregnant women or at any time during pregnancy. It is important to remember that the cause of the bleeding may not be determined in the field. Field priorities are the prevention, recognition, and treatment for shock (hypoperfusion). ■

■ Patient Care Vaginal Bleeding

Emergency Care Steps
1. Take body substance isolation precautions.
2. Assure an adequate airway and administer high-concentration oxygen.
3. Treat for shock and transport immediately. ■

Trauma to the External Genitalia

■ Patient Assessment Trauma to the External Genitalia

Traumatic injuries to the female external genitalia may result in profuse bleeding and severe pain.

Consider the patient's modesty when examining and caring for a wound to this area. ■

■ Patient Care Trauma to the External Genitalia

Emergency Care Steps
1. Control the airway and administer oxygen. Be alert for signs of shock.
2. Control any bleeding with direct pressure. Do not pack or insert anything into the vagina. ■

Sexual Assault

A patient who alleges sexual assault requires care for all physical wounds as well as compassionate psychological care. Consideration must also be given to preservation of evidence when possible.

■ Patient Assessment Sexual Assault

Since this is a crime scene, be sure it is safe before entering.

● Complete the normal assessment sequence, with consideration of the psychological needs of the patient. Assessment should be performed with preservation of evidence in mind. ■

■ Patient Care Sexual Assault

Emergency Care Steps
1. Maintain body substance isolation. Assure an open airway.
2. Maintain a nonjudgmental attitude during the history and physical examinations. Examine the external genitalia only if profuse bleeding is present. A female EMT-B attending may be helpful.
3. Take actions to preserve the crime scene. Discourage the patient from voiding, bathing, or cleaning wounds. However, actions to preserve the crime scene should never take precedence over life-saving care.
4. Follow local reporting requirements for assault/sexual assault cases. ■

CHAPTER REVIEW

■ SUMMARY

Obstetric and gynecologic complications will not be the most common emergency to which you will be called.

Pregnancy and childbirth are natural events. It is the primary role of the EMT-B to support the mother during the delivery and to care for the mother and newborn after birth. Sometimes there is more than one birth. There are also complications of delivery that you must be familiar with. These include prolapsed cord, breech birth, limb presentation, and premature birth. Babies may also be born with meconium (fecal matter) in the amniotic fluid.

Emergencies may also occur throughout the pregnancy. There may be a miscarriage, or spontaneous abortion. Later in the pregnancy there may be seizures or vaginal bleeding. There may be trauma to a pregnant woman at any time during the pregnancy. As an EMT-B, you will be required to provide care for all of these emergencies.

■ REVIEW QUESTIONS

1. Describe the anatomy of childbirth.
2. Define the following emergencies and how you would care for them:
   miscarriage
   seizure during pregnancy
   vaginal bleeding (late in pregnancy)
   trauma during pregnancy
3. Describe the events of a normal delivery and your role as an EMT-B assisting in the delivery.

4. What is the inverted pyramid? Describe when ventilations and ventilations plus compressions are required in resuscitation of the newborn.

5. Describe what you might see when assessing a healthy newborn for appearance, pulse, grimace, activity, and respiratory effort.

6. For the following complications of delivery explain how the infant would present and the emergency care you would provide:
prolapsed cord
breech presentation
limb presentation

7. Describe the care for a traumatic wound to the external female genitalia.

Lifting and Moving Patients

■ Lifting and moving patients is an important part of emergency care. The methods chosen to transport a patient will depend on location, terrain, patient condition, and more. A wide variety of patient-carrying devices are available, each with a specific purpose.

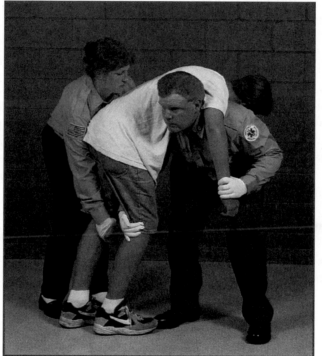

This chapter reviews the options available in lifting and moving patients. The chapter will also update the reader to the new EMT-B curriculum, which pays extra attention to safe lifting, as well as classifying emergent, urgent, and non-urgent moves.

MAKING THE TRANSITION

- Use of proper body mechanics during lifting and moving is explained.
- Safe lifting, reaching, pushing, and pulling are emphasized.
- Emergent, urgent, and non-urgent moves are classified.

Numbered objectives below are from the United States Department of Transportation 1994 EMT-Basic National Standard Curriculum. Objectives with colored bullets that follow in italics are from the EMT-Basic Transitional Program.

■ KNOWLEDGE AND ATTITUDE

At the completion of this chapter, you should be able to:

1. Define body mechanics. (p. 317)
2. Discuss the guidelines and safety precautions that need to be followed when lifting a patient. (pp. 317–318)
3. Describe the safe lifting of cots and stretchers. (pp. 319, 327, 328–329)
4. Describe the guidelines and safety precautions for carrying patients and/or equipment. (pp. 318–319)
5. Discuss one-handed carrying techniques. (p. 321)
6. Describe correct and safe carrying procedures on stairs. (pp. 327, 330)
7. State the guidelines for reaching and their application. (p. 318)
8. Describe correct reaching for log rolls. (pp. 318, 319)
9. State the guidelines for pushing and pulling. (p. 318)
10. Discuss the general considerations of moving patients. (p. 317)
11. State three situations that may require the use of an emergency move. (p. 319)

12. Identify the following patient-carrying devices: wheeled ambulance stretcher, portable ambulance stretcher, stair chair, scoop stretcher, long spine board, basket stretcher, and flexible stretcher. (pp. 319, 326–327, 330–331)
13. Explain the rationale for properly lifting and moving patients. (pp. 315, 317)
● *Relate the body mechanics associated with patient care and its impact on the EMT-Basic.* (pp. 315, 317–318)
● *Value the rationale for body mechanics playing an important role in the well-being of the EMT-Basic.* (pp. 315, 317–318)

■ SKILLS

1. Working with a partner, prepare each of the following devices for use, transfer a patient to the device, properly position the patient on the device, move the device to the ambulance, and load the patient into the ambulance: wheeled ambulance stretcher, portable ambulance stretcher, stair chair, scoop stretcher, long spine board, basket stretcher, flexible stretcher.
2. Working with a partner, the EMT-B will demonstrate techniques for the transfer of a patient from an ambulance stretcher to a hospital stretcher.
● *Demonstrate proper body mechanics.*

Your EMS unit is called to a patient with respiratory difficulty in an outlying part of your district. You arrive to find a long driveway and an intimidating set of stairs into the house. You begin a **scene size-up** and hope your patient is relatively light.

The dispatch information was correct. The patient is in considerable respiratory distress. After you and your partner finish the **initial assessment**, your partner, after contacting medical control, begins assisting with the patient's medication while you prepare for transport. Recalling the long set of stairs and incorporating the patient's condition into your plan, you decide to use a stair chair.

As you leave the house to get the chair, you notice some garden tools on the steps. You move them to prevent falling while carrying the patient. The stretcher is moved to a position on level ground where the patient can be transferred from the chair safely. Since it is chilly, you bring a blanket to cover the patient during her transfer down the stairs. You and your partner communicate as you carry the patient down the stairs. A few reassuring words to the patient help her to overcome her anxiety and feeling of being off balance.

The patient is moved safely and without worsening her feeling of respiratory distress. The remainder of the transportation to the hospital's emergency department is uneventful. Your care and planning in the transportation process has helped to bring the call to successful completion. ■

■ BODY MECHANICS

Body mechanics refers to how the body is used during the process of lifting and moving. Musculoskeletal injuries resulting from improper lifting are a significant cause of injury to EMS personnel, some of which result in permanent disability and shattered careers.

Even if you have been successfully lifting and moving patients for many years, it never hurts to review procedures for the proper moving of a patient. The actual process of lifting and moving can be broken down into two steps—decision making and planning and lifting and moving.

Decision Making and Planning

Decision making and planning are essential for any successful movement of a patient. This sets crucial groundwork that makes the actual movement more efficient. Consider these points:

- *What are the needs of the patient?* The condition of the patient will be an important part of transportation planning. Many patients with respiratory complaints will clearly be more comfortable sitting up. That same position will be improper for patients with spinal injuries.

- *What is the terrain like?* Elevators, stairs, narrow hallways, and other difficult places will affect transportation decisions. When possible, use wheeled devices such as the ambulance stretcher or stair chair to reduce the amount of carrying.

- *What is the weight of the patient?* What are the abilities and limitations of crew members? These questions must be answered as part of the decision-making process.

- *Communication* When planning or physically preparing to lift a patient, communication is essential. The communication process should include readiness, problems encountered during movement, and planning for the next phase. This becomes especially important when coordinating treatments such as CPR with the movements.

CHAPTER 16 Lifting and Moving Patients **317**

Lifting and Moving

Follow these steps when attempting to lift or move a patient.

- Position your feet properly.
- Use your legs, not your back, when lifting.
- Never twist your body while lifting. Attempting to turn or twist while lifting is a major cause of injury.
- Keep the weight you are lifting as close to your body as possible.
- Use an *even* number of people to lift. Uneven numbers may cause the lifting device to go off balance, causing injury to the EMT-B and patient.

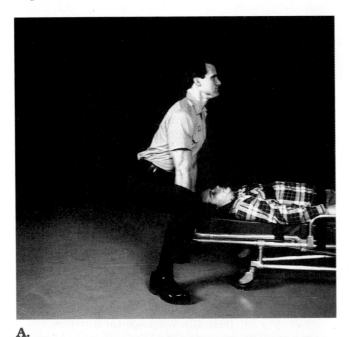

A.

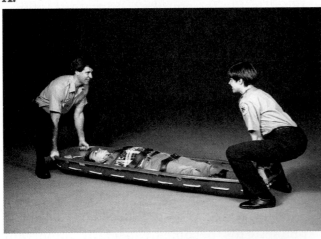

B.

FIGURE 16–1 The power lift, or squat lift.

The **power lift**, or squat lift (Figure 16–1), is recommended. By squatting instead of bending at the waist, the lifting is done primarily through the muscles of the legs rather than of the back. The position is called the power lift because it is used by weightlifters. The grip formed between your hand and the device is also important. As much of your fingers and hand should be in contact with the device as possible. Position your hands about ten inches apart when possible.

Reaching, Pushing, and Pulling

Simple lifting is not the only strenuous task performed by an EMT-B. Reaching, pushing, and pulling can cause injury as easily as lifting. These movements put the body at an unusual angle, which may cause injury.

Reaching Guidelines

- Keep your back in a locked-in position.
- Use caution when reaching overhead. Avoid hyperextended positions.
- Avoid twisting while reaching.
- Avoid reaching more than 15 to 20 inches in front of the body. Furthermore, avoid situations where prolonged reaching combined with lifting or other strenuous effort is required.

Reaching is commonly required when assisting in log rolling a patient to a backboard. When performing this activity remember to keep the back straight while leaning, lean from the hips, and use your shoulder muscles to help with the roll (Figure 16–2).

Pushing and Pulling Guidelines

- Push, rather than pull, wherever possible.
- Keep back locked-in. Push from the area between the waist and shoulder.
- If the weight is below waist level, use a kneeling position.
- Keep elbows bent with arm close to the sides.
- Avoid pushing or pulling from an overhead position when possible.

Preceptor Pearl

Few things are more important to the safety and longevity of an EMS provider than proper lifting and moving techniques. Habits that begin early are practiced throughout a career. Remember to emphasize proper lifting and moving techniques when working with new EMT-Bs—and be sure to practice these techniques yourself! ✦

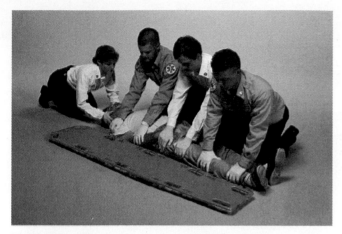

FIGURE 16–2 When doing a log roll, keep your back straight, lean from the hips, and use your shoulder muscles.

■ TYPES OF MOVES

The new EMT-B curriculum provides guidelines for emergency and non-emergency moves. This portion of the curriculum may differ from your current training or practice and will be covered in depth for this reason. As with many other portions of the EMT-B curriculum, the actual step-by-step procedure has not changed, but the situations where each is used are described in more detail and given increased structure.

Emergency Moves

Emergency moves are those which must be done immediately. The three basic situations where they may be required include the following:

1. Fire, explosives, or other hazardous materials threaten the life of the patient and the EMT-B.
2. A patient who requires immediate care cannot be accessed because another patient is in the way.
3. The patient requires immediate positioning in order to administer life-saving care (for example, placing a cardiac-arrest patient on a flat, firm surface).

The moves that are considered emergency moves are pictured in Skill Summaries 16–1, 16–2, and 16–3. The obvious problem with emergency moves is that these procedures provide minimal protection for patients with spinal injuries. However, since these moves are used in life-threatening situations, there are few choices. In order to minimize aggravation of spinal injury, move the patient along the long axis of the body.

Urgent Moves

Urgent moves are those that are required when the patient must be moved quickly, but with precautions for spinal injury. An example would be a trauma patient who requires treatment for inadequate breathing. The patient would be moved expeditiously, but with precautions for potential spinal injuries.

Rapid extrication is another example of an urgent move. A motor-vehicle accident patient who is breathing but who is in critical condition is a candidate for this procedure. The delay caused by taking the time to fully immobilize the patient could actually cause harm. The rapid extrication is an urgent move because it recognizes the need for spinal precautions but is quicker than standard extrication procedures. This procedure is reviewed in Chapter 13, Skill Summary 13–20.

Non-Urgent Moves

Non-urgent moves are generally those shown throughout the text. Non-urgent moves are performed when no harm will come to the patient due to the delay or the external environment. The patient will generally receive full assessment and care prior to being moved in a non-urgent manner.

A patient who was involved in a motor-vehicle accident who complains of neck pain, is not seriously injured, and is not in danger of injury from an unstable vehicle, fire, and so on would receive a full assessment, short-board immobilization, and transfer to a long spine board. Non-urgent moves are shown in Skill Summary 16–4.

■ PATIENT-CARRYING DEVICES

Many experienced EMT-Bs will be familiar with the types of patient-carrying devices and their use (Figure 16–3). Your choice of a patient-carrying device will depend on two main issues: terrain and patient condition. Stairs, elevators, hills, and other situations may require different devices. Also, patient conditions will affect your choices. Patients with cardiac and respiratory complaints feel more comfortable sitting up. If they are stable enough to do so, a stair chair is usually appropriate.

Emergency Moves—One Rescuer Drags

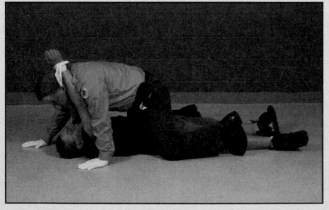

THE CLOTHES DRAG

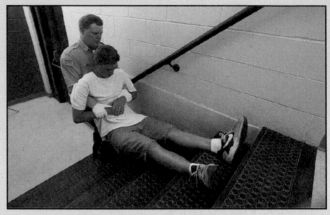

THE INCLINE DRAG Always head first.

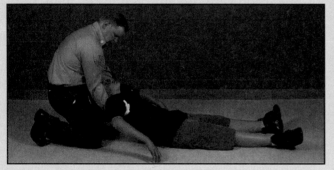

THE SHOULDER DRAG Be careful not to bump patient's head.

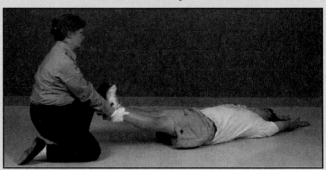

THE FOOT DRAG Be careful not to bump patient's head.

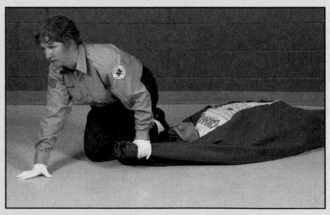

THE "FIREFIGHTER'S DRAG" Place patient on his back and tie hands together. Straddle the patient, facing his head; crouch and pass your head through his trussed arms and raise your body. Crawl on your hands and knees. Keep the patient's head as low as possible.

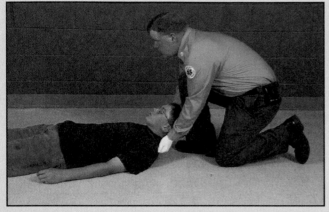

THE BLANKET DRAG Gather half of the blanket material up against the patient's side. Roll the patient toward your knees so that you can place the blanket under him. Gently roll the patient back onto the blanket. During the drag, keep the patient's head as low as possible.

Caution: Always pull in the direction of long axis of patient's body. Do not pull patient sideways. Avoid bending or twisting the trunk.

Emergency Moves—One Rescuer

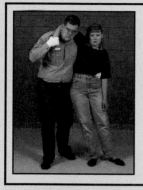

THE ONE-RESCUER ASSIST

Place patient's arm around your neck, grasping her hand in yours. Place your other arm around patient's waist. Help patient walk to safety. Be prepared to change movement technique if level of danger increases. Be sure to communicate with patient about obstacles, uneven terrain, and so on.

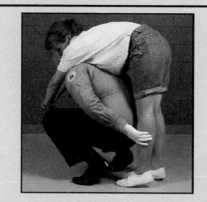

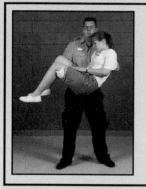

THE CRADLE CARRY

Place one arm across patient's back with your hand under her arm. Place your other arm under her knees and lift. If patient is conscious, have her place her near arm over your shoulder. **Note:** This carry places a lot of weight on the carrier's back. It is usually appropriate only for very light patients.

THE PIGGY-BACK CARRY

Assist the patient to stand. Place her arms over your shoulder so they cross your chest. Bend over and lift patient. While she holds on with her arms, crouch and grasp each leg. Use a lifting motion to move her onto your back. Pass your forearms under her knees and grasp her wrists.

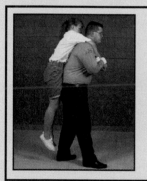

THE PACK STRAP CARRY

Have patient stand. Turn your back on her, bringing her arms over your shoulders to cross your chest. Keep her arms as straight as possible, her armpits over your shoulders. Hold patient's wrists, bend, and pull her onto your back.

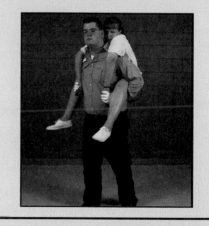

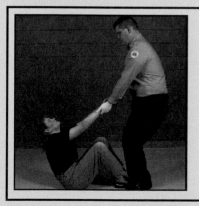

THE "FIREFIGHTER'S CARRY"

Place your feet against her feet and pull patient toward you. Bend at waist and flex knees. Duck and pull her across your shoulder, keeping hold of one of her wrists. Use your free arm to reach between her legs and grasp her thigh. Weight of patient falls onto your shoulders. Stand up. Transfer your grip on thigh to patient's wrist.

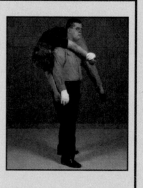

Emergency Moves—Two Rescuers

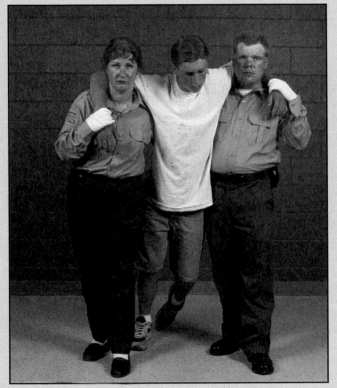

TWO-RESCUER ASSIST Patient's arms are placed around shoulders of both rescuers. They each grip a hand, place their free arms around patient's waist, then help him walk to safety.

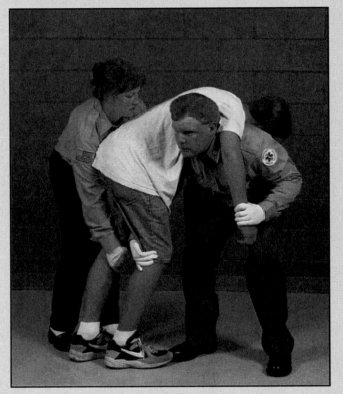

"FIREFIGHTER'S CARRY" WITH ASSIST Have someone help lift patient. The second rescuer helps to position patient.

Non-Urgent Moves, No Suspected Spine Injury

Extremity Carry

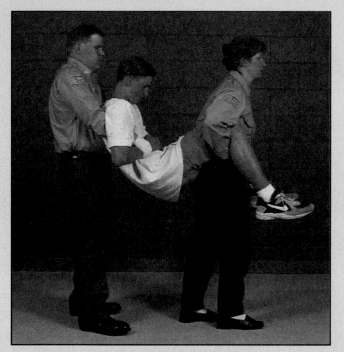

The extremity carry may be an emergency move or a non-urgent move for a patient with no suspected spine injury.

Place patient on back with knees flexed. Kneel at patient's head. Place your hands under his shoulders. Helper kneels at patient's feet and grasps patient's wrists. Helper lifts patient forward while you slip your arms under patient's armpits and grasp his wrists. Helper can grasp patient's knees while facing patient or turn and grasp patient's knees while facing away from patient. Direct helper so you both move to a crouch, then stand at the same time and move as a unit when carrying patient.

If patient is found sitting, crouch and slip your arms under patient's armpits and grasp his wrists. Helper crouches, then grasps patient's knees. Lift patient as a unit.

Draw Sheet Method

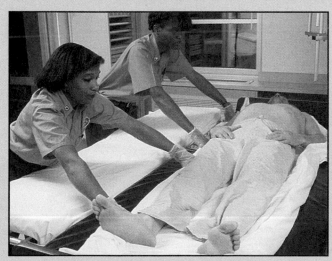

1. Loosen bottom sheet of bed and roll it from both sides toward patient. The stretcher, rails lowered, is place parallel to bed, touching side of bed. EMT-Bs use their body and feet to lock the stretcher against the bed.

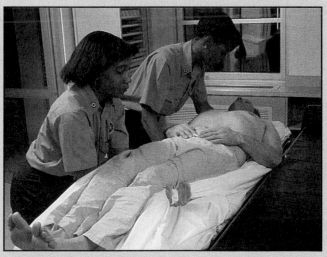

2. EMT-Bs pull on draw sheet to move patient to side of bed. They each use one hand to support patient while they reach under him to grasp draw sheet. EMT-Bs simultaneously draw patient onto stretcher.

Direct Ground Lift

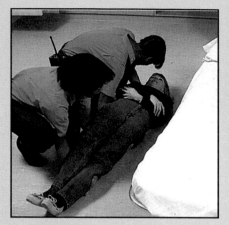

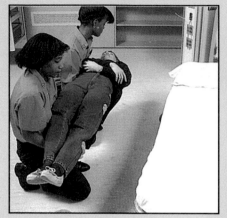

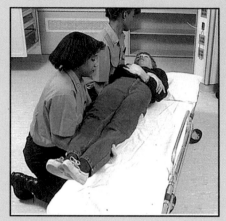

1. Stretcher is set in its lowest position and placed on opposite side of patient. EMT-Bs drop to one knee, facing patient. Patient's arms are placed on chest if possible. The head-end EMT-B cradles patient's head and neck by sliding one arm under patient's neck to grasp shoulder, the other arm under patient's lower back. The foot-end EMT-B slides one arm under the patient's knees and the other under the patient above the·buttocks.

2. On a signal, they lift patient to their knees.

3. On a signal, they stand and carry patient to stretcher, drop to one knee, and roll forward to place patient onto mattress.

Note: If a third rescuer is available, he should place both arms under patient's waist while the other two slide their arms up to the mid back or down to the buttocks as appropriate.

Direct Carry

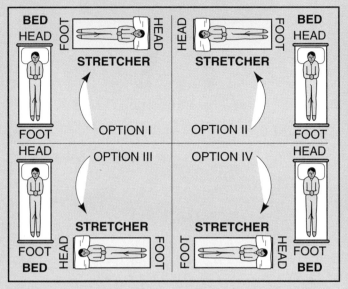

Stretcher is placed at 90° angle to bed, depending on room configuration. Prepare stretcher by lowering rails, unbuckling straps, and removing other items. Both EMT-Bs stand between stretcher and bed, facing patient.

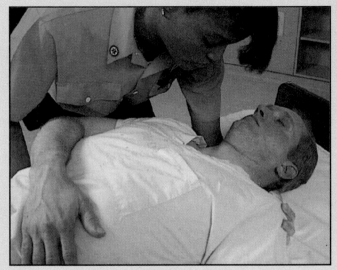

1. The head-end EMT-B cradles patient's head and neck by sliding one arm under patient's neck to grasp shoulder.

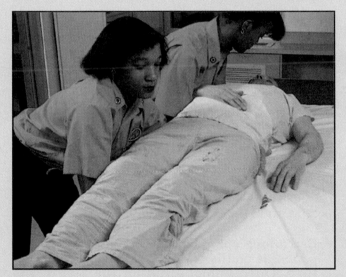

2. Foot-end EMT-B slides hand under patient's hip and lifts slightly. Head-end EMT-B slides other arm under patient's back. Foot-end EMT-B places arms under hips and calves.

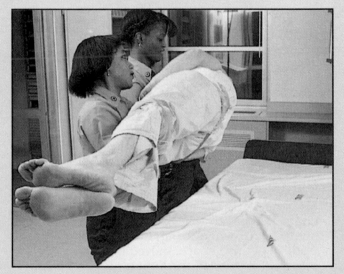

3. EMT-Bs slide patient to edge of bed and bend toward him with their knees slightly bent. They lift and curl patient to their chests and return to a standing position. They rotate and slide patient gently onto stretcher.

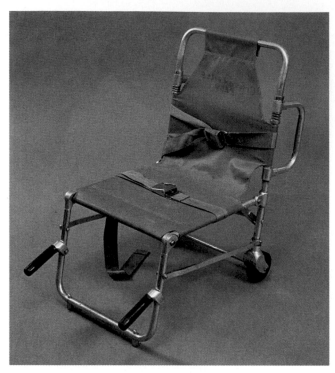

Stair Chair

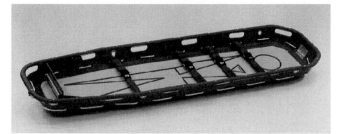

Vest-Type Extrication Device

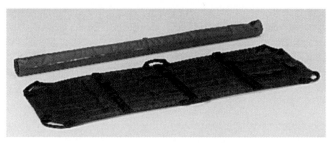

Basket Stretcher

Flexible Stretcher

FIGURE 16–3 Patient-carrying devices.

A spine-injured patient, however, must be transported immobilized and supine.

Use these general guidelines for selecting a patient-carrying device:

- Use the wheeled ambulance stretcher when there is an unrestricted pathway to the ambulance or a large elevator to an upper story.
- Use the portable ambulance stretcher, stair chair, Reeves stretcher, scoop stretcher, or long spine board when a patient must be removed from a confined space, moved through a narrow opening, or carried through a narrow hallway.
- Use a stair chair when it is impossible to carry a patient down stairs on a stretcher and when an elevator is too small for a stretcher.
- Use a basket (Stokes) stretcher to move a patient from one elevation to another by rope or ladder or when the patient must be carried over

debris, rough terrain, or uphill. Some Stokes stretchers can be fitted with a detachable wheel to facilitate movement over rough terrain.

When a person has a possible spinal injury, the patient-carrying device must provide straight-line neck and back immobilization. Selection of the device will be influenced by the location of the person and how the person must be moved.

- Use a long spine board when a spine-injured patient is on the ground or the floor of a structure. Once immobilized on the board, the patient can be carried directly to the ambulance or secured to the cot and wheeled there.
- Use a long spine board to immobilize a person who has already been immobilized with a short spine board or flexible, vest-type extrication device. Once a seated patient has been immo-

bilized on a short spine board or vest, he can be pivoted onto a long spine board.

- Use a long spine board to immobilize the patient and then secure the board and patient in a basket (Stokes) stretcher when the patient must be moved from one level to another and movement cannot be made over stairs or by elevator. Then use a rope, if you have been appropriately trained, to lower the stretcher or to slide it down the beams of a ladder.

The Ambulance Stretcher

The stretcher is the most commonly used patient-carrying device. However, if used improperly, it can be a source of injury to the EMT-B as well as a potential liability risk. In general, the principles of transfer for this device also apply to all others. In some cases, a patient may stand and help place himself on the stretcher. When moving a patient with no spinal injury from a vehicle, wreckage, or debris, you may need to adapt a moving technique to transfer the patient to the stretcher. For example, you might modify the cradle carry for someone seated and turned sideways in the front of an automobile. A patient with a suspected spinal injury should be secured to a long spine board before being transferred to the stretcher. The long board and the secured patient are lifted as a unit and secured to the wheeled ambulance stretcher.

The patient should then be covered by a top sheet and blankets, as required by weather. The side rails should be locked in the up position and the body straps fastened. Whenever you move a conscious patient, explain what you are doing and what obstacles you are maneuvering around, which will help comfort him.

The transfer of a bed-level or ground-level patient may require special lifting techniques such as the drawsheet or direct-carry method. Regardless of the method used, protect yourself from back injury and hernia. Do not position yourself too far from the patient and do not strain to lift the patient. Keep your balance to avoid possible injury to yourself, your partner, or the patient.

Regardless of the method used to move a patient, you and your partner should walk naturally at a smooth, fairly slow pace. Use two hands on the bed of the stretcher, rather than just pulling on the handles, to roll and maneuver the stretcher at a safe, constant speed. Turn corners slowly and squarely to keep the stretcher level and minimize discomfort to the patient. Lift the stretcher over thresholds and rugs. Use caution when maneuvering the stretcher to avoid bumping into and damaging walls and furniture.

The stretcher can be carried by the end-carry method or the side-carry method. The end carry is most widely used when moving the stretcher to the ambulance. The side carry is usually used to load the patient into the ambulance (Skill Summary 16–5). Often a stretcher is wheeled in the raised position by two EMT-Bs, one at the head end and one at the foot. The stretcher is guided by the EMT-B at the head. Never leave a patient unattended on a wheeled stretcher in the raised position for even a few seconds. The patient may shift position and the stretcher can easily topple over. Some services have policies that restrict moving the stretcher in the raised position. Other services simply require four hands on a raised stretcher at all times.

When you arrive at the hospital, you will move the patient from the ambulance stretcher to the hospital stretcher. See Skill Summary 16–6 for procedures.

The Folding Stair Chair

The folding stair chair is useful in narrow corridors, doorways, small elevators, and stairways. Since the device has wheels, it can be rolled on landings and other surfaces, thereby reducing strain on the EMT-Bs. A stair chair is not recommended for use with an unconscious or disoriented patient or a patient who has a possible spinal injury or fracture of the lower extremities. Unfold and secure the chair in the open position by the positive locking devices (not on all chairs). Unfasten and position the safety straps so they do not become tripping hazards. *Do not* use a patient's wheelchair when carrying the patient as it may collapse in your hands.

The direct-carry method can be modified when a bed-level or ground-level patient must be moved into a stair chair. The first part of the technique is the same as for transfer of a patient to a wheeled stretcher. However, the foot-end EMT slides his arm under the patient's thighs rather than under the midcalf. This maneuver allows the lower part of the patient's legs to drop down into a sitting position as he is eased into the chair.

The extremity transfer can be used to move a patient from the floor or ground to a stair chair or to any other patient-carrying device.

Loading the Wheeled Stretcher into the Ambulance

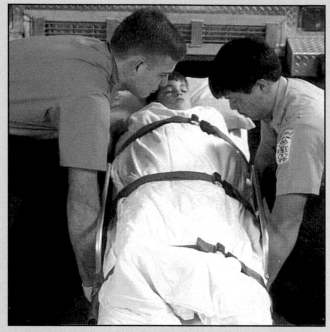

1. Clear interior of ambulance and lift rear step if necessary. Move stretcher as close to ambulance as possible. Lock stretcher in its lowest level before lifting. EMT-Bs position themselves on opposite sides of stretcher, bend at knees, and grasp lower bar of stretcher frame.

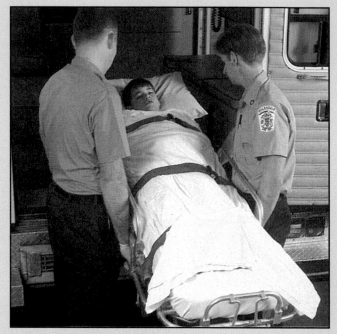

2. Both EMT-Bs come to a full standing position with their backs straight. Small sideways steps are used to move stretcher onto ambulance.

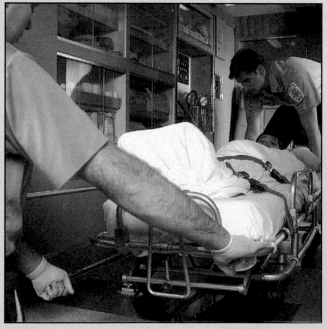

3. Stretcher is moved into securing device.

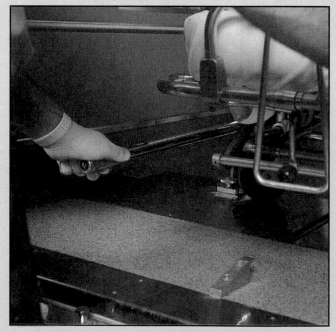

4. Both forward and rear catches are engaged.

Transfer to a Hospital Stretcher

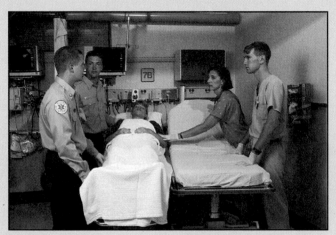

1. EMT-Bs position raised ambulance cot next to hospital stretcher. Hospital personnel adjust stretcher (raise or lower head) to receive patient from ambulance cot.

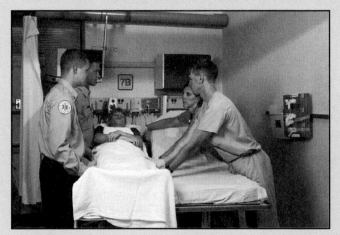

2. EMT-Bs and hospital personnel gather sheet on either side of patient and pull taut in order to transfer patient securely.

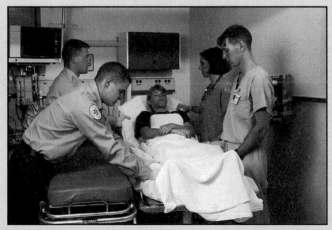

3. Holding gathered sheet at support points near shoulders, mid torso, hips, and knees, EMT-Bs and hospital personnel slide patient in one motion to hospital stretcher.

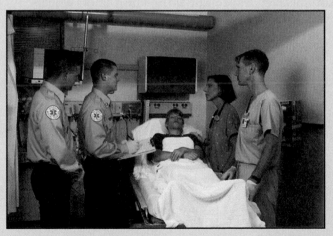

4. Assure patient is centered on stretcher. Make sure stretcher rails are raised before turning patient over to emergency department staff.

The procedure for using a stair chair is as follows:

1. One EMT-B assumes a head-end position, while the other EMT-B takes the foot-end position.
2. The EMT-B at the foot-end position assists the patient to a sitting position.
3. The head-end EMT-B reaches under the patient's armpits and grasps the patient's wrists, holding the arms to the patient's chest.
4. The foot-end EMT-B flexes the patient's knees and slides his hands into position under the knees.
5. Simultaneously, on the command of the head-end EMT-B, both move to a standing position, lifting the patient.
6. They carry the patient to the chair and lower him onto it.
7. The patient is draped with a sheet and a blanket is placed over his body and shoulders.
8. The patient is secured to the chair with three straps. One is fastened around the chest and the back of the chair. A second strap is placed across the thighs and around the seat of the chair. The third is fastened around the patient's legs and the lower portion of the chair.

A loaded stair chair is fairly easy to carry and maneuver, especially if the chair is on wheels. As with the ambulance stretcher, stair chairs should be rolled whenever possible; this reduces the risk of back strain for the EMT-Bs and injury to the patient. However, the following procedure is suggested when a stair chair must be carried over level ground.

1. When the chair and patient are to be moved, one EMT-B must be behind the chair to tilt the chair back. Always warn the patient that you are going to tilt the chair.
2. If the chair has wheels, tilt it carefully. The other EMT-B should stand at the patient's feet with his back to the patient. As the chair is tilted back, he should crouch and grasp the chair by its legs.
3. The two EMT-Bs should lift the chair simultaneously and carry the patient to the wheeled stretcher. Be sure the patient's feet are on the bar, not below it, so you don't set the chair on the patient's feet when you rest it on the ground.

4. Transfer the patient to the wheeled stretcher as soon as possible and *before* he is loaded onto the ambulance.

If a patient must be carried down stairs on a stair chair, the EMT-B at the foot-end should face the patient. A third person should spot the foot-end EMT-B while moving down steps. If the chair has wheels, do not allow them to touch the steps.

Preceptor Pearl

If you begin to lose your balance when carrying a patient down the stairs, if you are at the head end, sit down; if you are at the foot end, lean into the stairs to regain your balance. ❖

Scoop-Style (Orthopedic) Stretchers

The scoop-style stretcher is given its name because it splits in two. One piece is placed on each side of the patient. When brought together, it causes a scooping action, moving the patient onto the device. A scoop-style stretcher should not be used to transport a patient with a possible spinal injury. Always adjust the length of the stretcher to the patient's height. Separate the stretcher halves and place one half on each side of the patient. If the stretcher is the folding type, make sure the pins are properly set.

Slide the stretcher halves under the patient one at a time. This may be difficult since the stretcher may snag on clothing, grass, or debris. If necessary, roll the patient as a unit to either side to allow for proper positioning of the stretcher's parts. Mate the latch parts and make certain that the stretcher halves are securely locked together. Latching should be done from head to feet. Be careful not to pinch the patient when latching the two halves together. Adjust the head support.

Lift the scoop by the end-carry method. Move the patient to a long spine board as soon as possible. Secure the patient and long spine board as a unit to the wheeled ambulance stretcher by using three straps. Keep the stretcher as level as possible, even when moving down steps.

Special Transfer Devices

Some of the additional stretchers used in the field today are:

- *Basket-style (Stokes) stretcher*—Use the basket stretcher to move patients from one level to another or over rough terrain. *Do not* attempt to move a patient in a basket stretcher by rope or ladder unless you have been specifically trained in the techniques used for such moves.
- *Reeves sleeve*—This sleeve has an envelope configuration into which a regular long spine board can be inserted. Tabs with quick-hitch straps encapsulate the patient, providing security in almost any carrying position.
- *SKED®*—The SKED® stretcher comes rolled in a package. When opened, it can be quickly assembled and used to rescue someone from a confined space, a height, or a snow or water emergency.

Always remember to follow manufacturer's recommendations for inspection, cleaning, repair, and upkeep on all patient-carrying devices.

The selection and use of patient-carrying devices are important factors in the safety and condition of your patient. If transportation is not performed properly and taken seriously, you may harm your patient and incur liability for improper actions.

Packaging the Patient

Packaging refers to combining the patient and the patient-carrying device into a unit ready for transfer. A patient must be packaged so that his condition is not aggravated. For example, because laying a patient with shortness of breath flat may worsen his respiratory distress, move him sitting in a stair chair rather than laying him flat in a Reeves carrier. Before a low-priority patient is placed on the patient-carrying device, complete necessary care for wounds and fractures, stabilize impaled objects, and check all dressings and splints.

Preceptor Pearl

Do not waste time with extensive packaging of a badly traumatized patient. When a patient is categorized critical or unstable during the initial assessment, you should do resuscitative measures, immobilize the spine, and transport quickly. A neatly packaged corpse has not received optimal care! ❖

Cover and secure the properly packaged patient to the patient-carrying device. Covering a patient helps to maintain body temperature, prevents exposure to the elements, and helps assure privacy. A single blanket or perhaps just a sheet may be all that is required in warm weather. A sheet and blankets should be used in cold weather. When practical, cuff the blankets under the patient's chin with the top sheet outside. Do not leave sheets and blankets hanging loose; tuck them under the mattress at the foot and sides of the stretcher. In wet weather, a plastic cover should be placed over the blankets during transfer. Once the stretcher is in the ambulance, the cover can be removed to prevent the patient from overheating.

If a scoop-style stretcher or long spine board is used, fold a blanket once or twice lengthwise and carefully tuck the blanket under the patient. Cover the patient as best you can, place the patient and scoop-style stretcher on a wheeled ambulance stretcher, and then apply full covering. When using a basket (Stokes) stretcher, line the basket with a blanket prior to positioning the patient. If unable to do, cover the patient as you would when using the scoop-style stretcher.

Before seating a patient in a stair chair, place a sheet or blanket on the chair. This will facilitate transferring the nonambulatory patient later. Once seated on the chair, the patient should be covered. Have the patient sit upright with hands folded over the lap and legs together. Drape a sheet and then a blanket over the patient's body and shoulders. Carefully tuck in the sheet and blanket all around. In cold or wet weather, cover the patient's head, leaving the face exposed.

Many of today's devices for the transfer and transport of patients should have a minimum of three straps to secure the patient to the device. The first strap is at the chest level, the second at the hip or waist level, and the third on the lower extremities. Secure all patients, including those receiving CPR, to the patient-carrying device before attempting to transfer them to the ambulance.

If a patient is on the ambulance stretcher rather than on a carrying device, some services require shoulder harnesses. These harnesses secure the patient to the stretcher and prevent him from sliding forward in case of a quick stop.

CHAPTER REVIEW

■ SUMMARY

Lifting and moving patients is an important part of emergency care. When moving patients, whether lifting, reaching, pulling, or pushing, EMT-Bs must practice proper body mechanics in order to avoid injuring themselves. The types of moves used by an EMT-B can be classified into three groups: emergency moves (used when a patient must be moved immediately), urgent moves (used when a patient must be moved quickly, but with precautions for spinal injury), and non-urgent moves (used when no harm will come to the patient due to the delay or the external environment). The various patient-carrying devices used by EMT-Bs include stretchers (wheeled, scoop, flexible, specialty), stair chairs, and backboards. The choice of patient-carrying device is dependent on two issues: terrain and patient condition.

■ REVIEW QUESTIONS

1. Define body mechanics.
2. Describe or demonstrate the squat-lift (power-lift) technique.
3. Describe or demonstrate the power-grip technique.
4. Describe the considerations that go into planning how to lift or move a patient.
5. Define emergency moves, urgent moves, and non-urgent moves. Give an example of a patient and/or situation that fits each category.
6. List several patient-carrying devices and give a use for each.

17

Operations

■ *This chapter covers the "nuts and bolts" of an ambulance call, from the vehicle and its equipment, to emergency vehicle driving, to extrication and gaining access to multiple-casualty incident management. Your nonmedical operational responsibilities as an EMT-B may differ, depending on the type of service you work for. However, most of these responsibilities fall into*

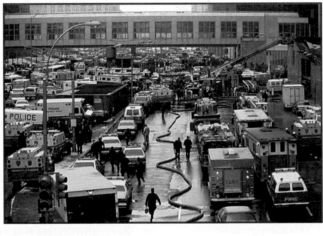

one of the five phases of an ambulance call: preparation, obtaining and responding, transferring the patient to the ambulance, transport to and arrival at the hospital, and terminating the call.

Since each service is different, this chapter discusses the common areas of operations of which all EMT-Bs should be aware. Each service, in its role as an employer, has the responsibility for providing additional training in its exposure-control plan, hazardous materials awareness, and the driving of its vehicles. In addition, your service should provide training in its regional multiple-casualty incident management plan, extrication and entrapment removal procedures, operating the stretcher and equipment, as well as its standard operating procedures (SOPs).

MAKING THE TRANSITION

- Carrying the right equipment to the patient's side to ensure proper initial assessment is emphasized.
- Ambulance collision risk factors are explained.
- Medical incident command is explained in detail.

The numbered objectives below are from the United States Department of Transportation 1994 EMT-Basic National Standard Curriculum.

■ KNOWLEDGE AND ATTITUDE

At the end of this chapter, you should be able to meet the following objectives:

Ambulance Operations

1. Discuss the medical and non-medical equipment needed to respond to a call. (pp. 335–338)
2. List the phases of an ambulance call. (pp. 340–349)
3. Describe the general provisions of state laws relating to the operation of the ambulance and privileges in any or all of the following categories: (pp. 341–346)
   - Speed
   - Warning lights
   - Sirens
   - Right-of-way
   - Parking
   - Turning
4. List contributing factors to unsafe driving conditions. (pp. 344–345, 346–347)
5. Describe the considerations that should be given to: (p. 345)
   - Request for escorts
   - Following an escort vehicle
   - Intersections
6. Discuss "Due Regard for Safety of All Others" while operating an emergency vehicle. (pp. 341–342)
7. State what information is essential in order to respond to a call. (pp. 340–341)
8. Discuss various situations that may affect response to a call. (pp. 345–346)
9. Differentiate between the various methods of moving a patient to the unit based upon injury or illness. (See Chapter 16)
10. Apply the components of the essential patient information in a written report. (pp. 348–349)
11. Summarize the importance of preparing the unit for the next response. (p. 349, see Chapter 3)
12. Identify what is essential for completion of a call. (p. 349, see Chapter 3)

13. Distinguish among the terms cleaning, disinfection, high-level disinfection, and sterilization. (See Chapter 3)
14. Describe how to clean or disinfect items following patient care. (See Chapter 3)
15. Explain the rationale for appropriate report of patient information. (pp. 348–349)
16. Explain the rationale for having the unit prepared to respond. (p. 349, see Chapter 3)

Gaining Access

1. Describe the purpose of extrication. (p. 351)
2. Discuss the role of the EMT-B in extrication. (pp. 351, 353–365)
3. Identify what equipment for personal safety is required for the EMT-B. (pp. 353–354)
4. Define the fundamental components of extrication. (p. 351)
5. State the steps that should be taken to protect the patient during extrication. (p. 355)
6. Evaluate various methods of gaining access to the patient. (pp. 358, 360–365)
7. Distinguish between simple and complex access. (pp. 358, 360)

Multiple-Casualty Situations

1. Describe the criteria for a multiple-casualty situation. (p. 365)
2. Evaluate the role of the EMT-B in the multiple-casualty situation. (pp. 367–370)
3. Summarize the components of basic triage. (pp. 365–367)
4. Define the role of the EMT-B in a disaster operation. (pp. 367–371)
5. Describe the basic concepts of incident management. (pp. 367–371)
6. Review the local mass-casualty incident plan. (pp. 365, 372)
7. Given a scenario of a mass-casualty incident, perform triage. (pp. 369–371)

■ SKILLS

1. Given a scenario of a mass-casualty incident, perform triage.

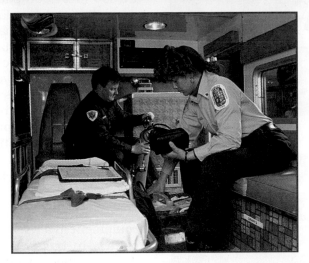

Since 06:00 is the change of shift at your ambulance service, at 05:45 you are ready to begin checking out the rig with your new partner. The night crew come out with coffee cups in hand and tell you about their busy shift: several patients with breathing difficulty, a minor injury from a slip on the ice, and an automobile collision involving an extrication. As the night shift leaves, one of them yells back, "Don't worry about the rig; it's in good shape!"

Your new partner: If the rig is in good shape, we can probably put off its check until after we eat breakfast.
You: Uh, uh! If they were busy all night, that's all the more reason for a good check this morning. Small items get used on each call. After a few calls in a row, items hardly ever get replaced. In fact, the types of calls they went on can be good predictors of the equipment they used. Let's take a few minutes and run through this together and maybe you'll see what I mean.
Your new partner: OK ... I suppose we should be extra careful to check the oxygen, nonrebreather masks, and the backboards since they had breathing calls and a bad collision.

Just as you suspected, you find the portable oxygen tank is around 500 psi, and there is only one nonrebreather mask left. Also there are no regular-sized Stiff-Neck™ cervical collars, and one of the Kansas™ board's head straps is missing. Checking the ambulance turns out to be a good idea because, just as you finish filling the oxygen tank and replacing supplies, the first call of the day comes in for a rollover collision involving a school bus. It looks like today will be even busier than last night. ∎

The strange thing about EMS is that because of variables such as traffic conditions, weather, population movement, and the general health of people in your community, it is often difficult to predict which day will be a busy one. Also, the occasional multiple-casualty incident stresses most EMS systems. Because you never really know when or what your next call will be, you should routinely replace used equipment and supplies after each call and conduct a thorough rig check at the beginning of every shift.

■ AMBULANCE OPERATIONS

Equipment Needed to Respond to a Call

The modern ambulance has come a long way from the "body wagons" used to transport the dead in medieval times. The ambulance is far more than just a vehicle for transporting a patient to the hospital. Today's ambulance is a well-equipped and efficiently organized mobile intensive care unit. Anyone who has been in this profession for fifteen or more years can tell you that, until the late 1960s, hearses were traditionally used as ambulances because they were the only vehicles in which a person could be transported lying down. It is likely that hearses would still be the vehicles of choice if it were not for the 1966 white paper, *Accidental Death and Disability: The Neglected Disease of Modern Society.* This paper called for vehicles that were better suited to the purpose of transporting the sick or injured to hospitals. Not long after, the U.S. DOT issued the modern ambulance specifications known as the KKK 1822(A), which are currently in their fourth (D) revision. These specs called for the Type I (pickup truck with a box back), Type II (van), and Type III (van front with a box back)—vehicles we all use today (Figure 17–1 A, B, and C).

However, due to the extra equipment placed on ambulances in the 1990s for specialty rescue operations and ALS, the gross vehicle weight was easily

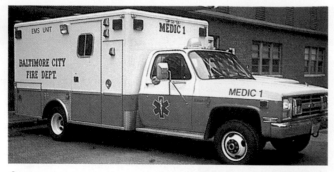

A.

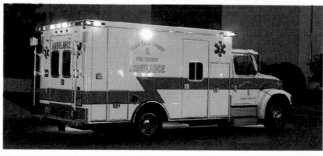

B.

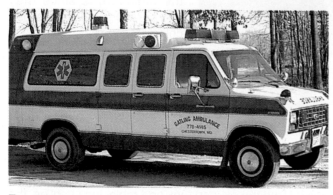

C.

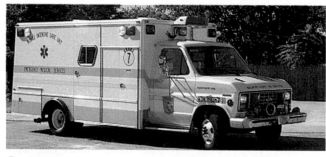

D.

FIGURE 17–1 A. Type I ambulance. **B.** Type II ambulance. **C.** Type III ambulance. **D.** Medium-duty ambulance.

exceeded. This paved the way for the medium-duty truck chassis (maximum gross vehicle weight 21,000 to 24,000 pounds) that is built for rugged durability and has large storage and work areas (Figure 17–1D). As patient care needs continue to expand and OSHA mandates evolve, the standards for ambulances will continue to change.

No matter what your region's vehicle is called, and even though it is especially designed and constructed, an ambulance is just another vehicle if it does not have the proper equipment for patient care and transportation.

Initial Assessment Bags

To decrease your scene time, carry the "right stuff" to the patient's side and package your supplies and equipment in a user-friendly manner. Portable kits or first-in bags come in all shapes, sizes, and designs. When setting up a first-in kit, keep in mind the steps of the initial assessment, focused medical history, and rapid trauma exam, which dictate the specific equipment needed at the patient's side in order to expedite care. In order to ensure proper care, your initial assessment bag should include:

Neck and spine stabilization and mental status check—set of rigid cervical collars

Airway—oral and nasal airways, suction unit and Yankauers, PPE, BSI

Breathing—adult and pediatric stethoscopes, BVM, oxygen tank and regulator, pocket mask with one-way valve, oxygen tubing, nonrebreather masks, and a pulse oximeter with adult and pediatric finger probes

Circulation—sphygmomanometer kit with separate cuffs for average-sized and obese adults as well as infant and child sizes; bandages and dressings; occlusive dressings; and PASG or MAST

Exposure—scissors to expose, as necessary, and a blanket to deal with exposure. In addition, carry a disposable thermometer and a hypothermia thermometer that goes down to at least 82°F, a penlight, and assessment cards.

In addition to these supplies, an AED and backboard and straps should be carried to the patient's side.

Typical emergency care equipment and supplies carried on a modern ambulance are shown in Figure 17–2.

Supplies: Infection Control, Patient Comfort, Protection

- ❒ 2 pillows
- ❒ 4 pillow cases
- ❒ 2 spare sheets
- ❒ 4 blankets
- ❒ 6 disposable emesis bags or basins
- ❒ 2 boxes of facial tissues
- ❒ 1 disposable bedpan, urinal, and toilet paper
- ❒ 1 package of drinking cups
- ❒ 1 package of wet wipes
- ❒ 4 liters of sterile water or saline
- ❒ 4 soft restraining devices
- ❒ 3 large and small red biohazard bags
- ❒ 3 large yellow bags
- ❒ 1 EPA registered intermediate-level disinfectant
- ❒ 1 EPA registered low-level disinfectant i.e., Lysol®
- ❒ 1 empty plastic spray bottle with a line at the 1:100 level
- ❒ 1 plastic bottle of water
- ❒ 1 plastic bottle of bleach
- ❒ 6 eye shields
- ❒ 1 large sharps container for vehicle
- ❒ 1 drug box sharps container for ALS unit
- ❒ 1 box (S/M/L) disposable latex/rubber gloves
- ❒ 6 disposable form-fitting masks in each size
- ❒ 6 disposable HEPA masks fitted for crew

Equipment: Patient Transfer

- ❒ 1 wheeled ambulance stretcher
- ❒ 1 Reeves stretcher
- ❒ 1 folding stair chair
- ❒ 1 scoop, or orthopedic, stretcher
- ❒ 1 Stokes, or basket, stretcher accessible on a rescue truck or supervisory vehicle
- ❒ 1 child safety seat for transporting infants and toddlers

Equipment: Airways, Ventilation, Resuscitation, Suction, O-2 Therapy

- ❒ OPAs in sizes suitable for adults, children, and infants
- ❒ soft rubber NPAs in sizes 14 to 30

- ❒ 1 infant, manually operated, self-filling, bag-valve-mask unit with reservoir
- ❒ 1 child, manually operated, self-filling, BVM with reservoir
- ❒ 1 adult, manually operated, self-filling, BVM unit with reservoir
- ❒ clear masks with air cushion (various sizes)
- ❒ 2 pocket face masks with one-way valves and disposable filters
- ❒ 2 commercially available jaw blocks
- ❒ 1 fixed oxygen delivery system. A typical installation consists of a minimum 3,000-liter reservoir, a two-stage regulator, and the necessary yokes, reducing valve, non-gravity-type flowmeter, and humidifier (for infants and children).
- ❒ 2 portable oxygen delivery systems that have a capacity of at least 350 liters. The system should have a regulator capable of delivering at least 15 liters of oxygen per minute. Many ambulances are equipped with multiple function regulators that can be used for liter flow oxygen, suctioning, and positive pressure ventilation as well as a demand valve.
- ❒ 2 spare D, E, or jumbo D oxygen cylinders (preferably aluminum) with a current hydrostat test date seal imprinted in the tank
- ❒ 6 adult and 4 pediatric nonrebreather masks
- ❒ 6 adult and 4 pediatric nasal cannula
- ❒ 1 automatic transport ventilator (optional)
- ❒ 1 plastic cartoon cup for administering blow-by oxygen to a child
- ❒ 1 fixed suction system that can provide an air flow of over 30 liters per minute at the end of the delivery tube. A vacuum of at least 300 mm Hg should be reached within 4 seconds after the suction tube is clamped. The installed system should have a large-diameter, nonkinking tube fitted with a rigid tip.
- ❒ 1 spare, nonbreakable, disposable suction bottle, and a container of water for rinsing the suction tubes
- ❒ an assortment of sterile catheters
- ❒ 1 portable suction unit fitted with a nonkinking tube and a large-bore Yankauer tip
- ❒ 3 spare rigid-tip Yankauers

(Continued on next page)

FIGURE 17–2 Typical ambulance equipment.

Supplies and Equipment: Immobilization of PSDEs

- ❏ 1 traction splint (i.e.: Sager or Hare)
- ❏ 2 padded 3" × 54" splints
- ❏ 2 padded 3" × 36" splints
- ❏ 2 padded 3" × 15" splints
- ❏ a variety of splints (air-inflatable splints, vacuum splints, wire ladder splints, cardboard splints, soft rubberized splints with aluminum stays and Velcro fasteners, padded aluminum [SAM] splints, and splints that are inflated with cryogenic [cold] gas)
- ❏ 12 tongue depressors for broken fingers
- ❏ 12 triangular bandages
- ❏ 6 rolls of Kling or self-adhering roller bandage
- ❏ 6 chemical cold packs
- ❏ 2 long spine boards (with speed clips or Velcro straps)
- ❏ 3 sets of rigid cervical collars in short/medium/tall/no-neck adult & child
- ❏ 2 KEDs, XP1s, Kansas boards, or LSP boards
- ❏ 6 9' × 2" web straps with aircraft-style buckles or D-rings
- ❏ 2 head immobilizers (i.e., Headbed, Bashaw CID, Ferno Head Immobilizer.)

Supplies: Wound Care and Shock (Hypoperfusion)

- ❏ 24 sterile 4" × 4" gauze pads
- ❏ 6 5" × 9" combine dressings
- ❏ 2 sterile multi-trauma 10" × 30" dressings
- ❏ 6 Kling bandages in 4" and 6" widths
- ❏ 6 occlusive dressings (Vaseline® gauze)
- ❏ aluminum foil (sterilized in separate package)
- ❏ 2 sterile burn sheets or burn kit
- ❏ adhesive strip bandages for minor wound care
- ❏ 6 rolls of 1" and 3" hypoallergenic adhesive tape
- ❏ 12 large safety pins
- ❏ 1 pair bandage scissors
- ❏ 2 pair PASG (MAST)
- ❏ 2 aluminum blankets (survival blankets)

Supplies for Emergency Childbirth

- ❏ 1 pair of surgical gloves
- ❏ 4 umbilical cord clamps or umbilical tape
- ❏ 1 rubber 3 oz bulb syringe
- ❏ 12 4" × 4" gauze pads
- ❏ 4 pairs of sterile disposable gloves
- ❏ 5 hand towels
- ❏ 2 baby receiving blankets
- ❏ 1 infant swaddler
- ❏ 4 sanitary napkins
- ❏ 2 large plastic bags
- ❏ 2 stockinette infant caps
- ❏ 2 surgical gowns
- ❏ 2 surgical caps
- ❏ 2 surgical masks
- ❏ 2 pairs of goggles or eye shields

Supplies and Equipment: Treatment of Poisoning and Altered Mental Status

- ❏ drinking water to dilute poisons
- ❏ activated charcoal
- ❏ paper drinking cups
- ❏ equipment for irrigating a patient's eyes with sterile water
- ❏ constriction bands for snakebites
- ❏ instant glucose paste

Equipment: Safety & Miscellaneous

- ❏ DOT *Emergency Response Guidebook*
- ❏ 1 pair binoculars
- ❏ 1 clipboard and prehospital care reports (PCRs)
- ❏ 1 ring cutter
- ❏ 25 assessment cards
- ❏ 1 portable radio
- ❏ 6 MCI management logs
- ❏ 50 triage tags and destination logs
- ❏ 1 each command vests (EMS Command, Triage, Treatment, Transport, Staging)
- ❏ 4 tarps in red, green, black, and yellow for MCI field treatment areas
- ❏ 6 disposable Tyvek® jumpsuits (optional)
- ❏ 6 flares
- ❏ 1 pair of jumper cables
- ❏ set of turnout gear: coat, helmet, goggles, gloves for each crew member
- ❏ 1 large floodlight/spotlight
- ❏ concentrated Gatorade® and a cooler for rehabilitation sector
- ❏ self-contained breathing apparatus (optional)
- ❏ 2 spring-loaded center punches
- ❏ 1 Glas-Master™ or flat-head axe
- ❏ 1 small sledge hammer, prybar, or Biel™ tool
- ❏ 2 wheel chocks
- ❏ 100' of utility rope
- ❏ 2 stuffed animals for pediatric patients

FIGURE 17–2 *(Continued)*

Ambulance Inspection: Engine Off	Ambulance Inspection: Engine On Outside Quarters
❑ Inspect the body of the vehicle.	*Set the emergency brake, put the transmission in "park," and have your partner chock the wheels before undertaking the following steps:*
❑ Inspect the wheels and tires for damage or proper inflation and wear. Don't forget to inspect the inside rear tires.	❑ Check the dash-mounted indicators.
❑ Inspect, adjust, and clean the windows and mirrors.	❑ Check dash-mounted gauges.
❑ Check the doors, latches, and locks.	❑ Depress the brake pedal and note if pedal travel seems correct or excessive.
❑ Inspect the cooling system. Allow the engine to cool first!	❑ Check air pressure as needed.
❑ Check all other fluid levels.	❑ Test the parking brake.
❑ Check the battery fluid level. If the battery is the sealed type, determine its condition by checking the indicator port.	❑ Turn the steering wheel from side to side.
❑ Inspect the interior surfaces and upholstery for damage and cleanliness.	❑ Check the operation of the windshield wipers and washers.
❑ Check the windows for operation and cleanliness.	❑ Turn on the vehicle's warning lights and check each flashing and revolving light.
❑ Test the horn and siren.	❑ Turn on the other vehicle lights and walk around the ambulance checking the headlights (high and low beams), turn signals, four-way flashers, brake lights, side- and rear-scene illumination lights, and box-marker lights.
❑ Check the safety belts and ensure that the latches and retractor mechanisms work.	❑ Check the operation of the heating and air-conditioning equipment.
❑ Adjust the seat for comfort and optimum steering wheel and pedal operation.	❑ Operate the communications equipment. Test portable as well as the fixed radios and any radio-telephone communications.
❑ Check the fuel level.	❑ Check the back-up alarm if you have one.

FIGURE 17–3 Ambulance inspection checklist.

Preceptor Pearl

The most modern, well-equipped ambulance is not worth the room it takes in the garage if it is not ready to respond. A state of readiness results from a planned preventive maintenance program, periodic servicing of the vehicle, and taking the daily shift checks very seriously. ✤

Ambulance Inspection

As soon as you report for duty, speak with the crew who are leaving. Determine whether they experienced any problems with the ambulance or its equipment during their shift. Make a thorough bumper-to-bumper inspection of the ambulance. Use the checklist provided by your service to do this. Examples of mechanical items to check include those in Figure 17–3.

Shut off the engine and complete your inspection by checking the patient compartment and all exterior cabinets (Figure 17–4). Check the interior of the patient compartment. Look for damage to the interior surfaces and upholstery. Be certain that any needed decontamination has been completed and that the compartment is clean (see Chapter 3). Check treatment supplies and rescue equipment. See that an item-by-item inspection of everything carried on the ambulance is done.

Not only should items be identified during the ambulance inspection, but also they should be checked for completeness, condition, and operation. The pressure of oxygen cylinders should be checked. Air splints should be inflated and examined for leaks. Oxygen and ventilation equipment should be tested for proper operation. Rescue tools should be examined for rust and dirt that may prevent them from working properly. Battery-powered devices should be operated to ensure that the batteries have a proper charge. Some equipment, such as the AED, may require additional testing.

When you are finished with your inspection of the ambulance and its equipment, complete the inspection report. Correct any deficiencies and replace missing items. Notify your supervisor of any deficiencies that cannot be immediately corrected.

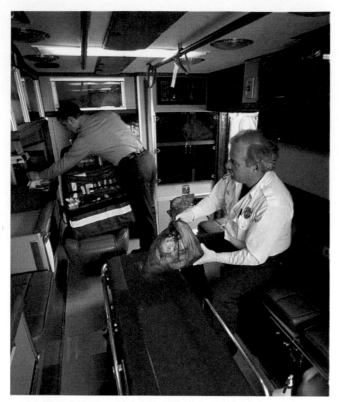

FIGURE 17–4 Checking the patient compartment in the ambulance.

Finally, clean the unit, if necessary, for infection control and appearance. Maintaining the ambulance's appearance enhances your service's image in the public's eye. If you take pride in your work, show it by taking pride in the appearance of your ambulance.

The Emergency Medical Dispatcher (EMD)

Many cities and communication centers have implemented training and certification based upon the **medical priority card system**, which originated in 1979 through the leadership of Jeffrey Clawson, MD. An Emergency Medical Dispatcher's responsibilities include:

- Interrogating callers and prioritizing the calls using a preplanned medically driven card system
- Providing medical prearrival instructions to callers and information to crews
- Dispatching and coordinating EMS resources
- Coordinating with other public safety agencies

The communications center should have central access such as enhanced 911 with 24-hour availability. When answering a call for help, the EMD must obtain as much information as possible about the situation in order to assist the responding crew. *The essential information is the nature of the call and location.* The questions the EMD will ask to obtain the dispatch information are:

1. *"What is the exact location of the patient?"* The EMD must ask for the house or building number and the apartment number, if any. It is important to ask the street name with the direction designator (e.g., North, East), the nearest cross street, the name of the development or subdivision, and the exact location of the emergency.

2. *"What is your call-back number? Stay on the line. Do not hang up until I (the EMD) tell you to."* In life-threatening situations, after the units have been dispatched, the EMD will offer instruction to the caller that the caller or others on the scene should follow until the units arrive. The call-back number is also important should there be any question about the location given. For example, several streets within a community may have the same name but a different direction designator, such as *North* Main or *South* Main.

3. *"What is the problem or nature of the call?"* This helps the EMD understand the caller's perception of the chief complaint. It also helps the EMD decide which line of questioning to follow and, according to preplanned medical response protocols, the priority of the response to send.

4. *"How old is the patient?"* This information will allow the EMS crew to be prepared with the pediatric kit if the patient is a child. Further, if pre-arrival CPR instructions are given, it is necessary to determine if the patient is an infant, child, or adult.

5. *"What's the patient's sex?"* This is asked if it is not already obvious by the caller's voice, or the caller is not the patient.

6. *"Is the patient conscious?"* An unconscious patient elicits the highest priority response.

7. *"Is the patient breathing?"* If the patient is conscious and breathing, the EMD often asks many additional questions relative to the chief complaint. This is done to determine the appropriate level of response, for example first response, paramedics, or ambulance responding COLD (at normal driving speed)—or HOT (an emergency, lights-and-siren mode). If the patient is not breathing, or the caller is not

sure, the EMD dispatches the maximum response and begins the appropriate pre-arrival instructions for a nonbreathing patient, which may also involve telephone directions for CPR if the patient is pulseless.

In addition, in trauma calls the EMD asks for the number of patients and about the severity of the injuries, as well as the name of the caller and details of any other special problems.

An EMD might dispatch an ambulance to the location of an injured person in this way:

"MEDCOM to Ambulance 621 and Medic 620, respond priority one to a 40-year-old unconscious male who fell from the roof of a house. The location is 165 Central Parkway, with Bridge Street on the cross. Time now is 16:45 hours."

The EMD will repeat the message to minimize any question about its content and to assure that the ambulance and medic receive the call.

Driving the Ambulance

No textbook can teach you how to drive an ambulance, nor can you become a good ambulance operator through experience alone. If you will be driving an ambulance, even occasionally, attend an emergency-vehicle-operator course that has both classroom and range practice.

In the course, you will learn how a vehicle operates, how it behaves on different types of roads, the proper use of audible and visual warning devices, and laws regarding the operation of emergency vehicles. You will learn how to prevent collisions by staying alert for problems caused by other motorists, changing road conditions, and hazards. You will then spend time behind the wheel as you are coached by an experienced ambulance driving instructor. On the driving range, you will learn how to use the vehicle's mirrors properly and to judge the vehicle's size, how to change lanes quickly and safely, how to recover from skids, and how to back and park the vehicle.

To be a safe ambulance operator, you must:

- Be physically fit. You should not have any impairment that prevents you from turning the steering wheel, operating the gearshift, or depressing the floor pedals. Nor should you have any medical condition that might disable

you while driving, such as a heart condition or epilepsy.

- Be mentally fit and have your emotions under control. Driving an ambulance is not a role for someone who gets turned on by lights and sirens!
- Be able to perform under stress.
- Have a positive attitude about your ability as a driver, but not be an overly confident risk taker.
- Be tolerant of other drivers. Always keep in mind that people react differently when they see an emergency vehicle. Accept and tolerate the bad habits of other drivers without flying into a rage.
- Never drive while under the influence of drugs or alcohol.
- Never drive with a suspended license.
- Always wear your glasses or contact lenses if required for driving.
- Evaluate your ability to drive based on personal stress, illness, fatigue, or sleepiness.

Understanding Driving Laws

Every state has statutes that regulate the operation of emergency vehicles. Although the provisions may vary, the intent of the laws is essentially the same. Emergency vehicle operators are generally granted certain exemptions with regard to speed, parking, passage through traffic signals, and direction of travel. However, the laws also clearly state: *If an emergency vehicle operator does not drive with due regard for the safety of others, he or she must be prepared to pay the consequences for his or her actions—consequences such as tickets, lawsuits, or even time in jail.*

Following are some points usually included in typical state laws that regulate the operation of ambulances. Be sure to review the actual laws in your state.

- An ambulance operator must have a valid driver's license and may be required to have completed a training program.
- Privileges granted under the law to the operators of ambulances apply when the vehicle is responding to an emergency or is involved in the emergency transport of a sick or injured person. When the ambulance is not on an emergency call, the laws that apply to the operation of nonemergency vehicles also apply to the ambulance.
- Even though certain privileges are granted during an emergency, the exemptions granted do not provide immunity to the operator in

cases of reckless driving or disregard for the safety of others.

- Privileges granted during emergency situations apply only if the operator uses warning devices in the manner prescribed by law.

- Park the vehicle anywhere, as long as it does not damage personal property or endanger lives.

- Proceed past red stop signals, flashing red stop signals, and stop signs. Some states require that emergency vehicle operators come to a full stop, then proceed with caution. Other states require only that an operator slow down and proceed with caution.

- Exceed the posted speed limit as long as life and property are not endangered.

- Pass other vehicles in designated no-passing zones after promptly signaling, ensuring that the way is clear, and taking precautions to avoid endangering life and property. This does not include passing a school bus with the red lights blinking. Wait for the driver to clear the children and to turn off the red lights.

- With proper caution and signals, disregard regulations that govern direction of travel and turning in specific directions.

Preceptor Pearl

Unfortunately, experience has shown that there is no such thing as a "rolling stop." Come to a complete stop, look all ways, then proceed with caution! ✢

Should you ever become involved in an ambulance collision (Figure 17–5), the laws will be interpreted by the court based upon two key issues. Did you use due regard for the safety of all others? Was it a true emergency? The requirement of due regard actually sets a higher standard for drivers of emergency vehicles than for the rest of the driving public. This is why it is not uncommon that, following a collision, an investigation by the district attorney or grand jury, as well as by the ambulance service, takes place.

Most states reserve emergency operation for a **true emergency**—a call in which the best information you have is that there is a possibility of loss of life or limb. A dispatch to a "collision" will usually get an emergency response. However, once you arrive and find that your patient has a minor injury, the call is no longer a true emergency. A lights-and-siren, high-speed response to the hospital in such a situation would be ruled illegal in most states.

Using Audio/Visual Warning Devices

Ambulance operators sometimes become so obsessed with the idea that sirens and flashing lights will clear the roads that they overlook hazards and take chances. Audible and visual warning devices do serve a purpose; however, safe emergency-vehicle operation can be achieved only when the proper use of warning devices is coupled with sound emergency and defensive driving practices. It is important to note that studies have shown that most other drivers do not see or hear your ambulance until it is within 50 to 100 feet of their vehicle.

Preceptor Pearl

Never allow the ambulance's lights and siren to give you a false sense of security! You cannot demand the right of way; the public needs to yield it to you. ✢

Using the Siren The siren is the most commonly used audible warning device. It is also the most abused. Consider the effects that sirens have on motorists, your patients, and ambulance operators.

- Motorists are less inclined to yield to ambulances when sirens are continually sounded.

- Many feel that the right-of-way privileges granted to ambulances by law are being abused when sirens are sounded.

- The continuous sound of a siren may cause a sick or injured person to suffer increased fear and anxiety, worsening the patient's condition.

- Ambulance operators themselves are affected by the continuous sound of a siren.

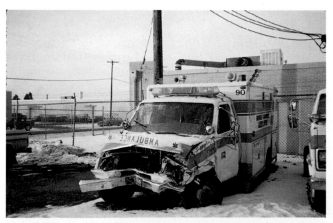

FIGURE 17–5 An ambulance collision.

Tests have shown that inexperienced ambulance operators tend to increase their driving speeds from 10 to 15 miles per hour while continually sounding the siren. In some reported cases, operators using a siren were unable to negotiate curves that they easily could pass through when not sounding the siren. Sirens can also affect your ability to hear other traffic.

Many states have laws that regulate the use of audible warning signals, and where there are no such statutes, ambulance organizations usually create their own SOPs. If your service does not have guidelines, the following suggestions may be helpful:

- *Use the siren sparingly, and only when you must.* Some states require the use of the siren at all times when the ambulance is responding in the emergency mode. Other states require it only when the operator is exercising any of the exemptions discussed above.

- *Never assume that all motorists will hear your signal.* Buildings, trees, and dense shrubbery may block siren sounds. Soundproofing keeps outside noises from entering vehicles, and radios, tape, or CD systems also decrease the likelihood that your siren will be heard.

- *Always assume that some motorists will hear your siren but ignore it.*

- *Be prepared for other drivers' panic and erratic maneuvers when they hear your siren.*

- *Do not pull up close to a vehicle and then sound your siren.* Such action may cause the driver to jam on the brakes so quickly that you will be unable to stop in time. Use the horn when you are close to a vehicle ahead.

- *Never use a siren to scare someone.*

Using Emergency Lights Whenever the ambulance is on the road, night or day, turn on the headlights to increase its visibility. In some states, the headlights of all vehicles must be turned on whenever the windshield wipers are being used. In most states it is illegal to drive at night with one headlight out, so alternating flashing headlights should be used only if they are secondary head lamps.

Probably the most useful light is the one in the center of the cowling on the front vehicle hood. This is easily seen in the rearview mirror of another vehicle and will get a driver's attention even if your siren fails to do so. Lights on the front bumper or in the grille are usually mounted too low to be effective warning signals. The large lights

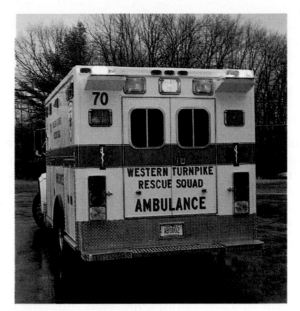

FIGURE 17–6 Yellow lights on the rear of the ambulance.

found in the upper, outermost corners of the patient compartment, or modular, should blink in tandem, or unison, rather than wigwagging or alternating. This helps the vehicle that is approaching from a distance identify the size of your ambulance.

There is a good deal of controversy over the use of strobes on ambulances. When planning the lighting package, refer to the latest research. Presently, researchers suggest combining single-beam bulbs and strobes rather than using either type of lighting system alone. When the ambulance is in the emergency response mode—either responding to the scene or responding to the hospital with a critical or unstable patient—all the emergency lights should be used. The vehicle should be easily seen from 360 degrees (Figure 17–6).

Using Four-way Flashers/Directional Signals
The four-way flashers and directional signals should not be used as emergency lights. This practice is very confusing to the driving public, as well as illegal in some states. Drivers expect a vehicle using four-way flashers to be traveling at a very slow rate of speed. Additionally, the flashers disrupt the function of the directional signals. In some communities, fire department ambulances returning to the station after calls still use their emergency lights. This "tradition" was established when firefighters rode on the back step of the vehicle. The lights were kept on to alert the public of their presence. According to OSHA regulations, it

is now illegal to build a fire truck with a back step for personnel. Avoid the practice of keeping emergency lights on when returning to station to prevent confusing the public.

Effect of Speed

When visibility is poor or when the road surface is slippery, drive slowly. Although your major concern is getting the patient to the hospital as quickly as you can, excessive speeding increases the probability of a collision. Speed also increases the ambulance's stopping distance, which reduces your chance of avoiding a hazardous situation.

Stopping distance is dependent on several factors, including the speed at which the vehicle is traveling, the vehicle's condition, road conditions, and the alertness of the operator. Stopping distance is the total of the reaction distance and the braking distance. Reaction distance is the number of feet the vehicle travels from the moment that the operator decides to stop until his foot applies pressure to the brake pedal. Braking distance is the number of feet the vehicle travels from the start of the braking action until the vehicle comes to a complete stop. Learn the stopping distances for a light truck, which is comparable to a typical (10,000 to 12,000 gross vehicle weight) Type I, II, or III ambulance. As you would expect, the medium-duty (21,000 to 24,000 gross vehicle weight) vehicles will have longer stopping distances. Perception distance is the number of feet the vehicle travels while the operator recognizes the hazard and decides how to react. Perception distance does, of course, add to stopping distance but is usually not included in stopping distance estimates because it varies with the individual.

What effect does speed have on an ambulance run? Consider a five-mile trip from an emergency scene to a hospital. Assuming that you will not have to stop or slow down, at 60 miles per hour you will be able to cover the five miles in 5 minutes. At 50 miles per hour it will take 6 minutes to reach the hospital. At 60 miles per hour the ambulance will travel 426 feet before the operator can bring the vehicle to a complete stop once he reacts to a dangerous situation; whereas, at 50 miles per hour the operator will be able to stop the ambulance in 280 feet. Clearly, the one minute gained in response time is not worth the risk of collision brought about by the 45% increase in stopping distance.

Drive Defensively

The ambulance operator must practice defensive driving at all times. Limit your perception distance by staying aware and alert and by scanning the road, your mirrors, and your speed every five seconds to maintain continual focus on your driving and the environment. Reaction distance can be decreased by recognizing potential hazards and instinctively "covering the brake"; if the potential hazard becomes an actual hazard, braking can be accomplished quickly. You can also decrease braking distance by maintaining a reasonable and prudent speed for the conditions as well as by driving a safe vehicle that is frequently checked and adequately maintained.

Let's compare a nondefensive and a defensive operator in a potentially hazardous situation. Assume that both drivers are experienced drivers and are in good physical and emotional condition, that the ambulance brakes have been well maintained, and that weather and road conditions are ideal.

The nondefensive operator is driving down a suburban street approaching three children playing ball close to the street, a potentially hazardous situation. Expecting the children to watch out for the ambulance, the driver does not take any special precautions. Typically, this nondefensive driver has the right foot on the accelerator while driving. When the potential hazard turns into an actual hazard, the driver must now move the right foot from the accelerator onto the brake pedal. The ambulance is traveling 30 miles per hour as it approaches the children. Suddenly, when one of the children chases the ball into the street, the operator recognizes the hazard and decides to apply the brake. While the operator is reacting, the ambulance continues to travel 33 feet until the brakes are applied. At this point, the braking distance begins and the ambulance travels 67 additional feet before coming to a complete stop. The total stopping distance is 100 feet. To get an accurate picture of this distance, use a tape measure and chalk to mark off 100 feet on the street.

Now consider the defensive ambulance operator who habitually "covers the brake" in potentially dangerous traffic situations. As soon as this driver sees the children playing and recognizes a potential hazard, he moves the foot from the accelerator to cover the brake, almost a reflex action. Like the nondefensive driver, our defensive driver is traveling at 30 miles per hour when first seeing the children. When the child runs into the street, the driver is ready to brake. The ambulance would travel 9 feet until the brake is depressed, but covering the brake gives this operator an additional benefit. Taking the foot off the accelerator slightly reduces the speed, bringing reaction distance down to about 8 feet. For the same reason, braking distance is reduced to about 66 feet. So the total stopping distance is 74 feet. This defensive driver, by being alert and covering the brake, saves 26 feet, which in this case could be just enough to save the child's life!

Escorts and Multiple Vehicles

When the police provide an escort for an ambulance, this creates additional hazards. Too often, the inexperienced ambulance operator follows the escort vehicle too closely and is unable to stop when the lead vehicle(s) make an emergency stop. Also, the inexperienced operator may assume that other drivers know that his vehicle is following the escort. In fact, other drivers will often pull out in front of the ambulance just after the escort vehicle passes.

Preceptor Pearl

Because of the dangers involved with escorts, most EMS systems recommend no escorts unless the operator is not familiar with the location of the patient (or hospital). ❖

Multiple-vehicle responses can be as dangerous as escorted responses, especially when the responding vehicles travel in the same direction, close together. In multiple-vehicle responses, when two vehicles approach the same intersection at the same time, not only may they fail to yield to each other, but other drivers may yield for the first vehicle but not the second. Extreme caution must be taken when approaching intersections.

Situations That Affect Response to a Call

A study conducted in New York State, based on 18 years of ambulance collisions, shows that the typical ambulance collision happens on a dry road (60%), with clear weather (55%), during daylight hours (67%), and in an intersection (72%). During this 18-year time period 5,782 ambulance collisions involving 7,267 injuries and 48 fatalities took place! Remember that the first rule of medicine is "Do no harm!"

An ambulance response can be affected by any of the following seven factors:

- *Day of the Week* Weekdays are usually the days of heaviest traffic flow because people are commuting to and from work. On weekends, commuter traffic generally diminishes, but traffic increases around urban and suburban shopping centers. Superhighways and interstate roads may be crowded on Friday and Sunday evenings. In resort areas, weekend traffic may be heavier than weekday traffic.

- *Time of Day* There was a time when traffic patterns were quite predictable by the time of the day. During morning rush hours, vehicles moved persons from suburbs to cities, and in the evening the traffic pattern was reversed. Today, downtown areas are still major employment centers, but so are suburban shopping malls, office complexes, and industrial parks. Accordingly, traffic over major arteries tends to be heavy in all directions during commuter hours. At these times, ambulance operators can expect gridlocked intersections, packed roads, and crawling vehicles regardless of the direction in which they must travel.

- *Weather* Adverse weather conditions reduce driving speeds and thus increase response times. A heavy snowfall can temporarily prevent any response at all. Always lengthen your following distance whenever there is decreased road grip due to inclement weather.

- *Road Construction* Road construction and maintenance activities can seriously impede the movement of vehicles. A detour usually has less effect on the movement of an emergency vehicle than the closing of one or more lanes of a multi-lane highway. An ambulance can continue to travel over a detour, but when several lanes of a highway are merged into one, there is often no way an ambulance can move around slow-moving or stopped vehicles or pull off the road in favor of an alternative route. There is no way to escape a traffic jam! Neither siren sounding nor light flashing can move vehicles out of the way when there is no place for them to go. Pay attention to the road construction in your district and plan responses accordingly.

- *Railroad Crossings* Although many road-grade crossings have been replaced with overpasses, there are still more than a quarter-million grade railroad crossings in the United States. Long, slow-moving freight trains often block traffic. Communities where this occurs should consider placing emergency response systems on both sides of the tracks to ensure that emergency response is not delayed.

- *Bridges and Tunnels*   Bridges and tunnels are erected to allow the flow of vehicles over and under natural and artificial dividers. However, the traffic over bridges and through tunnels slows during rush hours. When a collision occurs, the flow of vehicles, including emergency vehicles, may stop altogether. Unfortunately, drivers forget that bridges freeze before roadways, and collisions occur frequently.
- *Schools and School Buses*   An ambulance's response time is also affected by reduced speed limits in force during school hours, crossing guards, traffic, and drivers slowing down when an area is congested with children and school buses. When a school bus makes frequent stops along a two-lane road, traffic may back up behind the bus. Other vehicles cannot resume normal speed until the bus turns off or allows the traffic to pass. An emergency vehicle should never pass a stopped school bus with its lights flashing. Wait for the school bus driver to signal you to proceed by turning off the bus's lights. Unfortunately, emergency vehicles attract children, who often venture out into the street to see them. The operator of every emergency vehicle should slow down when approaching a school or playground.

When it appears that an ambulance will be delayed in reaching a sick or injured person because of these or other factors, the operator should consider taking an alternative route or requesting the response of another ambulance or first response unit. Always plan for times when changing conditions affect response. Obtain detailed maps of your service area. On the maps, indicate usually troublesome traffic spots such as schools, bridges, tunnels, railroad grade crossings, and heavily congested areas. Also indicate temporary problems such as road and building construction sites and long- and short-term detours. Using another color, indicate alternative routes to areas where normal routes are often blocked. Indicate snow routes, and so on. Hang one map in your quarters and place another map in the ambulance. If you follow these procedures, you will be able to select alternative routes that will get you to your destination quickly and safely.

Parking the Ambulance

Usually there is no problem parking the ambulance at the location of a sick or injured person. The unit can be parked at the curb or in a driveway. However, the parking task is not as easy at the scene of a collision (Skill Summary 17–1). The only way to ensure the safety of an ambulance at the scene of a vehicle collision is to park it completely off the roadway on a service road, shoulder, or driveway and utilize flares for traffic control.

Preceptor Pearl

Studies have shown that red revolving beacons attract intoxicated or tired drivers. Consider pulling off the road, turning off your headlights, and using just amber rear sealed beam blinkers that blink in tandem or unison to identify the size of your vehicle. ✤

There are two schools of thought about positioning an ambulance or other emergency vehicle on a road leading to a collision site. Some argue that the ambulance should be located beyond the wreckage (relative to the direction of traffic flow) to prevent it from being struck by oncoming traffic. Others favor placing the ambulance at the edge of the danger zone between the wreckage and approaching vehicles. The unit's warning lights will help alert oncoming traffic to the hazard ahead, although this does not reduce the need for other warning devices. Side beacons can be used for scene lighting. Once the ambulance is parked, set its emergency brake.

Transferring the Patient to the Ambulance

On most ambulance calls you will be able to reach a sick or injured person without difficulty, assess the patient's condition, carry out emergency-care procedures, and then transfer the patient to the ambulance. The patient's condition, the structure in which the patient is located, and the pathway over which you will carry the patient all affect your choice of a method for moving the patient.

Usually the transfer of a patient involves little more than placing the patient on a stretcher and moving it a short distance to the ambulance. The process can become more complicated if you think the patient may have spinal injuries. In this case, full spinal immobilization on a spine board must be done prior to placing the patient on the stretcher. If a traction splint has been applied to a tall patient, you need to assure that the patient is loaded properly to avoid slamming the door on the splint. You may need to place a patient with a traction splint into the ambulance feet first. In this case, if the patient also needs oxygen or suction,

Parking the Ambulance

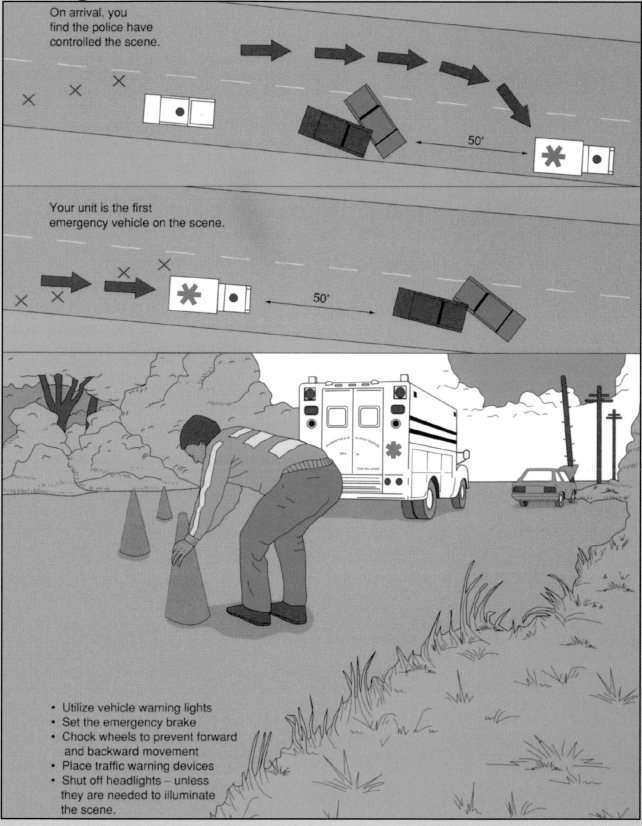

On arrival, you find the police have controlled the scene.

50'

Your unit is the first emergency vehicle on the scene.

50'

- Utilize vehicle warning lights
- Set the emergency brake
- Chock wheels to prevent forward and backward movement
- Place traffic warning devices
- Shut off headlights – unless they are needed to illuminate the scene.

use the portable oxygen and suction units since the permanent units are usually on the front wall of the compartment and will not reach the rear of the ambulance.

Transferring the patient to the ambulance is accomplished in these steps: (1) selecting the proper patient-carrying device, (2) packaging the patient for transfer, (3) moving the patient to the ambulance, and (4) loading the patient onto the ambulance (see Chapter 16).

En Route to the Hospital

While en route to the hospital, in most areas of the country, it is the responsibility of the EMT-B to contact and report to the hospital. The report should include the following information:

- Hospital identification
- Ambulance designation
- Brief description of the chief complaint and patient status or priority
- Facts learned during the subjective interview
- Facts learned during the objective exam (physical exam and vital signs)
- Your assessment of injuries or medical problems (what you suspect)
- Emergency care provided thus far
- Your estimated time of arrival (ETA) at the medical facility

Arrival at the Emergency Department

Definitive emergency care cannot be delivered by a single individual; it must come from a well-educated and competent team of EMDs, EMT-Bs, EMT-Ps, RNs, MDs, administrators, and allied health personnel. Although the responsibilities of each team member may vary, each person has an important role. Failure of any team member to do his or her job may mean the difference between rehabilitation and disability, a short-term or long-term hospital stay, even life or death to the victim of a sudden illness or injury. It is critical that all personnel responsible for some facet of life support and emergency care strive to provide optimum service at all times and in complete harmony with other persons within the system. Brief as it may be, the transfer is a crucial step during which your primary concern must be the continuation of patient-care activities.

It is usually the emergency department nurse to whom the EMT-B most directly relates, through both the ambulance-hospital communication and face-to-face contact upon arrival at the hospital.

In a routine admission or when an illness or injury is not life-threatening, check first to see where the patient is to go within the emergency department. If emergency department activity is particularly hectic, as it is when several seriously injured accident victims are admitted at the same time, it might be better to leave your patient in the relative security and comfort of the ambulance with one EMT-B, while your operator determines where the patient needs to be taken. Otherwise the patient may be subjected to distressing sights and sounds and even perhaps be in the way.

Preceptor Pearl

Under no circumstances should you simply wheel a non-emergency patient into a hospital, place him in a bed, and leave him! This is an important point. Unless you transfer care of your patient directly to a member of the hospital staff, you may be open to a charge of abandonment. ❖

Keep in mind that staff members may be treating other seriously ill and injured persons, so suppress any urge to demand attention for your patient. Simply continue emergency care measures until someone can assume responsibility for the patient. When properly directed, transfer the patient to a hospital stretcher.

Providing a Verbal and Written Report

Upon arrival at the ED, provide a verbal report to the emergency department personnel at your patient's bedside. Although similar to the radio report transmitted en route, this report stresses any changes you have observed in the patient's condition.

All EMT-Bs should participate in the early emergency department care of sick and injured persons. Even when the emergency department staff has taken over completely, it is often beneficial for you to remain in the area to be of assistance. This action promotes better patient care and also fosters improved communication and understanding between EMT-Bs and emergency department personnel. Working with the ED staff gives you the opportunity to learn more about definitive care procedures and, in turn, the ED staff gains respect for your abilities. Regrettably, this interaction may not be possible in an EMS system with a high volume of calls since it is more important for you to quickly prepare the ambulance for another call.

Remember that your job is not over until the paperwork is complete! Using your assessment card or notes and any additional changes you have observed in the patient's condition, you can now find a "quiet" spot and complete your prehospital care report. The essential patient information that should be on the prehospital care report (PCR) is the patient information gathered at the time of your initial contact with the patient on arrival at the scene, following all interventions, and on arrival at the facility. This **minimum data set** includes the following information: chief complaint, the level of consciousness in the AVPU format, the systolic blood pressure for all patients greater than three years old, skin perfusion or capillary refill for patients less than 6 years old, skin color and temperature, pulse rate, and respiratory rate and effort. In addition, the PCR should have the following administrative information: time incident reported, time your unit was notified, time of arrival at patient, time your unit left the scene, time of arrival at the hospital, and the time of transfer of care.

Be sure to complete all the boxes on the form and avoid stray marks, especially if your form is scanned into a computer. The narrative section of the form should describe your observations and not make conclusions. Pertinent negatives, such as the lack of chest or abdominal pain, the lack of shortness of breath, or the lack of an altered mental status, are important patient information to document. If you use abbreviations on the PCR, make sure they are standardized ones used by the medical profession and not "made up" ones. Spell the terms correctly and look up the spelling if necessary. Be sure to record the time and findings for every reassessment.

Since personal, sensitive information is written on the PCR, it is your responsibility to maintain confidentiality. Follow your state laws pertaining to confidentiality and the procedure for distribution of PCR copies in your region. Before handing in the PCR at the hospital, review it with your crew to make sure it is an accurate reflection of what was done and to ensure there is nothing on the form that might embarrass you.

If you make an error while writing out the PCR, you should draw only a single, straight line through the error and place your initials at the side of the correction.

Preceptor Pearl

Remember, the principle of medical documentation is, "If you didn't write it down you didn't do it!" Stress this point when working with new EMT-Bs. ✤

If a patient's valuables or other personal effects were entrusted to your care, transfer them to a responsible emergency department staff member. Some services have policies that involve obtaining a written receipt from emergency department personnel to protect the service from a charge of theft.

Terminating the Call

An ambulance run is not over until the personnel and equipment that comprise the prehospital emergency care delivery system are ready for the next response. This final phase of activity includes more than just changing the stretcher linen and cleaning the ambulance. A number of tasks must be accomplished at the hospital, during the return to quarters, and after arrival at the station (see Chapter 3).

En Route to and Back at Quarters

To ensure a safe return to quarters, an ambulance operator should practice every guideline for safe vehicle operation that was used while en route to the hospital. Defensive driving must be a full-time effort. Radio the EMD that you are returning to quarters and that you are available (or not available) for service. Refuel the ambulance per service policy.

When you return to quarters, a number of activities need to be completed before the ambulance can be placed in service and before it is ready for another call. The emphasis on protection from infectious diseases should not be underestimated; you need to take every precaution to protect yourself. It is essential that you follow your service's exposure control plan in accordance with OSHA regulations (see Chapter 3).

Use of Aeromedical Evacuation

In some circumstances, it is best for the patient to be transported by a helicopter or fixed-wing aircraft. These services are not available in all parts of the United States. Therefore, it is important that you know your local capabilities for air transport, when and whom to call, and what types of mission they will accept. Some programs do interhospital transfers only, while others do the complete range of missions from scene extrications to backcountry search-and-rescue operations.

Air rescue may be required for either operational or medical reasons.

Operational reasons for using a helicopter include:

- Ground transportation to the appropriate critical care facility will exceed 30 minutes.
- The helicopter can be airborne with a proper crew and can be at the scene quicker than an ambulance can transport the patient(s) to the nearest hospital.
- Extrication time at the scene is estimated to exceed 20 minutes.
- Ground transportation could be hazardous to the patient. Possible reasons are weather conditions and confirmed spinal cord injury.
- A helicopter landing site is available.
- A multiple-casualty incident threatens to overload local capabilities.
- Difficult access situations, such as wilderness rescue, access or egress impeded at the scene by road condition, weather, traffic, or search and rescue situations.
- A patient needs a higher level of ALS care than your agency can provide.

Medical reasons for using a helicopter include those in which the patient's condition is a "life or limb" threatening situation. A patient is high priority for rapid transport if he or she was injured in a collision in which evidence of any one of the following high-energy conditions exists or patient examination reveals that any of the following abnormal vital signs or physical findings exist:

- Fall of 15 feet or more
- Patient struck by a vehicle moving at 20 mph or faster
- Patient ejected from a vehicle
- Vehicle rollover with unrestrained passengers
- High-speed crash with 20 inches or more front-end deformity
- 15 inches or more of deformity into passenger compartment
- Patient was a survivor of an MVA where a death occurred in the same vehicle

- Glasgow coma scale of 13 or less
- Trauma score of 14 or less
- Sustained pulse rate of 120 per minute or more
- Head trauma with altered level of consciousness, hemiplegia
- Penetrating injuries of the head, neck, chest, abdomen, or groin
- Chest trauma with respiratory distress or signs and symptoms
- Two or more proximal long-bone fractures
- Amputations requiring reimplantation
- Facial/airway burns, burns of 15% body surface or greater
- Interhospital transfer of a critical patient
- Transport to a hyperbaric chamber

Note: Cardiac arrest patients are usually not transported by helicopter unless they are hypothermic. As always, follow your local protocols.

How to Call for a Helicopter

If your patient's situation meets local criteria for helicopter utilization, make sure you call for it as soon as possible so no time is lost in the ship's response. Contact the helicopter access point in your region and be prepared to give them the following information: your name and callback number, your agency name, nature of the situation, exact location of the incident including crossroads and major landmarks, exact location of a safe landing zone (LZ), communications frequency, and whom to contact as the helicopter approaches the scene.

How to Set Up a Landing Zone

A landing zone, or LZ, is approximately a 100' × 100' area, depending on the actual ship that is used in your region. To measure 100 feet walk out approximately 30 large paces (Figure 17–7). The LZ should be clear of wires, towers, vehicles, people, and loose objects. It must be on firm

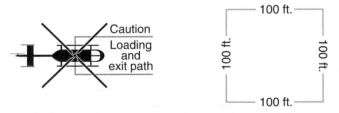

FIGURE 17–7 The air rescue helicopter landing zone.

ground with less than an eight-degree slope. In the LZ, keep emergency red lights on, but turn off any white or blue lights, which may obstruct the pilot's view. Do not allow traffic or smoking within 100' of the LZ. Place a flare on the upwind side of the LZ. Once the LZ is set and the helicopter is nearby, the LZ Officer should report the following to the pilot:

1. Describe the LZ relationship to terrain (i.e., in the valley, on top of the hill).
2. Describe major landmarks near the LZ (i.e., rivers, factories, water towers, major highways).
3. Estimate the distance between the LZ and the nearest town (i.e., LZ is located at the South Colonie High School; there are wires to the north and west side of the LZ, there are no other obstructions; the wind is out of the southeast).

How to Safely Approach a Helicopter

Standing nearby a "hot" or running helicopter can be extremely dangerous. Never approach a helicopter that has landed until the pilot or co-pilot has waved you to approach. Then it is important that you carefully approach from a safe zone. Never go near the tail rotor since it spins so fast that you cannot see it spinning. The information in Skill Summary 17–2 provides helpful information that could save your life.

■ THE EMT-B'S ROLE AT AN EXTRICATION

In some communities, there are at least ten types of special operations teams available. Each "special op" requires a significant amount of additional training over and above the EMT-B course. Examples of special operations include: vehicle rescue, water rescue, ice rescue, high-angle rescue, hazardous materials response, trench rescue, dive rescue, back country or wilderness rescue, farm rescue, and confined-space rescue. Training in each of these specialties is often a function of the types of emergency responses in your community. If there is a gorge in the middle of town, there often is a high angle team. Likewise if there is a river with low-head dams running through your district, a water-rescue team would be appropriate.

Extrication is the process by which entrapped patients are rescued from vehicles and other devices, buildings, tunnels, or other dangerous environments. Ten fundamental phases of the extrication process are:

1. Preparing for the rescue
2. Sizing up the situation
3. Recognizing and managing hazards
4. Stabilizing the vehicle or structure prior to entering
5. Gaining access to the patient
6. Providing initial patient assessment and a focused trauma exam
7. Disentangling of the patient
8. Immobilizing and extricating the patient
9. Providing ongoing assessment, triage, treatment, and transport
10. Terminating the rescue

Every step of this process needs to have medical input from the EMT-B acting as an advocate for the patient's medical needs with the Incident Commander, the Triage Sector Officer, and the Rescue Sector Officer. Safety is your highest priority; you need to minimize the potential for injury to yourself and other rescuers, as well as avoid additional injury to your patient. Although you may never have personally provided the disentanglement, since this is most often done by a fire department rescue squad in many communities, it is important for you to understand the process so you can keep your patient informed and anticipate any dangerous steps in the extrication action plan. Since extrication of a patient from a vehicle is the most common type of rescue across the United States, the next few pages focus on your role in this procedure. This section discusses phases 2, 3, 4, and 5 of the process, as well as the approach rescue teams should take for phase 7. Phases 1, 6, 8, and 9 have already been addressed in other chapters.

Sizing Up the Situation

It is important to have a keen eye as you arrive on the scene of a collision, because your first task is to evaluate hazards and calculate the need for additional BLS or ALS backup, police, fire, or specialty rescue response, or services such as would require a power company representative. Quickly determine how many patients are involved, their priority, and the mechanisms of injury. If you think additional ambulances will be needed, call for them immediately. You can always cancel your request for ambulances if they are not actually needed.

During the initial size-up, you must be able to "read" a collision vehicle and develop a plan of

Danger Areas Around Helicopters

A. The area around the tail rotor is extremely dangerous. A spinning rotor cannot be seen.

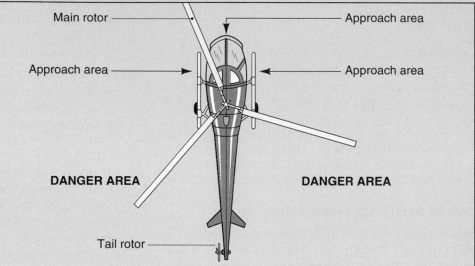

Main rotor

Approach area

Approach area

Approach area

DANGER AREA

DANGER AREA

Tail rotor

B. A sudden gust of wind can cause the main rotor of a helicopter to dip to a point as close as 4 feet from the ground. Always approach a helicopter in a crouch when the rotor is moving.

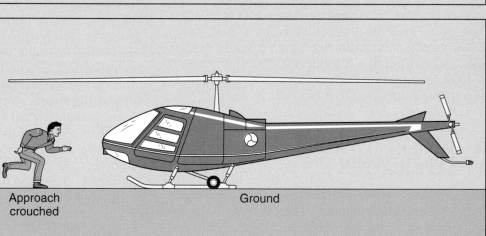

Approach crouched

Ground

C. Approach the aircraft from the downhill side when a helicopter is parked on a hillside.

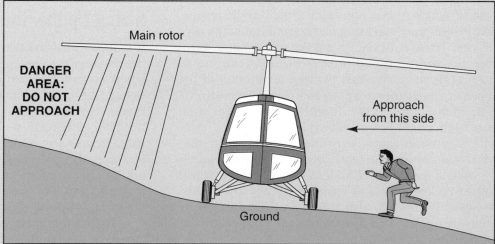

Main rotor

DANGER AREA: DO NOT APPROACH

Approach from this side

Ground

action based on your knowledge of rescue operations and your evaluation of the patient's status. Determine the extent of entrapment and the most appropriate means of egress for each patient. As soon as possible, evaluate the patient as high or low priority. Remember that a high-priority patient has only a "golden hour" at the maximum—the time from when the injury occurred to the time internal bleeding can be controlled in surgery at the hospital.

A low-priority patient can wait for rescue personnel to force open the doors, or remove the roof and/or displace the front end of the vehicle. For a low-priority patient, there is time to do a short-board or vest immobilization and careful transfer to the stretcher using the long board. However, if the patient is high priority, it may make more sense to use the rapid extrication technique, either for a vertical removal through the opened roof or for a horizontal removal through a doorway. The principles of spinal immobilization remain the same, but the requirements for speed of removal will dictate the specific technique you use.

During the size-up, check to see if the vehicle is equipped with air bags. A car with an air bag has a large, rectangular steering wheel hub. Special steps should be followed if the air bag has not deployed. (See, under Disentanglement Action Plan, "Step Three: Disentangle Occupants by Displacing the Front End" later in this chapter.) If the air bag has deployed, observers may have noticed "smoke" inside the vehicle during deployment. This is actually not smoke but dust from the cornstarch or talcum used to lubricate the bag, as well as the seal and particles from within the bag. The powder may contain sodium hydroxide, which can irritate the skin. For this reason, it is important to wear protective gloves and goggles when you gain access to the passenger compartment and to protect patients from getting additional dust in their eyes or wounds. The air-bag manufacturers recommend that you move the inflated bag and examine the steering wheel because damage to the wheel may indicate that the patient has a serious chest injury.

Recognizing and Managing Hazards

In some rural areas, fire departments have no rescue capabilities, so ambulance services are called upon to carry out vehicle rescue. In areas where rescue and fire units are available, the ambulance may nevertheless arrive at the scene first. Time and lives can be saved if you, after sizing up the situation and calling for the appropriate additional help, are able to recognize and initiate hazard management at least until personnel with more expertise arrive.

Hazards at a collision scene can range from nuisances—such as broken glass and debris, a slippery road, inclement weather, or darkness—to severe threats to safety—such as downed wires, spilled fuel, or fire. Also during size-up, watch out for loaded bumpers. Most cars are equipped with 5-mph bumpers designed to absorb low-speed front- and rear-end collision damage. If the bumpers were involved in the collision, you may notice that the bumper shock absorber system is compressed, or "loaded." Some rescue teams are trained to unload the shock absorber or to chain it to prevent an uncontrolled release.

Preceptor Pearl

Never stand in front of a loaded bumper. If it springs outward and strikes your knees, it will mostly likely break your legs! ❖

Traffic and spectators can become hazards if they are not controlled. A number of EMT-Bs have been killed at the scene of collisions by drivers who were watching the collision rather than the EMT-B crossing the street.

Safeguarding Yourself from Hazards

Collision-related hazards must be managed, if not eliminated, before any attempt is made to reach injured persons in damaged vehicles.

Collision sites can be dangerous workplaces. Jagged edges, flying glass, and fire are only a few of the hazards you may need to deal with. Remember that you are no good to your patient and crew if you become a patient yourself. It is vital that you take the time to properly protect yourself prior to engaging in any rescue activities. The unsafe act that contributes most to collision scene injuries is failure to wear protective gear during rescue operations. The following human factors can increase your potential for injury at a collision site:

- A careless attitude toward personal safety
- Lack of skill in tool use

Physical problems that impede strenuous effort

- Unsafe and improper acts

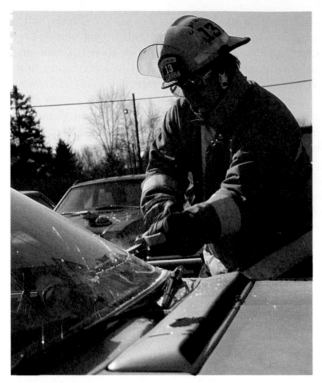

FIGURE 17–8 Dress for vehicle rescue.

- Failure to eliminate or control hazards
- Failure to select the proper tool for the task
- Using unsafe tools
- Failure to recognize mechanisms of injury and unsafe surroundings
- Lifting heavy objects improperly
- Deactivating safety devices designed to prevent injury
- Failure to wear highly visible outer clothing, especially when exposed to highway traffic

Figure 17–8 shows an EMT-B dressed for collision scene operations. Unfortunately, many services still allow their personnel to work around broken glass and the sharp metal of a collision in short-sleeve shirts or nylon jackets! This is a dangerous practice of simply not dressing for the work required at a collision scene. Any personnel allowed to work in the "inner circle" of a collision scene—the area immediately around and including the vehicle—should wear full protective gear to avoid being injured. Appropriate gear for a rescue operation includes: headgear, eye protection, hand protection, and body protection. Remember the value of protective gear; get your own if your service doesn't provide it (most states require it on ambulances), and use it!

Good head protection is essential. Trendy baseball caps, uniform hats, and wool watch caps do little except protect against sunlight, identify the wearer as a member of an emergency service, or keep the head warm. Plastic "bump caps" worn by butchers and warehouse workers also do not provide adequate protection. Headgear that offers adequate protection is the rescue helmet. The best rescue helmets do not have the firefighter's helmet rear brim, which can be awkward in tight spaces, although many EMT-Bs prefer and use firefighters' helmets. All helmets should be brightly colored, with reflective stripes and lettering, to make the wearer visible both day and night and should display the Star of Life on each side to identify the wearer as an EMS provider. Your level of training should also be indicated in order to facilitate management of a scene involving many EMS and rescue units.

Eye protection is vital. Hinged plastic helmet shields *do not* provide adequate protection; flying particles can strike the eyes from underneath or from the side. Wear safety goggles with a soft vinyl frame that conforms to the face and indirect venting to keep them fog-free. Or choose safety glasses with large lenses and side shields. These types of eyewear will also suffice for infection-control eye protection.

You should have optimal hand protection available. Wear disposable latex or rubber gloves underneath either firefighter's gloves or leather gloves. Firefighter's gloves will protect your hands from a variety of sharp, hot, cold, and dangerous surfaces. They are bulky, but can be worn in most rescue situations. If dexterity is impeded by firefighter's gloves, wear intermediate-weight leather gloves. Fabric garden or work gloves are too thin to offer adequate protection.

Often EMT-Bs protect their head, eyes, and hands, but leave their bodies virtually unprotected. Never wear light shirts or nylon jackets inside the inner circle because they do little to protect from jagged metal, broken glass, or flash fires. Wear either a short or midlength OSHA approved turnout coat to protect your body. Use a heavy-duty EMS or rescue jacket to protect you from inclement weather and minor injury. Bright colors and retro-reflective material help make your jacket more visible. To protect your lower body, wear either turnout pants with cuffs wide enough to pull over work shoes or fire-resistant trousers or jumpsuits. Also consider wearing high-top, steel-toe work shoes with extended tops to protect the ankles.

Safeguarding Patient from Hazards

It is your responsibility to ensure that further injuries are not inflicted on your patients during the rescue operations. The following items can be used to protect patients from heat, cold, flying particles, and other hazards.

- An aluminized rescue blanket offers protection from weather and, to a degree, from flying particles. A paper blanket does not afford this protection; it merely restricts the patient's view of the approaching glass or metal!
- A lightweight, vinyl-coated paper tarpaulin can protect from weather.
- A wool blanket protects the patient from cold. Cover the wool blanket with an aluminized blanket or a salvage cover whenever glass is being broken near a patient, since glass particles are almost impossible to remove from wool blankets.
- Short and long wood spine boards shield a patient from contact with tools and debris.
- Hard hats, safety goggles, industrial hearing protectors, disposable dust masks, and thermal masks (in cold weather—and unless the patient is on oxygen) protect a patient's head, eyes, ears, and respiratory passages.

Managing Traffic Hazards

Collisions almost always produce traffic problems. Often the wreckage blocks several lanes. Even if it doesn't, backups are caused when nosy drivers slow down to "rubberneck." Rescuers, firefighters, and police usually handle traffic control, but your ambulance may be the only responding unit or you may arrive ahead of other emergency service units.

Obviously, personal safety, rescue, and emergency care have priority. Because traffic is a natural predator of the EMT-B, an ambulance crew should still initiate basic traffic control, channeling vehicles past the scene. Your ambulance's warning lights will serve as the first form of traffic control; however, you should position other warning devices as soon as possible. Bad weather, darkness, vegetation, and curved or hilly roadways may prevent approaching motorists from seeing your ambulance.

Controlling Spectators

Spectators do more than just create problems for passing motorists. If allowed to wander freely, they will close in on the wreckage to get a better view. They may get so close that they interfere with rescue and emergency care efforts. Rescue squads, police, and fire units have personnel and equipment for crowd control; ambulances usually do not. However, you can usually initiate some crowd-control measures. If local policies permit it, ask for assistance from one or more responsible-looking bystanders. Ask the persons you recruit to keep the spectators away from the danger zone. Give them a roll of barricade tape if you have one. But remember not to put the recruited personnel in unsafe positions such as near spilled fuel or an unstable vehicle.

Electrical Utility Hazards

Electricity poses many dangers at vehicle collision scenes. When there is an electrical hazard, establish a danger zone and a safe zone. The danger zone should be entered only by individuals responsible for controlling the hazard, such as power company personnel or specialty rescue. The safe zone should be sufficiently far away to assure that an arcing or moving wire could not possibly injure any of the rescue personnel or bystanders. Keep these safety points in mind, as they may save your life someday:

- High voltages are not as uncommon on roadside utility poles as people often think.
- In some areas, wood poles support conductors of as much as 500,000 volts.
- Assume that the entire area is extremely dangerous. Conductors may have touched and energized any part of the system, including electrical, telephone, cable television, and other wires supported by the utility pole; guy wires; ground wires; the pole itself; the ground surrounding the pole; and nearby guardrails and fences.
- Assume that severed or displaced conductors may be energizing every conductor and wire at the highest voltage present. Dead wires may be reenergized at any moment. Energized conductors may arc to the ground.
- Ordinary protective clothing does not protect against electrocution.

A broken utility pole with wires down is very dangerous (Figure 17–9). You cannot work safely in the area until a power company representative assures you that the power is off and the scene is safe. If you discover that a utility pole is broken and wires are down, you should park the ambulance outside the danger zone. Before exiting the ambulance, be sure that no portion of the vehicle,

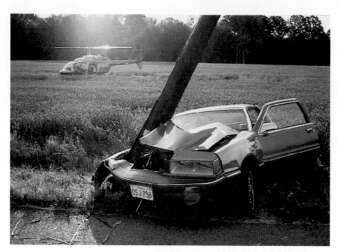

FIGURE 17–9 Damaged utility pole with wires down.

including the radio antenna, is contacting any sagging wires. Discourage occupants of the collision vehicle from leaving the wreckage, and use perimeter tape to set off a large safety zone. Keep bystanders outside the safety zone and prohibit traffic flow through the danger zone until the police can take over this responsibility. Determine the number of the nearest pole you can safely approach, and ask your dispatcher to advise the power company of the pole number and location. Stand in a safe place until the power company cuts the wires or disconnects the power.

Be especially careful when approaching a collision located in a dark area, such as a rural roadside at night. As you walk from the ambulance, sweep the area ahead of you to each side and overhead with the beam of a powerful hand light. An energized conductor may be dangling just at head level. If you discover that a wire is down, leave the area immediately and notify the power company. Even if wires are intact, a broken utility pole is still dangerous. Conductors supporting the pole can break at any time, dropping pole and wires onto the scene. Pad-mounted transformers and underground cables instead of utility poles and overhead wires supply electricity in many areas. When an above-ground transformer is struck and damaged, it poses a threat of electrocution. A vehicle may be energized by such a transformer.

Sometimes, especially in wet weather, a phenomenon known as *ground gradient* may provide your first clue that a wire is down. Voltage is greatest at the point where a conductor touches the ground, then diminishes as distance from the point of contact increases. That distance may be several inches or many feet. Being able to recog-

nize and respond properly to energized ground can save your life. Stop your approach immediately if you feel a tingling sensation in your legs and lower torso. This sensation means that you are on energized ground. Current is entering one foot, passing through your lower body, and exiting through your other foot. If you continue on, you could be electrocuted! Turn 180 degrees and take one of two escape measures. Bend one knee and grasp the foot of that leg with one hand; hop to a safe place on one foot. Or shuffle away from the danger area with both feet together, allowing no break in contact between your two feet or between your feet and the ground. Either technique helps prevent your body from completing a circuit with the energized ground.

Vehicle Fire Hazards

Extinguishing a vehicle fire is the responsibility of persons who are trained and equipped for the job: firefighters. When you find a vehicle on fire, always request their assistance. Never assume that someone else has called the fire department. A fire engine should always stand by at a vehicle rescue.

If you have been trained in the use of an extinguisher, there are some measures that you can take before fire units arrive (Figure 17–10). For small fires, a 15- or 20-pound class A:B:C dry chemical fire extinguisher can extinguish virtually anything that may be burning in a vehicle, including upholstery, fuel, and electrical components. Only burning magnesium and other flammable metals cannot be extinguished by an A:B:C extinguisher. Before attempting to put out a fire, always put on a full set of protective gear.

Many rescue units routinely disable the electrical system of every collision vehicle by cutting a

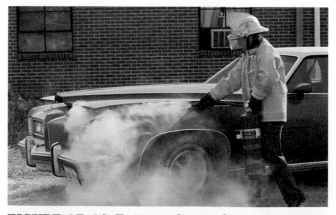

FIGURE 17–10 Extinguishing a fire in the engine compartment when the hood is partially open.

battery cable. This was a reasonable practice years ago when vehicles had more combustible materials and when wiring did not have self-extinguishing insulation. Today, however, the situation is different. Unless gasoline is pooled under a vehicle or undeployed air bags need to be disabled, cutting the battery out of the electrical system not only may be a waste of time, it may actually hinder the rescue operation!

Remember that many cars have electrically powered door locks, windows, and seat-adjustment mechanisms. Having the option of lowering a window rather than breaking it eliminates the likelihood of spraying the vehicle's occupants with glass. Being able to operate door locks may eliminate the need to force doors open. Also, if you are able to operate a powered seat, you can create space in front of an injured driver.

If there is reason to disrupt the electrical system, disconnect the ground cable from the battery. In this way, you will not be likely to produce a spark that can drop onto spilled fuel or ignite battery gases. Such a spark can be created when the positive cable is pulled away from the battery terminal or when a tool touches a metal component while in contact with the positive terminal or cable.

Stabilizing the Vehicle

Unstable collision vehicles pose a hazard to rescuers and patients alike. Rescuers often fail to stabilize collision vehicles because they *appear* to be stable. Rather than taking the chance of incorrectly "reading" a collision vehicle's stability, you should consider any collision vehicle from which patients need to be extricated to be unstable and act accordingly.

A vehicle may be found on its wheels, on its roof, or on its side. A collision vehicle that is upright on four inflated tires looks stable. However, it is easily rocked up and down, side to side, and back and forth as rescuers climb into and over it. These motions can seriously aggravate occupants' injuries. If you have access to the inside of the vehicle, make sure the engine is turned off, the gearshift is in park, the keys are removed from the ignition, and the parking brake is set. Use three step chocks (cribbing), one on each side and a third under the front or back of the vehicle, to stabilize a vehicle on its wheels. Then deflate all the tires. Simply pull the valve stems from their casing with pliers. Then tell a

TABLE 17–1 Supplies and Equipment for Vehicle Stabilization and Gaining Access

Quantity	Item
10	2 × 4 × 18-inch cribbing
10	4 × 4 × 18-inch cribbing
4	step chocks
6	wood wedges
2	vehicle wheel chocks
100 feet	nylon 1/2-inch utility rope
2	Hi-lift heavy duty jacks
1	"Door-and-window kit" with hand tools such as...

	1 pair	battery pliers
	1	12-inch adjustable wrench
	1	3- or 4-pound drilling hammer
	1	spring-loaded center punch
	2	hacksaws with spare blades
	1	10-inch locking-type pliers
	1	10-inch water-pump pliers
	several	12- to 15-inch flat pry bars
	1	8-inch flat blade screwdriver
	1	12-inch flat blade screwdriver
	1	spray container of power steering fluid as a lubricant

Quantity	Item
1	flat-head ax
1	Glas-Master™ windshield saw
1	combination forcible entry tool such as a Halligan or a Biel™ tool
500 feet	perimeter tape

police officer what you have done so investigators will not think that the tires are flat as a result of the collision. A listing of the equipment needed to accomplish vehicle stabilization and gaining access is listed in Table 17–1. If your ambulance is not equipped with step chocks, a degree of stabilization can be accomplished by placing wheel chocks or 2 × 4 cribbing in front and behind two tires on the same side.

If a car has rolled over several times and has come to rest on its wheels, the roof may be crushed, which prevents access through the windows. The roof may need to be raised with heavy-duty jacks before doors can be opened or the roof removed.

When a vehicle is on its side, there is a tendency for spectators to push it back onto its wheels. They fail to realize that this movement may injure, or more severely injure, occupants of the vehicle. Instead, the vehicle should be stabilized on its side, using ropes, hi-lift jacks, and/or cribbing. Do not attempt to gain access before this is accomplished. While a car on its side may appear stable, simply climbing onto one side in an attempt to open a door may cause the vehicle to drop onto its roof or wheels. Moreover, you can be trapped under the vehicle when it topples.

Position a safety guide at each end of the vehicle to "feel" the movement of the vehicle and quickly warn the rescuers placing cribbing, jacks, or ropes to get back if the vehicle begins to tip over. Some services will deploy two ropes looped around the same wheel in both directions so that personnel can temporarily hold the vehicle stable while jacks and/or cribbing are placed. The objective is to increase the number of contacts with the ground to make the vehicle on its side more stable, as shown in Skill Summary 17–3.

Preceptor Pearl

When placing cribbing, never kneel down. Always squat down, staying on both feet so you can quickly move away from the vehicle if necessary. ❖

There are many ways to stabilize a vehicle on its side—through sheer manpower or through the use of hydraulic rams and pneumatic jacks. If your ambulance is equipped with stabilization equipment, you should attend a formal vehicle rescue course that includes basic stabilization procedures, taught by a qualified instructor.

Once a vehicle is stabilized, if a door must be opened, tie it in the fully open position before you try to crawl inside. If the ambulance does not carry stabilization devices, or if you are not trained in their use, wait for a rescue squad to arrive before you try to enter the vehicle.

If the vehicle is resting on its roof, roof posts are intact, and the vehicle appears stable, it may be tempting to immediately try to reach the occupants by gaining access through window or door openings without stabilizing the vehicle. However, if the posts collapse, as is often the case when the windshield integrity has been broken, the vehicle may come crashing down and injure the EMT-B who is attempting the rescue. You *must* wait to gain access until the rescue crew has stabilized the vehicle. This is usually accomplished by building a box crib with 4 × 4s under the vehicle. If the vehicle is tilted with the engine, (its heaviest part) on the ground and the trunk in the air, you can try using two step chocks upside down under the trunk.

If the roof is crushed against the body of the vehicle, the vehicle is stable. It is, of course, impos-

sible to gain access through a window, door, or the roof. However, it may be possible to cut through the floor pan and either crawl inside, if the opening is big enough or the EMT-B small enough, or to reach through the opening to touch and offer emotional support to the occupants until rescue personnel can lift or open the vehicle.

Cribbing and jacks are usually used to stabilize an overturned car. If your ambulance has these devices, use them in the manner you were taught. If the ambulance is not equipped, or if you are not trained, stand by until a rescue unit has stabilized the vehicle, even if roof posts are intact and the vehicle appears stable.

When the roof is crushed flat against the body, as happens when all the roof posts have collapsed, the car is essentially a steel box resting on the ground with the occupants completely trapped inside. Unless the vehicle is on a hill or perched precariously on debris or another vehicle, this is the one time when stabilization is unnecessary. The structure is rigid. It will have to be lifted or opened by the rescue crew.

If the vehicle is unstable and cannot be safely approached, get as close as possible so you can talk or signal to the occupants to reassure them that help is on its way, and begin to get an idea of their conditions.

Gaining Access to the Patient

As an EMT-B, your responsibility is not the rescue of the vehicle but the rescue of the patient. You will usually assume that the occupant of a vehicle has sustained life-threatening injuries. At least one EMT-B needs to gain quick access to the patient, even while rescuers are working to gain a more wide-open access, create exitways, and disentangle the occupant.

After the vehicle is stable enough for you to approach it safely, check to see if a door can be opened or a window rolled down in the usual way *(Try Before You Pry!)*. Failing this, you may need to break a window to gain access even while the rescue crew is dismantling the vehicle for extrication of the occupants.

All automotive glass is one of two types: laminated or tempered. Windshields and some side and rear van and truck windows are laminated safety glass: two sheets of plate glass bonded to a sheet of tough plastic, like a glass-and-plastic sandwich. Most passenger car side and rear windows are tempered glass. They are very resilient,

Stabilizing Collision Vehicle with Cribbing

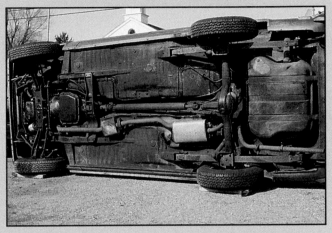

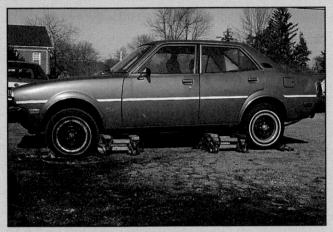

A. A car on its wheels can be stabilized by placing cribbing under the rocker panels to minimize rescuer-produced movements that may be harmful to the occupants. Deflate the vehicle's tires for maximum stability.

B. A car on its side can be stabilized by placing cribbing under the wheels, moving the car to the vertical position, and then ...

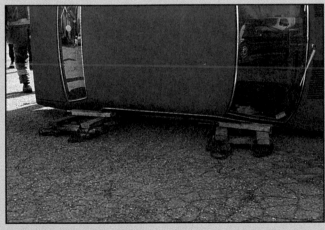

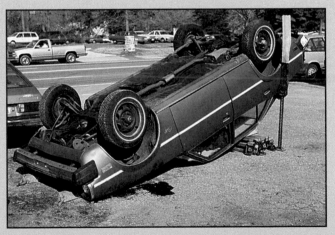

C. ... placing cribbing under the A- and C-posts. Stabilizing in this manner allows EMTs to pull the roof down to expose the entire interior of the car.

D. An overturned car can be stabilized by placing jacks and/or cribbing under the trunk, under the hood, or at both locations, depending on the position of the vehicle.

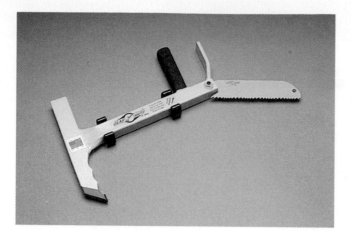

FIGURE 17–11 A Glas-Master™ saw can aid in windshield removal.

but when they do break, rather than shattering into sharp fragments they break into small, rounded pieces.

Try to gain access through a side or rear window as far away as possible from the occupants. Use a spring-loaded center punch against a lower corner to break the glass. Punch out fingerholds in the top of the window and use your gloved fingers to pull fragments away from the window.

A flathead ax is usually required to break through a windshield. However, it can also be done very quickly using a Glas-Master™ saw (Figure 17–11). A windshield is usually not broken to gain access, but the rescue squad may need to remove it if they plan to displace the dash or steering column or remove the roof. Before the windshield is broken, if possible, cover passengers with aluminized rescue blankets or tarps.

Once an entry point is gained, at least one properly dressed EMT-B should crawl inside the vehicle and begin an initial assessment and focused trauma exam as well as manual cervical stabilization. Don't forget to explain to the patient what is going on and provide emotional support by reassuring him or her that everything possible is being done.

Disentanglement Action Plan

In most instances, EMS personnel will not be directly involved in the disentanglement other than staying inside the vehicle and acting as the patient's advocate. The action plan that may be used by rescue personnel to free the trapped patient is a three-step procedure that can be carried out by fire, rescue, and EMS personnel with the appropriate equipment. The procedure is uncomplicated, requires minimal special equipment, and is not vehicle specific; that is, it can be used on virtually any car or truck. Therefore EMS personnel can be trained in a brief course and the ambulance compartments need not be overloaded with rescue equipment.

Step One: Gain Access by Removing the Roof

For more than 20 years, emergency service personnel have been trained to carry out a progression of procedures to reach the occupants of a wrecked vehicle: first try the doors; if that fails, unlock and unlatch the doors by nondestructive or destructive means; when all else fails, gain access through window openings. This multi-part procedure is time-consuming and requires a number of tools. A quicker and far more efficient procedure is to dispose of the roof of a collision vehicle as soon as hazards have been controlled and the vehicle is stable. Removing the roof makes the entire interior of the vehicle accessible. EMS personnel can stand beside or climb into the vehicle and pursue emergency care efforts while rescuers carry out disentanglement procedures. In addition, removing the roof creates a large exitway through which an occupant can be quickly removed when he has a life-threatening injury or when fire or another hazard is threatening the operation. It also provides fresh air and helps cool the patient when heat is a problem.

Skill Summary 17–4 illustrates the procedure for folding a collision vehicle's roof back like the roof of a convertible. While this is the most commonly used procedure, it is not the only way to dispose of a roof. A roof can be folded forward after cutting both C- and B-posts (rear and middle posts), folded to either side after cutting the posts of the opposite side, or removed altogether after severing all of the roof posts. If you lack a hydraulic rescue tool, you can accomplish all of these procedures with a hacksaw and a spray container of lubricant.

Step Two: Create Exitways by Removing Doors and Roof Posts

When rapid vertical extrication through the opened roof is not indicated, the next step is to open doors and remove roof posts. The benefits of this step are that EMS personnel can kneel beside the vehicle while carrying out patient care and immobilization procedures, and the immobilized patients can be easily rotated onto a long spine

Disposing of the Roof of a Car

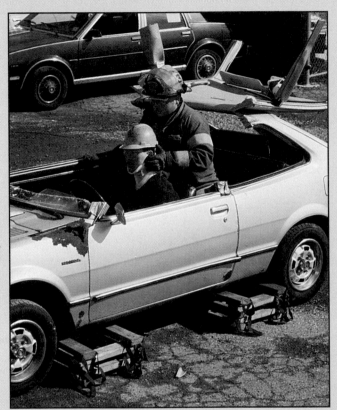

A. The traditional procedure for disposing of the roof is to sever the A- and B-posts, cut through the roof rails just ahead of the C-posts, and fold the roof back like the roof of a convertible. It is necessary either to remove or to cut the windshield, depending on the need for working space.

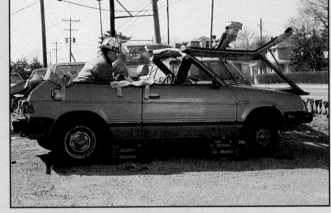

B. Folding the roof forward can be accomplished quickly when the C-posts are narrow. The roof is hinged either on the top or the bottom of the windshield, depending on the need for working space.

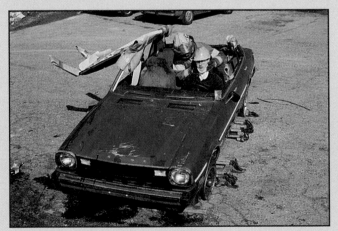

C. When a car has only one occupant, the roof can be folded to one side after severing the A-, B-, and C-posts of the opposite side.

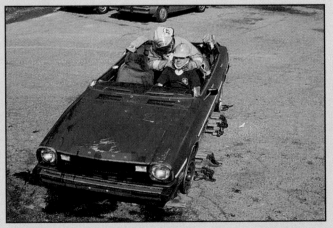

D. When a car has narrow C-posts, removing the roof altogether provides maximum working space.

CHAPTER 17 Operations   **361**

Displacing Doors and Roof Posts of a Car

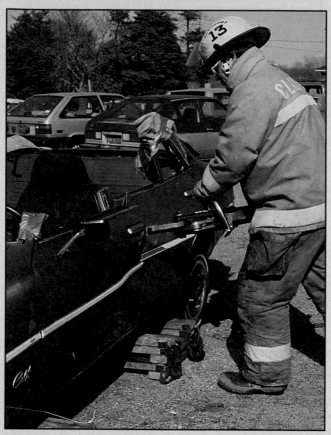

A. A collision vehicle's doors can be opened quickly with a hydraulic rescue tool. Doors can be opened at the latch or by breaking the hinges.

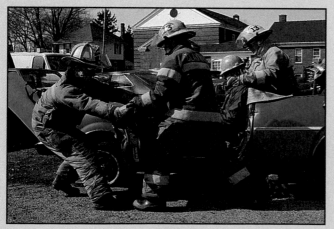

B. Once the front door has been opened, it can be moved beyond the normal range of motion by simply pushing on it. Seldom is there a need for removing a front door.

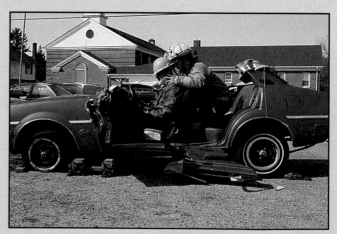

C. When the front doors of a four-door car have been opened at the latch side, the roof post and rear door can be pulled down simultaneously to expose the entire side of the vehicle.

Displacing the Front End of a Car

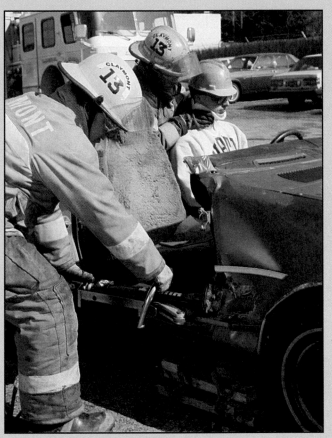

A. Relief cuts are made at the junction of the A-post with the rocker panel, and in the A-post between the door hinges.

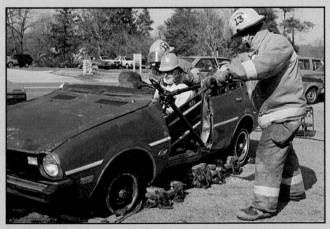

B. Heavy-duty jacks can be used to pivot the front end of the vehicle away from the relief cuts.

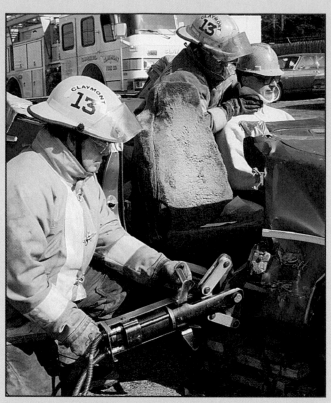

C. The combination hydraulic tool can be used in the spreading mode to displace the front end.

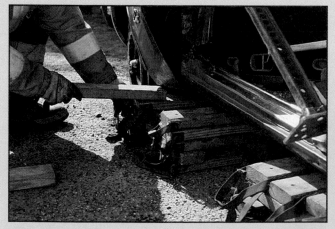

D. Displacing the front end will tend to lift the vehicle from the cribs. Cribbing must be added to the front cribs to prevent destabilization.

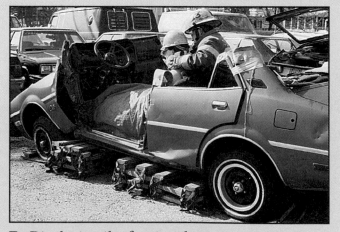

E. Displacing the front end creates working space by moving a number of mechanisms of entrapment away from the front seat occupants.

board. Skill Summary 17–5 shows a rescue team using a hydraulic rescue tool to open doors that cannot be unlatched and pulled open in the usual manner, as when doors are damaged or locks and latches jammed.

Step Three: Disentangle Occupants by Displacing the Front End

Most vehicle rescue training courses include procedures for displacing or removing seats, dash assemblies, steering wheels, steering columns, and pedals. A quicker and more efficient way to disentangle an injured driver and/or passenger from these mechanisms of entrapment is to displace the entire front end of the vehicle. While the task sounds difficult, it is not. Skill Summary 17–6 illustrates the procedure for displacing the front end of a passenger car with a combination hydraulic rescue tool. A dash displacement can also be accomplished with heavy-duty jacks and hacksaws.

If the steering wheel hub is large and rectangular, the car probably has an air bag or bags (the passenger-side bag is in the area of the glove compartment). If the bags have not deployed, they are not likely to deploy now unless extrication involves displacing the dash or steering wheel. If such displacement is to be done, air bag manufacturers recommend that you avoid placing your body or objects against an air bag module or in its path of deployment. Follow this recommendation *before* you disconnect the battery cables. *Air bag manufacturers strongly advise against displacement or cutting the steering column until the air bag system has been fully deactivated, cutting or drilling into an air bag module, or applying heat in the area of the steering wheel hub.*

Must this entire three-part procedure be used for all extrication operations and always be performed in the same order? Not necessarily! In some cases, it may be necessary only to force a door open to reach a single patient and create an exitway for his removal. In other cases, it may be prudent to open doors before disposing of the roof. In still other situations, there may not be a need to displace the front end of a collision vehicle.

Remember, the main purpose of your understanding of extrication procedures is so you can integrate them with your patient care plan.

■ MANAGING THE MULTIPLE-CASUALTY INCIDENT

A **multiple-casualty incident**, or **MCI**, is an event that places a great demand on EMS resources, be it equipment or personnel. A situation that involves more than one patient and requires an ambulance response of three or more vehicles is generally referred to as an MCI. However, the definition of an MCI differs from community to community and is based upon the resources that are available at any given moment.

A large-scale disaster can easily tax, if not overwhelm, a single agency. One way to minimize the operating difficulties of a large-scale MCI or disaster is for every EMT-B in the agency to become familiar with the local disaster plan. A **disaster plan** is a predetermined set of instructions that tells a community's various emergency responders what to do in specific emergencies. While no disaster plan can address every problem that could arise, there are several features common to every good disaster plan. The disaster plan should be:

- Written to address the events that are conceivable for a particular location.
- Well publicized so each emergency responder is familiar with the plan and how it is to be put into operation.
- Realistic and based upon the actual availability of resources.
- Rehearsed frequently to get all the "bugs" out. This is best done as an extension of what the EMT-Bs do every day. That is why many services declare a medical MCI for incidents requiring three or more ambulances and major collisions.

Components of an Incident Management System

An **incident management system**, or **IMS**, has been developed to assist with the control, direction, and coordination of emergency response resources. IMS has nine key components: strong visible command, common terminology, modular organization based upon incident needs, comprehensive resource management, manageable span of control, assurance of personnel safety and accountability, integrated communications, unified command, and consolidated action plans using goals and objectives.

When integrated, these components provide the basis for an effective operation. There is an essential need for **common terminology** in any emergency management system, which will potentially involve multiple agencies from different disciplines. Plain English always works best! Instead of trying to remember that the EMS Commander is unit 615 or car 2 or ambulance 7, simply refer to the individual by the name of the position—"EMS Command." This also facilitates transfer of command to supervisory personnel who may arrive later in the incident and assume command. The person in EMS Command should wear a clearly identifiable, bright-colored vest for easy identification, as should each of the sector officers.

At each incident, IMS organizational structure develops in a **modular fashion**. Since the development of the organization is top down, there is always at least an incident commander, or IC, identified at any incident. If the incident's needs dictate, the IC may delegate additional responsibilities to other personnel.

Management of communications at an incident requires **integrated communications**. An integrated communications plan includes standardized procedures, use of clear instruction with common terminology, two-way confirmation that messages are received, and status reports to update the IC on assignments that were delegated. Radio frequencies should be set up in advance to ensure that all arriving units have common frequencies and that these are tactical and command frequencies that can be used at the incident.

There are two methods of command: singular and unified. **Singular command** is used when all resources are specifically under the jurisdiction and control of one agency. In many communities, EMS is managed by fire services. Accordingly, singular command is often used at fire and rescue incidents. However, if police agencies have major involvement, if there is a separate EMS provider, or if other agencies are involved, **unified command** is more appropriate (Figure 17–12). In most communities unified command is the best way to manage resources since incidents tend to grow more complex and the right agency must take the lead at the appropriate time, with command officers from all agencies cooperating. In a unified command system, all agencies involved contribute to the command process by establishing a **consolidated action plan**. Complex incidents may require written

action plans that cover all strategic goals, all tactical objectives, and support activities for the incident's entire operational period. A unified command structure is best achieved by setting up one command post instead of separate ones for police, fire, and EMS.

Another important component of IMS is span of control. A **manageable span of control** spells out the number of subordinates that one supervisor can manage effectively. The desired range is three to seven, with five being optimum. It is very easy to lose track of your crew members at an incident if they are not assigned to smaller units.

IMS also designates incident facilities such as the **command post**, which is where each agency representative, the communications center, and the center of all planning and incident operations direction are located. Many communities utilize a **mobile command center**, which is a vehicle with desk space, maps, multiple radio frequencies, and enough room for the command officers from each agency. **Staging areas** are designated facilities designed to keep the scene from being clogged with equipment, vehicles, and personnel, yet keeping them within a few minutes of the incident so they can respond as directed.

Comprehensive resource management is attained by maximizing resource use, consolidating control of large numbers of ambulances, and reducing the communications load. Knowledge of the status of personnel and vehicles is critical to effective resource management.

The IMS Functional Areas

IMS has five major functional areas, or sections: command, operations, planning, logistics, and finance. In a major incident, each of the five may be a different person's responsibility; in a smaller incident these functional areas may be combined.

The **command** section is always staffed no matter what the size of the incident. The Incident Commander has overall responsibility for managing. The IC's responsibilities include assessing incident priorities, determining the strategic goals and tactical objectives, developing an incident action plan and the appropriate organizational structure, managing incident resources, ensuring personnel safety, coordinating activities of outside agencies, and authorizing release of information. With this long list of responsibilities, it is easy to see the need for delegation and establishment of various sector officers.

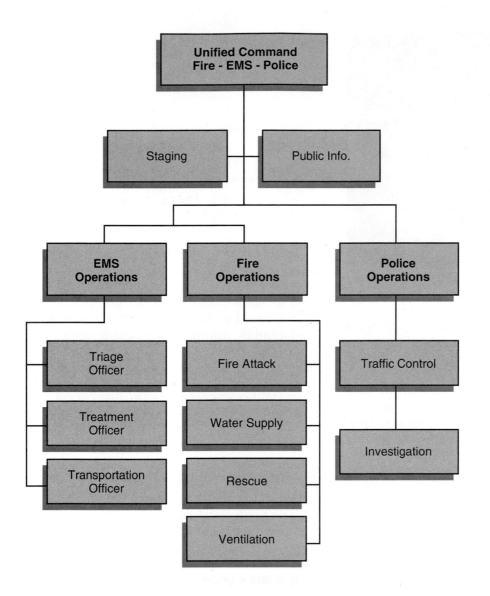

FIGURE 17–12
An organizational chart
for a unified command
method.

Unified Command
Fire - EMS - Police

Staging

Public Info.

EMS
Operations

Fire
Operations

Police
Operations

Triage
Officer

Fire Attack

Traffic Control

Treatment
Officer

Water Supply

Investigation

Transportation
Officer

Rescue

Ventilation

The **operations** section is responsible for all tactical operations at an incident, including those with which you are most familiar—patient care, firefighting, and hostage negotiations. The **planning** section is responsible for the collection, evaluation, dissemination, and use of information about the development of the incident and the status of resources. This includes situation status, resource status, and documentation and demobilization units, as well as technical specialists.

The **logistics** section is responsible for providing facilities, services, and materials for the incident. This includes the communications unit, medical unit, food unit, service branch, supply unit, facilities unit, and ground support units. The **finance** section is responsible for all costs and financial considerations at an extensive incident. This includes the time, procurement, compensations, claim, and cost units.

EMS Command at an MCI

In an incident that is primarily an EMS incident, the **EMS Command**, or Medical Command as some agencies refer to it, would often be the first crew leader on the first arriving EMS unit. The senior EMT-B's first responsibility includes confirming the incident by radio to the dispatcher. The EMS command describes the nature of the emergency, its exact location, and the best estimate of the number of patients. This crucial information is used by the dispatcher to send additional resources to the scene. The radio report also includes a request for any special resources that the EMT-Bs feel may be necessary.

Additional responsibilities of EMS command include sizing up resources and the need for additional EMS response, managing the EMS response, coordinating activities of all EMS personnel at the

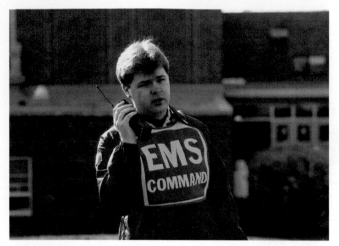

FIGURE 17–13 EMS command with a vest and radio.

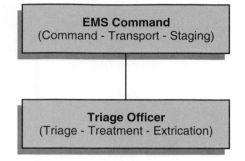

FIGURE 17–14 An organizational chart for a smaller incident.

incident, designating EMS sector officers, ensuring the safety of all EMS personnel, establishing communications contacts, and notifying hospitals. The EMS Commander dons the designated vest so that all units arriving on the scene can identify him (Figure 17–13). The EMS Commander may need to establish a Command Post and remain at that location. If a Command Post is already established, the EMS crew chief becomes the EMS representative at the Command Post. He or she works cooperatively with police and fire service commanders in the Command Post. The EMS sectors that are established as needed include:

- Staging sector
- Triage sector
- Treatment sector
- Transport sector
- Extrication sector (may be a fire-rescue responsibility)
- Mobile command center

At small incidents, it may only be necessary to designate command and the triage sector (Figure 17–14). At medium-sized incidents, command, triage, treatment, and transport may be designated (Figure 17–15). At larger incidents, EMS Command may designate all the sector officers and have an aide to assist with communications, a safety officer, and a public-information officer (Figure 17–16).

Preceptor Pearl

The EMS Commander who doesn't delegate, but attempts to wear all the vests, cannot possibly get the overall picture of the incident because he or she has taken on too much responsibility. ❖

Safety Officer and Staging Sector

When it becomes necessary, EMS Command may choose to designate a Safety Officer and a Staging Sector Officer. The **EMS Safety Officer** is responsible for ensuring scene safety for all EMS personnel. This officer pays close attention to details that EMS Command may not have the time to focus on, such as whether the personnel at the scene are identified adequately or are wearing the appropriate protective gear for the incident. The Safety Officer determines if personnel are about to encounter dangerous situations and takes responsibility for assuring compliance with OSHA regulations for the appropriate level of infection control follow-up for the incident.

FIGURE 17–15
An organizational chart for a medium-sized incident.

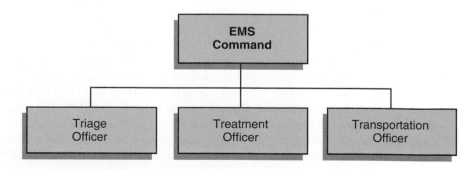

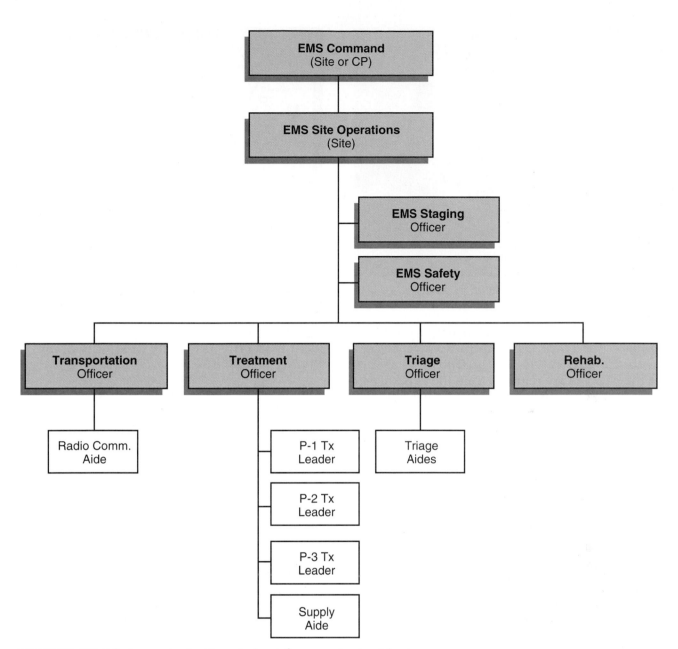

FIGURE 17–16 An organizational chart for a major incident.

The **EMS Staging Sector Officer** is responsible for establishing an assembly point and mobilization area for personnel and vehicles, releasing resources to the incident as requested by the Transport Sector Officer, and ensuring that the physiological needs of the personnel are being met. After an ambulance transports a patient to the hospital, it usually returns to the staging sector.

The Triage Sector

The **Triage Sector Officer** is responsible for establishing triage procedures as dictated by incident type. For easy identifications, the Triage Officer dons the appropriate vest (Figure 17–17). The first triage cut is done rapidly by using a bullhorn, PA system, or loud voice to direct all patients capable of walking (Priority 3) to move to a particular location. This action has a twofold purpose. It quickly identifies those individuals who have an open airway and adequate circulation, and it physically separates them from patients who need more care. In some cases, triage involves extrication of trapped patients; in other cases, it involves corralling all patients in order to funnel them to the treatment sector for medical evaluation.

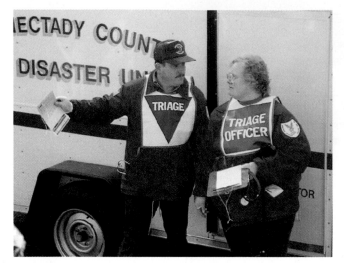

FIGURE 17-17 A triage officer in vest.

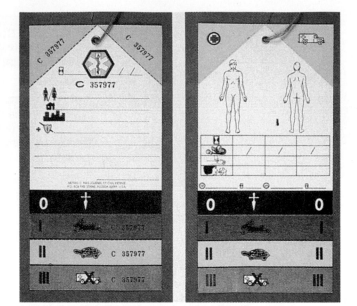

FIGURE 17-18 Typical triage tags used to identify Priority 1, Priority 2, Priority 3, and Priority 0 patients.

When extrication is needed or patients are entrapped, the Triage Officer must work very closely with the **Extrication Sector Officer** to assure that the patients are removed from the wreckage in the correct order. In instances in which patients are piled on top of one another, it may be necessary to remove a low-priority patient in order to access a higher priority patient. The triage officer is responsible for coordinating personnel and equipment usage and can appoint triage support personnel as needed to aid in the movement of patients to treatment and/or transportation sectors. Usually patients are immobilized on backboards if necessary and carried by "runners" to the appropriate treatment sector. Extensive treatment does not take place at the incident site because it is in a hazard zone and rescue and initial treatment of other patients could be impeded.

Triage is a French word which means "to sort." If you are assigned to work in the triage sector, you will need to do an initial triage and apply a **triage tag** to each patient (Figure 17–18). Different localities use different tagging systems. It is important that you know and understand the system used in your area. Because many MCIs are multiple-agency events, it is equally important that different services in the same region use the same coding system. If each agency were to use a different system, it would be impossible to correctly coordinate the order in which patients are to receive care.

Patients are usually divided into the following four categories:

- **Priority One (P-1)** The red color designation indicates that the patient has life-threatening critical injuries or illnesses such as airway and breathing difficulties, uncontrolled or severe bleeding, decreased mental status, patients with severe medical problems, shock (hypoperfusion), or severe burns. Whenever possible, these patients should be transported to the hospital first.

- **Priority Two (P-2)** The yellow color designation identifies patients with unstable or potentially unstable injuries such as burns without airway problems, major or multiple bone or joint injuries, back injuries with or without spinal cord damage. Whenever possible, these patients should be transported as soon as the P-1 patients have been removed from the scene.

- **Priority Three (P-3)** The green color designation identifies the "walking wounded," such as patients with minor painful, swollen, deformed extremities, minor soft tissue injuries, and psychological trauma. Whenever possible, isolate these patients from the P-1 and P-2 patients to limit their psychological trauma as well as to unclutter the scene. Many services routinely dispatch a school bus to transport the P-3 patients to a distant hospital for further evaluation and treatment. While this is helpful, ensure that these patients are reevaluated prior to allowing them to ride the bus and that medical personnel are placed on the bus in case a patient's condition changes.

- **Priority Zero (P-0)** The color black identifies the dead and includes victims with exposed brain matter, cardiac arrest for over 20 minutes except with cold-water drowning or severe hypothermia, decapitation, severed trunk, and incineration. In a situation where there is a limited amount of responders compared to the large number of patients, a patient with a critical injury may initially be prioritized as a P-3 and then, when ample help is available, either worked as a P-1 or left as a P-0. The basic principle of triage is to help as many of the seriously injured as possible. Dedicating an EMT-B crew to a cardiac arrest patient when there are many, many serious patients who need their help would violate the basic principle of triage.

The Treatment Sector

The **Treatment Sector Officer** is responsible for setting up treatment areas as requested and warranted by the site and transportation considerations. This officer supervises the area established to hold patients prior to transportation from the scene, as well as coordinates activities of all EMS personnel assigned to the sector.

The treatment officer and assistants triage the patients in that sector to determine the order in which they will receive treatment. During secondary triage, it may be necessary to recategorize to a higher or lower priority a patient whose condition has deteriorated or improved or who was incorrectly diagnosed. This necessitates moving the patient to the proper treatment sector as resources permit. During secondary triage, some services use a different tag on which more detailed information about the patient can be recorded. Other services set up their treatment sector by using red, yellow, green, and black tarps to separate the patients while they wait for transportation. The Treatment Officer appoints treatment personnel, directly oversees the patient care provided, determines the need for additional personnel and equipment, and coordinates movement of patients to ambulances with the transport sector.

The Transport Sector

The **Transport Sector Officer** establishes and maintains ambulance loading areas. This officer is responsible for supervising patient movement in conjunction with the treatment sector officer, accessing and monitoring local hospital capabilities, and determining patient destinations. The Transport Sector Officer also coordinates helicopter evacuations if they are used at the incident. No ambulance should proceed to a treatment sector without having been requested by the Transport Officer and directed by the Staging Officer. It is also vital that no ambulance transport any patient without the approval of the Transport Officer, since the Transport Officer maintains documentation of all patient destinations through a patient log or copies of the triage tags.

The Transport Officer also supervises the hospital communications network, which may involve appointing a hospital communicator to operate the hospital communications network, maintaining hospital status and capability, and providing patient information to hospitals via radio or cellular phone. During a major incident, individual ambulances should not communicate directly with the hospital. This will be done directly by the hospital communicator in an abbreviated manner. The hospital may be told only that they are receiving a Priority 1 patient with respiratory problems. The Transport Officer also appoints vehicle loaders to facilitate patient loading and ambulance movement from the scene.

Preceptor Pearl

Practice declaring EMS Command, establishing a triage sector, donning sector vests, giving an arrival report to dispatch, and applying triage tags at all incidents involving three or more ambulances! In this way, the procedures will be second nature to you at larger incidents. ❖

Freelancing

Individuals at the scene will be assigned to particular roles in one of the sectors. Upon arrival, you should report to the sector officer for specific duties. Once assigned a specific task, you should complete the task and report back to the sector officer. *At an MCI, never go off and do just anything you want. This is called "freelancing" and leads to confusion, lack of coordination of resources, and the potential for injury to the EMT-B.*

Psychological Aspects of MCIs

During MCIs, you often encounter psychologically stressed patients. While these patients may outwardly exhibit few signs of injury, they undoubtedly have been subjected to devastating circumstances that they are not prepared to cope with. Proper early management of the psychologically stressed patient supports later treatment and helps ensure a faster recovery. Some services will automatically dispatch a clergy member or a psychologist who has been oriented to emergency services work to assist these patients at the scene.

Adequately managing a patient during an MCI may require you to administer "psychological first aid." This may take the form of talking with a terrified parent, child, or witness. A compassionate, honest demeanor, as will listening to the patient and acknowledging his fears, can reassure him. Often this is all the patient needs.

Patients are not the only ones to sustain emotional scars during an MCI. Emergency responders do as well. Large-scale or horrific MCIs may affect rescuers as much as, if not more than, non-rescuers. No one gets "used to" walking through body parts at the scene of a plane crash! It is not a sign of weakness to talk about your feelings after a major incident.

Treat co-workers who become emotionally incapacitated as patients and remove them to an area where they can rest without viewing the scene. Ensure that these patients are monitored by an EMS provider until a clinically competent provider can take over. Do not allow these EMT-Bs to return to duty without first being evaluated by a psychologist. Critical incident stress debriefing (CISD) teams are a resource that can provide the emotional and psychological support needed by these patients. Intervention by a CISD team may help to prevent post-traumatic stress disorder and help put the individual "back in service" quicker.

CHAPTER REVIEW

■ SUMMARY

The five phases of an ambulance call include preparation, obtaining and responding, transferring the patient to the ambulance, transport to and arrival at the hospital, and terminating the call. Knowing which equipment should be brought to the patient's side and understanding the risk factors in responding to a call are paramount responsibilities of the EMT-B.

Since extrication of a patient from a vehicle is the most common type of rescue across the United States, it is important for the EMT-B to understand the process so he or she can keep the patient informed and anticipate any dangerous steps in the extrication action plan. You must not only safeguard the patient, but yourself as well by

choosing and wearing the proper protective gear. As an EMT-B your role in the extrication process is to rescue the *patient*, not the vehicle.

Knowledge and understanding of your agency's disaster plan can help minimize the operating difficulties of a large-scale MCI or disaster. A disaster plan should we written to address the events that are conceivable for a particular location, well publicized, realistic, and rehearsed. EMT-Bs should practice declaring EMS Command, establishing a triage sector, donning sector vests, giving an arrival report to dispatch, and applying triage tags at all incidents involving three or more ambulances, so the procedures will be second nature to them at larger incidents.

■ REVIEW QUESTIONS

1. List three kinds of ventilation devices that should be carried on the ambulance.

2. Write down a list of all the equipment that should routinely be brought to the patient's side to conduct the initial assessment and focused trauma exam.

3. Describe the typical ambulance collision: when, where, and how it most often occurs.

4. List three defensive driving techniques to help prevent ambulance collisions.

5. Discuss five factors that lead to increased driving time to calls.

6. List the phases of extrication.

7. Explain the role of the EMT-B in size-up of a motor-vehicle collision.

8. List the ten types of specialty operations teams and state who handles these incidents in your community.

9. Explain the role of the EMS Commander and the three sector officers that are designated at a medium-sized MCI.

10. List examples of patients who would be classified as high or low priority at an MCI scene and explain what to do with the "walking wounded."

CHAPTER 18

Hazmat Awareness

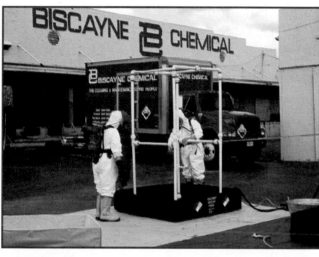

■ The amount of hazmat training needed by all EMT-Bs has been argued in many forums. Basically, the amount of training that you need is based on your local community's plan to deal with hazardous material incidents. If the plan calls for ambulance personnel to respond to a hazmat scene and to stage in the COLD ZONE waiting to transport decontaminated patients to the appropriate hospital, then experts argue that the first responder awareness level of training would be sufficient. However, if the plan designates that the EMT-Bs provide medical monitoring of a "hazmat team" or assist in decontamination of patients in the WARM ZONE, experts recommend that at least first responder operational, if not specialist or technician levels, would be needed. The latter, higher levels of training are beyond the scope of this text. However, this chapter is designed to help you meet the Occupational Safety and Health Administration (OSHA) training requirements at the first responder awareness level.

MAKING THE TRANSITION

■ Ongoing education of EMT-Bs should include hazmat first responder awareness level of training in compliance with OSHA regulations.

The objectives below state the OSHA training requirements at the first responder awareness level. To satisfy OSHA's requirements, a qualified instructor must present the hazmat material and test your understanding of it.

■ KNOWLEDGE AND ATTITUDE

At the completion of this lesson, you should be able to:

1. Define hazardous materials. (p. 375)
2. Describe the risks associated with a hazardous materials incident. (pp. 375–376)
3. Describe the potential outcomes associated with an emergency created when hazardous materials are present. (pp. 375–376)
4. Describe the content of the OSHA Rule 29 CFR Part 1910.120. (pp. 376–377)
5. Discuss the relationship between the NFPA Standards and the OSHA regulations in hazmat. (p. 377)
6. Identify five types of clues that might help the EMS provider recognize the presence of hazardous materials in an incident. (pp. 380–385)
7. Describe methods of identifying hazardous materials. (pp. 380–385)
8. Describe the role of the first responder awareness individual in the employer's (ambulance service) emergency response plan, including site security and control and use of the U.S. DOT *Emergency Response Guidebook.* (pp. 377–380)
9. Describe when additional resources are needed at a hazmat incident and how to notify the communications center of these needs. (pp. 377–378)
10. Define medical surveillance of a hazmat incident. (pp. 379–380)
11. Describe the medical monitoring of a hazmat incident. (p. 380)
12. Describe the refresher requirements of the OSHA hazmat training. (pp. 376–377)

ON THE SCENE

Freezing rain blanketed the highways during the Christmas holiday weekend. Due to poor road conditions, a tanker truck overturned on the state thruway. Fortunately, the driver was not seriously injured in the accident, but the tanker's contents were leaking onto the pavement. The police, fire department, and EMS had been called to assist in the situation. The dispatcher was originally alerted by a passing motorist on a cellular phone. The dispatcher did not know the identity of the leaking chemical, but he was able to advise the responders that the traffic was backed up for miles.

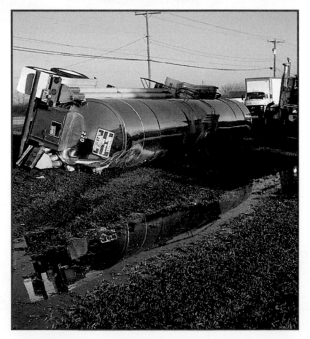

In the past, a first-emergency responder arriving at this incident might have walked through the spilled material to survey the situation—possibly confusing the product with rain on the ground. After calling for the fire department, he might have remained in his vehicle, attempting to warm up. While the specific chemical may not have been a hazard at the outside ambient temperature, at a warmer temperature it could vaporize into a gas that could be extremely hazardous. It's possible that the chemicals on the rescuer's shoes would be warmed by the vehicle's heater, and would be vaporized within the closed cab. The rescuer would then have become a victim.

The new approach to a similar hazardous materials incident would include the following actions: size up the situation and approach it with a high level of caution, identify the substances and hazards involved, secure the scene and establish medical command and control zones, obtain additional help from higher levels of personnel and resource agencies trained in hazardous materials, establish a rehab sector, assist with medical monitoring of the hazmat team members, treat decontaminated patients, and provide the Safety Officer and Incident Commander with medical insight about the chemicals involved in the situation. ■

■ WHAT IS A HAZARDOUS MATERIAL?

The definition of a hazardous material varies, depending on the regulations or standards of the defining agency. The U.S. Department of Transportation (DOT) defines a **hazardous material** as "any substance or material in a quantity or form which poses an unreasonable risk to health, safety, and property when transported in commerce." This definition is appropriate for DOT because it regulates commercial means of transportation. However, the Environmental Protection Agency (EPA), because it regulates the environment, defines a **hazardous substance** as "any substance designated under the Clean Water Act and Comprehensive Environmental Response Compensation and Liability Act as posing a threat to waterways and the environment when released." The EPA goes on to define **hazardous waste** as "any waste or combination of wastes which pose a substantial present or potential hazard to human health or living organisms because such wastes are nondegradable or persistent in nature, or because they can biologically magnify, or because they may otherwise cause or tend to cause detrimental cumulative effects."

Perhaps the most encompassing definition of a hazardous material is the National Fire Protection Association's (NFPA) in Standard #472. It defines it as "any substance that causes or may cause adverse effects on the health or safety of employees, the general public, or the environment: any biological agent and other disease-causing agent, or a waste or combination of wastes." Think about this definition the next time you consider throwing away a can of oil or some bloody bandages.

■ RECOGNIZING THE RISKS OF HAZARDOUS MATERIALS

Preparing to respond to a call that involves a hazardous material is more than having the money to buy protective encapsulated ("Gumby") suits. Hazmat training—as well as analyzing the hazmat risks in your community—is required by the Occupational Safety and Health Administration (OSHA). Hazardous materials are all around us, and the number of chemicals is constantly growing. Consider the case of a brewery in Golden, Colorado, where, in July of 1991, two anhydrous ammonia leaks occurred within a month, producing over 32 inhalation injuries. Could this happen in your area? Although there may not be a brewery in your district, what other manufacturers use anhydrous ammonia in the manufacture of their products?

Have you ever observed the trucks passing through your district? Consider the case of the tanker truck which, when one of its three cells split open on the New Jersey turnpike during rush-hour traffic, spilled 4,000 gallons of hydrochloric acid on the highway. In addition to the closing of 15 miles of packed highway, five police officers, seven firefighters, and more than a dozen motorists were hospitalized for severe respiratory burns.

Maybe your town is divided by a railroad and each year your service practices for a train multiple casualty incident (MCI). Watch as the trains go by and pay attention to the markings on the cars. To emphasize the importance of observing passing trains, consider this incident that took place in Murdock, Illinois. After a freight train carrying sulfuric acid, alcohol, and propane derailed, a fireball resulted that was visible for 20 miles. The explosion was so powerful that it threw a large portion of a tank car almost half a mile, and it required the evacuation of a four-mile area. Fortunately, only eight emergency workers required treatment for chemical exposure.

Take time to review what chemicals are manufactured and stored in or transported through your community. Do you have major interstate routes through your district? Does it have railroads, chemical plants, fertilizer storage facilities, waterways, airports, hospitals, water-treatment plants, refineries, nuclear plants, a nursery, or corner gas stations? What, exactly, is stored in those warehouses on the edge of town?

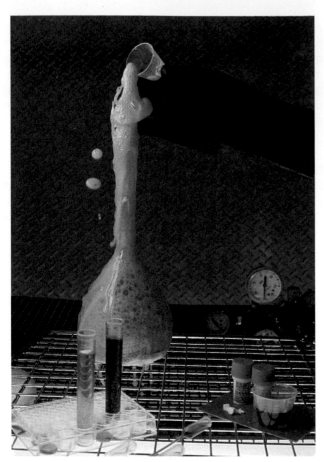

FIGURE 18-1 A chemistry laboratory can be the site of a hazmat incident.

However, don't mistakenly think that dangerous goods are carried only in 55-gallon drums, in tankers, or in rail cars. Some chemicals can be very hazardous in small quantities. Keep in mind that some small-package shippers in the United States, aware of the rules and regulations for shipping hazardous materials, very carefully and properly load their vehicles with less than the amount of chemical that would require a hazmat placard on the outside of their trucks. Even the local high-school chemistry class easily illustrates the volatility of small quantities of chemicals if they are improperly mixed (Figure 18-1). The local school lab can be very hazardous if not properly supervised. So be aware of the range of potential hazardous-material incident sites in your community.

■ HAZMAT RULES AND STANDARDS

Because of a few "high profile" incidents in the United States, the storage, transportation, and response to emergencies involving chemicals have come under the regulation of many government agencies.

SARA Title III: Planning Regulations

The **Superfund Amendments and Reauthorization Act of 1986 (SARA)** is a federal law. Title III of this law, the Emergency Planning and Community Right-to-Know Act, established hazardous chemical requirements for local, state, and federal governments, as well as industry, in the areas of emergency planning, emergency notification, community right-to-know reporting requirements, and toxic-chemical release reporting emissions inventory. The emergency planning section of SARA was designed to develop state and local preparedness and response capabilities through better coordination and planning. The governor of each state appointed a State Emergency Response Commission which, in turn, designated local emergency planning committees, or **LEPCs**. Your ambulance service may have some involvement in LEPCs, which are responsible for:

- Identifying facilities, transportation routes, and secondary facilities
- Establishing facility and community response procedures
- Designating facility and community emergency coordinators
- Developing facility and public notification procedures
- Developing methods for determining release and impact areas
- Describing emergency equipment and personnel at facilities and in the community
- Developing evacuation plans
- Developing training programs and schedules
- Designing methods and schedules for exercising plans

OSHA Regulations

In 1989, OSHA put in place 29 CFR Part 1910.120, which deals with the Emergency Response to Hazardous Substance Releases. These regulations:

- Spell out training requirements for five levels of responders to hazmat incidents
- Specify who can teach the training programs
- Set out refresher training requirements

- Specify medical surveillance and consultation requirements
- Specify chemical protective clothing and post-emergency response operations

These regulations were designed for the first response agencies to a hazardous materials incident, such as police departments, fire departments, and ambulance services. The regulations frequently use the terms "employer" and "employee." In some states, the courts have determined that volunteer agencies are employers and their members are employees, even if they do not receive remuneration for their services.

The training is broken into the following five levels:

- *First Responder Awareness* This recommended 4 to 6 hours of training is for rescuers who are likely to witness or discover a hazardous substance release. They are trained only to recognize the problem and initiate a response from the proper organizations.

- *First Responder Operations* This 8 hours of training is for those who initially respond to releases or potential releases of hazardous materials, in order to protect people, property, and the environment. These responders stay at a safe distance, keep the incident from spreading, and protect people from any exposures.

- *Hazardous Materials Technician* This 24 hours of training is for those who actually plug, patch, or stop the release of a hazardous material.

- *Hazardous Materials Specialist* This 24 hours of training is for those expected to respond with and provide support to hazardous material technicians. Their duties parallel those of the technician. However, specialists require a more directed or specific knowledge of the various substances they may be called upon to contain. They also act as the site liaison with federal, state, and local government authorities in regards to site activities.

- *On-Scene Incident Commander* This training level is for the rescuer who will assume control of the incident. Training includes the first-responder operations level in addition to competency in the following: 1) know and be able to implement the employer's incident command system, 2) know how to implement the employer's emergency response plan, 3) know and understand the hazards and risks associated with employees working in chemical-protective clothing, 4) know how to implement the local emergency response plan, 5) know the state emergency response plan and the plan of the

Federal Regional Response Team, and 6) know and understand the importance of contamination procedures.

Employees are expected to be adequately trained at the level in which they will participate prior to being involved in an incident. Each EMS agency is responsible for training its EMT-Bs in at least the awareness level if your original EMT-B training did not also include hazmat training. Some services show a video, run a drill, and review the hazmat plan. Then each employee is given a written test on the objectives they must pass, which is then inserted in the employee's file. In addition, OSHA requires that trainees at each level demonstrate their competencies annually.

National Fire Protection Association's Standards

The National Fire Protection Association (NFPA) sets voluntary standards for the fire service that are often adapted by local municipalities. Why is the NFPA writing safety standards for EMS? Because in the United States, more than 50% of the prehospital EMS is provided by the fire service. The NFPA standards most relevant to EMS are Standards 472, 473, and 704.

Standard 472: Professional Competence of Responders to Hazardous Materials Incidents preceded and set the stage for OSHA 1910.120. Standard 473: Competencies for EMS Personnel Responding to Hazardous Materials Incidents established two levels of EMS hazmat responder above the awareness level and was the first standard to specifically address the role of EMS personnel. This standard is also the best predictor of the next OSHA regulations for EMS personnel. Standard 704: This defines a method of classifying hazards discussed later in this chapter.

■ EMT-B'S FIRST RESPONDER ROLE

Establish Command and Control Zones

When you arrive on the scene of a hazmat emergency, take a defensive position in a safe place far enough from the site to ensure your safety. Try to

9-Station Decontamination Procedure

STEPS

Station 1. Rescuers enter decon areas and mechanically remove contaminants from victims. Tools are dropped in tool drop area. Rescuers are in SCBA and protective clothing. **Proceed to Station 2.**

Station 2. *Gross Decontamination*: Victims and rescue personnel are showered and/or scrubbed by decon personnel. Dilution is conducted inside diked area. Victims may be transported directly to Station 6. **Proceed to Station 6.**

Station 3. *Protective Clothing Removal*: Rescuers remove protective clothing, clothing is isolated and labeled for later disposal. Clothing is placed on contaminated side. **Proceed to Station 4.**

Station 4. *SCBA Removal*: Rescue personnel remove and isolate their SCBA. If re-entry is necessary, personnel don new SCBA from non-contaminated side. **Proceed to Station 5.**

Station 5. *Personal Clothing Removal*: All clothing and personal items are removed. Victims who have not been undressed are undressed here. All clothing and personal items are isolated in plastic bags and labeled for later disposal. **Proceed to Station 6.**

Station 6. *Body Washing*: Full body washing is performed using soft scrub brushes or sponges and soap or mild detergent. Cleaning tools are bagged for later disposal. **Proceed to Station 7.**

Station 7. *Dry Off*: Towels and sheets are used to dry off. Rescuers and victims are dressed in clean clothes. Towels/sheets are bagged for later disposal. **Proceed to Station 8.**

Station 8. *Medical Assessment*: Rapid patient assessment is conducted by rescuers. Necessary stabilization procedures are accomplished. **Proceed to Station 9.**

Station 9. *Transport*: Transfer of patient to hospital for medical attention or to recovery areas for rest and observation.

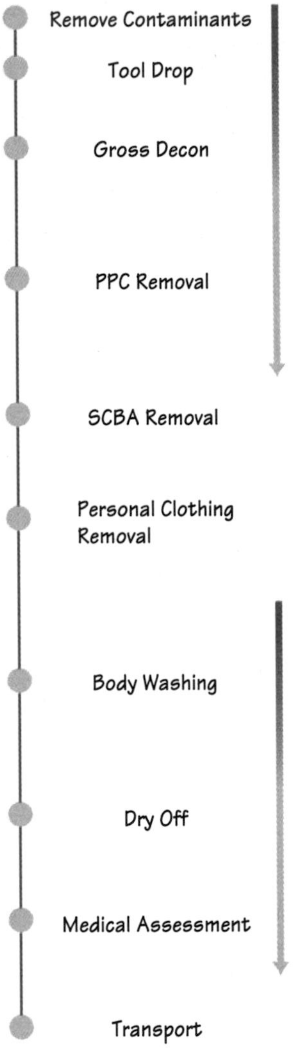

- Remove Contaminants
- Tool Drop
- Gross Decon
- PPC Removal
- SCBA Removal
- Personal Clothing Removal
- Body Washing
- Dry Off
- Medical Assessment
- Transport

FIGURE 18-2 An example of the field decontamination process.

position your vehicle upwind and at a higher level than the incident to avoid providing an ignition source for gases that stay near the ground and to prevent your inhaling potentially toxic fumes escaping from the area. Secure the scene without entering the area of contamination, commonly called the HOT ZONE. Do what you can to isolate the area, establish a perimeter, evacuate people if necessary, assure the safety of your crew, and direct bystanders to a safe area. Call for the hazmat team capable of entering the HOT ZONE to rescue the injured and control the incident.

Preceptor Pearl

Do not rescue people from the HOT ZONE unless you have been trained to the proper level and are dressed with the appropriate protection for the chemical involved. ✜

While help is on the way, implement your agency's incident management system and establish an EMS commander and a unified command post. Establish control zones, isolating a HOT ZONE, or area of contamination, as well as a decontamination corridor, or WARM ZONE. This

WARM ZONE provides the only way into and out of the HOT ZONE. It is in this zone that the hazmat team and all patients who have been removed from the HOT ZONE may need to be decontaminated, depending on the specific chemicals to which they were exposed. Properly dressed personnel in the decontamination corridor systematically remove the patients' clothing and bathe them with the appropriate agents for the chemical to which they were exposed. A sample of the stages in the decon corridor is illustrated in Figure 18–2.

Preceptor Pearl

It is important for you to ask if patients have been properly decontaminated and exactly how this was done *before* patients are loaded into your ambulance. The last thing you want to do is transport a contaminated patient to the hospital. This could lead to a shutdown of the entire emergency department in order to decontaminate the department's personnel. ✣

Equipment, other emergency rescuers, and the command post should be staged in the next adjacent area, called the COLD ZONE. Your responsibilities in the COLD ZONE will be discussed later in the chapter.

Identify the Substance Involved

An attempt must be made to identify the hazardous material and assess the severity of the situation. Until that is done, it will be difficult to determine the risk to the public, rescuers, patients, and the environment. (Sources that can assist you in identifying hazardous substances are provided in the last section of this chapter, "Sources for Identifying Hazardous Materials.") You must try to find out what the substance is and its properties and dangers; whether or not there is imminent danger of the contamination spreading; what you hear, see, and smell; how many victims are involved; and if there is any danger of secondary contamination from the victims. *Secondary contamination* occurs when a contaminated person makes contact with someone who previously was "clean."

An important piece of scene assessment equipment is a simple pair of binoculars (Figure 18–3). They may allow a visual inspection of the HOT ZONE from a safe distance so you can spot identifying labels, tank styles, and placards.

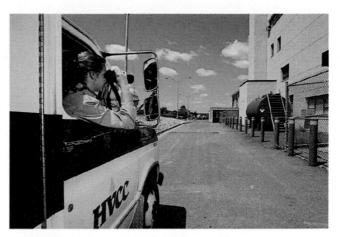

FIGURE 18–3 Binoculars may allow a visual inspection of the HOT ZONE from a safe distance.

If you are approached by victims leaving the HOT ZONE, listen very carefully to them, as they are a good source of information. Often these people have been ignored, only to discover, later in the incident, that one of the first people to exit the scene identified the hazardous material. Perhaps it was a chemist who knew exactly which chemicals were mixed or a factory worker who knew exactly the amount and type of bulk chemicals stored in a particular corner of the factory.

Be especially careful when something about the scene just doesn't add up or you get a funny feeling in your gut that something is wrong. As an EMT-B, you respond to many trauma scenes with multiple patients, yet it is unusual to respond to a medical call with multiple patients. Any time you arrive on the scene to find multiple patients with chest pain, breathing difficulty, or stomach cramps, stop and consider that they may have been poisoned in some manner. For example, it could be the air you are about to inhale that poisoned them: Thinking ahead will prevent you from becoming the next victim. The smart rescuer will size up the situation and call for and wear self-contained breathing apparatus (SCBA) *before* removing the patients to a safe spot for treatment.

Establish a Rehab Sector in the Cold Zone

In order to enter the HOT ZONE safely, the hazmat team will need to determine the most appropriate level of chemical-protective clothing. Any specialized hazmat clothing is very hot inside, causing its wearer to sweat excessively, which can lead to dehydration. The OSHA regulations require that medical surveillance and consultation be provided for the members of the hazmat team, as well as emergency response employees, who exhibit signs or symptoms that may have resulted from an exposure to a chemical. This surveillance and consultation takes place in the rehab sector located in the COLD ZONE.

The rehab sector should be protected from inclement weather conditions and be easily accessible to ambulances. The area should be upwind of the incident and free from exhaust fumes. Make sure the rehab sector has plenty of room in case it must be transformed into a treatment sector for a large number of injured or exhausted responders.

While treating decontaminated patients and hazmat team members in the COLD ZONE, you may be asked to assist in medical monitoring.

Medical monitoring involves a pre- and post-suiting up medical exam of the rescuers including: respiration, pulse, BP, mental status, ECG by ALS personnel, motor skills, hydration status, and weight (using a portable scale carried by the hazmat team). If a rescuer's heart rate exceeds 110 beats per minute, an oral temperature should be taken. If the rescuer's temperature exceeds 100.6°F or pulse exceeds 120, he must stay in the rehab sector until his temperature and pulse stabilize.

Advise the hazmat team of the specific dangers and early signs and symptoms of exposure. Make sure the team members are well informed about dehydration and heat exhaustion. Hazmat experts suggest encouraging team members to drink plenty of water prior to suiting up to help prevent dehydration. During periods of high heat stress and physical exertion, at least one quart of water per hour should be consumed. Electrolyte sport drinks are helpful but not essential; if used, they should be diluted to half their strength. Do not allow team members to drink caffeinated beverages, since these promote dehydration.

If the incident lasts for an extended period of time, rescuers should consider eating both fruits and foods that are low in salt and saturated fats. In cold environments, soups and stews are more easily eaten and digested than sandwiches, greasy hamburgers, or hot dogs.

If team members think they may have been exposed to a chemical, advise them to seek follow-up medical examinations per your local protocol. Carefully document all examinations you conduct on a prehospital care report (PCR). Your PCR may prove to be the only documentation of an exposure

when, years later, rescuers or patients suffer from medical problems that appear to have resulted from the particular incident. For example, this documentation may be needed in order for the rescuers to obtain workers' compensation.

EMS personnel should assist the Incident Commander or Safety Officer with the monitoring of team members via binoculars and radio. Look for central nervous system symptoms of exposure to the chemicals involved. Watch for, and listen for on the radio, signs such as clumsiness, disorientation, slurred speech, dizziness, or fatigue from heat exhaustion. Should any team member appear disoriented, both the team member and his partner should exit the incident and report to the decontamination corridor immediately. The suggested maximum period of work time before team members should report back to the rehab sector for rest is 45 minutes.

■ SOURCES FOR IDENTIFYING HAZARDOUS MATERIALS

There are at least five types of clues to help you detect and identify the presence of hazardous materials. They are container shapes, occupancy or location type, placards and labels, markings and colors, and shipping papers and documents.

Container Shapes

Knowledge of the typical shapes of tankers and rail cars can be a clue to how dangerous the substance inside or leaking out is. Study Figure 18–4, which shows the typical shapes of tankers and tells their content. Learning to recognize these types of tankers will give you a clue about the type of chemical inside the container.

- *MC-306 Atmospheric Pressure Cargo Tank*   The oval cross section of this tank indicates a non-pressurized tank of single-shell aluminum construction holding up to 9,000 gallons of petroleum products or class B poisons.

- *MC-307 Low Pressure Chemical Cargo Tank*   This low pressure tank has a circular cross section and typically a double-shell construction with an insulation layer and one or two sections. A cargo tank holds a maximum of 7,000 gallons of flammable or combustible liquids, mild corrosives, and most chemicals.

- *MC-312 Corrosive Cargo Tank* The corrosive cargo tank has a smaller-diameter circular cross section, with external ribs that are often visible. When insulated, the tank may not appear circular. The design includes overturn and splash protection at the dome cover valve locations. The tank carries up to a maximum of 6,000 gallons of strong corrosives.

- *MC-331 High Pressure Gas Cargo Tank* The high pressure tank has a circular cross section with rounded ends made of a single noninsulated shell. The upper two-thirds is usually painted white or a highly reflective color. The tank has an 11,500 gallon capacity of either LP gases or anhydrous ammonia.

- *MC-338 Cryogenic Liquid Tank* This well-insulated, double-shell tank has relief valve protection, which is often discharging vapors. The ends are flat. Such tanks usually transport liquid carbon dioxide, nitrogen, or argon.

- *Compressed Gas Trailer* This truck carries cylinders that are stacked and held together by a manifold on the rear of the trailer. It is not uncommon for the gases to be pressurized to 5,000 psi. These trailers usually carry oxygen, hydrogen, or nitrogen and are often found at construction or industrial sites.

Rail cars also come in pressurized, nonpressurized, and cryogenic tank cars carrying similar materials in larger quantities.

Occupancy or Location Type

By law, the facilities that store chemicals are required to inform the local fire department of the types of chemicals they use, the volume involved, and the specific location in their facility. Chemical plants, gardening supply stores, public pools, chemical labs, factories, and other industrial sites occur throughout our communities. So when planning for EMS at potential hazmat sites in your community, work with your fire department. Arrange for walk-through drills so you and other employees of your service can become familiar with potential hazmat sites that are local.

Suppose there is a warehouse store that sells pool supplies in your district. A can of chlorine is spilled and the store employees wet-mop the powder in an attempt to clean it up. Your ambulance is called because the chlorine fumes are throughout the building and both the employees and the customers are getting sick from inhaling

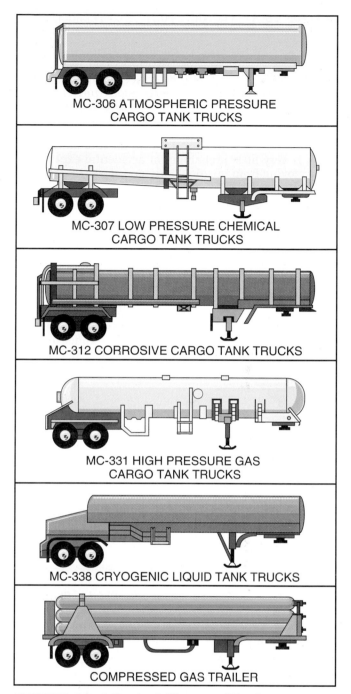

MC-306 ATMOSPHERIC PRESSURE CARGO TANK TRUCKS

MC-307 LOW PRESSURE CHEMICAL CARGO TANK TRUCKS

MC-312 CORROSIVE CARGO TANK TRUCKS

MC-331 HIGH PRESSURE GAS CARGO TANK TRUCKS

MC-338 CRYOGENIC LIQUID TANK TRUCKS

COMPRESSED GAS TRAILER

FIGURE 18–4 Typical Shapes of Tankers.

them. Think about how this hazmat might be handled in your community.

Preceptor Pearl

The point in preplanning is to prepare frequently for the small incidents. As you gain experience in planning, proceed to prepare for the mid-size incidents. These experiences will then prepare you for a large-size incident such as an overturned tanker truck spewing chemicals. Remember, you need to walk before you can run. ✚

CHART 18–1   The Nine Classes of Hazardous Materials

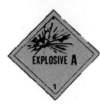

Class 1: Explosives/Blasting Agents Explosives are chemical compounds, mixtures, or devices designed to function by an explosion that creates an instantaneous release of gas or heat. Dynamite and black powder are examples. Blasting agents have been tested and found to be so insensitive that there is very little probability of accidental explosion or their moving from burning to detonation.

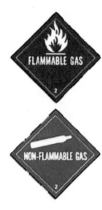

Class 2: Gases Which Are Compressed, Liquified, or Dissolved under Pressure These include flammable gases (red symbol) such as acetylene or hydrogen and nonflammable gases (green symbol) such as carbon dioxide and anhydrous ammonia. Corrosive gases like chlorine also fall under this class.

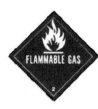

Class 3: Flammable and Combustible Liquids Acetone and gasoline are examples of flammables. Combustible liquids include fuel oils and ethylene glycols.

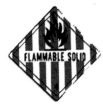

Class 4: Flammable Solids Flammable substances, other than explosives, are those that are liable to cause a fire that results from friction or heat retained from manufacturing. Such substances can be ignited easily and burn vigorously. Examples include pyroxylin plastics, magnesium aluminum powder, and products that are dangerous when wet, such as calcium carbide and phosphorous [the slashed "W" icon].

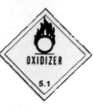

Class 5: Oxidizers/Organic Peroxides Oxidizers are substances that may react with other chemicals to generate heat or ignition. They usually accelerate fires to the point of explosion. Examples include ammonium nitrate fertilizer and calcium hypochlorite. Organic peroxides are derivatives of hydrogen peroxide in which one or more of the hydrogen atoms have been replaced by organic radicals such as benzoyl peroxide and peracetic acid solutions.

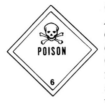

Class 6: Poisons, Irritants, and Etiologic Agents Class "A" poisons, such as cyanide gas or phosgene, are extremely dangerous if their vapors are inhaled. Class "B" poisons, such as arsenic and methyl bromide, are less dangerous substances, but can be a hazard to your health. Irritants, such as tear gas and xylol bromide, are liquid or solid substances that, in a fire, give off intensely irritating fumes. Etiologic agents include any microorganisms or their toxins which cause human disease. This also includes biohazards and organisms such as anthrax, rabies, tetanus, and botulism.

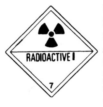

Class 7: Radiologic Materials Radiologic materials spontaneously emit ionizing radiation. Three levels of radiation—Alpha particles, Beta particles, and Gamma rays—can be emitted from products. Alpha particles do little damage since they can be absorbed (stopped) by a layer of clothing, a few inches of air, paper, or the outer layer of skin. Beta particles cannot be stopped by clothing (including turnout gear). Gamma rays are able to penetrate thick shielding and easily pass through clothing and the entire body.

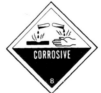

Class 8: Corrosives Corrosives are substances which, when handled improperly, can destroy body tissue. Examples include hydrochloric acid, sulfuric acid, and sodium hydroxide.

Class 9: Other Regulated Materials This is a catchall for potentially dangerous materials that do not fit into the above classes. Examples include hair sprays, shaving lotions, sawdust, magnetized materials, metallic mercury, and batteries.

Placards and Labels

There are two types of placards and labels generally used—the nine United Nation's (U.N.) classes of hazardous materials that are used in the transportation of chemicals, or the NFPA 704 system, which is generally reserved for fixed facilities or labels.

The U.N. placards are diamond shaped and 10¾" in size. A placard provides easy recognition through a combination of a colored background, a symbol on the top of the placard, and a U.N.

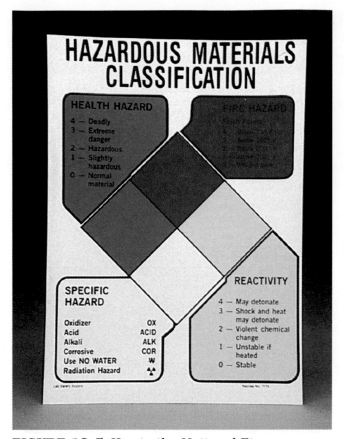

FIGURE 18–5 Key to the National Fire Protection Association (NFPA) 704 System of numeric and color codes.

class number on the bottom of the placard. There are also labels required by federal laws that are found on the containers of chemicals. The colors and symbols that appear each have a significance. The nine classes of hazardous materials found on both labels and placards are shown in Chart 18–1.

The NFPA 704 Hazard Classification System was originally developed for voluntary use but has since been adopted by many municipalities as the standard for classifying fixed facilities that contain hazardous materials. The system incorporates a diamond-shaped diagram (Figure 18–5) divided into four quadrants to identify the health or toxicity, the flammability, the reactivity, and any special warnings about a chemical. Although this system does not identify chemicals, it does provide valuable information through the use of the numbers 0 to 4 placed in each section of the placard or label. Study the placard as you read about each of the sections below:

- *Health "Blue Quadrant"* The assignment of numbers from 0 to 4 in this category illustrates

the effect of a single exposure on a person's health when firefighting over the time frame of a few seconds to an hour. The physical exertion demanded in firefighting or other emergency conditions may be expected to intensify the effects of any exposure. Only hazards arising out of an inherent property of the material are considered. For example, if there was a "2" in this section of the placard, it would indicate "Materials hazardous to health, but areas may be entered freely, with full-faced mask, self-contained breathing apparatus which provides eye protection."

- *Flammability "Red Quadrant"* Assignment of numbers from 0 to 4 in this category rates the susceptibility to burning. The method of attacking the fire is influenced by this susceptibility factor. For example, if there was a "4" in this section of the placard, it would indicate "Very flammable gases or very volatile flammable liquids. Shut off flow and keep cooling water streams on exposed tanks or containers."

- *Reactivity/Stability "Yellow Quadrant"* Assignment of numbers from 0 to 4 in this category illustrates the susceptibility of materials to release energy either by themselves or in combination with water. For example, if there was a "4" in this section of the placard, it would indicate "Materials that by themselves are readily capable of detonation or of explosive decomposition or explosive reaction at normal temperatures and pressures. Includes materials which are sensitive to mechanical or localized thermal shock." If a chemical with this hazard rating is in an advanced or massive fire, the area should be evacuated.

- *Specific Hazards "White Quadrant"* Specific hazards, such as "OX" (the chemical is an oxidizer), or a "W" with a line through it (do not add water to this chemical), or a radioactive symbol.

Markings and Colors

Since 1981, the United Nations' (UN) system for identifying hazardous materials has been required on all portable tanks, cargo tanks, and tank cars carrying hazardous materials. These four-digit identification numbers and symbols can be seen on the DOT chart in Figure 18–6. There are three methods of displaying the UN numbers:

- Orange panel adjacent to the placards. (Panel is 5 ⅞" by 15 ¾", with 4" high letters.)

- Center of appropriate placard. Combustible placards that display the number will have a

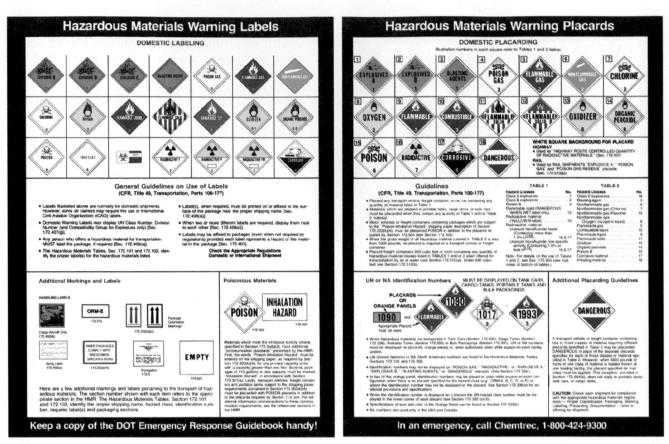

FIGURE 18–6 Examples of hazardous materials warning labels and placards.

white area under the number display to differentiate them from the flammable liquids.

- Center of a placard-sized white panel for hazardous substances and wastes not requiring a placard.

The color of portable gas tanks is also standardized. As an EMT-B, you are already familiar with the green steel tanks used for oxygen. Other pressurized gases are contained in tanks of specific colors also.

Shipping Papers and Documents

Shipping papers can be helpful in identifying the materials at a hazmat incident. A typical shipping paper must contain the following information:

1. proper shipping number
2. hazard classification
3. U.N. identification number
4. number of packages
5. type of packages

6. correct weight
7. the emergency response telephone number

The following emergency response information must be attached to the shipping papers:

1. description of the material
2. risks of fire or explosion
3. immediate hazards to health
4. immediate methods for handling small or large fires
5. immediate precautions to be taken in the event of an accident
6. initial methods for handling spills or leaks in the absence of a fire
7. preliminary first-aid measures

To find the shipping papers on a train, look for the waybill in the engine car. In a ship, check the mailbox, which is located on the bridge of the vessel. On an aircraft, the pilot is responsible for the shipping papers. The bill of lading can be found in the cab of a truck. If the shipping papers

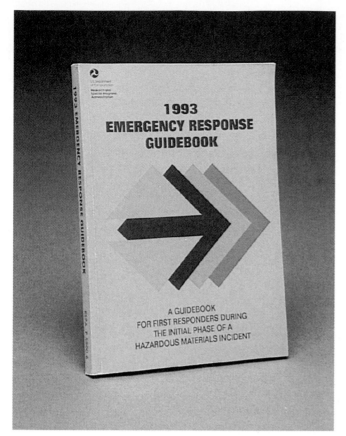

FIGURE 18-7 Have the latest edition of DOT's *Emergency Response Guidebook* in your vehicle at all times.

are not easily accessible, *never* put yourself or your crew members in danger trying to locate them.

Other Resources

Emergency Response Guidebook

All emergency vehicles should carry a copy of the U.S. DOT *Emergency Response Guidebook* (Figure 18–7). You may already be familiar with this book since it is often your first method of identifying a hazardous material. Over 2,500 chemicals are listed both alphabetically (blue section) and in numerical order by the UN identification number (yellow section). Once you locate a chemical in the book, it will refer you to a guide in the book's orange section, which gives general information about what to do in the first few minutes of a hazmat incident that involves the chemical and before additional assistance arrives. If a chemical listing is highlighted, you must immediately refer to the back of the book (green section) to obtain information about evacuation distance needed to protect people from being harmed by the chemical.

CHEMTREC

When shipping papers are not accessible or an emergency response number has not been listed on the papers, the incident commander should assign someone to contact the Chemical Transportation Emergency Center (CHEMTREC), which is a chemical industry service. CHEMTREC will give you immediate initial advice and contact the shipper of the materials involved for further advice. It is also able to provide state or federal resources for radiological incidents. When calling CHEMTREC, which is a 24-hour-a-day, 7-day-a-week toll-free number (1-800-424-9300), be prepared to provide the following information to the operator:

- Your name and call-back telephone number
- Location and nature of problem
- Name of material(s) involved
- Shipper or manufacturer
- Container type
- Rail car or truck number
- Carrier name
- Consignee
- Local conditions

Material Safety Data Sheets (MSDS)

Another section of OSHA regulations is the Hazard Communication standard, or CFR 1910.1200, which requires that employers must make available to employees information on the chemicals that are used in their workplaces. There are also annual training requirements in this regulation. Employers are required to post **material safety data sheets** (MSDSs) that provide information about the chemicals. These sheets can be helpful when you respond to a hazmat incident at a factory; so always request them. Unfortunately, there is no standardized format for the MSDS, although the manufacturer of the chemical is required to provide the name of the substance, its physical properties, fire and explosion hazard information, and emergency first-aid treatment.

Regional Poison Control Center

Another available resource is the regional poison control center. If contacted from the scene, it can help you determine the most appropriate course of treatment for patients exposed to specific chemicals.

CHAPTER REVIEW

■ SUMMARY

Hazardous materials (hazmats) are everywhere, and EMS frequently responds to incidents involving them. Because many incidents begin as routine EMS calls, it will be up to you, as a first-responder EMT-B, to recognize a hazmat incident early and follow your local plan for dealing with it. As a first responder to a hazmat incident, you must establish command and control zones, identify the substance involved, and establish a rehab sector in the COLD ZONE. In order to accomplish these tasks effectively, you should recognize the training required by law and become familiar with resources that can help you identify hazardous materials.

■ REVIEW QUESTIONS

1. Explain the major provisions in OSHA 1910.120.

2. Explain the relationship between NFPA 472 and OSHA 1910.120.

3. Define hazardous materials.

4. Describe the HOT ZONE, WARM ZONE, and COLD ZONE.

5. List what EMT-Bs may be expected to do in the COLD ZONE.

6. What are the medical monitoring requirements of the OSHA regulation?

7. Compare the UN placards to the NFPA placards.

8. List five sources that can be used to identify hazardous materials.

9. Explain how to use the U.S. DOT *Emergency Response Guidebook*.

10. State the function of CHEMTREC.

CHAPTER 19

Advanced Airway Management

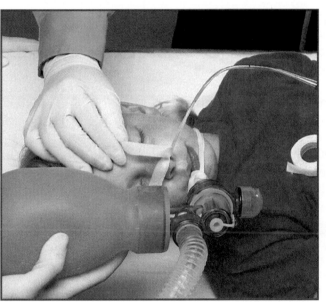

■ There is no skill more important for the EMT-Basic to master than the ability to assure that a patient has an adequate airway. Mastery of the airway is dependent on two separate skills: first, the ability to assess and recognize airway and breathing problems, and second, the ability to maintain an open airway by using both manual techniques and airway adjuncts. Assuring an adequate airway is the first assessment and treatment priority in both basic and advanced life support. Control of a patient's airway is recognized as so crucial a skill that airway skills which were always considered advanced are now included as an elective in the EMT-Basic curriculum. The potential benefit of teaching EMT-Bs advanced airway skills cannot be overstated, as EMT-Bs are frequently the first providers on the scene, and rapid and definitive control of the airway is essential to patient survival.

MAKING THE TRANSITION

- How to prepare for an intubation is explained.
- How to insert and assure the proper placement of an endotracheal tube are described.
- How to perform orotracheal suctioning is explained.
- How to use an indirect advanced airway such as an EOA or EGTA is described.

OBJECTIVES

The numbered objectives below are from the United States Department of Transportation 1994 EMT-Basic National Standards Curriculum.

■ KNOWLEDGE AND ATTITUDE

At the completion of this chapter, you should be able to:

1. Identify and describe the airway anatomy in the infant, child, and adult. (pp. 390–392)
2. Differentiate between the airway anatomy in the infant, child, and adult. (pp. 390–392)
3. Explain the pathophysiology of airway compromise. (pp. 390–392)
4. Describe the proper use of airway adjuncts. (p. 392, see Chapter 4)
5. Review the use of oxygen therapy in airway management. (see Chapter 4)
6. Describe the indications, contraindications, and technique for insertion of nasogastric tubes. (pp. 405–406)
7. Describe how to perform Sellick's maneuver (cricoid pressure). (pp. 398, 399, 401)
8. Describe the indications for advanced airway management. (pp. 390–392, 397, 407)
9. List the equipment required for orotracheal intubation. (pp. 394–397)
10. Describe the proper use of the curved blade for orotracheal intubation. (pp. 394–395)
11. Describe the proper use of the straight blade for orotracheal intubation. (pp. 394–395)
12. State the reasons for and proper use of the stylet in orotracheal intubation. (pp. 396, 397)
13. Describe the methods of choosing the appropriate size endotracheal tube in an adult patient. (pp. 395–396)
14. State the formula for sizing an infant or child endotracheal tube. (p. 403)
15. List complications associated with advanced airway management. (pp. 393, 407)
16. Define the various alternative methods for sizing the infant and child endotracheal tube. (pp. 403–404)
17. Describe the skill of orotracheal intubation in the adult patient. (pp. 397–402)
18. Describe the skill of orotracheal intubation in the infant and child patient. (pp. 403–405)
19. Describe the skill of confirming endotracheal tube placement in the adult, infant, and child patient. (pp. 399, 402, 404–405)
20. State the consequences of, and the need to recognize, unintentional esophageal intubation. (pp. 393, 399, 402)
21. Describe the skill of securing the endotracheal tube in the adult, infant, and child patient. (pp. 397, 399, 402, 404)
22. Recognize and respect the feelings of the patient and family during advanced airway procedures. (p. 402)
23. Explain the value of performing advanced airway procedures. (pp. 387, 390, 392)
24. Defend the need for the EMT-Basic to perform advanced airway procedures. (p. 387)
25. Explain the rationale for the use of a stylet. (p. 396)
26. Explain the rationale for having a suction unit immediately available during intubation attempts. (pp. 392–393)
27. Explain the rationale for confirming breath sounds. (pp. 398–399)
28. Explain the rationale for securing the endotracheal tube. (pp. 397, 404)

■ SKILLS

1. Demonstrate how to perform Sellick's maneuver (cricoid pressure).
2. Demonstrate the skill of orotracheal intubation in the adult patient.
3. Demonstrate the skill of orotracheal intubation in the infant and child patient.
4. Demonstrate the skill of confirming endotracheal tube placement in the adult patient.
5. Demonstrate the skill of confirming endotracheal tube placement in the infant and child patient.
6. Demonstrate the skill of securing the endotracheal tube in the adult patient.
7. Demonstrate the skill of securing the endotracheal tube in the infant and child patient.

Your rescue squad responds to a motor vehicle collision on a busy street.

On arrival, you **size up the scene** and note that the police have safely diverted traffic away from the crash site. There is only one car involved that has sustained extensive damage. The vehicle is upright and stable and there is no apparent fuel leak. Fire department first responders arrive on the scene at the same time as your unit. As the police officer directs your ambulance into the scene, she informs you that there is only one patient—a female who was ejected from the car. No purse has been found, and the police are in the process of trying to learn her identity by tracing the license plate.

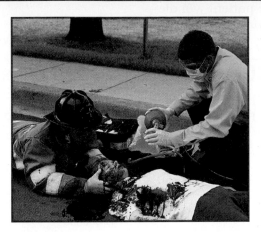

Approaching the patient to begin **initial assessment,** you and your partner find a female in her twenties, unconscious, face down in the street. You note her to be lying in a pool of blood and you hear gurgling respirations. You don gloves, mask, and goggles for BSI. While a fire department first responder maintains cervical stabilization, you and two first responders log-roll the patient onto her back. You see that she has sustained multiple facial lacerations and there is copious blood in the airway.

You begin to aggressively suction the patient's mouth with a large-bore, rigid-tip suction catheter and note that she has no gag reflex. You then insert an oropharyngeal airway, which she tolerates. The patient has some continued bleeding from the mouth, so you assign one of the first responders to suction the airway as needed and another to take over manual stabilization. Meanwhile you prepare to put oxygen on the patient and complete your initial assessment as your partner takes baseline vital signs. Assessment of the circulation has revealed strong radial pulses and no apparent major external blood loss. The patient remains completely unresponsive to any stimuli.

You quickly discuss the situation with your partner and decide—because of the urgency of getting control of this patient's airway—to delay the rapid trauma exam in order to go to the ambulance to set-up for orotracheal intubation while your partner and a first responder continue ventilation of the patient with the BVM.

Meanwhile your partner directs the other first responder and two police officers in maintaining manual stabilization while applying a rigid cervical collar and securing the patient to a backboard.

In the ambulance you select a 7mm endotracheal tube and a large curved laryngoscope blade and assure that both are functioning properly. Moments later the patient is loaded into the ambulance and you see that she is now fully immobilized. Your partner and the first responder continue to ventilate the patient with the BVM.

You turn on the on-board suction so it will be ready if needed and tuck the rigid catheter between the backboard and the stretcher to the right of the patient's head. Your partner hyperventilates the patient, giving her a series of ventilations at twice the usual rate. This will give the patient some extra oxygen to tide her through the moments when her oxygen intake will be interrupted while you insert an endotracheal tube.

You assign one of the first responders to again manually stabilize the patient's head while your partner opens the cervical collar and applies pressure to the cricoid cartilage. This will help suppress potential vomiting and help bring her glottic opening into your view. Using the laryngoscope, you then pass the endotracheal tube through the glottic opening into the trachea. After quickly inflating the endotracheal tube's cuff, you remove the mask from the BVM and attach the BVM bag directly to the endotracheal tube and begin ventilation. You listen for breath sounds and determine that the tube is properly placed. You secure the tube and initiate transport to the hospital. Your scene time was eleven minutes.

You perform the rapid trauma exam en route. Because of the need to monitor the patient's tube placement and ventilation, there is no time to conduct a **detailed physical exam**. You frequently auscultate for the presence of breath sounds and reconfirm that the tube is still properly placed. Your partner takes responsibility for conducting **ongoing assessment**, including monitoring the patient's vital signs, every five minutes en route. The patient begins to respond to pain by the time you arrive at the hospital. ■

Airway control is the highest priority in managing any critically ill or injured patient, because without an adequate airway the patient will die—no matter what other care you provide.

■ ANATOMY AND PHYSIOLOGY

There are specific aspects of both airway anatomy and physiology that the EMT-B who performs advanced airway skills must understand in greater depth in order to perform these skills effectively and successfully.

Anatomy

Air that enters the respiratory tract through the nose then passes through the **nasopharynx**; air that enters through the mouth passes through the **oropharynx**. The **hypopharynx** is the area directly above the openings of both the **trachea** and the **esophagus**. The leaf-shaped **epiglottis** protects the airway by covering the entrance to the trachea when swallowing occurs. Anterior to the epiglottis is a groovelike structure called the **vallecula**.

The epiglottis allows air to pass into the opening of the trachea and through the **larynx**, or voice box. The larynx contains the two **vocal cords**.

Giving support to the larynx and trachea are several rigid pieces of cartilage. The thyroid cartilage is a shield-shaped structure at the anterior of the larynx. Multiple horseshoe-shaped cartilages give support to the trachea. The **cricoid cartilage** is a cartilage at the lower portion of the larynx. It is unique in that it is the only cartilage that completely surrounds the trachea.

Once air has passed through the larynx, it proceeds through the trachea until the trachea bifurcates, or splits, into the two **mainstem bronchi** at the level of the **carina**. The right mainstem bronchus splits off the carina at less of an angle than the left mainstem bronchus. Because of the angle of the right mainstem bronchus, objects that pass all the way down the trachea (such as aspirated food) tend to lodge in the right rather than the left mainstem bronchus. The mainstem bronchi subsequently divide into smaller air passages until reaching the level of the **alveoli**, where the exchange of oxygen and carbon dioxide takes place.

When learning the anatomy of the airway, remember that the majority of the time you are managing a critical airway problem the patient

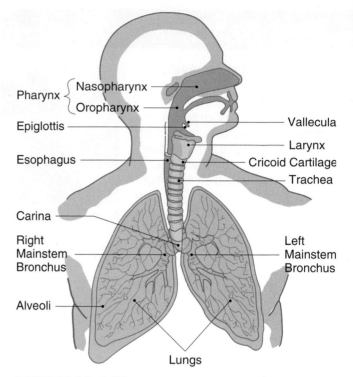

FIGURE 19–1 The airway, anatomical position.

will be supine, or lying flat. For this reason it is important to visualize the anatomy in both the traditional upright "anatomical position" (Figure 19–1) and in the supine position (Figure 19–2).

Physiology

The most important aspect of respiratory physiology for the EMT-B who uses advanced airways is an understanding of what can cause the respiratory system to fail so severely that an advanced airway is necessary.

When the respiratory system functions properly, adequate breathing is the result of many factors including the following:

- A functioning brain stem, where the brain's centers of respiratory control are located
- An open airway
- An intact chest wall
- The ability of gas exchange to take place at the alveoli

Injuries or illnesses that affect any of these components can result in inadequate breathing and respiratory failure. For example, a massive head injury could result in both brain stem injury

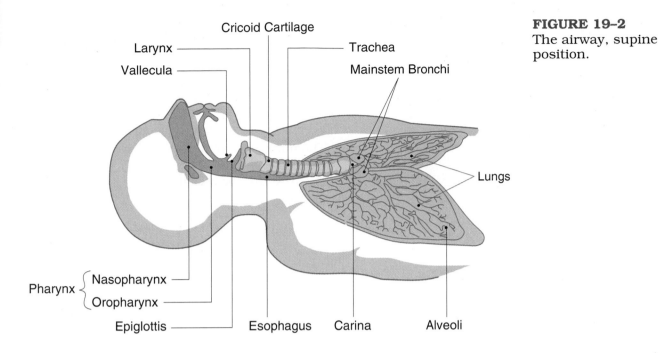

FIGURE 19–2
The airway, supine
position.

Cricoid Cartilage

Larynx

Trachea

Vallecula

Mainstem Bronchi

Lungs

Pharynx { Nasopharynx

Oropharynx }

Epiglottis

Esophagus

Carina

Alveoli

and an airway obstructed by blood and broken teeth. Similarly, a patient with massive pulmonary edema from congestive heart failure can go into respiratory failure because edema prevents adequate gas exchange at the level of the alveoli.

Assessing the adequacy of a patient's breathing is an essential skill when making decisions about what basic and advanced airway management is indicated. A patient's respiratory status can range anywhere from normal, unlabored breathing to respiratory arrest. Recognition of adequate breathing and respiratory arrest is rarely a challenge for the EMT-B. It is recognizing the more subtle signs and symptoms of inadequate breathing that is an essential skill for the EMT-B.

In general, when assessing the adequacy of breathing you should carefully observe the rate, rhythm, quality, and depth of the patient's respirations. The normal rate of breathing is dependent on the age of the patient (Table 19–1). An adequately breathing patient will normally be breathing in a regular rather than an irregular rhythm. The quality of a patient's breathing should be

assessed by listening for breath sounds and observing chest expansion and effort of breathing. The adequately breathing patient will have breath sounds that are equal and present bilaterally. In addition, when observing the patient's chest during normal breathing you will note equal and full expansion of the chest and a lack of any accessory muscle use in the chest or neck during inspiration. Finally, the depth of breathing (tidal volume) will normally be sufficient not only to expand the lungs, but to assure adequate delivery of oxygen and removal of carbon dioxide at the level of the alveoli.

When a patient is in respiratory distress because of inadequate breathing, the following variations in rate, rhythm, quality, and depth of breathing will be noted.

- *Rate*—Outside the normal range: either too fast or too slow
- *Rhythm*—Irregular pattern of breathing
- *Quality*—
  - Breath sounds: diminished, unequal or absent
  - Chest expansion: unequal or inadequate
  - Effort of breathing: increased effort—use of accessory muscles and inability to speak in full sentences
- *Depth*—Shallow

In addition, you may also note the following signs and symptoms in the patient with inadequate breathing.

TABLE 19–1 Normal Rates of Breathing

Normal Rates of Breathing
Adult — 12–20 breaths per minute
Child — 15–30 breaths per minute
Infant — 25–50 breaths per minute

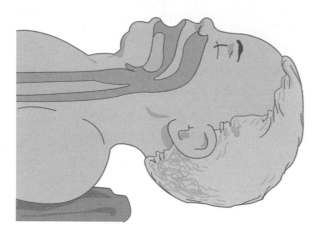

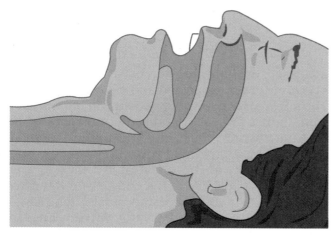

FIGURE 19–3 Adult and child airways compared.

- Cyanosis in the lips, nail beds, and finger tips
- Cool and clammy skin
- Agonal breathing (gasping breaths just prior to respiratory arrest).

Pediatric Airway Anatomy and Physiology

As you reviewed in Chapter 14, the anatomy and physiology of the pediatric respiratory systems differ from those of adults (Figure 19–3). Younger patients may also have different signs and symptoms of respiratory failure than adults. Unique features of the pediatric versus the adult airway include the following:

- All structures in the mouth and nose are smaller in the child and can be more easily obstructed.

- The tongue is proportionately larger, occupying more of the mouth and pharynx.
- The trachea is softer and more flexible, allowing the airway to be closed off if the neck is extended too far when opening the airway.
- The trachea is narrower, allowing the airway to become more easily obstructed if swelling occurs.
- The narrowest area in the airway is at the level of the cricoid cartilage.
- Because the chest wall is softer, the diaphragm is relied on heavily for the work of breathing.

Although infants and children may manifest inadequate breathing with the signs and symptoms mentioned above, they also frequently show respiratory distress in other ways, including:

- A slower than normal heart rate
- Weak or absent peripheral pulses
- Retractions between and below the ribs, above the clavicles and sternal notch
- Nasal flaring, in which the nostrils "flare" open with exhalation and clamp almost shut with inhalation
- So-called "seesaw" breathing, in which the chest and abdomen move in opposite directions during breathing

PEDIATRIC HIGHLIGHT

Recognition of respiratory distress and inadequate breathing is especially critical in pediatrics, since respiratory failure is the leading cause of cardiac arrest in this age group. ■

■ MANAGEMENT OF THE AIRWAY

Although this chapter is about advanced airway management, it cannot be overemphasized that the primary management of any airway is done with basic techniques such as opening and suctioning the airway, administering oxygen, and using oro- and nasopharyngeal airways (see Chapter 4).

Oropharyngeal Suctioning

The goal of airway management is keeping the airway open and free of obstructions. If the airway is obstructed with secretions, blood, or foreign materials, the airway will have to be suctioned. Suction equipment should always be within easy reach when managing any critical patient. If the patient is being managed outside the ambulance, a suctioning device should be brought to the patient's side. If the patient is in the ambulance, the on-board suction system should be set up and ready for immediate use.

Preceptor Pearl

Nothing is more embarrassing for the EMT-B, or harmful for the patient, than fumbling around to get a suction unit working when the airway is filled with vomit or blood. A working rigid-tip suction catheter is an essential piece of equipment for suctioning the mouth and pharynx, which must be done before performing orotracheal intubation. ❖

Orotracheal Intubation

An **endotracheal tube** is a tube designed to be inserted into the trachea (*endo* meaning "into," *tracheal* referring to the trachea). Oxygen, medication, or a suction catheter can be directed into the trachea through the endotracheal tube. **Intubation** means the insertion of a tube. **Orotracheal intubation** is the placement of an endotracheal tube orally, that is, by way of the mouth (*oro* means "mouth"), then through the vocal cords and into the trachea.

Orotracheal intubation allows direct ventilation of the lungs through the endotracheal tube, by-passing the entire upper airway. The endotracheal tube is placed through the vocal cords with direct *visualization* of the process. A **laryngoscope** is an illuminating instrument that is inserted into the pharynx and allows you to visualize the pharynx and larynx.

The advantages of orotracheal intubation of the apneic patient include:

- Allows complete control of the airway by inserting the tube directly into the trachea; this prevents the tongue, blood, or debris that may be present in the upper airway from interfering with the passage of air into the trachea and lungs.
- Minimizes the risk of aspiration by blocking vomitus or foreign matter from being aspirated.
- Allows for direct oxygen delivery to the lungs
- Allows for deep suctioning of the airway by passing a flexible suction catheter through the endotracheal tube to suction the trachea to the level of the carina

Complications

Although orotracheal intubation is frequently a life-saving procedure, it has many potential complications. Orotracheal intubation is considered an "invasive" technique because it requires placement of equipment inside the body cavity. Whenever you perform an invasive procedure you must be aware of the potential complications and be prepared to recognize and treat them should they arise. These concerns about invasive procedures are never more critical than in orotracheal intubation, since improper placement of the endotracheal tube in the apneic patient, if it is not immediately detected and corrected, can rapidly result in the patient's death.

Specific complications of orotracheal intubation include:

- *Slowing of the heart rate* Stimulation of the airway with the laryngoscope and the ET tube can lead to a slowing of the heart. The patient's heart rate should be monitored throughout the intubation.

- *Soft tissue trauma to the teeth, lips, tongue, gums, and airway structures.*

- *Hypoxia* Prolonged attempts at intubation may lead to inadequate oxygenation, or oxygen starvation, known as **hypoxia**. To prevent this, you should **hyperventilate** the patient with high-concentration oxygen (ventilations provided at about double the normal rate, or 24 ventilations per minute) prior to intubation, and intubation attempts should be limited to 30 seconds from the time ventilations cease until the patient is ventilated through the ET tube.

- *Vomiting* Stimulation of the airway may cause the patient to gag and vomit.

- *Right mainstem intubation* The ET tube has to remain superior to the carina (before the point where the right and left mainstem bronchi branch off) in order to send air into both lungs. If the tube is advanced too far, the tube is likely to go down the steep right mainstem bronchus. Mainstem intubation results in only one lung being ventilated and the development of hypoxia.

- *Esophageal intubation* This is the most serious complication since the unrecognized placement of the tube in the esophagus rather than the trachea will rapidly result in death.

- *Accidental extubation* Even if the ET tube is properly placed initially, the tube can become dislodged while moving the patient, or by the patient himself if he regains consciousness. Be sure to reassess chest wall movement and breath sounds after every major move with the intubated patient such as down the stairs or from the floor to the stretcher.

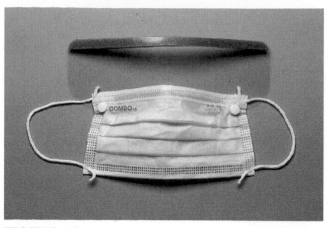

FIGURE 19-4 Body substance isolation precautions must include gloves, mask, and protective eyewear when managing the airway.

Equipment

Orotracheal intubation requires specialized equipment.

Mask and Goggles Due to the high risk of splattering of sputum or blood during intubation, it is essential that body substance isolation precautions be taken. This means that a mask and goggles or other protective eyewear be worn in addition to gloves (Figure 19-4). This is mandatory, since your face will be in direct line with the path of secretions, blood, and vomit coming from the mouth while you attempt to visualize the airway.

Laryngoscope A laryngoscope is made up of two components: the handle that contains the batteries, and the blade that is inserted in the airway and illuminates the airway. In most laryngoscopes the handle and the blades are two separate pieces that need to be assembled with each use. In these devices the blade is placed parallel to the handle and the notch at the base of the blade is attached to the bar on the handle. The blade is then lifted to a 90-degree angle with the handle and, as the blade locks into place, the light at the tip of the blade illuminates (Figure 19-5).

Always check the light at the end of the blade to assure that it illuminates with a bright white color and that the bulb is tightly secured to the blade. Some disposable laryngoscopes are pre-assembled with the handle and blade as a single fixed unit. No matter what type of laryngoscope you use, it is essential that you conduct a daily check of the device to assure that it is working properly. Spare batteries and bulbs should always be stored with the laryngoscope.

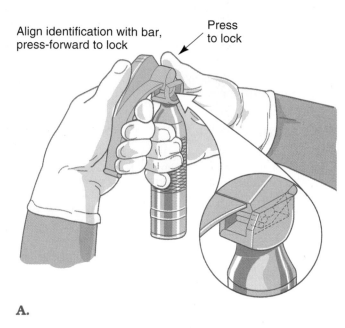

Align identification with bar, press-forward to lock

Press to lock

A.

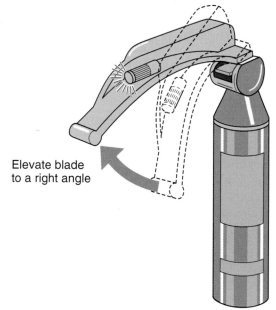

Elevate blade to a right angle

B.

FIGURE 19-5 A. Affix the laryngoscope blade. **B.** Elevate the laryngoscope blade.

Laryngoscope blades are specifically designed to fit into the anatomy of the airway and provide optimal illumination of the vocal cords to enable you to pass the ET tube between them. Most commercially available blades are designed with the light on the right side of the blade. This requires that the handle of the scope be held in the left hand to provide optimal illumination of the airway.

There are two general types of blades: straight and curved. Both types of blades come in assort-

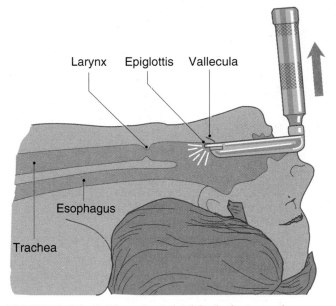

FIGURE 19–6 The straight blade brings the glottic opening and vocal cords into view by lifting the epiglottis.

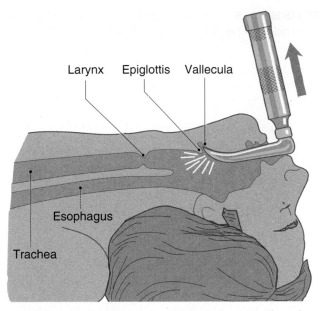

FIGURE 19–7 The curved blade brings the glottic opening and vocal cords into view by lifting the vallecula.

ed sizes ranging from the smallest size, 0, to the largest, 4. The size of the blade used depends on the size of the patient. Most adult patients can be intubated using a size 2 or 3 straight blade or a size 3 curved blade (pediatric blade sizes will be discussed later in this chapter). The decision as to whether to use a straight or curved blade depends on individual preference; however, straight blades are preferred for pediatric orotracheal intubations.

Each blade type is designed to enable you to visualize the cords by taking advantage of different anatomical mechanisms. The straight blade is designed so that the tip of the blade is placed under the epiglottis to lift the epiglottis upward and bring the **glottic opening** (the entrance to the trachea) and the vocal cords into view (Figure 19–6). The curved blade is designed so that the tip of the blade is inserted into the vallecula and lifting of the laryngoscope handle in an upward fashion brings the glottic opening and the vocal cords into view (Figure 19–7).

Endotracheal Tube The endotracheal tube (Figure 19–8) is comprised of a single lumen (tube) through which air and supplemental oxygen are delivered. At the proximal end of the tube (the end that will remain outside the patient, nearest to you) is a standard 15 millimeter adapter for connection to the bag valve.

At the distal end of the tube (the end farthest from you that will go into the patient) is a cuff. The cuff is designed to be inflated after the tube is placed to prevent leakage of air and fluid around the tip of tube. The cuff holds approximately 10 cc of air and should be inflated only enough to prevent air from leaking around the tube. The cuff of the tube is filled with a 10 cc syringe at the inflation valve. Just below the inflation valve is the pilot balloon, which fills with air when the cuff is inflated. Since the cuff is inside the patient's trachea, you won't be able to see if it is inflated, but the inflation of the pilot balloon will verify that there is air in the cuff. If the pilot balloon does not hold air, then you must assume that the cuff at the end of the tube has also failed.

ET tubes used on infants and children less than eight years old do not have a cuff (see Orotracheal Intubation of an Infant or Child later in this chapter). Many ET tubes have a small hole on the left side of the tube on the opposite side of the bevel, known as a Murphy eye. This feature is designed to lessen the chances of tube obstruction.

Endotracheal tubes come in various diameters, from 2.0 millimeters (used on premature infants) to 10.0 millimeters (used on large adults). The diameter measured is the distance from one internal wall of the tube to the other: called the internal diameter or "i.d." No matter what the internal diameter of the tube, the standard 15 millimeter adapter is affixed to the end of the tube. When determining the proper size of the endotracheal tube in the adult patient, the rule of thumb

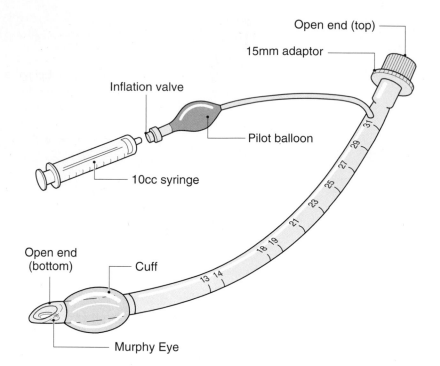

FIGURE 19-8
The endotracheal tube.

Open end (top)

15mm adaptor

Inflation valve

Pilot balloon

10cc syringe

Open end
(bottom)

Cuff

Murphy Eye

is: In an emergency use a 7.5 mm tube. For more precise sizing of the endotracheal tube, it is generally accepted that the adult male should receive either an 8.0 or an 8.5 mm tube and the adult female should receive from a 7.0 to an 8.0 mm tube. The sizing of pediatric endotracheal tubes will be discussed later in this chapter.

The adult endotracheal tube is a standard length of 33 centimeters. The side of the tube is marked in centimeters starting from the tip of the tube. The most important measurement to remember is that, as a general rule, a properly placed endotracheal tube will have the 22 centimeter mark at the teeth. This position assures that the tip of the tube is in the trachea above the carina. (As you will learn, assuring proper placement of the tube is a critical skill, and checking the length marking is only a small part of this procedure.) It may be helpful to envision the depth of tube placement by reviewing the following distances in the average adult.

- 15 centimeters from the teeth to the vocal cords
- 20 centimeters from the teeth to the sternal notch
- 25 centimeters from the teeth to the carina

As you can see, there is very little room for error when placing the ET tube, since only a few centimeters can mean the difference between the proper placement and the tube being placed past the carina into the mainstem bronchus.

Accessories to the Endotracheal Tube There are several accessories to the ET tube with which you need to be familiar. These include the stylet, lubricant, a 10 cc syringe, devices for securing the tube once it is placed, and a suction device.

Because the endotracheal tube is made of relatively flexible plastic, it is generally recommended that a **stylet**—a long, thin, bendable metal probe—be inserted into the tube prior to intubation to help stiffen the tube and provide it with a shape that will ease its insertion through the vocal cords. It is recommended that the stylet be lubricated with water-soluble lubricant, such as K-Y® jelly, Lubifax®, or Surgilube®, prior to insertion into the tube to allow for a smooth withdrawal of the stylet once the tube is successfully placed. A silicone-based lubricant or a petroleum-based lubricant such as Vaseline® must not be used because it will cause aspiration pneumonia.

Once the lubricated stylet is inserted, the endotracheal tube should be shaped into a "hockey stick" configuration. To avoid trauma to the airway, the stylet should *not* be inserted past the tip of the tube. Since all stylets are longer than the ET tube it is easy to inadvertently allow the tip to extend beyond the end of the tube. Such an error, however, could cause a puncture of the trachea. To avoid this complication, the tip of the stylet should not be inserted beyond the proximal end of the Murphy eye and the excess length bent over the 15 mm adapter (Figure 19–9).

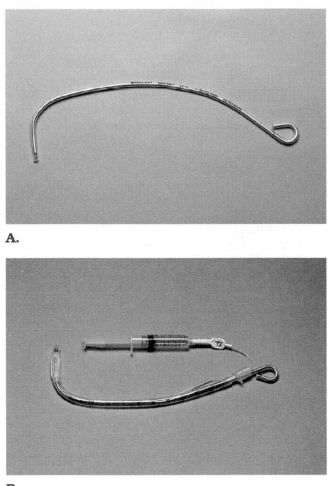

A.

B.

FIGURE 19-9 A. The stylet.   **B.** The stylet in place.

When performing orotracheal intubation, excessive oral secretions often obstruct an adequate view of the vocal cords. Paradoxically, airways are sometimes very dry, thus making insertion of the tube difficult because of friction between the end of the tube and the patient's pharynx and glottis. For these reasons, it is important both that a wide-bore suction device be operational and within easy reach during intubation attempts, and that water-soluble lubricant be applied to the outside of the distal portion of the tube. The suction device should be turned on and placed by your right hand. In general, you can use half a packet of lubricant on the stylet and the other half of the packet on the outside of the tube.

Another piece of essential equipment for use with the endotracheal tube is a 10 cc syringe. As mentioned above, the syringe is used to inflate the cuff through the inflation valve. The syringe should also be used to test that the cuff is intact and holds air prior to inserting the tube. Once the integrity of the cuff has been assured, the air should be withdrawn, but the syringe should remain attached to the tube so that it is easily found when it is time to reinflate the cuff after the patient is intubated. It should be noted that, following final inflation of the cuff, the 10 cc syringe should be detached from the inflation valve to prevent any subsequent leakage of air out of the cuff and back into the syringe.

One of the final steps in orotracheal intubation is securing the tube to the patient so that it does not move or become dislodged. This is especially important in the prehospital setting where the tube can easily be dislodged during patient movement. Prior to securing the endotracheal tube, an oral airway or similar device should be inserted as a bite block in case the patient becomes responsive and gnaws at the tube. There are a number of methods for securing endotracheal tubes. These range from cloth tape to commercially available devices. The manner in which tubes are secured is usually dictated by the medical control authorities of the EMS system you work in. Whatever system you use, make sure the tube is firmly secured in place and able to withstand the tugs and pulls that are routine during moves of critically ill patients.

Indications

When properly performed, orotracheal intubation is clearly a life-saving technique. It is essential, however, that you know under what conditions a patient needs to be intubated. The following is a listing of indications for when to perform orotracheal intubation.

- With inability to ventilate the apneic patient
- To protect the airway of a patient without a gag reflex or cough
- To protect the airway of a patient unresponsive to any painful stimuli
- In cardiac arrest

Technique of Insertion—The Adult Patient

Orotracheal intubation is the most complicated and difficult procedure the EMT-B is expected to perform. Properly performed, it is truly a life-saving procedure. Incorrectly performed, the EMT-B's actions can easily result in the patient's death. Because many EMT-Bs will only rarely perform orotracheal intubation, it is essential that you not only learn and practice the technique extensively during your training but also practice the technique on a regular basis.

The following is a step-by-step guide to orotracheal intubation of the adult patient (Skill Summary 19–1).

Preparation

1. Assure body substance isolation precautions. This should include gloves, goggles or other protective eyewear, and a mask.

2. Assure that adequate ventilation with a BVM and high-concentration oxygen is being performed.

3. Hyperventilate the patient at a rate of 24 breaths per minute prior to any intubation attempts.

4. Assemble, prepare, and test all equipment including:
   - A suction unit with a large-bore rigid tip should be functional and positioned so that it is within easy reach of the intubater's right hand should it be needed
   - The cuff on the ET tube should be tested and then deflated, with the 10 cc syringe left attached to the inflation valve.
   - The assembled laryngoscope with a bright and constant light
   - The device that will be used to secure the tube after successful intubation

5. Position yourself at the patient's head so that, during intubation, *left* and *right* are your left and right as well as the patient's left and right.

Visualizing the Glottic Opening and Vocal Cords

6. Preposition the patient's head to assure good visualization of the vocal cords.
   - If trauma is not suspected, tilt the head, lift the chin, and attempt visualization of the cords. If the cords cannot be seen, raise the patient's shoulders approximately one inch by placing a towel beneath them and attempt visualization again.
   - If trauma is suspected, the patient will have to be intubated with the head and neck in a neutral position with a second rescuer maintaining in-line stabilization of the neck and head.

7. Hold the laryngoscope in your left hand and insert the laryngoscope into the right corner of the patient's mouth.

8. Use a sweeping motion to lift the tongue upward and to the left, out of the way, to enable visualization of the glottis.

9. Insert the blade into the proper anatomical location:

- Curved blade into the vallecula
- Straight blade lifts the epiglottis

10. Lift the scope up and away from the patient.

11. Avoid using the teeth as a fulcrum.

12. Application of the cricoid pressure (Sellick's maneuver) during intubation attempts may be beneficial. Sellick's maneuver is performed by a second rescuer who uses his index finger and thumb to exert direct pressure on the patient's cricoid cartilage (Figure 19–10). Since the cricoid cartilage is the only cartilage in the neck that completely encircles the trachea, direct pressure helps to compress the esophagus, which is anterior to (behind) the trachea, lowering the risk of vomiting. In addition, the pressure often brings the vocal cords into better view. Cricoid pressure should be maintained until the patient is intubated.

13. Visualize the glottic opening and vocal cords. Once the cords come into view do not lose site of them!

Inserting the Endotracheal Tube

14. With the right hand, carefully insert the ET tube through the vocal cords. The tube should be inserted just deep enough that the cuff material is past the cords. Verify that the ET tube is at about 22 cm at the gums and teeth.

15. Remove the laryngoscope and extinguish the lamp.

16. Remove the stylet, if used.

17. Inflate the cuff with 5 to 10 cc of air and remove the syringe.

18. Continue to hold onto the ET tube. Never let go of the tube until it is secured in place.

19. Have a partner attach the bag valve to the ET tube and deliver artificial ventilations.

Assuring Correct Tube Placement

20. The single most accurate way of assuring proper tube placement is visualizing the ET tube passing through the vocal cords. All the following methods are for verification of tube placement.
   - Observe the patient's chest rise and fall with each ventilation.
   - Auscultate for the presence of breath sounds as follows.
     a. Begin over the epigastrium. No breath sounds should be heard here during ventilations.
     b. Listen over the left apex (top of the left lung area). Compare the breath sounds with those at the right apex. Breath sounds should be heard equally on both sides.

The Cricoid Cartilage

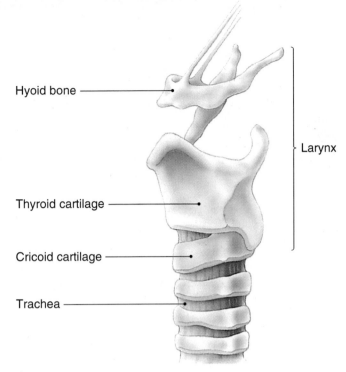

Hyoid bone

Larynx

Thyroid cartilage

Cricoid cartilage

Trachea

A.

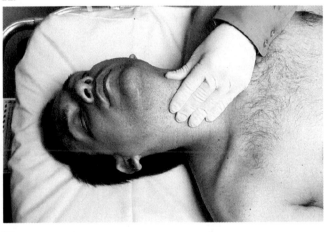

B.

FIGURE 19–10 A. The cricoid cartilage rings the trachea at the lower end of the larynx.
B. Sellick's maneuver is placing pressure on the cricoid cartilage to help suppress vomiting and to help bring the glottic opening into view.

    c. Listen over the left base (bottom of the lung area). Compare the breath sounds with those at the right base. Breath sounds should be heard equally on both sides.
• Observe the patient for signs of deterioration after tube placement—for example becoming combative or developing cyanosis. Both

are signs of hypoxia (oxygen starvation) and probable incorrect tube placement.
• Use other objective measures such as pulse oximetry or end tidal carbon dioxide detectors if allowed by local protocol.

Detecting and Correcting Incorrect Tube Placements

21. If breath sounds are diminished or absent on the left but present on the right, it is likely the tube has advanced beyond the carina and intubated the right mainstem bronchus. If this occurs
• Deflate the cuff and gently withdraw the tube while artificially ventilating and while auscultating over the left apex of the chest.
• Take care not to completely remove the endotracheal tube.
• When the breath sounds become equal at both the left and right apex, reinflate the cuff and follow the above directions for securing the tube.

22. If breath sounds are present only in the epigastrium, the esophagus has been intubated and air is being sent into the stomach instead of the lungs. Since esophageal intubation is a fatal occurrence, immediately deflate the cuff and withdraw the tube. The patient should then be hyperventilated for at least 2 to 5 minutes prior to your second attempt to intubate.

23. The EMT-B should make only two attempts at orotracheal intubation. If both attempts fail, insert an oral airway, continue to ventilate the patient with high-concentration oxygen via BVM, and aggressively suction the airway.

Securing the Tube

24. If breath sounds are heard bilaterally and no sounds are heard over the epigastrium, the endotracheal tube should be secured in place using tape or whatever system is approved by your medical director. An oral airway may be inserted as a bite block to protect the tube. Note the depth of the tube at the teeth, both before and after securing it, to assure the tube has not been dislodged during the procedure.

Ongoing Assessment

25. Be sure to assess and reassess the breath sounds following every major move with the patient.

Preceptor Pearl

It cannot be overemphasized that inadvertent esophageal intubation will likely result in the patient's death. Because of the magnitude of this complication, if at any time—despite your efforts to properly assess tube placement—you are in doubt of proper tube placement, immediately withdraw the tube, and manage the airway with basic airway adjuncts. ✥

Orotracheal Intubation—Adult Patient

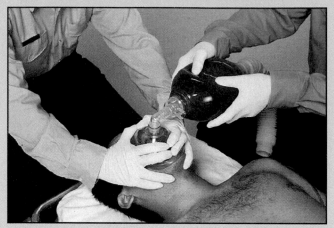

1. Hyperventilate the patient.

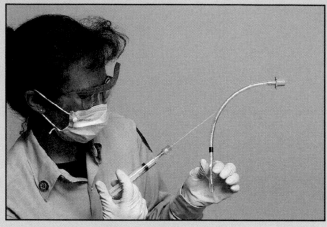

2. Assemble, prepare, and test all equipment.

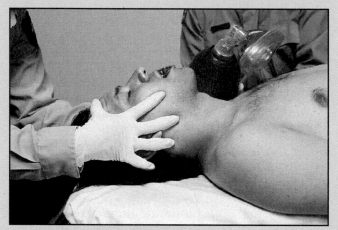

3. Position the patient's head.

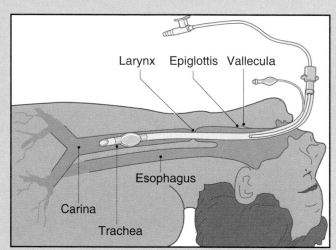

Larynx   Epiglottis   Vallecula

Esophagus

Carina

Trachea

4. Make sure the airway is aligned. (If trauma is suspected, keep patient's head and neck in a neutral position with manual stabilization.)

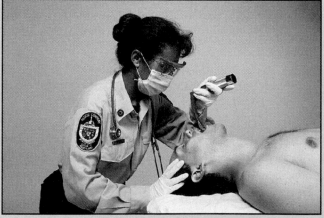

5. Prepare to insert laryngoscope blade.

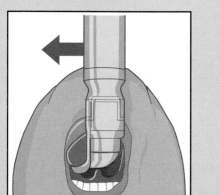

6. Lift the tongue out of the way.

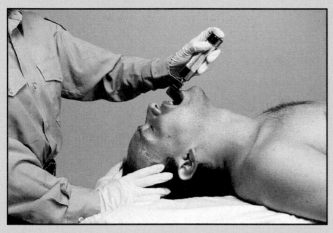

7. Insert the blade (curved blade into vallecula, straight blade under epiglottis) and lift to bring glottic opening into view.

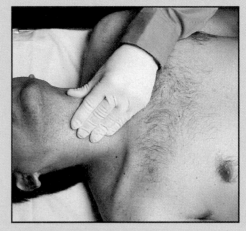

8. A second rescuer may perform Sellick's maneuver (cricoid pressure) during intubation to suppress vomiting and aid visualization.

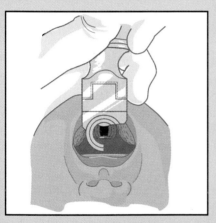

9. Visualize the glottic opening.

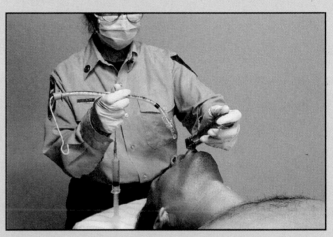

10. Insert endotracheal tube with stylet.

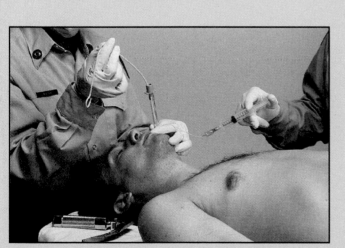

11. Remove laryngoscope and stylet. Inflate the cuff with 5–10 ccs of air.

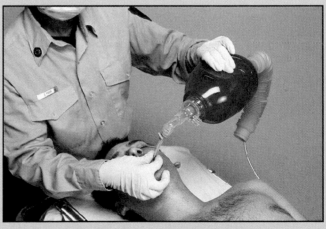

12. Attach bag-valve unit or other ventilation device to tube.

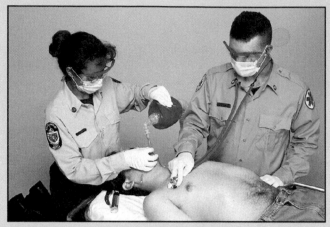

13. Auscultate both epigastrium and lung fields to confirm correct placement.

CONFIRM CORRECT PLACEMENT OF TUBE.

• Observe rise and fall of chest.
• Auscultate epigastrium for absence of breath sounds.
• Auscultate over both lungs for breath sounds. The sounds should be equal when comparing the left and right sides.
• Observe patient for signs of deterioration, e.g., cyanosis.
• Use measures such as pulse oximetry or end tidal carbon dioxide detectors per local protocols.

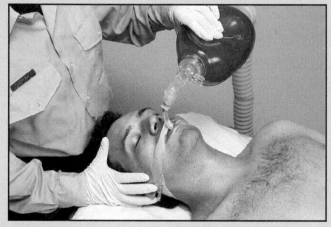

14. If correct placement is confirmed, secure tube in place.

CORRECT ANY INCORRECT PLACEMENT OF TUBE.

• Breath sounds present on right, diminished or absent on left—right mainstem bronchus probably intubated. Deflate cuff, gently withdraw tube (continue ventilation) until breath sounds are equal right and left.
• Breath sounds in epigastrium—esophagus intubated. Withdraw tube. Hyperventilate 2–5 minutes.

Note: Make only two attempts at intubation. If both attempts fail, insert an oral airway and continue to ventilate with bag-valve mask. Aggressively suction the airway. If tube has been correctly placed and secured, reassess breath sounds and placement after every major move with patient. Offer reassurance and emotional support to the patient and family.

Orotracheal Intubation of an Infant or Child

Although the goal of orotracheal intubation is identical in both adult and pediatric patients, intubation of the infant and child requires special training because of various considerations of anatomy, physiology, and size.

The specific anatomy and physiology of the pediatric airway has been discussed earlier in this chapter. The importance of these factors as they relate to orotracheal intubation are as follows:

1. It is often difficult to create a single clear visual plane from the mouth through the pharynx and into the glottis for orotracheal intubation because of such factors as the relatively large size of the tongue of the infant and child.
2. Because of size differences among infants and children as well as the fact that the narrowest portion of the airway is at the level of the cricoid ring, the proper sizing of the endotracheal tube is crucial.
3. Because infants and children tend to develop hypoxia (oxygen starvation) and bradycardia (slowed heartbeat) easily during intubation attempts, pediatric intubations require careful monitoring coupled with swift and accurate technique.

The indications for orotracheal intubation of the infant and child are similar to those for the adult patient.

- When prolonged artificial ventilation is required
- When adequate artificial ventilation cannot be achieved by other means
- To ventilate the clearly apneic patient
- To ventilate the cardiac arrest patient
- To control the airway of unresponsive patients without a cough or gag reflex

The laryngoscope blades and the endotracheal tubes necessary for the orotracheal intubation of infants and children must be carefully sized to the patient. In general the straight blade, usually a size 1, is preferred in infants and small children because it provides for greater displacement of the tongue and better visualization of the glottis. As in adults, the blade lifts the epiglottis bringing the vocal cords into view. In older children the curved blade is often preferred because the blade's broad base displaces the tongue better, allowing improved visualization of the vocal cords once the blade is placed into the vallecula and lifted.

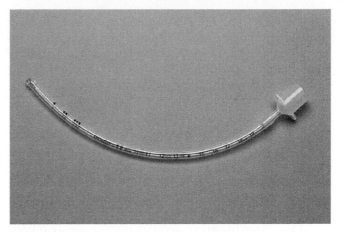

FIGURE 19–11 An uncuffed endotracheal tube is used for patients under 8 years of age.

Assorted sizes of endotracheal tubes should always be stocked in the pediatric airway kit. As previously mentioned, the proper sizing of the tube is essential in children.

Preceptor Pearl

Ideally a chart should be placed in the airway kit to assist you in determining what size tube is generally used for a certain age patient. As an alternative there are commercially available measuring tapes that estimate tube size based on the height of the patient. ✤

A formula—(patient's age + 16)/4 = tube size—can also be used to estimate the proper size. Finally, using the diameter of the patient's little finger or the diameter of the nasal opening are alternative techniques for estimating correct tube size.

Because infants are often the pediatric patients who require orotracheal intubation, it is helpful to simply memorize that newborns and small infants generally require a 3.0 to a 3.5 tube, and a 4.0 tube can be used for older infants up to the age of one year. No matter what system you use in determining tube size, it is always prudent to have one half-size larger tube and one half-size smaller tube on stand-by, since the size of the glottic structures does vary in infants and children.

Endotracheal tubes come in both cuffed and uncuffed versions. Cuffed tubes are always used in adult patients. In the pediatric population, cuffed tubes are reserved for children 8 years of age and older. For younger children and infants, uncuffed tubes are used since the narrowing of the airway at the level of the cricoid cartilage serves as a functional cuff, snugging the tube in the airway. Uncuffed tubes (Figure 19–11) should display a vocal cord marker to assure proper placement of the tube. This marker is designed so that the vocal cords are at the level of the translucent marker-break in the tube. If the child is old enough to get a cuffed tube it should be inserted, like the adult tube, just deep enough that the cuff material is distal to the cords.

The depth of proper tube placement at the teeth to assure that the endotracheal tube is at the level of the mid-trachea can also be approximated by age (Table 19–2). **However, direct visualization of the tube being placed properly is the best measure of tube depth.**

The step-by-step procedure for orotracheal intubation of infants and children is very similar to the procedure outlined for adults (above and in Skill Summary 19–1).

There are, however, some important differences that you must keep in mind when performing a pediatric intubation.

1. The rate of hyperventilation both before and after intubation must be adjusted to the patient's age.

2. The patient's heart rate must be continuously monitored during intubation attempts since mechanical stimulation of the airway and hypoxia can both slow the heart rate. If the heart rate is noted to slow during intubation, the blade should immediately be withdrawn and the infant or child reventilated with high-concentration oxygen.

3. The optimal positioning of the patient's head is to gently tilt the head forward and lift the chin into the "sniffing position" (Figure 19–12).

4. Very little force is needed to intubate the infant or child. Gentle finesse is the rule, not the exception.

5. Sellick's maneuver is also often beneficial, but the landmarks may be difficult to locate in the

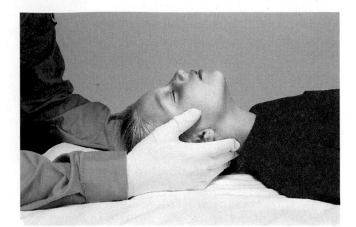

FIGURE 19–12 Place the pediatric patient's head in the "sniffing position" for intubation.

infant and child. In addition, excessive pressure on the relatively soft cartilage may cause tracheal obstruction.

6. When using a straight blade, remember that the epiglottis in infants and children is not as stiff as in adults and may partially obscure a clear view of the vocal cords.

7. Since distances in the infant and child are small, be certain to hold onto the tube until you are assured it is well secured. As with adults, reassess tube placement every time you move the patient.

8. In infants and children, the best indicator of tube placement is symmetrical rise and fall of the chest during ventilation.

9. Breath sounds in infants and children can often be misleading since the chest is small and sounds are easily transmitted from one area to another.

10. Observe the patient for increase in heart rate and improving color after intubation. An infant or child who becomes dusky in color and whose heart rate slows after intubation is likely not to be properly intubated.

11. Once tube placement is confirmed, the patient should be secured to an appropriate device to prevent any head movement from dislodging the tube.

12. If the tube is properly placed but there is inadequate chest expansion, seek out one of the following causes:
    • The tube is too small and there is an air leak around the tube at the glottic opening. This is detected by auscultating over the neck. The tube should be replaced by a larger tube.
    • The pop-off valve on the bag-valve device has not been deactivated.

TABLE 19–2 Length of Endotracheal Tubes in Pediatrics

Measurement of Endotracheal Tube at the Teeth
6 months to 1 year: 12 cm teeth to midtrachea
2 years: 14 cm teeth to midtrachea
4–6 years: 16 cm teeth to midtrachea
6–10 years: 18 cm teeth to midtrachea
10–12 years: 20 cm teeth to midtrachea

- There is a leak in the bag-valve device.
- The ventilator is delivering an inadequate volume of air/oxygen.
- The tube is blocked with secretions. This can be treated initially with endotracheal suctioning. If suctioning fails, the tube should be removed.

13. Infants and children are at risk for the same complications of orotracheal intubation as adult patients. Inadvertent esophageal intubation is perhaps even more rapidly fatal in infants and children than adults. In addition, barotrauma from overinflation of the lungs can result in collapse of the lung, which can further compromise your ability to ventilate the patient.

Nasogastric Intubation of a Pediatric Patient

An additional procedure you will have to master in conjunction with orotracheal intubation of an infant or child is the placement of a nasogastric tube (NG tube). A **nasogastric tube** is inserted through the nose into the infant's or child's stomach. The most common use of the NG tube in advanced airway management is to decompress the stomach and proximal bowel of air. In infants and children, air frequently fills the stomach and bowel after overly aggressive artificial ventilation or as a result of air swallowing. The NG tube provides an escape route for excess air. The NG tube can also be used to drain the stomach of blood or other substances. In the hospital setting, NG tubes can be used to give medication and provide a route for nutrition as well.

The indications for insertion of the NG tube in pediatric patients are as follows:

- Inability to adequately ventilate the patient because of distention of the stomach
- An unresponsive patient with gastric distention

Many experts believe that the NG tube should be inserted only after the trachea has been secured with an endotracheal tube to prevent incorrectly placing the NG tube into the trachea instead of the esophagus. Other possible complications of NG intubation include trauma to the nose, triggering vomiting, and—in very rare cases—passing the tube into the cranium through a basilar skull fracture. *Because of the risk of cra-*

TABLE 19–3   Equipment for Nasogastric Intubation

Equipment for Nasogastric Intubation

Nasogastric tubes of various sizes—
    Newborn/infant: 8.0 French
    Toddler/preschool: 10.0 French
    School age: 12 French
    Adolescent: 14–16 French

20 cc syringe
Water soluble lubricant
Emesis basin
Tape
Stethoscope
Suction unit with connecting tubing

nial intubation with the NG tube, the presence of major facial trauma or head trauma is considered a contraindication to the nasogastric tube. In such cases, should the infant or child require gastric decompression, the insertion of the tube through the mouth (orogastric technique) is preferred if allowed by local protocol.

The equipment required for nasogastric tube insertion is listed in Table 19–3.

The procedure for insertion of the nasogastric tube is illustrated in Skill Summary 19–2 and is as follows:

1. Prepare and assemble all equipment.
2. Assure that the patient is well oxygenated prior to the procedure.
3. Measure the tube from the tip of the nose and around the ear to below the xiphoid process. (If the tube will be inserted by the orogastric technique, measure from the lips.) This length will determine the depth the tube will be inserted.
4. Lubricate the end of the tube.
5. Pass the tube gently downward along the nasal floor.
6. Confirm that the tube is in the stomach by
   - Aspirating stomach contents
   - Auscultating a rush of air over the epigastrium while injecting 10 to 20 cc of air into the tube
7. Aspirate gastric contents by attaching the tube to suction.
8. Secure the tube in place with tape.

Nasogastric Intubation of the Pediatric Patient

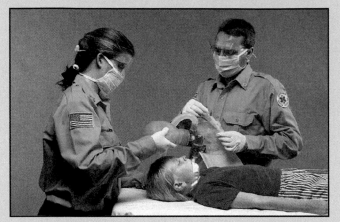

1. Oxygenate patient.

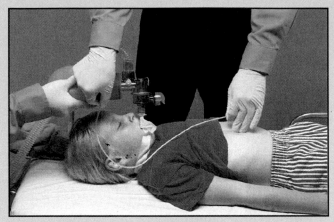

2. Measure tube from tip of nose, over ear, to below xiphoid process.

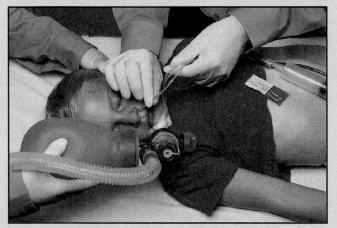

3. Pass lubricated tube gently downward along nasal floor into stomach.

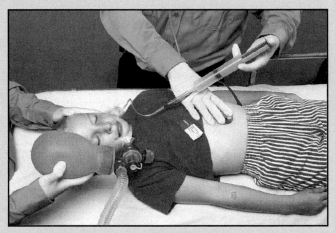

4. To confirm correct placement, auscultate over epigastrium. Listen for bubbling while injecting 10–20 cc air into tube.

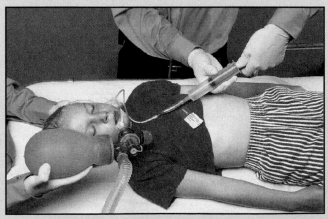

5. Use suction to aspirate stomach contents.

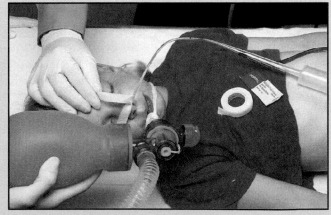

6. Secure tube in place.

Orotracheal Suctioning

In conjunction with your training in advanced airway management, you may also be trained in the techniques of orotracheal suctioning. For this procedure, a flexible soft suction catheter is used to suction the trachea, usually down to the level of the carina in the artificially ventilated patient. This procedure is sometimes referred to as "deep suctioning" to set it apart from the basic airway management procedure—suctioning of the oropharynx (mouth and pharynx), in which suctioning does not advance as far as the trachea.

The indications for orotracheal suctioning are as follows:

- *Obvious secretions in the airway* This may be detected by either moist bubbling sounds during ventilation with the bag valve mask or by visible secretions inside the endotracheal tube after the patient has been intubated.
- *Poor compliance with bag-valve-mask ventilation* Resistance to ventilation may be caused by secretions below the level of the larynx in the trachea.

The technique for orotracheal suctioning is shown in Skill Summary 19–3. Specific steps in the procedure include:

1. Observe body substance isolation precautions. Be especially mindful to have eye protection, as splattering during deep suctioning is common.
2. Pre-oxygenate the patient with high-concentration oxygen prior to attempting suction.
3. Hyperventilate the patient prior to suctioning.
4. Check that all equipment is operating correctly.
5. Use sterile technique.
6. Approximate the desired length of the catheter to be inserted by measuring from the lips to the ear to the nipple line. This will approximate the level of the carina.
7. Advance the catheter to the desired location.
8. Apply suction and withdraw the catheter in a twisting motion.
9. Resume ventilations.
10. To prevent hypoxia, attempts at deep suctioning should not exceed 15 seconds.

Deep suctioning techniques are not without potential complications. Most of the serious complications relate to the fact that the ventilated patient is deprived of oxygen during suctioning.

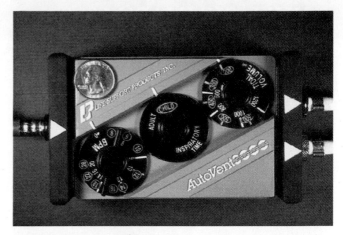

FIGURE 19–13 The automatic transport ventilator (ATV).

Hyperventilation prior to suctioning, careful technique, and limiting suctioning to 15 seconds can help prevent the following complications of deep suctioning.

- Cardiac arrhythmias
- Hypoxia
- Coughing
- Damage to the lining (mucosa) of the airway
- Spasm of the bronchioles (bronchospasm) if catheter extends past the carina
- Spasm of the vocal cords (laryngospasm) during orotracheal suctioning

Automatic Transport Ventilators

Automatic transport ventilators (ATVs) (Figure 19–13) have been used extensively in Europe for a number of years. The devices are rapidly gaining popularity in the United States, as recent studies have demonstrated them to be superior in some respects to manual ventilation with the BVM.

ATVs are compact devices with controls that set both the rate of ventilation and the tidal volume. Tidal volumes are determined by the patient's weight. A number of different ATV models are commercially available. The American Heart Association recommends that ATVs should meet certain minimal standards. They should:

- Have the ability to deliver 100% oxygen
- Be able to provide at least two rates of ventilation—10 breaths per minute for adults and 20 breaths per minute for children
- Be lightweight (2 to 5 kg) and rugged

Orotracheal Suctioning

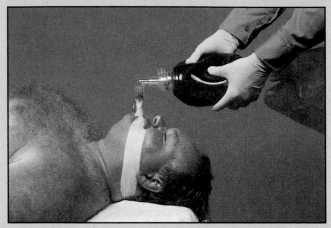

1. Hyperventilate patient.

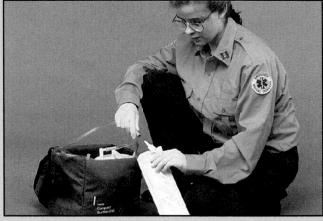

2. Carefully check equipment.

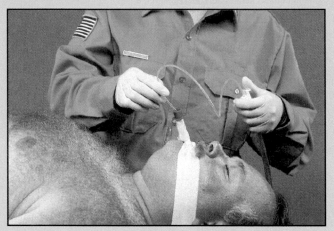

3. Insert catheter without applying suction.

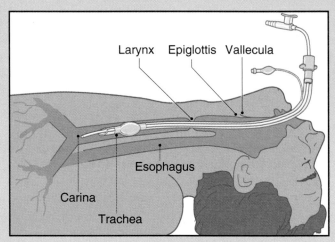

Larynx   Epiglottis   Vallecula

Esophagus

Carina

Trachea

4. Catheter may be advanced as far as carina level.

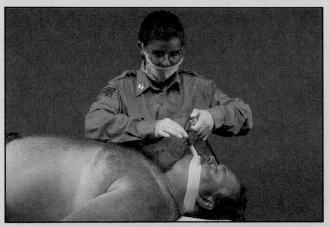

5. Advance catheter to desired level, apply suction, and withdraw catheter with a twisting motion.

6. Resume ventilation. Suctioning procedure should interrupt ventilation for not more than 15 seconds.

- Be equipped with an audible alarm to alert the user to problems in ventilation
- Have a standard 15 mm/22 mm coupling to connect with a mask or endotracheal tube

Although some units are marketed for pediatric use with controls for lower tidal volumes, the device is not suitable for children less than 5 years of age.

Because ATVs do require some additional training for safe use, the decision to use ATVs in an EMS system and the establishment of ATV protocols should be made by the medical director.

Esophageal and Multilumen Airways

In some EMS systems medical direction may elect to allow the EMT-B to use esophageal and/or multilumen airways such as the PtL® or the Combitube®. Although these devices do not provide the definitive airway control of an endotracheal tube, when properly used they provide superior ventilation of the apneic patient as compared with a simple oral airway adjunct.

The EOA and EGTA Airways

For over twenty years, alternative methods of intubating the patient using the esophageal obturator airway (EOA) and its close cousin, the esophageal gastric tube airway (EGTA), have been available. They can be passed "blindly" into the pharynx, eliminating the need to use a laryngoscope to visualize the process as it is happening, and they do not need to be maneuvered between the vocal cords into the trachea, so many of the problems of improper placement are eliminated.

The ease of use and simplicity of both these devices have probably been overemphasized. It is true that they are easier to insert than the endotracheal tube. Nevertheless, they are invasive procedures, and the EMT using either device must be well versed in its complications, indications, and contraindications.

The major feature of the EOA or EGTA is an inflatable cuff that allows the trachea to be open but closes off the esophagus. The device is usually used during CPR or rescue breathing to "seal the meal," or prevent regurgitation (bringing up stomach contents that can be aspirated into the lungs) and prevent gastric distention (blowing air meant for the lungs into the stomach, which in turn tends to cause vomiting or regurgitation).

Both the EOA and the EGTA are usually connected to a BVM unit that blows air or oxygen through the mask port. (As noted above, the EOA or EGTA tube doesn't go into the trachea, but since the esophagus is sealed off by the inflatable cuff, the only place for the ventilation to go is into the trachea and the lungs.)

Although the EOA or EGTA is less often misplaced than an endotracheal tube, it does sometimes get pushed into the trachea instead of the esophagus. When this happens—if the error is not quickly recognized through listening for lung sounds—it can be fatal.

There are certain contraindications to the use of the EOA or the EGTA. Neither should be used in:

- A patient who is alert, verbally responsive, or who responds to painful stimuli and also still has a gag reflex. Vomiting and aspiration are likely.
- A patient who is under the age of 16 or who is less than 5 feet tall. The devices come in only one size and are too long for the anatomy of a small patient.
- A patient who has ingested a corrosive substance. A corrosive could perforate the tip of the device, or may weaken the esophagus so that the device could perforate the esophagus wall.
- A patient with a known esophageal disease such as cancer or esophageal varicose, which weaken the wall of the esophagus and increase the chance for a ruptured esophagus.
- A patient with significant upper airway bleeding. Blood flowing from the nose or mouth will pass directly into the lungs once the inflated cuff has closed off the esophagus.

Although the EOA and EGTA have much in common, the differences are important to learn. Both have an air-cushion-inflatable mask and a 16-inch tube with a 35 cc inflatable air cuff on the distal end. The EOA has a closed distal end to the tube and series of air holes on the proximal end of the tube. As air is ventilated into the tube with the mask sealed against the face, the air exits the holes into the pharynx. Since the tube has a blind end and the cuff is inflated after insertion, no air gets into the esophagus (Figure 19–14).

The EGTA has an open end to the tube, or a valve at the end through which a tube can be inserted into the esophagus and the stomach. In this way, stomach contents can be suctioned or medications administered to the stomach. Ventilations are not blown through the tube port

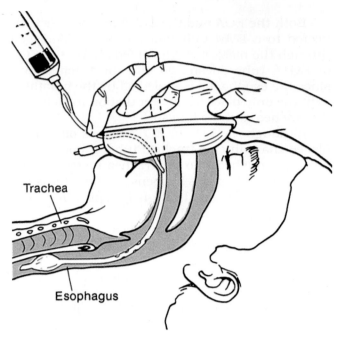

Check the positioning of the EOA by ventilating it by a bag-valve device and then watching for bilateral expansion of the chest and auscultating for bilateral breath sounds. If the chest does not rise on both sides and breath sounds are not heard, withdraw the tube, hyperventilate the patient, and reinsert the EOA. When the tube is correctly positioned, the cuff will lie below the carina. To avert possible esophageal rupture, inflate the cuff in the esophagus with nor more than 35 ml of air.

FIGURE 19–14 The esophageal obturator airway (EOA).

(indeed, this port is designed so that a BVM coupling will not fit, thus avoiding ventilating the stomach by mistake). Instead, the ventilations enter through a second port which, like the first and only EOA port, is a standard 15 mm ventilation device adapter. These ventilations, of course, do not travel through the tube at all but flow freely under the mask and into the mouth and pharynx on the outside of the tube. In other words, the EGTA provides access to the stomach while still protecting the trachea; the EOA only protects the trachea.

To attach the mask to the tube of either device, insert the tube into the port 180 degrees from the desired normal anatomical position, then twist the tube 180 degrees until it snaps into place in the mask. To detach the mask from the tube, simply squeeze the plastic tips that protrude through the mask and pull out the tube from the opposite direction from which it was inserted. Both devices should be stored in the position of function. They should never be stored flat or rolled into a coil, as the shape of the tube will be lost and

will decrease your chances of correctly intubating the esophagus.

To insert either device, you will first need to assemble all the correct supplies.

- An EOA or EGTA tube with the proper mask (*the masks are not interchangeable* and will fit only the correct tube)
- A water-soluble lubricant
- A BVM with reservoir
- A stethoscope
- A suction unit and rigid Yankauer tip
- A supply of 4 × 4 gauze pads
- A 35 cc syringe
- Gloves, goggles, and mask

Then perform the following procedures.

1. One EMT hyperventilates the patient with the BVM. Meanwhile ...
2. A second EMT lubricates the tube with the water-soluble lubricant.
3. Stop the resuscitation momentarily and lift the jaw and tongue straight upward without hyperextending the neck. This is best accomplished with the neck in the neutral or slightly flexed position.
4. Pass the tube following the pharyngeal curvature until the mask is seated against the face (Figure 19–15).
5. Give one ventilation with the BVM and watch for the chest to rise. This is the way to check that the tube has been correctly placed in the esophagus and has not been incorrectly inserted in the trachea (which would block off

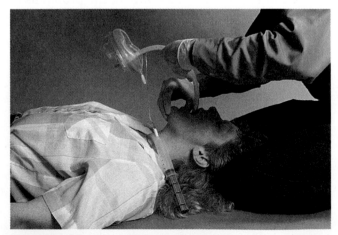

FIGURE 19–15 Advance the EOA or EGTA tube carefully behind tongue and into pharynx and esophagus.

410   CHAPTER 19 Advanced Airway Management

the trachea and air passage into the lungs). Once you are certain that the tube is correctly placed in the esophagus...

6. Inflate the cuff using the 35 cc syringe. (You must be certain the tube is in the esophagus. Inflation of the cuff in the trachea could cause serious damage.)

7. Use the stethoscope to listen to both lung fields (sounds of air intake into the lungs should be present) and the epigastrium. Having assured correct placement of the device...

8. Ventilate the patient using the BVM or flow-restricted, oxygen-powered ventilation device.

Preceptor Pearl

The key point to remember is that the EOA or EGTA mask must be sealed in the same manner as a BVM mask. The AHA Emergency Cardiac Care Guidelines recommend that ventilation with a mask be a two-person, four-handed skill: two hands on the mask attending to the seal, two hands squeezing the bag. Otherwise, a sufficient ventilation volume is unlikely to be delivered. ❖

When working with the EOA or EGTA, keep the following in mind:

• Remove the bag from the mask prior to each defibrillation to prevent its weight from pulling out the tube.

• Be alert for vomitus in the airway and the need for suction, since regurgitation *can* occur even with the EOA or EGTA in place. If you need to suction, temporarily remove the mask from the tube.

• If using a CPR board, which has an indentation to hyperextend the neck, be especially careful as hyperextension can increase the chances of misplacing the EOA or EGTA in the trachea. To guard against this possibility, it is wise to place a towel under the back of the patient's head to put it in the neutral or flexed position. The importance of listening to lung sounds to confirm correct placement cannot be overemphasized.

If the patient becomes conscious, you must remove the tube. Remember that extubation is likely to cause vomiting. Follow these guidelines for removing the EOA or EGTA.

• Always have the suction unit with a rigid Yankauer tip standing by.

• Do not deflate the EOA or EGTA cuff until the patient has resumed breathing and an ET tube has been inserted and its cuff is inflated in the trachea. If you are using an EGTA, a gastric tube can be inserted through it to decompress the stomach or evacuate its contents to reduce the chances of regurgitation or vomiting.

• Provided there is no possibility of a spinal injury, or if the patient is secured to a spine board, turn the patient on his side, insert the syringe into the one-way valve, and withdraw air slowly from the EOA or EGTA cuff.

• Carefully remove the tube, staying alert for vomiting.

The Pharyngo-tracheal Lumen Airway (PtL®)

One problem with airway devices such as the endotracheal tube, the EOA, and the EGTA is that they must be correctly placed into the intended passageway, the trachea or the esophagus. The Pharyngo-tracheal Lumen Airway (PtL®) has been constructed to get around this problem. It can easily be inserted into either the trachea or esophagus with minimum skill, and it will work no matter which passageway it is in.

The PtL® has two lumens (tubes), one inside the other, and for this reason it is sometimes referred to as a double-lumen airway. A long endotracheal-type tube is located within a short, large-diameter tube. The long tube can be inserted into either the trachea or the esophagus, while the shorter tube opens into the pharynx above the epiglottis. Both tubes have low-pressure cuffs at their distal ends. On the long tube, the cuff, when inflated, provides a seal for the trachea or esophagus, depending on which of the two passageways it is resting in. On the short tube, the larger-volume cuff, when fully inflated, seals off the oropharynx.

When the long, inner tube of the PtL® is placed in the esophagus and its cuff is inflated to seal off the esophagus, air delivered through the short outer tube is diverted into the trachea and the lungs. When the long, inner tube is placed in the trachea, air is delivered through that tube, not the short outer tube, to the lungs. Whether it is in the esophagus or the trachea, the longer tube's cuff prevents air from leaking into the esophagus and stomach.

The PtL® also solves the problem of needing extra hands to provide a seal for a face mask. The cuff on the short, outer tube seals the pharynx and prevents delivered air from escaping through the mouth and nose, as well as preventing blood and debris from entering the airway from above. Both tubes of the PtL® have a 15 mm adapter to which a BVM or other ventilation device can be attached.

The PtL® also includes inflation lines so that the cuffs can be inflated. A metal stylet is provided to facilitate guiding the tubes into position. A plastic bite block prevents the patient's teeth from occluding the airway. A neck strap secures the airway to the patient's head.

As with the EOA or EGTA, the PtL® should *not* be used on:

- A conscious patient or one with an active gag reflex
- A patient under the age of 16
- A patient who has swallowed a corrosive substance
- A patient with a known esophageal disease

The procedure to insert the PtL® starts with preparing the equipment. Ensure that both cuffs are fully deflated, that the long, clear, inner #3 tube (see Figure 19–16) has a bend in the middle, and that the white cap is securely in place over the deflation port located under the #1 inflation valve. Lubricate the long #3 tube with a water-soluble lubricant.

If the patient has facial trauma, quickly sweep out the mouth with your gloved fingers and remove any broken teeth, dentures, or other debris that could damage the air cuffs or interfere with passing the tube.

When the patient and the airway are ready, insertion should be accomplished quickly between ventilations.

1. Open the airway. In a patient with potential spinal trauma, have a partner stabilize the head in a neutral in-line position while you pass the airway with minimal cervical manipulation. Use a thumb-in-mouth jaw-lift or tongue-lift method to open the airway. If you have ruled out spinal trauma, hyperextend the patient's head with one hand, insert your thumb deep into the patient's mouth, grasp the tongue and lower jaw between your thumb and index finger, and lift straight upward.

2. Hold the PtL® in your free hand so that it curves in the same direction as the natural curvature of the pharynx. Then insert the tip of the airway into the patient's mouth and advance it carefully behind the tongue until the teeth strap contacts the lips and teeth. (Positioning the airway in this manner with the teeth strap against the lips and teeth is proper for an average-sized adult. If the patient is very small, it may be necessary to

withdraw the airway so that the teeth strap is as much as one inch from the teeth. When the patient is very large, it may be necessary to insert the airway beyond the normal depth so that the teeth strap is actually inside the patient's mouth, past the teeth.)

3. When the tube is at the proper depth, flip the neck strap over the patient's head and tighten it with the hook-and-tape closures located on both sides of the strap.

4. Inflate the small cuff that seals either the esophagus or the trachea and the large cuff that seals the oropharynx, first making sure that the white cap is in place over the deflation port located under the inflation valve. To inflate both cuffs simultaneously, deliver a sustained ventilation into the inflation valve. Failure to inflate the cuffs properly can be detected by the failure of the exterior pilot balloon to inflate or by hearing or feeling air escaping from the patient's mouth and nose. In this case one of the cuffs, probably the large one, may be torn. Quickly remove the airway and replace it with a new one. When you see by the pilot balloon that the two cuffs are inflated, deliver puffs of air to increase pressure in the cuffs and improve the seal.

5. Is the long, clear #3 tube in the esophagus or the trachea? Determine its location by ventilating the short, green #2 tube. If the chest rises, the long tube is in the esophagus and air is, obviously, being diverted through the trachea into the lungs. In this case, deliver ventilations with breaths or with air or oxygen delivered from a BVM or positive-pressure ventilator through the short, green #2 tube.

6. If the chest does not rise when the short, green #2 tube is ventilated, the long, clear #3 tube is probably in the trachea. In this case, remove the stylet and deliver ventilations through the #3 tube. Verify proper delivery of ventilations by listening to both lung fields (for sounds of air entering both lungs) and the epigastrium (where there should be *no* sounds of air entering the esophagus and stomach). Also verify chest rise with each breath.

7. Continue ventilations through the airway until the patient regains consciousness or protective airway gag reflexes return, or the patient is transferred to the ED.

Continually monitor the appearance of the pilot balloon during ventilation efforts. Loss of pressure in the balloon will signal a loss of pressure in the cuffs. If you suspect that a cuff is leaking, increase cuff pressure by blowing forcefully

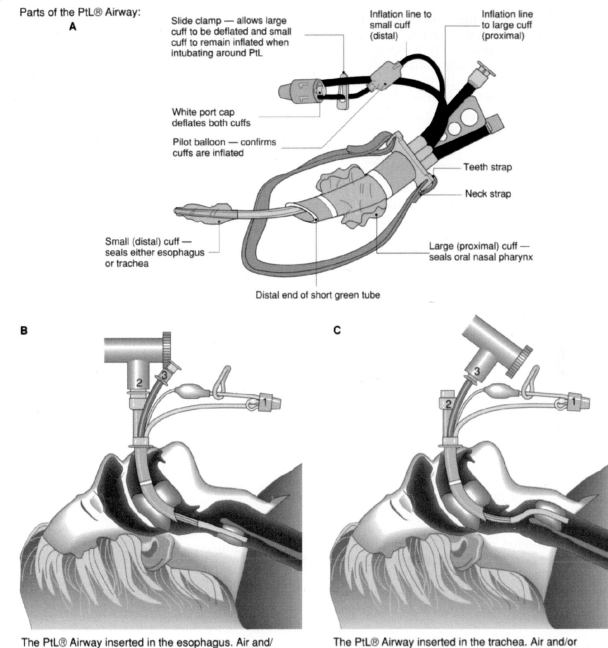

Parts of the PtL® Airway:
A

Slide clamp — allows large cuff to be deflated and small cuff to remain inflated when intubating around PtL

Inflation line to small cuff (distal)

Inflation line to large cuff (proximal)

White port cap deflates both cuffs

Pilot balloon — confirms cuffs are inflated

Teeth strap

Neck strap

Small (distal) cuff — seals either esophagus or trachea

Large (proximal) cuff — seals oral nasal pharynx

Distal end of short green tube

B

The PtL® Airway inserted in the esophagus. Air and/or oxygen delivered into the short #2 tube passes into the lungs. An inflated cuff at the end of the long #3 tube seals the esophagus, while another inflated cuff seals the oropharynx and prevents air loss from the mouth and nose.

C

The PtL® Airway inserted in the trachea. Air and/or oxygen is delivered into the long #3 tube after the stylet is removed. The inflated cuff at the end of the long tube keeps air from leaking from the trachea into the esophagus. The large cuff that is sealing the oropharynx serves as a secondary seal.

FIGURE 19–16 A. The PtL® airway.   **B.** The PtL® in place in the esophagus.   **C.** The PtL® in place in the trachea.

into the #1 inflation valve, or replace the airway. Repositioning the PtL® to ensure that the teeth strap is snug against the patient's teeth is another way of reducing leakage.

As with the EOA or EGTA, if the patient becomes conscious, you must remove the PtL®.

Remember that extubation is likely to cause vomiting. Follow these guidelines for removing the PtL®:

• If there is no possibility of trauma, or if the patient is secured to a spine board, turn the patient onto his side and make sure that the stomach has been decompressed and that gastric contents have been evacuated. This can be accomplished by passing a #18 French Levine suction catheter into the non-airway tube.

- Remove the white cap from the deflation port to simultaneously deflate both cuffs.
- Carefully withdraw the airway and discard it.
- Stay alert for vomiting.

The Esophageal Tracheal "Combitube®"

The most recent alternative to the EOA, EGTA, and PtL® airways is called the esophageal tracheal combitube or, more commonly, "Combitube®." Like the PtL® airway, the Combitube® is a double lumen airway and functions very much like a PtL®. With the Combitube®, however, one lumen is not inside the other. Rather, the two lumens are separated by a partition wall.

In one lumen of the Combitube®, the distal end is sealed and there are perforations in the area that would be in the pharynx. When the tube is in the esophagus, ventilations are delivered through this tube. The sealed end prevents the ventilations from entering the esophagus and stomach and diverts them through the perforations into the pharynx, from which they flow into the trachea and the lungs.

In the other lumen of the Combitube®, the distal end is open. When the tube is in the trachea, ventilations are delivered through this tube.

The Combitube® has a distal cuff that inflates to seal the esophagus or trachea, depending on which passageway it is in. When the trachea is sealed, the cuff prevents stomach contents from being aspirated, but it does not prevent ventilations from entering the trachea via the tube that passes through the cuff.

There is also a pharyngeal balloon that, as with the PtL®, seals the pharynx, preventing air from escaping the mouth and nose and blood and debris from entering the airway.

As with the EOA or EGTA, the PtL® should not be used on:

- A conscious patient or one with an active gag reflex
- A patient under the age of 16
- A patient who has swallowed a corrosive substance
- A patient with a known esophageal disease

Follow these steps to insert the Combitube®:

1. Insert the device blindly, watching for the two black rings on the Combitube® that are used for measuring the depth of insertion. These rings should be positioned between the teeth and the bony cavities where the teeth have their roots.
2. Use the large syringe to inflate the pharyngeal cuff with 100 cc of air. On inflation, the device will seat itself in the posterior pharynx behind the hard palate.
3. Use the smaller syringe to fill the distal cuff with 10 cc to 15 cc of air.
4. Usually the tube will have been placed in the esophagus. On this assumption, ventilate through the esophageal connector. It is the external tube that is the longer of the two and is marked #1. As with the PtL®, you must listen for the presence of breath sounds in the lungs and the absence of sounds from the epigastrium in order to be sure that the tube is, in fact, placed in the esophagus.
5. If there is an absence of lung sounds and presence of sounds in the epigastrium, the tube has been placed in the trachea. In this case, change the ventilator to the shorter tracheal connector, which is marked #2. Listen again to be sure of proper placement of the tube.

An advantage of the Combitube® over the PtL® is that no stylet must be withdrawn from the open-ended esophageal lumen before suctioning of the stomach can take place, making this process quicker. Another advantage is the automatic seating of the pharyngeal cuff.

The biggest advantage of the Combitube® is that rapid intubation is possible independent of the position of the patient, which is helpful for trauma patients requiring limited cervical spine movement.

As with the EOA, EGTA, or PtL®, if the patient becomes conscious, you must remove the Combitube®. Remember that extubation is likely to cause vomiting. Have suction equipment ready. Follow the same guidelines as for removal of the other airway devices.

Preceptor Pearl

Whenever a Combitube®, PtL®, EOA or EGTA is inserted or extubated, gloves, mask, and goggles should be worn to protect the EMT-B from the potential spraying of body fluids. ❖

CHAPTER REVIEW

■ SUMMARY

Airway control is the highest priority in managing any critically ill or injured patient, because without an adequate airway the patient will die—no matter what other care you provide. Control of a patient's airway is recognized as so crucial a skill that advanced airway skills are now included as an elective in the EMT-B curriculum. Advanced airway management centers on the skill of orotracheal intubation, the placement of an endotracheal tube in the patient's trachea. This permits complete control of the airway, minimizes the risk of aspiration, allows for better oxygen delivery, and allows for deep suctioning of the trachea.

Endotracheal intubation of pediatric patients is similar to the procedure for adults, with differences in the airways of infants and children as follows: All structures in the mouth and nose are smaller; the tongue is proportionately larger; the trachea is softer, more flexible, and narrower; the airway is especially narrow at the cricoid cartilage; and the chest wall is softer. These differences result in the airways of infants and children being more easily obstructed, in the use of uncuffed endotracheal tubes under the age of 8 because the narrow cricoid acts as a cuff, and in distinctive breathing patterns. Pediatric patients are more susceptible to damage from incorrect placement of a tube and to interruptions of the supply of oxygen and must be monitored especially carefully during intubation and suctioning procedures.

■ REVIEW QUESTIONS

1. Explain why it is important for EMT-Bs to be able to perform orotracheal intubation.

2. List and explain the intubation errors that can lead to a patient's death.

3. Explain the procedures for assuring correct placement of an ET tube.

4. Explain the reasons and describe the procedure for insertion of a nasogastric tube in a pediatric patient.

5. Explain how orotracheal suctioning differs from oropharyngeal suctioning.

6. Explain the reasons why orotracheal suctioning may be advisable.

7. List the steps in the insertion of an EOA or EGTA.

8. Explain why the ET tube is the preferred device over the EOA, EGTA, PtL®, or Combitube®.

9. List the steps in the insertion of the PtL®.

10. List the steps in the insertion of the Combitube®.

National Registry of Emergency Medical Technicians Skill Sheets

The National Registry of Emergency Medical Technicians is an organization founded in 1970, one of whose goals is to establish nationwide professional standards for EMTs. Many state EMS systems use examinations developed by the National Registry to establish certification of EMTs.

The National Registry has prepared a certification examination correlated to the 1994 Department of Transportation Emergency Medical Technician-Basic: National Standard Curriculum. The examination includes both a written portion and a practical portion that consists of a series of performance-based skill stations.

To assist students in preparing for the skill stations that are part of the EMT-Basic examination, as well as to establish guidelines and parameters for those who will evaluate students' performance at the skill stations, the National Registry has developed a series of skill sheets. Each skill sheet contains a set of directions, the skill criteria, and the critical criteria that if not met by the student result in immediate failure of the station.

In studying for the National Registry examination, you should use these skills sheets in conjunction with the material presented in the textbook and not as the sole means of learning the individual skills. The skill sheets will aid you in organizing the steps necessary to perform each skill and in identifying the criteria that will be used to evaluate your performance. You can use these sheets to evaluate your own performance when practicing these skills and preparing for your practical skills evaluation.

Note: Three skill sheets regarding advanced airway management are included. The use of these skills will vary based on your medical director, training program, and local protocol.

■ ORGANIZATION OF THE NATIONAL REGISTRY EXAMINATION

The practical examination consists of six stations, five mandatory stations and one random basic skill station consisting of both skill-based and scenario-based testing. The random skill station is conducted so the candidate is totally unaware of the skill to be tested until he or she arrives at the test site.

The candidate will be tested individually in each station and will be expected to direct the actions of any assistant EMTs who may be present in the station. The candidate should pass or fail the examination based solely on his or her actions and decisions.

On the next page is a list of the stations and their established time limits. The maximum time is determined by the number and difficulty of tasks to be completed.

INSTRUCTIONS TO THE CANDIDATE

PATIENT ASSESSMENT/MANAGEMENT—TRAUMA

This station is designed to test your ability to perform a patient assessment of a victim of multisystem trauma and voice-treat all conditions and injuries discovered. You must conduct your assessment as you would in the field, including communicating with your patient. You may remove the patient's clothing down to shorts or swimsuit if you feel it is necessary. As you conduct your assessment, you should state everything you are assessing. Clinical information not obtainable by visual or physical inspection, for example, blood pressure, will be given to you after you demonstrate how you would normally gain that information. You may assume that you have two EMTs working with you and that they are correctly carrying out the verbal treatments you indicate. You have (10) ten minutes to complete this skill station. Do you have any questions?

PATIENT ASSESSMENT/MANAGEMENT—MEDICAL

This station is designed to test your ability to perform a patient assessment of a victim with a chief complaint of a medical nature and voice-treat all conditions and injuries discovered. You must con-

duct your assessment as you would in the field, including communicating with your patient. As you conduct your assessment, you should state everything you are assessing. Clinical information not obtainable by visual or physical inspection, for example, blood pressure, will be given to you after you demonstrate how you would normally gain that information. You may assume that you have two EMTs working with you and that they are correctly carrying out the verbal treatments you indicate. You have (10) ten minutes to complete this skill station. Do you have any questions?

CARDIAC ARREST MANAGEMENT/AED

This station is designed to test your ability to manage a pre-hospital cardiac arrest by integrating CPR skills, defibrillation, airway adjuncts, and patient/scene management skills. There will be an EMT assistant in this station. The EMT assistant will only do as you instruct him. As you arrive on the scene you will encounter a patient in cardiac arrest. A first responder will be present performing single rescuer CPR. You must immediately establish control of the scene and begin resuscitation of the patient with an automated external defibrillator. At the appropriate time, you must control the airway and ventilate the victim using adjunctive equipment. You may not delegate this action to the EMT assistant. You may use any of the supplies available in this room. You have (15) fifteen minutes to complete this skill station. Do you have any questions?

AIRWAY, OXYGEN, VENTILATION SKILLS BAG-VALVE-MASK APNEIC PATIENT WITH PULSE

This station is designed to test your ability to ventilate a patient using a bag-valve mask. As you enter the station you will find an apneic patient with a palpable central pulse. There are no bystanders and artificial ventilation has not been initiated. The only patient intervention required is airway management and ventilatory support using a bag-valve mask. You must initially ventilate the patient for a minimum of 30 seconds. You will be evaluated on the appropriateness of ventilator volumes. I will inform you that a second rescuer has arrived and will instruct you that you must control the airway and the mask seal while the second rescuer provides ventilation. You may use only the equipment available in this room. You have (10) ten minutes to complete this procedure. Do you have any questions?

SPINAL IMMOBILIZATION—SUPINE PATIENT

This station is designed to test your ability to provide spinal immobilization on a patient using a long spine immobilization device. You arrive on the scene with an EMT assistant. The assistant EMT has completed the scene size-up as well as the initial and focused assessments. As you begin the station there are no airway, breathing, or circulatory problems. You are required to treat the specific, isolated problem of an unstable spine using a long spine immobilization device. When moving the patient to the device, you should use the help of the assistant EMT and the evaluator. The assistant EMT should control the head and cervical spine of the patient while you and the evaluator move the patient to the immobilization device. You are responsible for the direction and subsequent action of the EMT assistant. You may use any equipment available in this room. You have (10) ten minutes to complete this procedure. Do you have any questions?

SPINAL IMMOBILIZATION—SEATED PATIENT

This station is designed to test your ability to provide spinal immobilization on a patient using a half spine immobilization device. You arrive on the scene with an EMT assistant. The assistant EMT has completed the scene size-up, initial and focused assessments. As you begin the station, there are no airway, breathing, or circulatory problems. You are required to treat the specific, isolated problem of an unstable spine using a half spine immobilization device. Continued assessment of airway, breathing, and central circulation is not necessary. You are responsible for the direction and subsequent actions of the EMT assistant.

Transferring the patient to the long spine board should be accomplished verbally. You may use any equipment available in this room. You have (10) ten minutes to complete this procedure. Do you have any questions?

IMMOBILIZATION—LONG BONE INJURY

This station is designed to test your ability to properly immobilize a closed, non-angulated long bone injury. You are required to treat only the specific, isolated injury. The scene size-up and initial assessment have been completed and during the focused assessment a closed, non-angulated injury of the _____ (radius, ulna, tibia, fibula) was detected. Ongoing assessment of the patient's airway, breathing, and central circulation is not necessary. You may use any equipment available in this room. You have (5) five minutes to complete this procedure. Do you have any questions?

IMMOBILIZATION—JOINT INJURY

This station is designed to test your ability to properly immobilize a non-complicated shoulder injury. You are required to treat only the specific, isolated injury. The scene size-up and initial assessment have been accomplished on the victim and during the focused assessment a shoulder injury was detected. Ongoing assessment of the patient's airway, breathing, and central circulation is not necessary. You may use any equipment available in this room. You have (5) five minutes to complete this procedure. Do you have any questions?

IMMOBILIZATION—TRACTION SPLINTING

This station is designed to test your ability to properly immobilize a mid-shaft femur injury with a traction splint. You will have an EMT assistant to help you in the application of the device by applying manual traction when directed to do so. You are required to treat only the specific, isolated injury. The scene size-up and initial assessment have been accomplished on the victim, and during the focused assessment a mid-shaft femur deformity was detected. Ongoing assessment of the patient's airway, breathing, and central circulation is not necessary. You may use any equipment available in this room. You have (10) ten minutes to complete this procedure. Do you have any questions?

BLEEDING CONTROL/SHOCK MANAGEMENT

This station is designed to test your ability to control hemorrhage. This is a scenario-based testing station. As you progress through the scenario, you will be offered various signs and symptoms appropriate for the patient's condition. You will be required to manage the patient based on these signs and symptoms. A scenario will be read aloud to you, and you will be given an opportunity to ask clarifying questions about the scenario; however, you will not receive answers to any questions about the actual steps of the procedures to be performed. You may use any of the supplies and equipment available in this room. You have (10) ten minutes to complete this skill station. Do you have any questions?

AIRWAY, OXYGEN, VENTILATION SKILLS UPPER AIRWAY ADJUNCTS AND SUCTION

This station is designed to test your ability to properly measure, insert, and remove an oropharyngeal and a nasopharyngeal airway as well as suction a patient's upper airway. This is an isolated skills test comprised of three separate skills. You may use any equipment available in this room. You have (5) five minutes to complete this skill station. Do you have any questions?

AIRWAY, OXYGEN, VENTILATION SKILLS MOUTH-TO-MASK WITH SUPPLEMENTAL OXYGEN

This station is designed to test your ability to ventilate a patient with supplemental oxygen using a mouth-to-mask technique. This is an isolated skills test. You may assume that mouth-to-mouth ventilation is in progress and that the patient has a central pulse. The only patient management required is ventilatory support using a mouth-to-mask technique with supplemental oxygen. You must ventilate the patient for at least 30 seconds. You will be evaluated on the appropriateness of ventilatory volumes. You may use any equipment available in this room. You have (5) five minutes to complete this skill station. Do you have any questions?

AIRWAY, OXYGEN, VENTILATION SKILLS SUPPLEMENTAL OXYGEN ADMINISTRATION

This station is designed to test your ability to correctly assemble the equipment needed to administer supplemental oxygen in the pre-hospital setting. This is an isolated skills test. You will be required to assemble an oxygen tank and regulator and administer oxygen to a patient using a nonrebreather mask. At this point you will be instructed to discontinue oxygen administration by the nonrebreather mask because the patient cannot tolerate the mask and start oxygen administration using a nasal cannula. Once you have initiated oxygen administration using a nasal cannula, you will be instructed to discontinue oxygen administration completely. You may use only the equipment available in this room. You have (5) five minutes to complete this skill station. Do you have any questions?

PATIENT ASSESSMENT/MANAGEMENT—TRAUMA

		Points Possible	Points Awarded
Takes or verbalizes body substance isolation precautions		1	
SCENE SIZE-UP			
Determines the scene is safe		1	
Determines the mechanism of injury		1	
Determines the number of patients		1	
Requests additional help if necessary		1	
Considers stabilization of spine		1	
INITIAL ASSESSMENT			
Verbalizes general impression of patient		1	
Determines responsiveness		1	
Determines chief complaint/apparent life threats		1	
Assesses airway and breathing	Assessment	1	
	Initiates appropriate oxygen therapy	1	
	Assures adequate ventilation	1	
	Injury management	1	
Assesses Circulation	Assesses for and controls major bleeding	1	
	Assesses pulse	1	
	Assesses skin (color, temperature, and condition)	1	
Identifies priority patients/makes transport decision		1	
FOCUSED HISTORY AND PHYSICAL EXAM/RAPID TRAUMA ASSESSMENT			
Selects appropriate assessment (focused or rapid assessment)		1	
Obtains or directs assistant to obtain baseline vital signs		1	
Obtains SAMPLE history		1	
DETAILED PHYSICAL EXAMINATION			
Assesses the head	Inspects and palpates the scalp and ears	1	
	Assesses the eyes	1	
	Assesses the facial area including oral and nasal area	1	
Assesses the neck	Inspects and palpates the neck	1	
	Assesses for JVD	1	
	Assesses for tracheal deviation	1	
Assesses the chest	Inspects	1	
	Palpates	1	
	Auscultates the chest	1	
Assesses the abdomen/pelvis	Assesses the abdomen	1	
	Assesses the pelvis	1	
	Verbalizes assessment of genitalia/perineum as needed	1	
Assesses the extremities	1 point for each extremity includes inspection, palpation, and assessment of pulses, sensory and motor activity	4	
Assesses the posterior	Assesses thorax	1	
	Assesses lumbar	1	
Manages secondary injuries and wounds appropriately **1 point for appropriate management of secondary injury/wound**		1	
Verbalizes reassessment of the vital signs		1	
	TOTAL:	40	

CRITICAL CRITERIA

___ Did not take or verbalize body substance isolation precautions
___ Did not assess for spinal protection
___ Did not provide for spinal protection when indicated
___ Did not provide high concentration of oxygen
___ Did not find or manage problems associated with airway, breathing, hemorrhage, or shock (hypoperfusion)
___ Did not differentiate patients needing transportation versus continued on scene assessment
___ Did other detailed physical examination before assessing airway, breathing, and circulation
___ Did not transport patient within ten (10) minute time limit

PATIENT ASSESSMENT/MANAGEMENT—MEDICAL

	Points Possible	Points Awarded
Takes or verbalizes body substance isolation precautions	1	

SCENE SIZE-UP

Determines the scene is safe	1	
Determines the mechanism of injury/nature of illness	1	
Determines the number of patients	1	
Requests additional help if necessary	1	
Considers stabilization of spine	1	

INITIAL ASSESSMENT

Verbalizes general impression of patient		1	
Determines responsiveness/level of consciousness		1	
Determines chief complaint/apparent life threats		1	
Assesses airway and breathing	Assessment	1	
	Initiates appropriate oxygen therapy	1	
	Assures adequate ventilation	1	
Assesses Circulation	Assesses/controls major bleeding	1	
	Assesses pulse	1	
	Assesses skin (color, temperature, and condition)	1	
Identifies priority patients/makes transport decision		1	

FOCUSED HISTORY AND PHYSICAL EXAM/RAPID ASSESSMENT

Signs and Symptoms (Assesses history of present illness)	4	

Respiratory	Cardiac	Altered Mental Status	Allergic Reaction	Poisoning/ Overdose	Environmental Emergency	Obstetrics	Behavioral
•Onset? •Provokes? •Quality? •Radiates? •Severity? •Time? •Interventions?	•Onset? •Provokes? •Quality? •Radiates? •Severity? •Time? •Interventions?	•Description of the episode •Onset? •Duration? •Associated symptoms? •Evidence of trauma? •Interventions? •Seizures? •Fever?	•History of allergies? •What were you exposed to? •How were you exposed? •Effects? •Progression? •Interventions?	•Substance? •When did you ingest/become exposed? •How much did you ingest? •Over what time period? •Interventions? •Estimated weight? •Effects?	•Source? •Environment? •Duration? •Loss of consciousness? •Effects— General or local?	•Are you pregnant? •How long have you been pregnant? •Pain or contractions? •Bleeding or discharge? •Do you feel the need to push? •Last menstrual period? •Crowning?	•How do you feel? •Determine suicidal tendencies •Is the patient a threat to self or others? •Is there a medical problem? •Interventions?

Allergies	1	
Medications	1	
Past pertinent history	1	
Last oral intake	1	
Events leading to present illness (rule out trauma)	1	
Performs focused physical examination Assesses affected body part/system or, if indicated, completes rapid assessment	1	
VITALS (Obtains baseline vital signs)	1	
INTERVENTIONS Obtains medical direction or verbalizes standing order for medication interventions and verbalizes proper additional intervention/treatment	1	
TRANSPORT (Re-evaluates transport decision)	1	
Verbalizes the consideration for completing a detailed physical examination	1	

ONGOING ASSESSMENT (verbalized)

Repeats initial assessment	1	
Repeats vital signs	1	
Repeats focused assessment regarding patient complaint or injuries	1	
Checks interventions	1	
TOTAL:	34	

CRITICAL CRITERIA

___ Did not take or verbalize body substance isolation precautions if necessary
___ Did not determine scene safety
___ Did not obtain medical direction or verbalize standing orders for medication interventions
___ Did not provide high concentration of oxygen
___ Did not evaluate and find conditions of airway, breathing, circulation
___ Did not find or manage problems associated with airway, breathing, hemorrhage, or shock (hypoperfusion)
___ Did not differentiate patients needing transportation versus continued assessment at the scene
___ Did detailed or focused history/physical examination before assessing airway, breathing, and circulation
___ Did not ask questions about the present illness
___ Administered a dangerous or inappropriate intervention

CARDIAC ARREST MANAGEMENT/AED

	Points Possible	Points Awarded
ASSESSMENT		
Takes or verbalizes body substance isolation precautions	1	
Briefly questions rescuer about arrest events	1	
Directs rescuer to stop CPR	1	
Verifies absence of spontaneous pulse *(skill station examiner states "no pulse")*	1	
Turns on defibrillator power	1	
Attaches automated defibrillator to patient	1	
Ensures all individuals are standing clear of the patient	1	
Initiates analysis of rhythm	1	
Delivers shock (up to three successive shocks)	1	
Verifies absence of spontaneous pulse *(skill station examiner states "no pulse")*	1	
TRANSITION		
Directs resumption of CPR	1	
Gathers additional information on arrest event	1	
Confirms effectiveness of CPR (ventilation and compressions)	1	
INTEGRATION		
Directs insertion of a simple airway adjunct (oropharyngeal/nasopharyngeal)	1	
Directs ventilation of patient	1	
Assures high concentration of oxygen connected to the ventilatory adjunct	1	
Assures CPR continues without unnecessary/prolonged interruption	1	
Re-evaluates patient/CPR in approximately one minute	1	
Repeats defibrillator sequence	1	
TRANSPORTATION		
Verbalizes transportation of patient	1	
TOTAL:	20	

CRITICAL CRITERIA

___ Did not take or verbalize body substance isolation precautions
___ Did not evaluate the need for immediate use of the AED
___ Did not direct initiation/resumption of ventilation/compressions at appropriate times
___ Did not assure all individuals were clear of patient before delivering each shock
___ Did not operate the AED properly (inability to deliver shock)

	Points Possible	Points Awarded
Takes or verbalizes body substance isolation precautions	1	
Voices opening the airway	1	
Voices inserting an airway adjunct	1	
Selects appropriate size mask	1	
Creates a proper mask-to-face seal	1	
Ventilates patient at no less than 800 ml volume *(The examiner must witness for at least 30 seconds)*	1	
Connects reservoir and oxygen	1	
Adjusts liter flow to 15 liters/minute or greater	1	
The examiner indicates the arrival of second EMT. The second EMT is instructed to ventilate the patient while the candidate controls the mask and the airway.		
Voices re-opening the airway	1	
Creates a proper mask-to-face seal	1	
Instructs assistant to resume ventilation at proper volume per breath *(The examiner must witness for at least 30 seconds)*	1	
TOTAL:	11	

CRITICAL CRITERIA

___ Did not take or verbalize body substance isolation precautions
___ Did not immediately ventilate the patient
___ Interrupted ventilations for more than 20 seconds
___ Did not provide high concentration of oxygen
___ Did not provide or direct assistant to provide proper volume/breath
    (more than 2 ventilations per minute are below 800 ml)
___ Did not allow adequate exhalation

	Points Possible	Points Awarded
Takes or verbalizes body substance isolation precautions	1	
Directs assistant to place/maintain head in neutral in-line position	1	
Directs assistant to maintain manual immobilization of the head	1	
Assesses motor, sensory, and distal circulation in extremities	1	
Applies appropriate size extrication collar	1	
Positions the immobilization device appropriately	1	
Directs movement of the patient onto device without compromising the integrity of the spine	1	
Applies padding to voids between the torso and the board as necessary	1	
Immobilizes the patient's torso to the device	1	
Evaluates the pads behind the patient's head as necessary	1	
Immobilizes the patient's head to the device	1	
Secures the patient's legs to the device	1	
Secures the patient's arms to the device	1	
Reassesses motor, sensory, and distal circulation in extremities	1	
TOTAL:	14	

CRITICAL CRITERIA

___ Did not immediately direct or take manual immobilization of the head
___ Released or ordered release of manual immobilization before it was maintained mechanically
___ Patient manipulated or moved excessively, causing potential spinal compromise
___ Patient moves excessively up, down, left, or right on the device
___ Head immobilization allows for excessive movement
___ Upon completion of immobilization, head is not in the neutral in-line position
___ Did not reassess motor, sensory, and distal circulation after immobilization to the device
___ Immobilized head to the board before securing torso

SPINAL IMMOBILIZATION
SEATED PATIENT

	Points Possible	Points Awarded
Takes or verbalizes body substance isolation precautions	1	
Directs assistant to place/maintain head in neutral in-line position	1	
Directs assistant to maintain manual immobilization of the head	1	
Reassesses motor, sensory, and distal circulation in extremities	1	
Applies appropriate size extrication collar	1	
Positions the immobilization device behind the patient	1	
Secures the device to the patient's torso	1	
Evaluates torso fixation and adjusts as necessary	1	
Evaluates and pads behind the patient's head as necessary	1	
Secures the patient's head to the device	1	
Verbalizes moving the patient to a long board	1	
Reassesses motor, sensory, and distal circulation in extremities	1	
TOTAL:	12	

CRITICAL CRITERIA

___ Did not immediately direct or take manual immobilization of the head

___ Released or ordered release of manual immobilization before it was maintained mechanically

___ Patient manipulated or moved excessively, causing potential spinal compromise

___ Device moves excessively up, down, left, or right on patient's torso

___ Head immobilization allows for excessive movement

___ Torso fixation inhibits chest rise, resulting in respiratory compromise

___ Upon completion of immobilization, head is not in the neutral position

___ Did not reassess motor, sensory, and distal circulation after voicing immobilization to the long board

___ Immobilized head to the board before securing the torso

IMMOBILIZATION SKILLS
LONG BONE

	Points Possible	Points Awarded
Takes or verbalizes body substance isolation precautions	1	
Directs application of manual stabilization	1	
Assesses motor, sensory, and distal circulation	1	
NOTE: The examiner acknowledges present and normal.		
Measures splint	1	
Applies splint	1	
Immobilizes the joint above the injury site	1	
Immobilizes the joint below the injury site	1	
Secures the entire injured extremity	1	
Immobilizes hand/foot in the position of function	1	
Reassesses motor, sensory, and distal circulation	1	
NOTE: The examiner acknowledges present and normal.		
TOTAL:	10	

CRITICAL CRITERIA

___ Grossly moves injured extremity
___ Did not immobilize adjacent joints
___ Did not assess motor, sensory, and distal circulation before and after splinting

IMMOBILIZATION SKILLS
JOINT INJURY

	Points Possible	Points Awarded
Takes or verbalizes body substance isolation precautions	1	
Directs application of manual stabilization of the injury	1	
Assesses motor, sensory, and distal circulation	1	
NOTE: The examiner acknowledges present and normal.		
Selects proper splinting material	1	
Immobilizes the site of the injury	1	
Immobilizes bone above injured joint	1	
Immobilizes bone below injured joint	1	
Reassesses motor, sensory, and distal circulation	1	
NOTE: The examiner acknowledges present and normal.		
TOTAL:	8	

CRITICAL CRITERIA

___ Did not support the joint so that the joint did not bear distal weight
___ Did not immobilize bone above and below injured joint
___ Did not reassess motor, sensory, and distal circulation before and after splinting

IMMOBILIZATION SKILLS
TRACTION SPLINTING

	Points Possible	Points Awarded
Takes or verbalizes body substance isolation precautions	1	
Directs application of manual stabilization of the injured leg	1	
Directs the application of manual traction	1	
Assesses motor, sensory, and distal circulation	1	
NOTE: The examiner acknowledges present and normal.		
Prepares/adjusts splint to the proper length	1	
Positions the splint on the injured leg	1	
Applies the proximal securing device (e.g., ischial strap)	1	
Applies the distal securing device (e.g., ankle hitch)	1	
Applies mechanical traction	1	
Positions/secures the support straps	1	
Re-evaluates the proximal/distal securing devices	1	
Reassesses motor, sensory, and distal circulation	1	
NOTE: The examiner acknowledges present and normal.		
NOTE: The examiner must ask candidate how he/she would prepare the patient for transportation.		
Verbalizes securing the torso to the long board to immobilize the hip	1	
Verbalizes securing the splint to the long board to prevent movement of the splint	1	
TOTAL:	14	

CRITICAL CRITERIA

____ Loss of traction at any point after it is assumed
____ Did not reassess motor, sensory, and distal circulation before and after splinting
____ The foot is excessively rotated or extended after splinting
____ Did not secure the ischial strap before taking traction
____ Final immobilization failed to support the femur or prevent rotation of the injured leg
____ Secured leg to splint before applying mechanical traction

NOTE: If the Sager splint or Kendrick Traction Device is used without elevating the patient's leg, application of manual traction is not necessary. The candidate should be awarded 1 point as if manual traction were applied.

NOTE: If the leg is elevated at all, manual traction must be applied before elevating the leg. The ankle hitch may be applied before elevating the leg and used to provide manual traction.

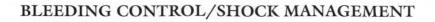

BLEEDING CONTROL/SHOCK MANAGEMENT

	Points Possible	Points Awarded
Takes or verbalizes body substance isolation precautions	1	
Applies direct pressure to the wound	1	
Elevates the extremity	1	
NOTE: The examiner must now inform the candidate that the wound continues to bleed.		
Applies an additional dressing to the wound	1	
NOTE: The examiner must now inform the candidate that the wound still continues to bleed. The second dressing does not control the bleeding.		
Locates and applies pressure to appropriate arterial pressure point	1	
NOTE: The examiner must now inform the candidate that the bleeding is controlled.		
Bandages the wound	1	
NOTE: The examiner must now inform the candidate that the patient is showing signs and symptoms indicative of hypoperfusion.		
Properly positions the patient	1	
Applies high-concentration oxygen	1	
Initiates steps to prevent heat loss from the patient	1	
Indicates need for immediate transportation	1	
TOTAL:	10	

CRITICAL CRITERIA

___ Did not take or verbalize body substance isolation precautions

___ Did not apply high concentration of oxygen

___ Applied tourniquet before attempting other methods of bleeding control

___ Did not control hemorrhage in a timely manner

___ Did not indicate a need for immediate transportation

AIRWAY, OXYGEN, AND VENTILATION SKILLS
UPPER AIRWAY ADJUNCTS AND SUCTION

OROPHARYNGEAL AIRWAY

	Points Possible	Points Awarded
Takes or verbalizes body substance isolation precautions	1	
Selects appropriate size airway	1	
Measures airway	1	
Inserts airway without pushing the tongue posteriorly	1	
NOTE: The examiner must advise the candidate that the patient is gagging and becoming conscious.		
Removes oropharyngeal airway	1	

SUCTION

	Points Possible	Points Awarded
NOTE: The examiner must advise the candidate to suction the patient's oropharynx/nasopharynx.		
Turns on/prepares suction device	1	
Assures presence of mechanical suction	1	
Inserts suction tip without suction	1	
Applies suction to the oropharynx/nasopharynx	1	

NASOPHARYNGEAL AIRWAY

	Points Possible	Points Awarded
NOTE: The examiner must advise the candidate to insert a nasopharyngeal airway.		
Selects appropriate airway	1	
Measures airway	1	
Verbalizes lubrication of the nasal airway	1	
Fully inserts the airway with the bevel facing toward the septum	1	
TOTAL:	13	

CRITICAL CRITERIA

___ Did not take or verbalize body substance isolation precautions
___ Did not obtain a patent airway with the oropharyngeal airway
___ Did not obtain a patent airway with the nasopharyngeal airway
___ Did not demonstrate an acceptable suction technique
___ Inserted any adjunct in a manner dangerous to the patient

MOUTH-TO-MASK WITH SUPPLEMENTAL OXYGEN

	Points Possible	Points Awarded
Takes or verbalizes body substance isolation precautions	1	
Connects one-way valve to mask	1	
Opens patient's airway or confirms patient's airway is open (manually or with adjunct)	1	
Establishes and maintains a proper mask to face seal	1	
Ventilates the patient at the proper volume and rate *(800–1200 ml per breath/10–20 breaths per minute)*	1	
Connects mask to high-concentration oxygen	1	
Adjusts flow rate to 15 liters/minute or greater	1	
Continues ventilation at proper volume and rate *(800–1200 ml per breath/10–20 breaths per minute)*	1	
NOTE: The examiner must witness ventilations for at least 30 seconds.		
TOTAL:	8	

CRITICAL CRITERIA

___ Did not take or verbalize body substance isolation precautions
___ Did not adjust liter flow to 15 L/min or greater
___ Did not provide proper volume per breath
    (more than 2 ventilations per minute are below 800 ml)
___ Did not ventilate the patient at 10–20 breaths per minute
___ Did not allow for complete exhalation

OXYGEN ADMINISTRATION

	Points Possible	Points Awarded
Takes or verbalizes body substance isolation precautions	1	
Assembles regulator to tank	1	
Opens tank	1	
Checks for leaks	1	
Checks tank pressure	1	
Attaches nonrebreather mask	1	
Prefills reservoir	1	
Adjusts liter flow to 12 liters/minute or greater	1	
Applies and adjusts mask to the patient's face	1	
NOTE: The examiner must advise the candidate that the patient is not tolerating the nonrebreather mask. Medical direction has ordered you to apply a nasal cannula to the patient.		
Attaches nasal cannula to oxygen	1	
Adjusts liter flow to 6 liters/minute or less	1	
Applies nasal cannula to the patient	1	
NOTE: The examiner must advise the candidate to discontinue oxygen therapy.		
Removes the nasal cannula	1	
Shuts off the regulator	1	
Relieves the pressure within the regulator	1	
TOTAL:	15	

CRITICAL CRITERIA

___ Did not take or verbalize body substance isolation precautions

___ Did not assemble the tank and regulator without leaks

___ Did not prefill the reservoir bag

___ Did not adjust the device to the correct liter flow for the nonrebreather mask (12 L/min or greater)

___ Did not adjust the device to the correct liter flow for the nasal cannula (up to 6 L/min)

VENTILATORY MANAGEMENT
ENDOTRACHEAL INTUBATION

NOTE: If a candidate elects to initially ventilate with a BVM attached to a reservoir and oxygen, full credit must be awarded for steps denoted by "**" if the first ventilation is delivered within the initial 30 seconds

	Points Possible	Points Awarded
Takes or verbalizes body substance isolation precautions	1	
Opens airway manually	1	
Elevates tongue and inserts simple airway adjunct (oropharyngeal or nasopharyngeal airway)	1	
NOTE: The examiner now informs the candidate no gag reflex is present and the patient accepts the adjunct.		
**Ventilates the patient immediately using a BVM device unattached to oxygen	1	
**Hyperventilates the patient with room air	1	
Note: The examiner now informs the candidate that ventilation is being performed without difficulty.		
Attaches the oxygen reservoir to the BVM	1	
Attaches BVM to high-flow oxygen	1	
Ventilates the patient at the proper volume and rate *(800–1200 ml per breath/10–20 breaths per minute)*	1	
NOTE: After 30 seconds, the examiner auscultates and reports breath sounds are present and equal bilaterally and medical direction has ordered intubation. The examiner must now take over ventilation.		
Directs assistant to hyperventilate patient	1	
Identifies/selects proper equipment for intubation	1	
Checks equipment — Checks for cuff leaks	1	
— Checks laryngoscope operation and bulb tightness	1	
NOTE: The examiner must remove the OPA and move out of the way when the candidate is prepared to intubate.		
Positions the head properly	1	
Inserts the laryngoscope blade while displacing the tongue	1	
Elevates the mandible with the laryngoscope	1	
Introduces the ET tube and advances it to the proper depth	1	
Inflates the cuff to the proper pressure	1	
Disconnects the syringe from the cuff inlet port	1	
Directs ventilation of the patient	1	
Confirms proper placement by auscultation bilaterally and over the epigastrium	1	
NOTE: The examiner must ask, "If you had proper placement, what would you expect to hear?"		
Secures the ET tube *(may be verbalized)*	1	
TOTAL:	21	

CRITICAL CRITERIA

___ Did not take or verbalize body substance isolation precautions

___ Did not initiate ventilations within 30 seconds after applying gloves or interrupts ventilations for greater than 30 seconds at any time

___ Did not voice or provide high oxygen concentrations (15 L/min or greater)

___ Did not ventilate patient at a rate of at least 10/minute

___ Did not provide adequate volume per breath (maximum of 2 errors/minute permissible)

___ Did not hyperventilate the patient prior to intubation

___ Did not successfully intubate within 3 attempts

___ Used the patient's teeth as a fulcrum

___ Did not assure proper tube placement by auscultation bilaterally and over the epigastrium

___ If used, the stylette extended beyond the end of the ET tube

___ Inserted any adjunct in a manner that would be dangerous to the patient

___ Did not disconnect syringe from cuff inlet port

VENTILATORY MANAGEMENT
DUAL LUMEN AIRWAY DEVICE (PTL OR COMBI-TUBE) INSERTION
FOLLOWING AN UNSUCCESSFUL ENDOTRACHEAL INTUBATION ATTEMPT

	Points Possible	Points Awarded
Continues body substance isolation precautions	1	
Confirms the patient is being properly ventilated with high-percentage oxygen	1	
Directs assistant to hyperventilate the patient	1	
Checks/prepares airway device	1	
Lubricates distal tip of the device (*may be verbalized*)	1	
Removes the oropharyngeal airway	1	
Positions the head properly	1	
Performs a tongue-jaw lift	1	
Inserts airway device to proper depth	1	
COMBI-TUBE	PTL		
Inflates pharyngeal cuff and removes syringe	Secures strap	1	
Inflates distal cuff and removes syringe	Blows into tube #1 to inflate both cuffs	1	
Ventilates through proper first lumen		1	
Confirms placement by observing chest rise and auscultating over the epigastrium and bilaterally over the chest		1	
NOTE: *The examiner states: "You do not see rise and fall of the chest and hear sounds only over the epigastrium."*			
Ventilates through the alternate lumen		1	
Confirms placement by observing chest rise and auscultating over the epigastrium and bilaterally over the chest		1	
NOTE: *The examiner confirms adequate chest rise, bilateral breath sounds, and absent sounds over the epigastrium.*			
Secures tube at appropriate step in sequence		1	
TOTAL:		16	

CRITICAL CRITERIA
___ Did not take or verbalize body substance isolation precautions
___ Interrupted ventilation for greater than 30 seconds
___ Did not direct hyperventilation of the patient prior to placement of the device
___ Did not assure proper placement of the device
___ Did not successfully ventilate patient
___ Did not provide high-flow oxygen (15 L/min or greater)
___ Inserted any adjunct in a manner that would be dangerous to the patient

	Points Possible	Points Awarded
Continues body substance isolation precautions	1	
Confirms the patient is being properly ventilated	1	
Directs assistant to hyperventilate the patient	1	
Identifies/selects proper equipment	1	
Assembles airway	1	
Tests cuff	1	
Inflates mask	1	
Lubricates tube (*may be verbalized*)	1	
Removes the oropharyngeal airway	1	
Positions head properly with neck in the neutral or slightly flexed position	1	
Grasps and elevates tongue and mandible	1	
Inserts tube in the same direction as the curvature of the pharynx	1	
Advances tube until the mask is sealed against the face	1	
Ventilates the patient while maintaining a tight mask seal	1	
Confirms placement by observing chest rise and auscultating over the epigastrium and bilaterally over the chest	1	
NOTE: The examiner confirms adequate chest rise, bilateral breath sounds, and absent sounds over the epigastrium.		
Inflates the cuff to the proper pressure	1	
Disconnects the syringe	1	
Continues ventilation of the patient	1	
TOTAL:	18	

CRITICAL CRITERIA

___ Did not take or verbalize body substance isolation precautions
___ Interrupted ventilation for more than 30 seconds
___ Did not direct hyperventilation of the patient prior to placement of the device
___ Did not assure proper placement of the device
___ Did not successfully ventilate the patient
___ Did not provide high-flow oxygen (15 L/min or greater)
___ Inserted any adjunct in a manner that would be dangerous to the patient

Pretest/Posttest

PRETEST

1. Which of the following is a level of training set forth in the National EMS Education and Practice Blueprint?
   A. EMT-Intermediate
   B. First Responder
   C. EMT-Basic
   D. All of the above.

2. Which of the following would <u>not</u> be considered off-line medical direction?
   A. radio contact with a physician
   B. standing orders
   C. protocols
   D. medical director's involvement in quality improvement

3. Which of the following statements about Do Not Resuscitate (DNR) orders is false?
   A. Generally, mentally competent patients may refuse care.
   B. A DNR order usually requires a signature from a physician.
   C. You do not need to actually see the order; verbal confirmation from a family member is sufficient.
   D. All of the above.

4. Abandonment is best defined as
   A. treating a patient against his will.
   B. deviation from the accepted standard of care.
   C. terminating care without assuring the patient is turned over to a qualified provider.
   D. failing to have the patient sign a waiver or release.

5. Which of the following is <u>not</u> a component of negligence?
   A. a duty to act
   B. breaching or failing to perform a duty
   C. criminal intent
   D. causing physical or psychological injury

6. Which of the following is <u>not</u> part of the scene size-up?
   A. initial assessment
   B. body substance isolation
   C. scene safety
   D. mechanism of injury determination

7. Which statement about mechanism of injury (MOI) is false?
   A. MOI may help determine what care will be given.
   B. A patient complaining of neck pain without a significant MOI does not require a cervical collar.
   C. A thorough MOI determination may reveal hidden injuries.
   D. Some information about MOI can be determined by the type of motor vehicle collision.

8. Usually the emotional stages a dying person goes through occur in the following order:
   A. denial, anger, bargaining, depression, acceptance.
   B. acceptance, rage, depression, bargaining, denial.
   C. denial, acceptance, anger, bargaining, and depression.
   D. depression, bargaining, acceptance, denial rage.

9. Which of the following statements regarding critical incident stress debriefings is false?
   A. Many of the counselors are peers.
   B. It is usually held within 24 to 72 hours of the incident.
   C. Critique and investigation can promote psychological healing.
   D. The discussion is confidential.

10. All of the following are recommended for dealing with EMS stress except
    A. requesting assignment to a less busy area.
    B. increasing caffeine intake.
    C. avoiding fatty foods.
    D. seeking professional mental health assistance if necessary.

11. The regulations regarding bloodborne pathogens are developed by
    A. The Department of Transportation (DOT).
    B. The Occupational Safety and Health Administration (OSHA).
    C. The National Registry of EMTs.
    D. U.S. Department of Health and Human Services (USDHHS).

12. Organisms that cause infections are called
    A. pathogens.
    B. allergens.
    C. histamines.
    D. auto-immune.

13. A disease spread by contact with a patient's open wound is called
    A. bloodborne.
    B. airborne.
    C. Hepatitis A.
    D. None of the above.

14. An occupational exposure is best described as
    A. any time you come in contact with blood or other body fluids.
    B. contact with blood or other body fluids on intact skin areas.
    C. contact with blood or other body fluids in an open wound.
    D. blood or other body fluids splashed on an impervious gown.

15. If a patient is thought to have TB, you should wear the normal BSI personal protective equipment plus a
    A. surgeon's mask.
    B. HEPA mask.
    C. Tyvek suit.
    D. gown.

16. Your patient is found at the base of a stairway. Due to the mechanism of injury, which method would you use to open the airway?
    A. modified jaw thrust
    B. triple airway maneuver
    C. jaw thrust
    D. chin lift

17. If your unresponsive patient just vomited and has chunks of pasta in the mouth, you should
    A. suction his mouth.
    B. sweep out his mouth with your gloved fingers.
    C. ventilate as soon as possible.
    D. None of the above.

18. Which of the following is not an advantage of using the pocket mask to ventilate a non-breathing patient?
    A. A one-way valve prevents exhaled air from contacting you.
    B. The device can be easily sealed with one hand.
    C. There is no direct contact with the patient.
    D. Oxygen may be connected to the mask.

19. The American Heart Association (AHA) strongly recommends EMT-Bs use a _____ if they are ventilating alone.
    A. bag-valve mask
    B. pocket mask
    C. positive pressure ventilator
    D. None of the above.

20. A patient who presents in shock and who is adequately breathing on his own should be given
    A. ventilations with a pocket mask.
    B. oxygen with a nonrebreather.
    C. oxygen with a nasal cannula.
    D. ventilations with a BVM.

21. Another name for a rigid tip suction device is
    A. Yankauer.
    B. tonsil tip.
    C. tonsil sucker.
    D. All of the above.

22. You should administer high-concentration oxygen by nonrebreather mask to a responsive patient who has a respiratory rate faster than
    A. 8.
    B. 12.
    C. 16.
    D. 24.

23. The "Q" in OPQRST stands for
    A. quality.
    B. quantity.
    C. quickness.
    D. qualifiers.

24. An adult at rest typically has a respiratory rate between
    A. 8 and 16.
    B. 12 and 20.
    C. 16 and 24.
    D. 20 and 28.

25. The normal systolic blood pressure of a child is usually around
    A. 60 plus twice the age.
    B. 80 plus twice the age.
    C. 60 plus four times the age.
    D. 80 plus four times the age.

26. The proper order of steps in the evaluation of the unresponsive medical patient is initial assessment, then
    A. rapid physical exam, vital signs, history of present illness, SAMPLE history.
    B. vital signs, history of present illness, SAMPLE history, rapid physical exam.
    C. history of present illness, SAMPLE history, rapid physical exam, vital signs.
    D. SAMPLE history, rapid physical exam, vital signs, history of present illness.

27. The general impression includes all of the following except
    A. approximating patient's age.
    B. distinguishing medical from trauma.
    C. judging severity of condition.
    D. assessing mental status.

28. The "A" in DCAP-BTLS stands for
    A. abrasions.
    B. avulsions.
    C. amputations.
    D. airway.

29. Which of the following lists steps of the rapid trauma exam in the proper order?
    A. neck, chest, extremities, abdomen
    B. head, neck, chest, abdomen
    C. chest, abdomen, extremities, pelvis
    D. head, neck, chest, posterior

30. When assessing the chest, you should search for DCAP-BTLS plus
    A. crepitation and breath sounds.
    B. breath sounds and distention.
    C. distention and deformity.
    D. deformity and crepitation.

31. The "P" in SAMPLE history stands for
    A. provokes.
    B. punctures.
    C. pulse.
    D. pertinent past history.

32. A general principle to follow when communicating with a patient is to
    A. avoid eye contact so that you don't appear too threatening.
    B. use medical terms so that the patient sees that you are knowledgeable.
    C. behave in a confident manner so that the patient gains trust in you.
    D. position yourself slightly higher than the patient to show you are in charge.

33. Which of the following might be appropriate to use in a radio report?
    A. "thank you"
    B. "sixty, six-zero"
    C. patient's name
    D. findings and suspected diagnosis

34. Which of the following lists radio report information in the proper order?
    A. estimated time of arrival, age and sex, mental status, emergency care
    B. estimated time of arrival, age and sex, emergency care, mental status
    C. age and sex, mental status, emergency care, estimated time of arrival
    D. age and sex, emergency care, mental status, estimated time of arrival

35. An important principle to remember when completing the prehospital care report (PCR) is
    A. include your conclusions with a description of your findings.
    B. list only signs and symptoms about which the patient complained.
    C. use radio codes to save space and time.
    D. record the time with your reassessment findings.

36. If a patient refuses treatment and transport, you should
    A. complete just a refusal form without a PCR.
    B. make sure the patient is competent.
    C. tell the patient this is the only chance he will get for ambulance transportation.
    D. ask the police to put the patient in protective custody so you can transport him.

37. The EMT-B may assist the patient in taking
    A. aspirin.
    B. insulin.
    C. codeine.
    D. nitroglycerin.

38. Epinephrine is a _____ drug name.
    A. brand
    B. generic
    C. trade
    D. registered

39. Oral glucose comes in what type of medication form?
    A. gel
    B. a slurry
    C. fine powder
    D. sublingual spray

40. Which medication is used to treat patients who are hypoxic?
    A. activated charcoal
    B. nitroglycerin
    C. oxygen
    D. oral glucose

41. When administering medication to the patient, make sure it is the right
    A. dose.
    B. route of administration.
    C. medication.
    D. All of the above.

42. A patient should be treated for cardiac compromise if she has
    A. an automatic implanted cardiac defibrillator (AICD).
    B. a pacemaker.
    C. a headache.
    D. epigastric discomfort.

43. The most ominous side effect of nitroglycerin is
    A. headache.
    B. euphoria.
    C. hypotension.
    D. nausea.

44. When treating a patient in cardiac arrest, how many stacked shocks should you administer initially?
    A. two   B. three   C. four   D. six

45. After you give two shocks with the AED, your patient regains a spontaneous pulse. Your next step should be to
    A. give oxygen by nonrebreather mask.
    B. evaluate the adequacy of breathing.
    C. evaluate the blood pressure.
    D. transport immediately.

46. You are transporting a patient with chest pain to the hospital when he suddenly loses consciousness. Your partner is in the patient compartment with you. After you confirm the patient has no pulse, you should next
    A. begin CPR.
    B. suction the airway.
    C. deliver a shock.
    D. tell your driver to pull over and stop.

47. Which of the following statements best describes how the body's muscles work during normal inhalation?
    A. The diaphragm relaxes and the intercostal muscles contract.
    B. The diaphragm contracts and the intercostal muscles contract.
    C. The diaphragm relaxes and the intercostal muscles relax.
    D. The diaphragm contracts and the intercostal muscles relax.

48. To use an inhaler properly, the patient must do what before triggering the spray?
    A. exhale deeply
    B. inhale deeply
    C. take a normal breath
    D. hold his breath for 15 seconds

49. Which of the following conditions must a patient meet for an EMT-B to assist in the use of an epinephrine auto-injector?
    A. shock or respiratory distress
    B. respiratory distress or weakness
    C. weakness or itching
    D. itching or shock

50. A patient who is submerged in cold water loses significant amounts of heat through
    A. evaporation.
    B. convection.
    C. conduction.
    D. respiration.

51. If you are going to rewarm a frostbitten area, what temperature water should you use?
    A. 80 to 85°F   C. 100 to 105°F
    B. 90 to 95°F   D. 110 to 115°F

52. What is the pharmacological effect of oral glucose?
    A. increases the sugar level in the blood
    B. increases the insulin level in the body
    C. increases absorption of toxic substances
    D. None of the above.

53. What is the pharmacological effect of activated charcoal?
    A. stimulates the brain center to cause vomiting
    B. binds to certain poisons and prevents absorption
    C. works as an antidote against certain poisons
    D. None of the above.

54. You complete a focused history and physical exam on your diabetic patient. He tells you he takes insulin. Your patient has an altered mental status, has a history of diabetes, and a gag reflex. How should you treat this patient?
    A. Administer glucose.
    B. Assist patient with his insulin.
    C. Give oxygen only and transport.
    D. Transport. No medical intervention necessary.

55. Your two-year-old patient has ingested some type of mushroom. During the initial assessment, you determine the patient is unconscious, airway is patent, breathing rate is 6 times per minute, and pulse is weak and rapid. You should next
    A. continue with your focused history and physical exam.
    B. assist ventilations with a bag valve mask and supplemental oxygen.
    C. administer activated charcoal.
    D. administer oxygen with a nonrebreather mask.

56. When caring for the behavioral emergency, all of the following are true except
    A. check the availability of advanced life support.
    B. calm the patient.
    C. move quickly.
    D. make good eye contact.

57. While assessing a trauma patient, you discover bright-red, spurting blood. What type of bleeding is this?
    A. venous bleeding
    B. arterial bleeding
    C. capillary bleeding
    D. All of the above.

58. Given the above patient, during which assessment would this type of bleeding be detected and treated?
    A. ongoing assessment
    B. scene size-up
    C. focused physical exam
    D. initial assessment

59. Given the above patient, what would be the first step in controlling bleeding?
    A. Use a "pressure" point.
    B. Use direct pressure.
    C. Use a tourniquet.
    D. Use elevation only.

60. Early stages of shock (hypoperfusion) include all of the following except
    A. feeling of impending doom.
    B. low blood pressure.
    C. restlessness and anxiety.
    D. altered mental status.

61. Partial-thickness burn injuries are best characterized by
    A. pink to red skin with no blisters.
    B. dry, tough, and leathery skin.
    C. white to waxy or charred skin.
    D. white to red skin with blisters.

62. A sound or feeling caused by broken bone ends rubbing together is called
    A. crepitus.
    B. swelling.
    C. angulation.
    D. None of the above.

63. If a patient's bone ends are protruding, the EMT-B should
    A. carefully push them back in.
    B. realign the extremity so it is in a splint.
    C. splint the long bone in its angulated position.
    D. None of the above.

64. The objective(s) of splinting include
    A. immobilizing the distal joint.
    B. immobilizing the bone ends.
    C. immobilizing the proximal joint.
    D. All of the above.

65. The earliest sign of brain injury is
   A. altered level of consciousness.
   B. obvious bruising.
   C. unequal pupils.
   D. All of the above.

66. A bruise of the brain is referred to as a
   A. dislocation.
   B. major compromise.
   C. contusion.
   D. concussion.

67. When comparing the child's airway to that of the adult, the
   A. adult's is smallest at the vocal cords.
   B. child's is smallest in diameter at the cricoid ring.
   C. child's trachea is easier to obstruct.
   D. All of the above.

68. A good way to provide oxygen to a toddler in respiratory distress would be to
   A. use a nonrebreather mask.
   B. limit the liter flow to less than 6 lpm.
   C. use blow-by with a plastic cup.
   D. use a nasal cannula.

69. Common causes of seizures in pediatric patients include
   A. infection and epilepsy.
   B. hypoglycemia and poisoning.
   C. high fever and head trauma.
   D. All of the above.

70. Of the following injury locations on pediatric patients, which would you suspect were inflicted rather than accidental?
   A. shins
   B. knees
   C. upper arms
   D. spinal prominence

71. After a call in which numerous children were injured, the EMT-B should consider
   A. conducting a critique.
   B. informing the Medical Director.
   C. preplanning for the next pediatric call.
   D. stress debriefing.

72. A viral illness that may cause inflammation of the larynx of an infant or toddler is called
   A. bronchitis.
   B. croup.
   C. asthma.
   D. epiglottitis.

73. The "presenting" part in a breech birth is the
   A. buttocks or legs.
   B. arm.
   C. head.
   D. umbilical cord.

74. The condition in which an EMT-B may place a gloved hand into the vagina is called
   A. placenta previa.
   B. toxemia of pregnancy.
   C. prolapsed cord.
   D. premature birth.

75. Meconium is
   A. blood.
   B. fecal matter from the fetus.
   C. the outer covering of the placenta.
   D. the area between the vagina and the anus.

76. The first clamp put on the umbilical cord after delivery should be at least how many inches from the infant?
   A. 1
   B. 2 to 4
   C. 8 to 12
   D. 12

77. Which of the following statements is false?
   A. After a birth, the mother can tolerate a blood loss of 1500 cc.
   B. Uterine massage may help control vaginal bleeding.
   C. A woman may develop shock after delivery if bleeding is not controlled.
   D. Oxygen may be administered to the mother after birth.

78. Which statement regarding body mechanics is false?
   A. Lift with your legs, not your back.
   B. When lifting, keep the stretcher as far from the body as possible.
   C. Communicate clearly with your partner while lifting.
   D. Lifting partners should have similar strength and height when possible.

79. Which of the following patients should be moved using an emergency move?
   A. a conscious patient with spinal injury inside a vehicle
   B. a patient with inadequate breathing inside a vehicle
   C. a patient with a fractured arm
   D. None of the above.

80. Choose the correct statement regarding patient positioning.
    A. Spine-injured patients should be transported on their side to prevent aspiration.
    B. Shock patients should have their legs elevated 24 inches to combat shock.
    C. Pregnant women with hypotension should be placed on their left side when possible.
    D. A patient with chest pain must lie supine for airway maintenance.

81. You have a patient who is conscious, alert, and appears stable. He was involved in a motor vehicle accident and is complaining of neck pain. Choose the most appropriate course of treatment.
    A. rapid extrication to long board and transport
    B. short board to long board and transport
    C. no immobilization required—patient is stable
    D. short board only and transport

82. When transferring a patient from bed to bed or stretcher to bed, the move commonly used is the
    A. drag method.
    B. power lift.
    C. draw sheet method.
    D. log roll method.

83. The recommended policy about police escorts is to
    A. request them whenever you are in a rush.
    B. only use them if you are lost.
    C. avoid using them as they are very dangerous.
    D. None of the above.

84. Components of the extrication process include
    A. sizing up the situation.
    B. disentangling the patient.
    C. gaining access.
    D. All of the above.

85. Why is it important to stay away from the bumpers of a crushed car?
    A. They will need to be pulled out first.
    B. They may be used to investigate the cause.
    C. They may be loaded and could cause serious injury.
    D. All of the above.

86. The unsafe act that contributes most to collision scene injuries is
    A. using unsafe tools.
    B. failure to wear protective gear.
    C. deactivating safety devices.
    D. lifting heavy objects improperly.

87. A disaster plan should be
    A. realistic and based upon available resources.
    B. written to address incidents conceivable for your community.
    C. well publicized with the emergency responders.
    D. All of the above.

88. The EMS Sector Officer who is responsible for communicating with the hospital and arranging for helicopters is
    A. transport.
    B. extrication.
    C. triage.
    D. staging.

89. Which of the following is not an EMT-B's first responder role at a hazmat incident?
    A. entering the HOT ZONE to rescue the injured
    B. securing the scene without entering the area of contamination
    C. establishing an EMS commander and unified command post
    D. establishing control zones

90. Equipment and personnel at a hazmat scene should be staged in the _____ zone.
    A. COLD
    B. WARM
    C. HOT
    D. DECON

91. The rehab sector should be located in the _____ zone.
    A. HOT
    B. WARM
    C. COLD
    D. DECON

92. Medical monitoring of hazmat personnel involves
    A. evaluating hydration status.
    B. taking presuiting-up vital signs.
    C. taking weight using a portable scale.
    D. All of the above.

93. If the heart rate exceeds _____, an oral temperature should be taken during medical monitoring.
A. 60
B. 80
C. 100
D. 110

94. Decontamination should be done in the _____ zone.
A. COLD
B. WARM
C. HOT
D. REHAB

95. The leaf-shaped structure that covers the glottic opening is the
A. vallecula.
B. esophagus.
C. cricoid.
D. epiglottis.

96. The best pediatric ET tube diameter is
A. a quarter of the child's wrist size.
B. twice the child's age divided by four.
C. the diameter of the child's smallest finger.
D. None of the above.

97. Advanced airway management is indicated for which patients?
A. cardiac arrest
B. those that respond to painful stimuli
C. those requiring high-concentration oxygen
D. All of the above.

98. The straight laryngoscope blade used during orotracheal intubation
A. fits into the vallecula.
B. is inserted into the glottic opening.
C. lifts the epiglottis.
D. None of the above.

99. Complications of orotracheal intubation include
A. slowing of the heart rate.
B. hypoxia.
C. soft-tissue trauma.
D. All of the above.

100. Why is it important to frequently reassess lung sounds after placing an ET tube?
A. Sometimes they will disappear.
B. The tube may become accidentally dislodged.
C. The tube frequently moves into the left mainstem.
D. All of the above.

POSTTEST

1. Which statement regarding the attributes of an EMT-B is false?
   A. The EMT-B will maintain a clean and neat appearance.
   B. The EMT-B will place the safety of the patient before his or her own safety.
   C. The EMT-B will maintain knowledge and skills proficiency.
   D. The EMT-B will maintain knowledge of local, state, and national issues affecting EMS.

2. Which of the following is considered part of the EMT-B's role in quality improvement?
   A. documentation
   B. conducting preventive maintenance
   C. continuing education
   D. All of the above.

3. Battery is best defined as
   A. touching the patient without his consent.
   B. an assumption that an unconscious patient would accept your care.
   C. the result of a breach of duty to act.
   D. failure to inform the patient of risks involved in his care.

4. The concept which allows you to provide care for an unconscious patient is called
   A. patient refusal.
   B. implied consent.
   C. scope of practice.
   D. battery.

5. Which of the following is not an authorized release of patient care information?
   A. judicial subpoena
   B. report to the receiving hospital
   C. authorized insurance requests
   D. warning other providers about a patient's HIV status

6. Which of the following is a hazard that may be detected in the scene size-up?
   A. violence
   B. downed wires
   C. hazardous materials
   D. All of the above.

7. The difference between mechanism of injury and nature of illness is
   A. mechanism of injury is used primarily on medical calls.
   B. nature of illness is used primarily on trauma calls.
   C. mechanism of injury is used in trauma calls.
   D. both terms are interchangeable.

8. Signs and symptoms of EMS stress include all of the following except
   A. nightmares and difficulty sleeping.
   B. delusional thoughts.
   C. inability to concentrate.
   D. irritability.

9. When dealing with dying patients or their families, appropriate actions include all of the following except
   A. tolerance of angry or emotional behavior.
   B. treating the patient and family with dignity.
   C. not offering false reassurance.
   D. not speaking in front of the patient.

10. Which of the following is the most appropriate action if you are faced with a violent scene?
    A. Attempt to stop the violence.
    B. Be sure to wear body armor; then enter the scene.
    C. Retreat to a safe place and call police.
    D. Enter only with 2 to 3 additional EMT-Bs.

11. What governmental agency established guidelines for bloodborne pathogens?
    A. National Institute of Mental Health (NIMH)
    B. Environmental Protection Agency (EPA)
    C. Federal Trade Commission (FTC)
    D. The Occupational Safety and Health Administration (OSHA)

12. The purpose of an exposure control plan is to
    A. make it more difficult for EMS agencies to perform patient care activities.
    B. establish procedures for dealing with bloodborne pathogens.
    C. protect the employer from litigation when employees come in contact with blood or other body fluids.
    D. increase the fines OSHA can assess to employers for infractions.

13. Pathogens may enter your body through
    A. non-intact skin.
    B. your mouth or nose.
    C. your eyes.
    D. All of the above.

14. Which of the following statements is true?
    A. Not all blood or other body fluids are considered infectious.
    B. All blood and other body fluids should be considered infectious.
    C. Blood is the only body fluid that is considered infectious.
    D. Blood and other body fluids spread airborne pathogens.

15. A law which defines procedures by which EMT-Bs and other emergency workers may find out if they have been exposed to a potentially infectious disease is
    A. Tuberculosis mandate.
    B. OSHA 1910.1030.
    C. Ryan White CARE Act.
    D. NFPA 479.

16. The most reliable sign that your patient is being adequately ventilated is the patient's
    A. color returns to normal.
    B. pupils constrict.
    C. capillary refill becomes delayed.
    D. All of the above.

17. To select the proper size oral airway, you should measure from your patient's
    A. nose to earlobe.
    B. nose to the tip of the chin.
    C. center of the mouth to the angle of the jaw.
    D. None of the above.

18. When placing a nasal airway, be sure to
    A. lubricate with a water-based jelly.
    B. insert the bevel side away from the septum.
    C. measure from the nose to the jugular notch.
    D. All of the above.

19. The proper oxygen flow rate for a nonrebreather mask is _____ liters per minute.
    A. 2   B. 6   C. 10   D. 15

20. When a "D" size oxygen tank is half full, the gauge should read
    A. 500.
    B. 1000.
    C. 1500.
    D. 2000.

21. Pop-off valves on BVMs should
    A. be ignored.
    B. always be used.
    C. be removed or replaced.
    D. None of the above.

22. Which of the following is an example of a high-priority condition?
    A. simple childbirth
    B. intoxication
    C. spinal cord injury
    D. difficulty breathing

23. An adult at rest typically has a pulse between
    A. 40 and 80.   C.   60 and 100.
    B. 50 and 90.   D.   70 and 110.

24. When listening to breath sounds, you should listen for
    A. presence and crackles.
    B. presence and equality.
    C. wheezes and stridor.
    D. wheezes and crackles.

25. The ongoing assessment consists of repeating the initial assessment,
    A. repeating the focused history, checking interventions, repeating the detailed physical exam.
    B. repeating vital signs, checking interventions, repeating the detailed physical exam.
    C. repeating vital signs, repeating the focused history, repeating the detailed physical exam.
    D. repeating vital signs, repeating the focused history, checking interventions.

26. The proper order of steps in the evaluation of the responsive medical patient is initial assessment, then
    A. focused physical exam, vital signs, history of present illness, SAMPLE history.
    B. vital signs, history of present illness, SAMPLE history, focused physical exam.
    C. history of present illness, SAMPLE history, focused physical exam, vital signs.
    D. SAMPLE history, focused physical exam, vital signs, history of present illness.

27. The best way to open the airway of a trauma patient who has snoring respirations is the
    A. head-tilt, chin-lift maneuver.
    B. jaw-thrust maneuver.
    C. abdominal thrust.
    D. use of suction.

28. Your patient is complaining of pain in his pelvis after he was struck by a car. How should this affect your patient assessment?
   A. Refrain from compressing the pelvis.
   B. Assess the pelvis during the rapid trauma exam but not the detailed physical exam.
   C. Assess the pelvis during the rapid trauma exam and the detailed physical exam.
   D. Assess the pelvis during the detailed physical exam but not the rapid trauma exam.

29. Areas you assess during the detailed physical exam that you do not assess during the rapid trauma exam include
   A. neck veins.
   B. breath sounds.
   C. ears.
   D. pupils.

30. Which of the following is an example of a significant mechanism of injury?
   A. stab wound to the forearm
   B. bicycle-pedestrian collision
   C. fall of eighteen feet
   D. earthquake

31. Which of the following is not a high-priority condition?
   A. difficulty breathing
   B. poor general impression
   C. car crash
   D. severe pain

32. Which of the following might be appropriate radio report terminology?
   A. "be advised"
   B. "ambulance 2 to dispatcher"
   C. "you're welcome"
   D. "we" instead of "I"

33. Which of the following lists radio report information in the proper order?
   A. chief complaint, major past illnesses, baseline vital signs, general impression
   B. chief complaint, baseline vital signs, general impression, major past illnesses
   C. baseline vital signs, general impression, chief complaint, major past illnesses
   D. general impression, chief complaint, major past illnesses, baseline vital signs

34. Your verbal report to the medical or nursing staff at the hospital should include
   A. introduction of patient, summary of radio transmission, additional vital signs.
   B. summary of radio transmission, additional vital signs, insurance information.
   C. additional vital signs, suspected diagnosis, introduction of patient.
   D. just a repetition of the radio transmission.

35. An important principle to remember when completing the prehospital care report (PCR) is
   A. record important observations about the scene.
   B. refrain from clutter by omitting pertinent negatives.
   C. use personal abbreviations to save time and space.
   D. spelling is not important as long as the intent of the writer is clear.

36. If you make an error while completing the PCR, you should
   A. scratch the error out so that no words are recognizable.
   B. add a note with the correct information.
   C. initial the error and correct it.
   D. put parentheses around the error and finish the report.

37. You carry three medications on your ambulance. Which are they?
   A. lidocaine, atropine, and nitroglycerin
   B. aspirin, dextrose 50%, and sterile water
   C. activated charcoal, oxygen, and oral glucose
   D. albuterol, nitroglycerin, and epinephrine

38. An auto-injector is best given in the
   A. mouth.   C. thigh.
   B. forearm.   D. neck.

39. Why do we assist the patient with a prescribed inhaler?
   A. to dilate the coronary arteries
   B. to constrict the bronchial tree
   C. to constrict the blood vessels
   D. to dilate the bronchial tree

40. Many patients who suffer from severe allergic reactions carry
   A. a bronchodilator.
   B. an epinephrine auto-injector.
   C. an oxygen tank.
   D. All of the above.

41. In most EMS systems, before you help a patient self-administer prescribed nitroglycerin for chest pain, you will need permission from
A. medical direction.
B. the patient's personal physician.
C. the family.
D. All of the above.

42. The EMT-B may assist patients in taking prescribed
A. blood pressure medications.
B. water pills for pulmonary edema.
C. inhalers for breathing difficulty.
D. insulin for diabetes.

43. The preferred position for a patient with cardiac compromise is
A. position of comfort, usually sitting.
B. position of comfort, usually supine.
C. on the left side.
D. Trendelenburg.

44. To be effective, nitroglycerin should be administered
A. orally with no water.
B. orally with water.
C. sublingually with swallowing.
D. sublingually without swallowing.

45. If the AED gives a "no shock" message, you should
A. press the analyze button again immediately.
B. check the pulse.
C. resume CPR.
D. transport immediately.

46. How often should an AED's operation and supplies be checked?
A. every shift
B. every three days
C. every week
D. only after every use

47. A patient in cardiac arrest came back with a spontaneous pulse after you gave two shocks with the AED. En route to the hospital, he goes back into cardiac arrest with a shockable rhythm. How many stacked shocks should you now deliver?
A. one
B. two
C. three
D. six

48. Where will the retractions of a child with severe difficulty breathing be most evident?
A. intercostal and periumbilical
B. periumbilical and substernal
C. substernal and suprasternal
D. suprasternal and intercostal

49. The skin of a patient with a severe allergic (anaphylactic) reaction typically is
A. flushed and itchy.
B. pale and sweaty.
C. warm and dry.
D. jaundiced and mottled.

50. After you have activated an epinephrine auto-injector by pressing it firmly against the patient's thigh, you should
A. remove it immediately and save it for a second dose.
B. remove it immediately and dispose of it properly.
C. hold it in place for at least 10 seconds and save it for a second dose.
D. hold it in place for at least 10 seconds and dispose of it properly.

51. Active rewarming of a hypothermic patient is appropriate when the patient is
A. responding appropriately.
B. unresponsive.
C. responsive to painful stimuli.
D. responsive to verbal stimuli.

52. You should cool a heat exposure patient if
A. she is unresponsive.
B. she complains of being hot.
C. her skin is hot.
D. she responds to painful stimuli.

53. How should you administer oral glucose?
A. Place a tongue depressor between cheek and gum.
B. Ask the patient to drink glucose after mixing with water.
C. Use an auto-injectable pen.
D. None of the above.

54. Your 20-year-old patient has taken 25 aspirin tablets. He refuses your request to drink the activated charcoal. How should you respond?
A. Advise the patient that he will die.
B. Restrain the patient and administer.
C. Acknowledge the patient's feelings and attempt to change his mind.
D. Give him a mixture of water and salt.

55. Which one of the following patients should receive activated charcoal?
    A. an elderly woman who has taken 20 sleeping pills and who is nearly asleep
    B. a young man who has accidently swallowed gasoline
    C. an infant who has ingested drain cleaner.
    D. None of the above.

56. You respond to a possible suicide attempt. You should next
    A. conduct a detailed physical exam.
    B. make sure the scene is safe.
    C. conduct an initial assessment.
    D. conduct a focused history and physical exam.

57. Which of the following is a typical term you would use to describe a behavioral emergency patient?
    A. schizophrenic emergency
    B. psychotic emergency
    C. neurotic emergency
    D. emotional emergency

58. Blood loss would be considered severe if a one-year-old infant lost ____ cc of blood.
    A. 65
    B. 35
    C. 100
    D. All of the above.

59. Lacerations are best characterized by
    A. complete or incomplete detachment.
    B. rubbing or shearing of first layer of skin.
    C. tearing of skin by sharp object.
    D. accumulation of blood beneath the skin.

60. A high index of suspicion for internal injuries would first take place during the
    A. ongoing assessment.
    B. scene size-up.
    C. focused physical exam.
    D. initial assessment.

61. All of the following are characteristic of a critical burn injury, except
    A. partial-thickness burn over 20% BSA.
    B. full-thickness burn over 10% BSA.
    C. partial-thickness burn of the hands.
    D. partial-thickness burn encircling the leg.

62. A characteristic of a minor burn injury in a child less than five years old is a
    A. partial-thickness burn over 25% of BSA.
    B. full-thickness burn over 20% of BSA.
    C. partial-thickness burn over 5% of BSA.
    D. partial-thickness burn over 15% of BSA.

63. In the first two hours of an uncomplicated simple fracture of the tibia and fibula the patient can lose
    A. a pint of blood.
    B. two pints of blood.
    C. three pints of blood.
    D. None of the above.

64. Always evaluate the ____ before and after the splint is applied.
    A. distal circulation
    B. swelling
    C. blood pressure
    D. All of the above.

65. In which type of injury should the patient not be log rolled?
    A. tibia   C. cervical spine
    B. pelvic   D. lumbar

66. When the head of the femur is out of its socket, this is called a
    A. dislocated hip.
    B. dislocated femur.
    C. fractured femur.
    D. fractured pelvis.

67. A patient who struck her head and has a bruise behind the ears has
    A. Battle's sign.
    B. a concussion.
    C. raccoon's eyes.
    D. a contusion.

68. When opening the airway of the unconscious trauma patient, always
    A. assess mental status.
    B. use the drowning program.
    C. use the jaw thrust.
    D. None of the above.

69. The spinal immobilization of a child less than seven years old should include each of the following except
    A. padding behind the shoulders.
    B. torso straps.
    C. padding behind the head.
    D. head blocks and collar.

70. The anterior fontanelle usually seals up within _____ months of age.
A. 6   B. 12   C. 18   D. 24

71. When managing a foreign body airway obstruction in an infant,
A. sweep out the mouth right away.
B. provide a series of five abdominal thrusts.
C. alternate backblows with chest thrusts.
D. hyperextend the neck twice at once.

72. The usual cause of cardiac arrest in infants is due to
A. poisoning.
B. respiratory failure.
C. heart attack.
D. stroke.

73. How can the EMT-B minimize stress from dealing with children?
A. Learn as much as possible about pediatric illness.
B. Learn how healthy children react.
C. Practice pediatric skills.
D. All of the above.

74. A tube inserted in a child to help drain excessive fluid in the brain is called a
A. central line.
B. tracheotomy.
C. shunt.
D. gastrostomy.

75. The "presenting" part in a prolapsed cord is the
A. buttocks or legs.
B. arm.
C. head.
D. umbilical cord.

76. The skin between the vagina and the anus is called the
A. birth canal.
B. peritoneum.
C. meconium.
D. perineum.

77. If you deliver and suction the airway of an infant and breathing does not begin simultaneously, the next step is
A. mouth-to-mouth resuscitation.
B. rub the baby's back or flick the soles of the feet as stimulus.
C. begin CPR immediately.
D. do nothing at this time.

78. The "bag of waters" is actually the
A. placenta.
B. umbilical cord.
C. meconium.
D. amniotic sac.

79. Infection control equipment that is appropriate for childbirth includes
A. gloves and mask.
B. gloves, mask, gown.
C. gloves, mask, gown, and eyewear.
D. gloves only.

80. Which lifting and moving device would be most appropriate for a medical patient with difficulty breathing who needs to be moved from a second-floor bedroom?
A. scoop stretcher
B. basket stretcher
C. flexible stretcher
D. stair chair

81. Which of the following statements regarding emergency moves is true?
A. If necessary, try to pull or drag with the long axis of the body.
B. Emergency moves should never be performed because spinal injuries may result.
C. Emergency moves should be used only when there is no threat to life.
D. Short backboards must be used for emergency moves.

82. Which of the following statements regarding wheeled stretchers is true?
A. The stretcher should be used only on uneven terrain.
B. The device is designed to be used by one person at all times.
C. Wheeled stretchers require preventive maintenance and cleaning.
D. It is best to use odd numbers of people to lift stretchers to maintain balance.

83. If you must move a patient to get to a second patient who is in cardiac arrest, you should use a(n) _____ move.
A. emergency
B. non-emergency
C. urgent
D. standing take-down

84. The procedure used by weightlifters that includes bending at the knees and using your legs to lift is called the
A. squat lift.
B. weight lift.
C. two-hand lift.
D. power grip.

85. The consequences of an ambulance operator failing to drive with due regard for the safety of others include
A. tickets.
B. lawsuits.
C. time in jail
D. All of the above.

86. A key principle of medical documentation is
A. use as much medical terminology as possible.
B. if you didn't write it down, you didn't do it.
C. abbreviate each term so your report fits on one page.
D. All of the above.

87. Which is the correct sequence for a rescue?
A. disentanglement, hazard management, and gaining access
B. gaining access, size up, and extrication
C. size up, hazard management, and disentanglement
D. termination of rescue, disentanglement, and size up

88. The functional area that is always staffed at a multiple casualty incident is called
A. finance.
B. operations.
C. planning.
D. command.

89. The EMS Sector Officer at an MCI responsible for categorizing patients by priority is
A. treatment.
B. triage.
C. transport.
D. staging.

90. When arriving at the scene of a hazmat incident, the first-responding EMT-B should
A. take a defensive position in a safe place far enough from the site to ensure his own safety.
B. position his vehicle downwind from the incident.
C. enter the HOT ZONE to rescue the injured.
D. None of the above.

91. Equipment and personnel at a hazmat incident should be staged in the _____ zone.
A. DECON
B. WARM
C. HOT
D. None of the above.

92. OSHA says the incident commander at a hazmat incident must
A. know how to implement the employer's emergency response plan.
B. be able to implement the employer's incident command system.
C. understand the hazards and risks associated with employees working in chemical protective clothing.
D. All of the above.

93. A flat ended tanker truck that is well insulated with a double shell and that has a pressure relief valve that is frequently discharging vapors is probably carrying
A. a compressed gas.
B. a cryogenic liquid.
C. gasoline.
D. a corrosive liquid.

94. The orange section of the DOT *Emergency Response Guidebook* contains
A. evacuation distances.
B. general information about what to do in the first few minutes of a hazmat incident.
C. a listing of chemicals in alphabetical order.
D. a listing of chemicals in numerical order.

95. Endotracheal tubes come in various sizes. When intubating an adult female, you should use a size
A. 6.0 to 6.5 mm tube.
B. 7.0 to 8.0 mm tube.
C. 8.0 to 8.5 mm tube.
D. 9.0 to 10.0 mm tube.

96. A properly placed ET tube in an adult will have the _____ centimeter mark at the teeth.
A. 18
B. 20
C. 22
D. 24

97. Once the lubricated stylet is inserted in the tube, the ET tube should be bent into a(n)
   A. "L" shape.
   B. hockey stick shape.
   C. "J" shape.
   D. None of the above.

98. The application of cricoid pressure during intubation is referred to as the
   A. Adam's apple maneuver.
   B. cricoid puncture.
   C. tracheal pressure.
   D. Sellick maneuver.

99. Generally, uncuffed ET tubes are used for children below the age of
   A. 4.
   B. 6.
   C. 8.
   D. 10.

100. Alternative methods to advanced airway management include the
   A. EOA or EGTA.
   B. PtL® airway.
   C. Combitube®.
   D. All of the above.

Answer Key

Pretest Answers

(Note: Page numbers in parentheses ( ) refer to page numbers in this textbook where answers can be found or supported.)

1. D (p. 6); **2. A** (pp. 9–10); **3. C** (p. 12);
4. C (p. 14); **5. C** (pp. 14, 16); **6. A** (pp. 24–25);
7. B (p. 25); **8. A** (p. 23); **9. C** (p. 22);
10. B (p. 22); **11. B** (p. 33); **12. A** (p. 33);
13. A (pp. 33–34); **14. A** (p. 34);
15. B (pp. 37–38); **16. C** (p. 51); **17. B** (p. 57);
18. B (p. 57); **19. B** (p. 58); **20. B** (pp. 63, 66);
21. D (p. 56); **22. D** (p. 74); **23. A** (p. 76);
24. B (p. 81); **25. B** (p. 84); **26. A** (pp. 87–90);
27. D (p. 87); **28. A** (pp. 96, 97);
29. B (pp. 96, 97, 98); **30. A** (p. 97);
31. D (pp. 96, 99); **32. C** (p. 110);
33. B (p. 111); **34. A** (p. 112); **35. D** (p. 113);
36. B (p. 116); **37. D** (p. 124); **38. B** (p. 125);
39. A (p. 123); **40. C** (p. 123); **41. D** (p. 126);
42. D (p. 133); **43. C** (p. 134); **44. B** (p. 141);
45. B (p. 144); **46. D** (p. 146);
47. B (pp. 154, 155); **48. A** (pp. 157, 158);
49. A (p. 161); **50. C** (p. 165); **51. C** (p. 170);
52. A (p. 181); **53. B** (p. 182); **54. A** (p. 182);
55. B (p. 184); **56. C** (p. 190); **57. B** (p. 198);
58. D (p. 199); **59. B** (p. 200); **60. B** (p. 204);
61. D (p. 211); **62. A** (p. 228); **63. B** (p. 229);
64. D (p. 229); **65. A** (pp. 256, 257);
66. C (p. 255); **67. D** (pp. 288–289);
68. C (p. 293); **69. D** (p. 296); **70. C** (p. 295);
71. D (p. 300); **72. B** (p. 297); **73. A** (p. 311);
74. C (p. 311); **75. B** (p. 311); **76. B** (p. 309);
77. A (p. 309); **78. B** (p. 318); **79. B** (p. 319);
80. C (p. 305); **81. B** (p. 326); **82. C** (p. 323);
83. C (p. 345); **84. D** (p. 351); **85. C** (p. 353);
86. B (p. 353); **87. D** (p. 365); **88. A** (p. 371);
89. A (pp. 377–378); **90. A** (p. 379);
91. C (p. 380); **92. D** (p. 380); **93. D** (p. 380);
94. B (pp. 378–379); **95. D** (p. 390);
96. C (p. 403); **97. A** (p. 397); **98. C** (p. 395);
99. D (p. 393); **100. B** (p. 399)

Posttest Answers

(Note: Page numbers in parentheses ( ) refer to page numbers in this textbook where answers can be found or supported.)

1. B (p. 7); **2. D** (p. 10); **3. A** (p. 16);
4. B (p. 14); **5. D** (p. 16); **6. D** (p. 24);
7. C (p. 24); **8. B** (p. 22); **9. D** (p. 23);
10. C (p. 27); **11. D** (p. 33); **12. B** (p. 33);
13. D (pp. 33–34); **14. B** (p. 34); **15. C** (p. 36);
16. A (p. 49); **17. C** (p. 52); **18. A** (p. 55);
19. D (p. 66); **20. B** (p. 64); **21. C** (p. 59);
22. D (p. 77); **23. C** (p. 76); **24. B** (p. 80);
25. D (p. 84); **26. C** (pp. 78–79); **27. B** (p. 95);
28. A (p. 91); **29. C** (p. 104); **30. C** (p. 94);
31. D (p. 96); **32. D** (p. 111); **33. A** (p. 112);
34. A (p. 112); **35. A** (p. 113);
36. C (pp. 116, 118); **37. C** (p. 123);
38. C (p. 125); **39. D** (p. 124); **40. B** (p. 125);
41. A (p. 125); **42. C** (p. 124); **43. A** (p. 134);
44. D (pp. 136, 138); **45. B** (p. 145);
46. A (p. 147); **47. C** (pp. 141, 147);
48. D (p. 160); **49. A** (p. 160); **50. D** (p. 164);
51. A (p. 167); **52. C** (pp. 172–173);
53. A (p. 181); **54. C** (p. 184); **55. D** (p. 182);
56. B (p. 186); **57. D** (p. 186);
58. C (pp. 198–199); **59. C** (p. 207);
60. B (p. 203); **61. A** (p. 215); **62. C** (p. 215);
63. A (p. 229); **64. A** (p. 229); **65. B** (p. 240);
66. A (p. 240); **67. A** (p. 256); **68. C** (p. 258);
69. C (pp. 279, 280); **70. C** (p. 288);
71. C (p. 290); **72. B** (p. 292); **73. D** (p. 299);
74. C (p. 299); **75. D** (p. 311); **76. D** (p. 303);
77. B (p. 310); **78. D** (p. 306); **79. C** (p. 307);
80. D (p. 327); **81. A** (p. 319); **82. C** (p. 331);
83. A (p. 319); **84. A** (p. 318); **85. D** (p. 341);
86. B (p. 349); **87. C** (p. 351); **88. D** (p. 366);
89. B (p. 369); **90. A** (p. 377); **91. D** (p. 379);
92. D (p. 377); **93. B** (p. 381); **94. B** (p. 385);
95. B (p. 396); **96. C** (p. 396); **97. B** (p. 396);
98. D (p. 398); **99. C** (p. 403); **100. D** (p. 409)

Chapter Review Answers

(Note: Page numbers in parentheses ( ) refer to page numbers in this textbook where answers can be found or supported.)

Chapter 1
1. pp. 5–6; **2.** pp. 6–8; **3.** pp. 9–10;
4. pp. 10–11; **5.** pp. 12–13, 16; **6.** p. 17

Chapter 2
1. p. 21; **2.** p. 22; **3.** p. 23; **4.** p. 23; **5.** p. 24;
6. p. 25; **7.** p. 25; **8.** pp. 26–27; **9.** pp. 27–28;
10. pp. 28–29

Chapter 3
1. pp. 33–34; **2.** p. 33; **3.** pp. 33–36;
4. pp. 37–38; **5.** pp. 36–37; **6.** pp. 38–41

Chapter 4
1. p. 49; **2.** pp. 49–50; **3.** pp. 50–51;
4. pp. 52–54; **5.** pp. 54–55; **6.** pp. 55–57;
7. p. 59; **8.** pp. 63–64; **9.** pp. 64–65; **10.** p. 66

Chapter 5
1. pp. 71–76; **2.** p. 74; **3.** pp. 74, 75; **4.** p. 74;
5. pp. 76, 80; **6.** pp. 80–84; **7.** pp.84–85; **8.** p. 87

Chapter 6
1. pp. 94, 96; **2.** pp. 94–95; **3.** pp. 96, 104–105;
4. p. 97; **5.** p. 97; **6.** pp. 96–99; **7.** p. 104

Chapter 7
1. pp. 109–110; **2.** p. 110; **3.** p. 112; **4.** p. 111;
5. p. 113; **6.** pp. 116, 118; **7.** pp. 116, 117

Chapter 8
1. pp. 123–124; **2.** pp. 124–125; **3.** p. 126;
4. p. 126; **5.** p. 126; **6.** p. 127; **7.** pp. 126–127;
8. p. 127; **9.** p. 127; **10.** p. 127

Chapter 9
1. p. 132; **2.** pp. 134–137; **3.** pp. 137, 138;
4. pp. 137, 139; **5.** pp. 141, 142, 146;
6. p. 141; **7.** p. 146

Chapter 10
1. pp. 156–157; **2.** pp. 157, 158;
3. pp. 160–161; **4.** pp. 161, 162; **5.** p. 169;
6. p. 172; **7.** p. 173

Chapter 11
1. pp. 180, 183; **2.** p. 182; **3.** p. 181; **4.** p. 181;
5. pp. 181, 183; **6.** pp. 184, 185; **7.** p. 182;
8. p. 186; **9.** pp. 186, 190

Chapter 12
1. p. 198; **2.** p. 198; **3.** pp. 199–202;
4. pp. 203–204; **5.** pp. 204, 206, 207; **6.** p. 213;
7. p. 220

Chapter 13
1. pp. 226, 227; **2.** p. 225; **3.** p. 228; **4.** p. 229;
5. pp. 229–252; **6.** p. 253; **7.** pp. 256–257;
8. p. 258; **9.** pp. 260, 261; **10.** pp. 261–262

Chapter 14
1. pp. 287–289; **2.** pp. 286–287; **3.** p. 290;
4. pp. 295–296; **5.** p. 295; **6.** p. 295;
7. pp. 297–298; **8.** p. 297; **9.** p. 298; **10.** p. 299

Chapter 15
1. pp. 303, 304; **2.** pp. 304–306, 312;
3. pp. 306–309; **4.** p. 310; **5.** pp. 309–310;
6. p. 311; **7.** p. 313

Chapter 16
1. p. 317; **2.** p. 318; **3.** p. 318; **4.** pp. 317–318;
5. p. 319, 320–325; **6.** pp. 326–331

Chapter 17
1. p. 337; **2.** p. 336; **3.** p. 345; **4.** pp. 344–345;
5. pp. 345–346; **6.** p. 351; **7.** p. 351; **8.** p. 351;
9. pp. 368–371; **10.** pp. 370–371

Chapter 18
1. pp. 376–377; **2.** p. 377; **3.** p. 375;
4. pp. 378–379, 380; **5.** pp. 379–380; **6.** p. 380;
7. pp. 382–384; **8.** pp. 380–385; **9.** p. 385;
10. p. 385

Chapter 19
1. p. 393; **2.** p. 393; **3.** pp. 398–399;
4. pp. 405–406; **5.** pp. 392–393, 407; **6.** p. 407;
7. pp. 410–411; **8.** pp. 393, 409;
9. pp. 412–413; **10.** p. 414

Index